W9-CFI-913

MEDICAL TERMINOLOGY
Specialties

A Medical Specialties Approach With Patient Records

F. A. DAVIS COMPANY • Philadelphia

MEDICAL TERMINOLOGY
Specialties

A Medical Specialties Approach With Patient Records

Regina M. Masters, CMA, RN, BSN, MEd
Director of Medical Education
Olympic Consulting Group, Ltd., Toledo, Ohio
Psychiatric Nursing Services, Flower Hospital,
Sylvania, Ohio

Barbara A. Gylys, CMA, BS, MEd
Professor Emerita of Health and Human Services
University of Toledo Community and Technical College
Toledo, Ohio

F. A. Davis Company
1915 Arch Street
Philadelphia, PA 19103

Copyright © 2003 by F. A. Davis Company

All rights reserved. This book is protected by copyright. No part of it may be reproduced, stored in a retrieval system, or transmitted in any form or by any means, electronic, mechanical, photocopying, recording, or otherwise, without written permission from the publisher.

Printed in the United States of America

Last digit indicates print number: 10 9 8 7 6 5 4 3 2 1

Acquisitions Editor: Andy McPhee
Developmental Editor: Elena Coler
Cover Design: Christine Cantera
Interior Design: Melissa Walter

As new scientific information becomes available through basic and clinical research, recommended treatments and drug therapies undergo changes. The author(s) and publisher have done everything possible to make this book accurate, up to date, and in accord with accepted standards at the time of publication. The authors, editors, and publisher are not responsible for errors or omissions or for consequences from application of the book, and make no warranty, expressed or implied, in regard to the contents of the book. Any practice described in this book should be applied by the reader in accordance with professional standards of care used in regard to the unique circumstances that may apply in each situation. The reader is advised always to check product information (package inserts) for changes and new information regarding dose and contraindications before administering any drug. Caution is especially urged when using new or infrequently ordered drugs.

Library of Congress Cataloging-in-Publication Data

Masters, Regina M., 1959–
   Medical terminology specialties : a medical specialties approach with
patient records / Regina M. Masters, Barbara A. Gylys.—1st ed.
     p. ; cm.
  Includes indexes.
   ISBN 0-8036-0907-8 (alk. paper)
   1. Medicine—Terminology—Problems, exercises, etc.
   [DNLM: 1. Terminology—Problems and Exercises.   2. Medical
Records—Problems and Exercises.   3. Specialties, Medical. W 15 M423m
2003] I. Gylys, Barbara. A.   II. Title.
   R123 .M346 2003
   610'. 1'4—dc21

                       2002074172

Authorization to photocopy items for internal or personal use, or the internal or personal use of specific clients, is granted by F. A. Davis Company for users registered with the Copyright Clearance Center (CCC) Transactional Reporting Service, provided that the fee of $.10 per copy is paid directly to CCC, 222 Rosewood Drive, Danvers, MA 01923. For those organizations that have been granted a photocopy license by CCC, a separate system of payment has been arranged. The fee code for users of the Transactional Reporting Service is: 8036-0907/03 + $.10.

*To my coauthor, whose endless hours of
collaboration, immense patience, and encouragement
were always there when needed.*

*To my father, for giving me continuous drive
and confidence.*

*To my husband and my children Andrew, Julia, and Caitlin—
all of whom have supported me in numerous ways in this most
important endeavor.*

R.M.M.

*To my husband, who happens to be my colleague
and best friend.*

*To Regina Maria, Julius II, Andrew, Julia,
Caitlin, and Anthony.*

B.A.G.

Preface

Medical Terminology Specialties: A Medical Specialties Approach with Patient Records offers an innovative and realistic approach for learning medical terminology in a new and exciting way. Medicine today revolves around areas of specialization. The book's content and organization take full advantage of that reality by helping you to apply medical terminology concepts to the real clinical world.

This approach, combined with the practical application of medical records, will strengthen your ability to read and interpret various types of records encountered in health-care settings. It will also foster greater understanding of medical reports and their legal implications.

Organization and Content

Although the book is designed as a classroom teaching text for programs that require medical terminology, its organization incorporates many instructional features that can help you work through the material at your own pace.

Chapters 1, 3, and 4 include basic rules of medical word building. These chapters are devoted to the introduction of major medical suffixes and prefixes and to the structural organization of the human body. Chapter 2 discusses major medical specialties and the role of health-care practitioners. It includes an introduction to medical records and provides a basic foundation for understanding the purpose and styles of various types of medical reports. The information presented in these initial chapters will be essential to your understanding and mastery of the material covered in subsequent chapters. We strongly recommend that you complete the first four chapters before proceeding to the chapters that follow.

Chapters 5 through 17 offer detailed discussions of medical terminology as it relates to medical specialties. Each chapter provides an overview of a medical specialty, along with its respective body system, and introduces terminology related to that particular specialty. The chapter outline highlights the structure of the chapter. Each chapter also includes competency verification activities (with answer keys to provide immediate student feedback), word analyses to reinforce how medical terms are formed, and authentic medical records and critical thinking questions to help you interpret medical records.

Chapters 18–20 do not address any specific body system, yet each chapter covers a medical specialty.

Chapter 21 contains extensive coverage of medical records along with critical-thinking activities.

Chapter Components

Each chapter includes:

- Learning objectives to identify tasks you'll be able to perform and knowledge you'll gain after successfully completing the chapter.

- At-a-glance overviews of the main functions of each particular body system and a preview of the facts and concepts discussed in the chapter.

- Selected key terms, which are listed at the beginning of each chapter and define the meanings of medical terms relevant to that body system. Bold face is used for clinically significant terms, as well as for terms used to label anatomical illustrations.

- Phonetic pronunciation of medical terms. See the pronunciation guide on the inside back cover of the textbook.

- Descriptive explanations of pathological conditions, diagnostic procedures and tests, surgical and therapeutic procedures and tests, and pharmacology related to each medical specialty.

- Practical applications designed as competency-based verification activities, to help you apply the information you have acquired and to monitor your own progress.

- Interactive workbook format with sufficient space to write answers.

- Plentiful medical illustrations to help you locate structures being discussed and visualize a clear image of physiological events, disease processes, and techniques.

- Audio recordings on an accompanying CD-ROM to help you learn proper pronunciation.

- Authentic medical records to help you apply terms you learn to the real world. Note that patient and physician names have been changed, as have other standard pieces of information such as hospital names. This information has been changed to preserve the confidentiality of patients and physicians. However, other than personal information, we have essentially left the records alone. We have, in fact, made a concerted effort to maintain the language and tone of the original documents. We wanted you to see an accurate reflection of real-world medical records.

Appendixes

The comprehensive group of appendixes we've developed provide information essential to your training in the language of medicine. These user-friendly resources are designed to accommodate a variety of learning and resource needs. We believe you'll find great value in the appendixes as study, review, and reference aids.

Supplemental Materials

A comprehensive *Instructor's Guide* is available to instructors who adopt *Medical Terminology Specialties* for use in their courses. The *Instructor's Guide* can help the teacher make the best possible use of the textbook and its accompanying products. It contains useful information about the special features of the textbook, suggested course outlines that can be used to teach a 10- or 15-week course, and suggestions for developing a contemporary learning package that integrates the latest technological tools for a self-paced distance learning course.

Other supplementary materials include a Brownstone computerized test bank, which allows the instructor to create custom-generated or random-selected tests from more than 1,800 items, a printable version of all multiple-choice test items and anatomy activities, and a PowerPoint® presentation that can be used to supplement classroom study of the book's chapters.

We believe that the medical specialties approach we've developed, in concert with the wide array of supplementary materials we've created, give *Medical Terminology Specialties* the power you need to learn medical terminology and, ultimately, to succeed as a health-care professional.

Acknowledgments

We thank Jean-Francois Vilain, former Publisher of Health Professions, who was instrumental in initiating this project. He orchestrated a significant part of its development but retired shortly before the textbook was placed into production. We are grateful for his guidance not only with this book but also with the many other successful projects we were involved in during his tenure at FA Davis. We will miss him as a publisher and as a friend, and we wish him the best in the years to come.

This book was finally brought to its final form due to the collaborative efforts of many skilled and dedicated individuals. Margaret Biblis, Publisher; Andy McPhee, Acquisitions Editor; and Susan Rhyner, Manager of Creative Development came on board just in time to provide a microscopic examination of the entire project and guide it into its final stages of production. Both Margaret and Susan made it manifestly clear that they wanted our medical terminology book to be the best that it can be—pedagogically sound, accurate, user-friendly, and visually attractive. Needless to say, this required profound dedication to incorporate changes by both the authors and numerous individuals involved in the production of the book. The end result of our efforts shows an improved, user-friendly presentation of both the material and illustrations throughout the entire textbook.

We are particularly thankful to Dr. Julius A. Gylys, who provided the framework for developing the structure and functions of many body systems chapters. He methodically reviewed and edited numerous chapters throughout the entire development of the book.

We are especially grateful to Michelle Bishop, Department of Medicine, University of Florida for her contributions in the development of the Neurology and Psychiatry chapters. She also provided useful suggestions in other chapters that led to accurate changes in the manuscript. Her support and dedication provided a great deal of support during the various stages of development.

For the meticulous editing and constructive suggestions in their areas of expertise, we sincerely thank:

Victoria Gylys-Morin, MD
Associate Professor, Children's Hospital Medical Center
Cincinnati, OH

Robert Morin, MD, FACE
Senior Research Scientist, Proctor and Gamble Pharmaceuticals
Cincinnati, OH

Julius A. Gylys, PhD
Department of Clinical & Health Psychology
University of Florida
Veteran's Affairs Medical Center
Gainesville, FL

No writing project could be undertaken without a knowledgeable and hard-working panel of reviewers. We acknowledge and express our gratitude to our reviewers who read either portions or all of the manuscript as it was being prepared. Their forthright criticisms and helpful suggestions for improving the narrative and illustrations added immeasurably to the quality of the finished product. The review panel for the first edition included:

Michelle M. Bishop, PhD
Dept of Medicine
Division of Hematology/Oncology
Univ of Florida Health Science Center

Donald Everett Crews, MEd, CMA
Southwest Georgia Technical College
Thomasville, Georgia

Michael Fugate, MEd, RT(R)
Santa Fe Community College
Gainsville, FL

Gylys, Karen, RN, PhD
Assistant Professor
UCLA School of Nursing

Sue A. Hunt, MA, RN, CMA
Middlesex Community College
Lowell, MA

Trudi James-Parks, AART, RT(R)
Lorain County Community College
Elyria, OH

Carol Masker, BS
Morris County School of Technology
Denville, NJ

Patricia McLane, RRA, MA
Henry Ford Community College
Dearborn, MI

Roberta J. Miller, RT-RM
Medical College of Ohio, Dept of Radiology
Toledo, OH

Karen Minchella, PhD, CMA
Consulting Management Association
Fraser, MI

Paulette Nitkiewicz, RN
Westmoreland County Community College
Youngwood, PA

Lydia D. Schafer, PhD
Assistant Professor
Depts of Pathology and Physician Assistant Studies
Medical College of Ohio
Toledo, OH

Susan King Strasinger, DA, MT (ASCP)
University of West Florida
Pensacola, FL

Richard Weidman, RRA
Tacoma Community College
Tacoma, WA

Victoria Wetle, RN, CMSC, EdD
Chemeketa Community College
Salem, OR

We are especially grateful to the editorial and production staff at FA Davis Co., who guided, inspired, and shaped this enormous project into a dynamic learning tool.

Elena Coler, Developmental Editor, systematically and meticulously read the manuscript, helping it along at every stage. Her patience, creativity, and support are evident throughout the textbook.

Jack Brandt, Illustrations Specialist, and Louis Forgione, Art and Design Manager—for the quality illustrations that are found throughout the book.

Michael W. Bailey, Director of Production, Robert Butler, Production Manager, and Bette Haitsch, Managing Editor—all of whom provided their expertise to make the production of this book possible.

In today's textbook market, it is imperative that medical terminology textbooks include ancillary products (such as CDs, electronic test banks, web sites) that enable the instructor and student to absorb the materials presented in the book using the latest state-of-the-art technology. We are very fortunate and extremely appreciative of the dedication and expertise provided by Ralph Zickgraf, Manager, Electronic Publishing, and Kirk Pedrick, Senior Developmental Editor, Electronic Publishing. Their patience, untiring efforts, creativity, and determination to produce a "program of excellence" is evident in the quality of the finished product.

We would also like to acknowledge Carol Richards, CMA, and Karen Minchella, PhD, CMA, both of whom assisted in developing questions for the electronic test bank and interactive software.

We are grateful to Andrew R. Masters, student at Miami University in Oxford, Ohio, who spent endless hours working through the final copy of the text. Our thanks also go to Barbara Blank, CMT, Instructor at Stautpzenberger College, Toledo, Ohio and medical transcriptionist at The Toledo Hospital for reviewing, formatting, and editing the medical reports. Last but not least, we appreciate Patricia Acerra, AP, LMT who reviewed some of the chapters.

CONTENTS AT A GLANCE

APPENDIXES

TABLE OF CONTENTS

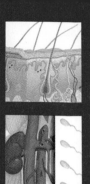
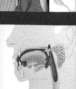
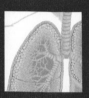

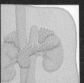

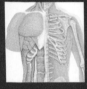

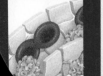

chapter

1

Medical Word Components

Chapter Outline

Objectives

Upon completion of this chapter, you will be able to:

- Identify the four component parts used to form medical words.
- Understand how to divide medical words into their component parts.
- Find and use the guidelines to define and build medical words correctly.
- Demonstrate your knowledge of this chapter by successfully completing the activities.

To understand the meaning of medical words, it is important to learn how to divide them into their component parts: the *word root*, the *suffix*, the *prefix*, and the *combining form*.

MEDICAL WORD COMPONENTS

Word Roots

Medical words contain at least one or more word roots. The word root is the foundation of the word. The word root frequently, but not always, indicates a body part and usually stems from the Greek or Latin language. Examine *tonsillitis*, *tonsillectomy*, *colitis*, and *colectomy* to determine their components (roots and suffixes) and meanings. You will note that the meaning of the word changes whenever you change a component.

In the examples that follow, the arrows designating the word roots are bolded in black type, whereas those indicating suffixes are highlighted in blue.

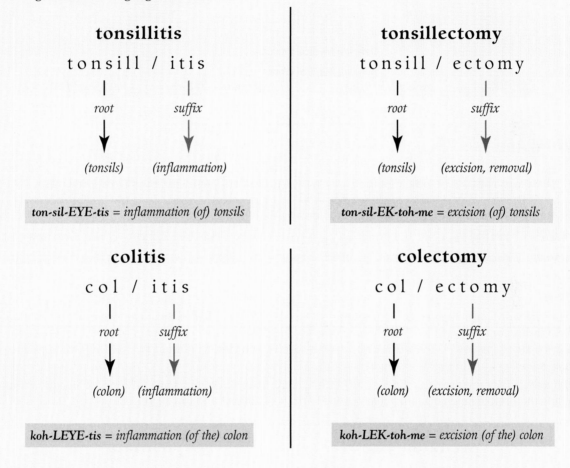

tonsillitis

t o n s i l l / i t i s

root — suffix

(tonsils) — (inflammation)

ton-sil-EYE-tis = *inflammation (of) tonsils*

tonsillectomy

t o n s i l l / e c t o m y

root — suffix

(tonsils) — (excision, removal)

ton-sil-EK-toh-me = *excision (of) tonsils*

colitis

c o l / i t i s

root — suffix

(colon) — (inflammation)

koh-LEYE-tis = *inflammation (of the) colon*

colectomy

c o l / e c t o m y

root — suffix

(colon) — (excision, removal)

koh-LEK-toh-me = *excision (of the) colon*

Word Analysis

The roots *tonsill* and *col* indicate body parts, the tonsils and colon, respectively. *Tonsill* stems from the Latin term *tonsilla* (almond); *col* stems from the Greek term *kolon* (colon). The suffix *-itis* means "inflammation"; the suffix *-ectomy* means "excision," "removal." By adding a different suffix to the root, the meaning of the word is changed as shown in the previous examples. It is not necessary to know whether a word is of Latin or Greek origin. This information is provided to illustrate that numerous medical words are derived from as early as the 1st century BC.

Suffixes

Suffixes are word endings. In the previous examples, *-itis* and *-ectomy* are suffixes attached to the root *tonsill.* In the following examples, examine the terms *mastectomy* and *mastitis* to determine their components and their meanings.

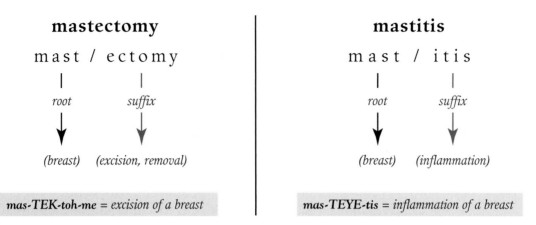

Word Analysis

The word root *mast* indicates the body part, the breast. The root stems from the Greek term *mastos* (breast). The suffix *-ectomy* means "excision," "removal"; the suffix *-itis* means "inflammation." By adding different suffixes to the root *mast,* the meaning of the word is changed.

Prefixes

Prefixes are word parts located at the beginning of words. Prefixes change the meanings of words, but not all medical terms contain prefixes. Prefixes are connected directly to the beginning of a word and do not require adding a connecting vowel. You will recognize many prefixes in medical terms because they are the same prefixes as the ones used in everyday English.

Prefixes usually indicate a position, number, measurement, direction, sense of time, or negation. Simply changing the prefix can change the meaning of a word. Consider the following terms:

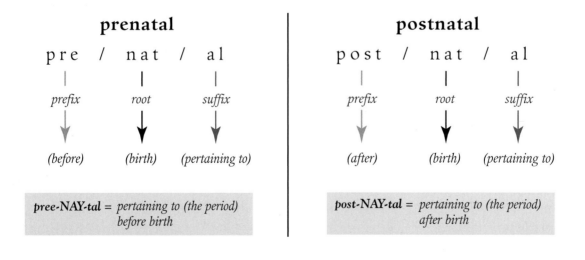

Both prefixes indicate a sense of time: *pre-* means "before"; *post-* means "after." The prefixes are attached directly to the medical term that follows. In the previous examples, *pre-* and *pro-* are attached to the medical term *natal*. In this text, whenever a prefix stands alone it will be followed by a hyphen, as in *pre-* and *post-*. Whenever a suffix stands alone it will be preceded by a hyphen, as in *-al*.

Word Analysis

The root *nat* means "birth"; the suffix *-al* means "pertaining to" or "relating to."

Combining Forms

The combining form is a word root plus a vowel, which is usually an *o*. The difficulty of pronouncing certain combinations of word roots requires the insertion of a vowel. Like the word root, the combining form usually indicates a body part. In this text, a combining form will be listed word root/vowel as illustrated in the following examples.

Examples of Combining Forms

WORD ROOT	+	COMBINING VOWEL	=	COMBINING FORM	MEANING
arthr	+	o	=	arthr/o	joint
gastr	+	o	=	gastr/o	stomach
nephr	+	o	=	nephr/o	kidney
neur	+	o	=	neur/o	nerve
oste	+	o	=	oste/o	bone

Multiple roots in medical words are linked together with a combining vowel. In the first example following, the two roots *oste* and *arthr* are linked together with one combining vowel. In the second example, two roots *gastr* and *enter* are also linked together with one combining vowel. Both *oste/o/arthr/itis* and *gastr/o/enter/itis* have two roots that are connected with one combining vowel, the *o*. Review the word components in the following examples.

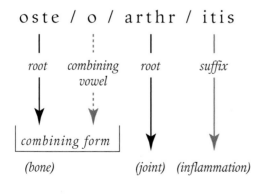

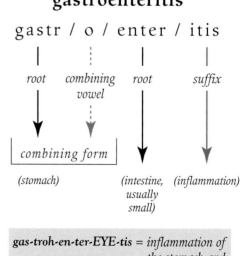

A combining vowel is used to link a root to a suffix that begins with a consonant as illustrated with *arthr/o/centesis* and *gastr/o/pathy.*

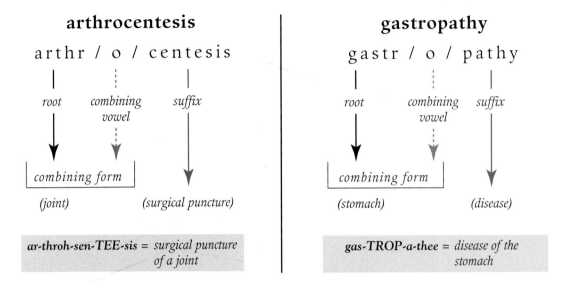

A combining vowel is not used to link a root to a suffix that begins with a vowel as illustrated with *arthr/itis* and *gastr/ectomy.*

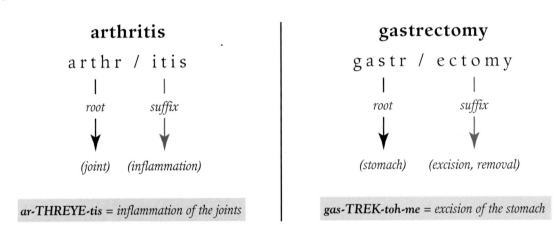

Word Analysis

The roots *oste, gastr,* and *arthr* indicate body parts and are of Greek origin. *Oste* stems from the word *osteon* (bone). *Gastr* stems from the word *gaster* (belly); *arthr* stems from the word *arthron* (joint). The suffix *-itis* means "inflammation"; *-centesis* means "puncture"; *-pathy* means "disease"; and *-ectomy* means "excision," "removal."

When studying medical terminology, learn the combining form rather than the root because the combining form makes most words easier to pronounce. In the previous example, the root without a connecting vowel would be written *arthrcentesis* (ar-thr-sen-TEE-sis). This is almost a tongue twister and is difficult to pronounce. By adding the vowel after the root, the word *arthrocentesis* (ar-throh-sen-TEE-sis) is much easier to pronounce.

Activity 1–1: Competency Verification
Medical Word Components

Match the numbered list items with those in the right-hand column:

1. _j_ pre-

2. _d_ basic components of words

3. _g_ combining form

4. _h_ combining vowel(s)

5. _i_ post-

6. _f_ compound word

7. _e_ Greek and Latin languages

8. _c_ location of prefixes

9. _b_ location of suffixes

10. _a_ word roots

a. foundation of words (e.g., *cardi, arthr*)

b. end of a word

c. beginning of a word

d. word root, suffix, combining form, and prefix

e. origin of most medical words

f. contains two or more word roots

g. *arthr/o*

h. *o* and *i*

i. after

j. before

Correct Answers _____ × 10 = _____ **% Score**

Activity 1–2: Competency Verification
Word Roots, Combining Forms, Suffixes, and Prefixes

Check the box [✓] as you complete each numbered section.

[   ] **1.** Pronounce each medical word listed below aloud.

[   ] **2.** Review all the words below, and underline the combining form(s). Use the abbreviation "CF" to label it (them).

[   ] **3.** Identify the roots, suffixes, and prefixes.

[   ] **4.** Give the meaning of each component by referring to the material in the previous sections, or use a medical dictionary. You are not expected to know the meaning of all the component parts.

Example			
os-tee-oh-ar-THREYE-tis	oste / o /	arthr /	itis
Identify roots, combining forms (CF), suffixes, and prefixes	CF	root	suffix
Meaning	bone	joint	inflammation

1. *mas-TEYE-tis* mast / itis

Identify roots, combining forms (CF), suffixes, and prefixes	
Meaning	

2. *ton-sil-EK-toh-mee* tonsill / ectomy

Identify roots, combining forms (CF), suffixes, and prefixes	
Meaning	

3. *ar-throh-sen-TEE-sis* arthr / o / centesis

Identify roots, combining forms (CF), suffixes, and prefixes	
Meaning	

4. *post-NAY-tal* post / nat / al

Identify roots, combining forms (CF), suffixes, and prefixes	
Meaning	

5. *gas-troh-en-ter-EYE-tis*   g a s t r / o / e n t e r / i t i s

Identify roots, combining forms (CF), suffixes, and prefixes	
Meaning	

6. *mas-TEK-toh-mee*   m a s t / e c t o m y

Identify roots, combining forms (CF), suffixes, and prefixes	
Meaning	

7. *ar-THREYE-tis*   a r t h r / i t i s

Identify roots, combining forms (CF), suffixes, and prefixes	
Meaning	

8. *koh-LEYE-tis*   c o l / i t i s

Identify roots, combining forms (CF), suffixes, and prefixes	
Meaning	

9. *ar-THROP-a-thee*   a r t h r / o / p a t h y

Identify roots, combining forms (CF), suffixes, and prefixes	
Meaning	

10. | *koh-LEK-toh-mee* | c o l / e c t o m y

| Identify roots, combining forms (CF), suffixes, and prefixes | |
| Meaning | |

Correct Answers _____ × 10 = _____ **% Score**

GUIDELINES FOR DEFINING AND BUILDING MEDICAL WORDS

Defining Medical Words

There are three basic steps for defining medical words. First, define the suffix, or last part of the word. Second, define the prefix, or the word part attached to the beginning of the word. Last, define the middle of the word.

Here is an example: oste/o/arthr/itis
　　　　　　　　　(2)　(3)　(1)

1. Define the suffix first; *-itis* means "inflammation."

2. Define the beginning of the word; *oste/o* means "bone."

3. Define the middle of the word; *arthr* means "joint."

The meaning of *oste/o/arthr/itis* is inflammation (of) bone and joint. By understanding the components of this word, you can sense its basic meaning. A quick check of the dictionary further explains that the term refers to a type of arthritis marked by progressive cartilage deterioration in synovial joints and vertebrae.

Building Medical Words

To learn how to build medical words correctly, follow three rules:

Rule 1: A word root is used before a suffix that begins with a vowel.

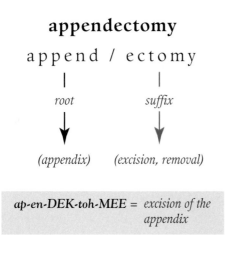

appendectomy

append / ectomy

root　　　suffix

(appendix)　(excision, removal)

ap-en-DEK-toh-MEE = excision of the appendix

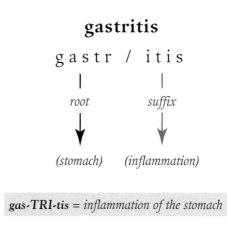

gastritis

gastr / itis

root　　　suffix

(stomach)　(inflammation)

gas-TRI-tis = inflammation of the stomach

Rule 2: A combining form (root + *o*) is used before a suffix that begins with a consonant.

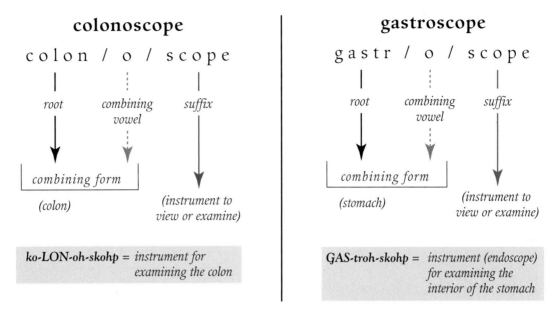

colonoscope

c o l o n / o / s c o p e

| | | |
| root | combining vowel | suffix |

combining form

(colon) (instrument to view or examine)

ko-LON-oh-skohp = *instrument for examining the colon*

gastroscope

g a s t r / o / s c o p e

| | | |
| root | combining vowel | suffix |

combining form

(stomach) (instrument to view or examine)

GAS-troh-skohp = *instrument (endoscope) for examining the interior of the stomach*

Rule 3: A combining form (root + *o*) can be used to link multiple roots even when the root begins with a vowel.

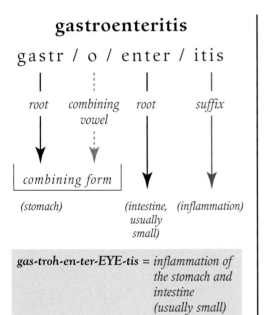

gastroenteritis

gastr / o / enter / itis

| | | | |
| root | combining vowel | root | suffix |

combining form

(stomach) (intestine, usually small) (inflammation)

gas-troh-en-ter-EYE-tis = *inflammation of the stomach and intestine (usually small)*

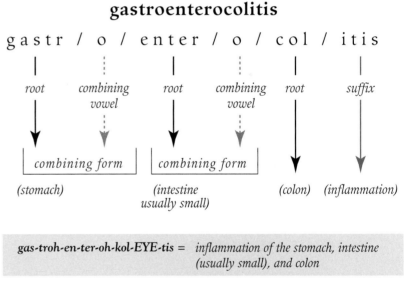

gastroenterocolitis

gastr / o / enter / o / col / itis

| | | | | | |
| root | combining vowel | root | combining vowel | root | suffix |

combining form   combining form

(stomach) (intestine usually small) (colon) (inflammation)

gas-troh-en-ter-oh-kol-EYE-tis = *inflammation of the stomach, intestine (usually small), and colon*

Activity 1–3: Competency Verification
Define and Build Medical Words

Define the following words by applying the definition guidelines that were introduced earlier. First, define the suffix, then define the first prefix. Last, define the middle of the word.

Review the examples in the previous section before writing your answer:

1. tonsill/itis   inflammation (of) tonsils

2. tonsill/ectomy   _____

3. pre/nat/al   _____

4. col/itis   _____

5. gastr/o/scope   _____

Apply the three basic rules for medical word building. The first word is completed for you. You are not expected to know these rules from memory. Refer to the guidelines for defining and building medical words as you complete the following questions. Use the abbreviation CF to designate combining form; use WR to designate word root.

6. gastr/itis   **Rule 1:** A WR is used to link a suffix that begins with a vowel.

7. arthr/o/centesis   _____

8. col/ectomy   _____

9. gastr/o/scope   _____

10. enter/o/col/itis   _____

11. append/ectomy   _____

12. gastr/o/enter/o/col/itis   _____

13. arthr/o/pathy   _____

14. colon/o/scope   _____

15. oste/o/arthr/itis _____

Correct Answers _____ × 6.67 = _____ % Score

PRONUNCIATION OF MEDICAL WORDS

Although the pronunciation of medical words usually follows the same rules that govern the pronunciation of ordinary English words, they may be difficult to pronounce when you first encounter them. To master the pronunciations, study the basic rules of pronunciation, listen to the audio recordings, and repeat the words after you have been introduced to them. Pronunciation guidelines are located in the inside front cover of this textbook. When in doubt about a pronunciation, refer to the guide or use a medical dictionary.

Activity 1–4: Competency Verification
Pronunciation Guidelines

Check the box [✓] as you complete each numbered section.

[   ] **1.** Review the pronunciation guidelines located in the inside front cover of this textbook.

[   ] **2.** Refer to the pronunciation guidelines to complete the following exercise.

Underline one of the items within the parentheses to complete the sentence:

1. The macron (ˉ) above a vowel is used to indicate (short, long) vowel pronunciations.

2. The breve (˘) above a vowel is used to indicate (short, long) vowel pronunciations.

3. When *pn* is in the middle of a word, it is pronounced with a (hard, soft) *p* and a (hard, soft) *n*.

   Examples are ortho*pn*ea, hyper*pn*ea.

4. The letters *c* and *g* have a (hard, soft) sound before other letters.

   Examples are *c*ardiac, *c*ast, *g*astric, *g*onad.

5. When *pn* is at the beginning of a word, it is pronounced only with the sound of (*p, n*).

   Examples are *pn*eumonia, *pn*eumotoxin.

6. Words with *ps* are pronounced with the sound of (*p, s*).

   Examples are *ps*ychology, *ps*ychosis.

7. The combination *ch* is sometimes pronounced like (*k, chiy*).

   Examples are *ch*olesterol, *ch*olera.

8. When *i* is at the end of a word (to form a plural), it is pronounced like (*eye, ee*).

   Examples are bronch*i*, fung*i*, nucle*i*.

9. For *ae* and *oe*, only the (first, second) vowel is pronounced.

   Examples are burs*ae*, pleur*ae*, r*oe*ntgen.

10. When *e* and *es* form the final letter or letters of a word, they are often pronounced as (combined, separate) syllables.

    Examples are syncop*e*, systol*e*, appendic*es*.

| Correct Answers _____ × 10 = _____ % Score |

FORMING PLURALS

When a word changes from singular to plural form, the ending (or suffix) of the word changes as well. For example, the medical report may list one diagno*sis* or several diagno*ses*. The rules for forming plurals starting from the singular forms of the words are given in the inside back cover of the textbook. When in doubt about singular and plural word formations, refer to the rules located on the inside back cover or use a medical dictionary.

Activity 1–5: Competency Verification
Forming Plural Words

Review the rules for forming plurals, located on the inside back cover of this textbook, and use them to complete this activity. The first item is completed for you.

Singular	Plural	Rule
1. sarco*ma*	sarco*mata*	Retain the *ma* and add *ta*.
2. thromb*us*	_____	_____
3. append*ix*	_____	_____
4. diverticul*um*	_____	_____
5. ovar*y*	_____	_____
6. diagno*sis*	_____	_____
7. lum*en*	_____	_____
8. vertebr*a*	_____	_____
9. thor*ax*	_____	_____
10. spermatozo*on*	_____	_____

Correct Answers _____ × 10 = _____ **% Score**

Activity 1–6: Competency Verification
Medical Word Components

Identify the components of each word in the appropriate box. Write the suffix first. Then write the element in the first part of the word. Finally, write the element in the middle. In this review, it is not important for you to know the meaning of the words, but you should understand how to divide them into their component parts. The first word is an example that is completed for you.

Medical Word and Meaning	Components of Medical Words			
	Prefix	Combining Form (root + vowel)	Word Root (s)	Suffix
peri / dent / al around teeth pertaining to pĕr-ĭ-DĔN-tăl	peri-		dent	-al
1. tonsill / ectomy tonsils excision tŏn-sĭl-ĔK-tō-mē				
2. post / nat / al after birth pertaining to pōst-NĀ-tăl				
3. mast / itis breast inflammation măs-TĪ-tĭs				
4. gastr / o / scope stomach instrument to view GĂS-trō-skōp				
5. enter / o / col / itis intestine colon inflammation *(usually small intestine)* ĕn-tĕr-ō-kō-LĪ-tĭs				
6. pre / nat / al before birth pertaining to prē-NĀ-tăl				
7. oste / o / arthr / itis bone joint inflammation ŏs-tē-ō-ăr-THRĪ-tĭs				
8. append / ectomy appendix excision, removal ăp-ĕn-DĔK-tō-mē				
9. gastr / ectomy stomach excision, removal găs-TRĔK-tō-mē				
10. arthr / o / centesis joint surgical puncture ar-thrō-sĕn-TĒ-sĭs				

Activity 1–7: Competency Verification
Defining Medical Terms

Use the following table to complete the statements below:

Combining Forms	Suffixes and Prefixes	Meaning
append/o		appendix
arthr/o		joint
col/o		colon
enter/o		intestine (usually small)
gastr/o		stomach
mast/o		breast
oste/o		bone
	-centesis	puncture
	-itis	inflammation
	-pathy	disease
	-scope	instrument to view or examine
	pre-	before
	post-	after

1. Mast/ectomy is an excision of a(n) _____.

2. Tonsill/itis is a(n) _____ of the tonsils.

3. A colon/o/scope is an instrument to examine the _____.

4. Oste/o/malacia is a softening of _____ (singular).

5. Post/nat/al means "pertaining to (the period) _____ birth."

6. Arthr/o/centesis is a surgical puncture of a _____.

7. Arthr/o/pathy is a _____ of the joints.

8. A prefix that means "before" is _____-.

9. The combining form for stomach is _____ / ___.

10. The suffix for disease is -_____.

11. The combining form for the breast is _____ / ____.

12. The suffix meaning "instrument to examine" is -_____.

13. The combining form append/o refers to the _____.

14. Gastro/enter/itis is an inflammation of the stomach and the _____.

15. The suffix for surgical puncture is -_____.

| **Correct Answers** _____ × **6.67** = _____% **Score** |

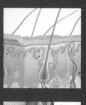

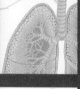

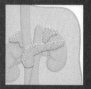

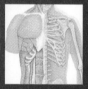

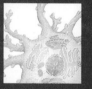

chapter

2

Medical Specialties and Medical Records

Objectives

Upon completion of this chapter, you will be able to:

- Understand the importance of an accurate and comprehensive medical record.

- Identify and describe several medical specialties.

- Explain how the medical record is used in the health-care system.

- Differentiate between and describe different types of medical reports found in the medical record.

- Demonstrate your knowledge of this chapter by successfully completing the activities.

MEDICAL SPECIALTIES AND MEDICAL RECORDS AT A GLANCE

Learning medical terminology using the medical specialty approach provides a realistic and practical application of the various components of medical care in the health-care system. Hospitals, outpatient clinics, medical group practices, and surgical centers employ health-care practitioners to assist physicians in one or more medical specialties. Thus, a health-care practitioner, such as a nurse, physician assistant, or medical assistant may assist several physicians in providing patient care in several different specialty areas. Although there are numerous medical specialties, only the major ones are covered in this textbook (see the Table of Contents).

In the health-care industry, the medical record provides a means of documenting patient care and is one of the main forms of communication between health-care practitioners. Various types of medical reports are included in the medical record: The progress notes, the history and physical examination, the consultation, the discharge summary, the operative report, diagnostic studies, and so forth. Authentic medical reports are found in subsequent chapters throughout this textbook. All names have been changed to maintain patient confidentiality. The purpose of the reports is to provide you with an understanding of how the language of medicine is applied in the health-care system and to reinforce the terminology covered in the chapter. For a more comprehensive examination of the medical record, refer to Chapter 21.

HEALTH-CARE PRACTITIONERS

The health-care system comprises many different medical and allied health professionals, all of whom provide direct or indirect services related to medical care. The medical doctor (MD), or physician, is the primary health-care practitioner. Working under the direct supervision of the physician, other health-care practitioners (e.g., the physician assistant, nurse practitioner, medical assistant, etc.) complement the physician's goals in providing quality medical care. These health-care practitioners form the medical team and implement the plan of treatment designed to improve or maintain the health and well-being of the patient. Other professionals working as part of the medical team include the receptionist, medical secretary, laboratory technician, and all other support members who have direct or indirect contact with the patient. Working as a team member is an important element in providing quality medical care for all patients.

In addition to the MD, the doctor of osteopathic medicine (DO) is also a primary health-care practitioner. Like the MD, the DO provides state-of-the-art methods of treatment, including prescribing drugs and performing surgeries. Unlike the MD, the DO places special emphasis on the body's musculoskeletal system. The osteopathic philosophy maintains that good health requires proper alignment of bones, muscles, ligaments, and nerves.

To earn the MD degree, one must first successfully complete 4 years of study from an accredited medical school. The MD may then begin postgraduate training, which lasts at least 3 years, and in some instances longer. Postgraduate training is called *residency*. Upon completion of each residency program, examinations are administered to certify competency in a specialty area of medicine.

After residency, a doctor may then want to further specialize by fulfilling a *fellowship* training. Fellowships last from 2 to 5 years and train doctors in clinical (patient) care and research skills. For example, a pediatrician may choose to do a fellowship in cardiology. Upon successful completion of fellowship training and examinations, the doctor is then a recognized specialist in pediatric cardiology.

Besides obtaining the degree, the MD must be licensed to practice medicine. Each state has a medical board that establishes a licensing examination and any other requirements that candidates must pass before they can practice medicine.

MEDICAL SPECIALTIES

As various medical specialties emerge, doctors spend more years in training to develop expertise in a specialty of medicine. The physician's medical specialty evolves around providing medical care for a particular body system. For example, a cardiologist provides medical care for patients with heart and vascular disorders, whereas a pulmonologist provides medical care for patients with lung and breathing problems. The major areas of medical specialties are summarized in Table 2–1. Whenever medical care extends beyond the scope of a physician's practice the patient is referred to a different specialist for additional treatment. For example, a patient may be treated by the family physician for back pain. If the family physician cannot resolve the problem, the patient may be referred to an orthopedic doctor for additional care. Unlike in other medical practices, specialists in family practice, internal medicine, and pediatrics are the first links of providing medical care in the health-care system. First-link physicians are often referred to as *primary care providers* because they are the first health-care practitioners patients usually consult. These physicians tend to see patients on a regular basis for a variety of ailments and preventive treatments. As stated previously, when the primary care provider does not possess the expertise to treat a patient's health-care problem, the primary care provider refers the patient to a specialist who is best suited to treat the patient.

TABLE 2–1: Medical Specialties

MEDICAL SPECIALTY	SPECIALIST	SCOPE OF MEDICAL PRACTICE
Anesthesiology an=without esthesio= feeling logy=study of	Anesthesiologist	Treatment of pain and the administration of medication to relieve pain during surgery
Cardiology cardio=heart logy=study of	Cardiologist	Treatment of heart and vascular disorders
Cardiovascular Surgery cardio=heart vascul=vessel ar=pertaining to	Cardiovascular surgeon	Surgical treatment of heart and blood vessels
Dermatology dermato=skin logy=study of	Dermatologist	Diagnosis and treatment of skin disorder
Emergency Medicine	Emergency physician	Emergency evaluation and treatment of conditions caused by trauma or sudden illness
Endocrinology endo=within crino=secrete logy=study of	Endocrinologist	Diagnosis and treatment of endocrine gland disorders
Family Practice	Family practitioner	Primary care and treatment of children and adults on a continuing basis
Gastroenterology gastro=stomach entero=intestines logy=study of	Gastroenterologist	Treatment of diseases involving the stomach, intestines, gallbladder, and bile duct
Gerontology geronto=old age logy=study of	Gerontologist	Diagnosis and treatment of diseases affecting the elderly
Hematology hemato=blood logy=study of	Hematologist	Treatment of blood disorders
Immunology immuno=immune, immunity logy=study of	Immunologist	Treatment of allergic disorders and the management of the body's immune system
Internal Medicine	Internist	Diagnosis and nonsurgical treatment of disorders in adults
Neurology neuro=nerve logy=study of	Neurologist	Diagnosis and nonsurgical treatment of the nervous system and its disorders
Neurosurgery	Neurosurgeon	Diagnosis and surgical treatment of the central nervous system and its disorders

Obstetrics and Gynecology (OB-GYN)
  Obstetrics
  obstetro=midwife
	Obstetrician	Treatment of pregnant women and the fetus during the pregnancy, childbirth, and postpartum periods

Gynecology
  gyneco=woman, female
  logy=study of
	Gynecologist	Surgery and treatment of the female reproductive system

Oncology onco=tumor logy=study of	Oncologist	Diagnosis and treatment of cancer

Table continued on following page.

TABLE 2–1: Medical Specialties (*Continued*)

MEDICAL SPECIALTY	SPECIALIST	SCOPE OF MEDICAL PRACTICE
Ophthalmology ophthalmo=eye logy=study of	Ophthalmologist	Medical and surgical treatment of eye disorders
Orthopedics ortho=straight ped=foot ics=pertaining to	Orthopedist, orthopedic surgeon	Medical and surgical treatment of the musculoskeletal system (bones, muscles, and joints)
Otorhinolaryngology oto=ear rhino=nose laryngo=larynx logy=study of	Otorhinolaryngologist, otolaryngologist	Medical and surgical treatment of diseases and injuries of the ear, nose, and throat
Pathology patho=disease logy=study of	Pathologist	Diagnosis of diseases by analyzing cells obtained at biopsy or autopsy
Pediatrics ped=child iatric=treatment, medicine, physician	Pediatrician	Care and treatment of children
Plastic Surgery	Plastic surgeon	Surgery for alteration, replacement, and restoration of body structures due to a defect or for cosmetic reasons
Proctology procto=anus, rectum logy=study of	Proctologist	Treatment of disorders of the colon, the rectum, and the anus
Psychiatry psych=mind -iatry=medicine, physician, treatment	Psychiatrist	Diagnosis, treatment, and prevention of mental, emotional, and behavioral disorders
Pulmonology pulmono=lung logy=study of	Pulmonologist	Treatment of lung diseases and breathing disorders
Radiology radio=radiation, x-ray logy=study of	Radiologist	Use of x-rays to diagnose and treat diseases
Rheumatology rheumato=watery flow logy=study of	Rheumatologist	Treatment of joint and muscle disorders
Urology uro=urine logy=study of	Urologist	Surgical and nonsurgical treatment of the male urinary and reproductive systems and the female urinary system

Activity 2–1: Competency Verification

Medical Practice Information

1. What are the requirements to receive the MD degree in the United States?

_____

_____

2. Besides the MD degree, what are the other requirements to practice medicine?

_____

_____

3. Define *fellowship training.*

_____

_____

4. Define the role of the primary care provider.

_____

_____

5. What types of specialists are considered primary care providers?

_____

Correct Answers _____ × **20** = _____ **% Score**

THE MEDICAL RECORD

The medical record is initiated at the time of the patient's first appointment with a health-care practitioner. It is a compilation of written documents that provide information and insight into the patient's health history. The majority of these written documents consist of various types of medical reports. Nonmedical information, such as occupation, address, telephone number and so forth, as well as demographic information, such as race, gender, and age, are also part of the medical record. Because there are many different types of services or procedures performed on a patient, various health-care practitioners contribute reports and other information in the medical record. Thus, it is an important method of communication between the physician and the health-care team involved in caring for the patient. The primary purpose of a medical record is to document and compile a database of relevant facts related to the patient's health history, illness, and treatment. The medical record also serves as a legal document. Accurate, documented information not only ensures quality medical care for the patient but also provides evidence to protect the legal interests of the health-care facility, the physician, and the patient if needed in a court of law. Because letters are frequently used to communicate patient information to other physicians, government offices, as well as the patient, they become part of the patient's medical record. There are several standard business letter formats (styles), and one such format is illustrated in Medical Record 2–1. This correspondence is from the doctor to the patient and in this case, it becomes part of the patient's medical record. The letter provides evidence that Mrs. Mung neglected to follow the physician's recommendations of obtaining a Holter moniter that would help determine the extent of her palpitations. A review of the medical record provides a clear description of exactly what occurred during the physician's supervision of a patient. The medical record is also used to justify insurance reimbursements.

MEDICAL REPORTS

There are numerous types and styles of medical reports. Some of the most common medical reports found within the medical record are discussed in this chapter.

Progress Notes

Progress notes, also called *chart notes*, contain information entered by various health-care practitioners after examining, talking, or meeting with a patient. Progress notes contain a description of the patient's problem or chief complaint (CC), physical findings, physician's treatment plan, and results of any diagnostic tests. The physician, nurse, or other health-care practitioner who contributes some type of medical service to the patient usually enters progress notes in the chart. This form of documentation is found in the medical records of all health-care facilities. Health-care practitioners in hospitals, clinics, and doctors' offices all write progress notes. Usually, the notes are hand-written. The notes may remain handwritten or they may be dictated and then later typed by a medical transcriptionist, medical secretary, or medical assistant. Medical Record 2–2 is an example of progress notes recorded in an outpatient clinic. These progress notes appear in the SOAP (subjective, objective, assessment, plan) format. Chapter 21 discusses the SOAP format in detail.

History and Physical Examination

The history and physical examination (H&P) is a comprehensive document generated by the physician or other examiner at the patient's first office visit. The H&P documents important data related to the patient's medical history, social history, and the com-plaint or illness that prompted the patient to seek medical attention. The primary purpose of the H&P is to compile information that the physician needs to determine a diagnosis and a treatment plan for the patient. Medical Record 2–3 contains the H&P for Mary Draper who presented in the emergency room complaining of difficulty in breathing. Read the H&P (Medical Record 2–3) to become familiar with this type of medical report.

Consultation

A consultation is the written correspondence of a physician who requests and then receives further medical evaluation of his or her patients from specialists or other physicians. In Medical Record 2–4, the cardiovascular specialist, Dr. Ford, completes an examination requested by the patient's primary physician. Most consultation reports usually contain a brief history of the patient's illness, the physician's findings, pertinent laboratory and x-ray results, a preliminary diagnosis, and a suggested course of treatment. The consultation may be in a letter format, as shown in Medical Record 2–4, or written on a consultation request form.

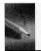

Activity 2–2: Competency Verification
Medical Records

1. When is the medical record initiated?

   _____

2. How would a medical record be advantageous as a legal document if a patient sues the physician?

   _____

3. Besides medical information, what other type of information is contained in the medical record?

   _____

   _____

   _____

4. What is the primary purpose of the history and physical?

   _____

   _____

5. What is a consultation report?

_____

_____

Correct Answers _____ × 20 = _____ **% Score**

Imaging Report

An imaging report contains the findings and diagnostic impressions from conventional radiographs or other imaging procedures. Numerous types of diagnostic imaging procedures are available to establish or confirm a diagnosis. These procedures are discussed extensively in Chapter 18, Radiology and Nuclear Medicine. The imaging report shown in Medical Record 2–5 is an illustration of one such radiographic procedure called magnetic resonance imaging (MRI). Unlike x-rays, MRI uses magnetic waves to produce a cross-sectional multiplanar image of the entire body or specific body part. It also has the ability to produce images through bone tissue and fluid-filled soft tissues. The physician ordered this diagnostic imaging procedure for Timothy Anders, an automobile accident victim, to determine whether there was any evidence of spinal cord injury.

Laboratory Report

Laboratory reports summarize documented findings of tests performed on tissue samples, blood, and other body fluids. The laboratory test is a valuable diagnostic tool. Specific laboratory tests can be used to diagnose a particular disease; for example, an abnormal glucose level may indicate diabetes mellitus. Test results that deviate from normal values can be indicative of a particular disease state or health problem. Medical Record 2–6 summarizes the findings of a chemistry profile and a urinalysis (UA). A profile can be designed to screen several of the body's 12 systems or one particular function, such as liver function. The chemistry profile (blood test) in Medical Record 2–6 shows Joleen Smythers'

potassium level at 3.8 mmol/L. The normal range is 3.5 to 5.0 mmol/L. When you review the laboratory report, you will find that all of the normal ranges of the tests performed are listed on this report. Although her level is a bit low, it still falls within the normal range. However, an abnormally low level may be indicative of loss of body fluids, whereas a high level may be indicative of renal failure or diabetic ketoacidosis—a type of acidosis caused by an accumulation of ketone bodies in advanced stages of uncontrolled diabetes mellitus. When the results of a laboratory test are abnormal, the physician can further investigate the abnormal result. The laboratory test known as a urinalysis (urine test) is used to detect kidney and urinary tract abnormalities. The physician ordered a chemistry profile and urinalysis preoperatively (before surgery) for Joleen Smythers to obtain information about the patient's state of health and to determine the presence of any abnormalities. The report format of the tests is designed by the General Hospital and Medical Center and may differ from the format of other hospitals. Additionally, some of the abbreviations may be unique to General Hospital and do not necessarily represent the standard universal abbreviations that are listed in medical references, dictionaries, and throughout this textbook. Other types and styles of laboratory reports are included in Chapter 21.

It is not necessary for you to understand the reports at this time, but you should review them to familiarize yourself with the general content of such reports. Abbreviations and definitions are listed at the end of the chapter and in Appendix A.

Medical Record 2–1. Letter
_____

GENERAL HOSPITAL AND MEDICAL CENTER
2211 Fifth Avenue North • Healthy City, USA 12345 • (321) 123-4567
_____

February 22, 20xx

Mrs. Anna Mung
4397 George Street
Healthy City, USA 12345

Dear Mrs. Mung:

I have tried to reach you multiple times by phone. Our office staff has left several messages for you to call, and you have not yet returned the phone calls. When you were in the office on February 9, 20xx, you were having problems with palpitations, and I had discussed obtaining a Holter monitor. I told you at that time that we would contact you with an appointment date and time.

Since you have not returned our calls, we have been unable to schedule this important test. Please contact my office at your earliest convenience.

Sincerely,

Bruce Burkhart, MD

BB/sl

Medical Record 2–2. Progress Notes

GENERAL HOSPITAL AND MEDICAL CENTER
2211 Fifth Avenue North • Healthy City, USA 12345 • (321) 123-4567

Progress Notes

Patient Name: Joan Carroll
Birth Date: 12/23/xx

Patient Number: 34-46-92
Room Number: OP

Date: March 5, xxxx

SUBJECTIVE
Patient presents with a 2–3 day history of upper respiratory sinus congestion and increasing bilateral otalgia, sore throat, dry cough. She has no history of hay fever. She is allergic to amoxicillin. Only medicine is Wellbutrin. She is taking a family vacation to Puerto Rico and is flying tomorrow.

OBJECTIVE
Physical examination shows her to be well developed, well nourished, and in no acute distress. There is serous otitis on the right. The left tympanic membrane is benign. The oropharynx is mildly erythematous. Rapid-Strep is negative. Neck is supple without lymphadenopathy. Lungs are clear to auscultation bilaterally.

ASSESSMENT
Upper respiratory infection versus allergic rhinits.

PLAN
As she is flying, we will treat very aggressively. We will try to decrease inflammation and open the eustachian tubes. I have given her Claritin-D as well as Flonase nasal inhaler. We will treat her with ibuprofen and Afrin prior to flying, and she will take erythromycin if needed for increasing symptoms. I have given her a prescription as she is going out of town. If she is worsening, she will fill this prescription.   She will follow up if worsening or failing to improve.

_____
Robert Scott, MD

RS/lm
D: 03/05/xx
T: 03/06/xx

>>> MEDICAL RECORD 2-3: HISTORY AND PHYSICAL EXAMINATION

Term	Pronunciation	Meaning
pulmonary	*PŬL-mō-nĕ-rē*	_____
intubation	*ĭn-tū-BĀ-shŭn*	_____
prednisone	*PRĔD-nĭ-zōn*	_____
hypertension	*hī-pĕr-TĔN-shŭn*	_____
Xanax	*ZĂ-năks*	_____
Proventil	*prō-VĔNT-ĭl*	_____
Paxil	*PĂK-sĭl*	_____
Adalat	*ĂD-ă-lăt*	_____
Accupril	*Ă-kū-prĭl*	_____
nausea	*NAW-sē-ă*	_____
diarrhea	*dī-ă-RĒ-ă*	_____
melena	*MĔL-ĕ-nă*	_____
hematochezia	*hĕm-ă-tō-KĒ-zē-ă*	_____
bruit	*brwē*	_____
thyromegaly	*thī-rō-MĔG-ă-lē*	_____
tachycardia	*tăk-ē-KĂR-dē-ă*	_____
hepatosplenomegaly	*hĕp-ă-tō-splē-nō-MĔG-ă-lē*	_____
edema	*ĕ-DĒ-mă*	_____
Cefizox	*SĔ-fĭ-zŏks*	_____
Solu-Medrol	*Sŏ-lū-MĔD-rŏl*	_____

>>> MEDICAL RECORD 2-4: CONSULTATION

Term	Pronunciation	Meaning
retrosternal	*rĕt-rō-STĔR-năl*	_____

pericarditis	*pĕr-ĭ-kăr-DĪ-tĭs*	_____
claudication	*klăw-dĭ-KĀ-shŭn*	_____
pleuritic pain	*ploo-RĬT-ĭk păn*	_____
paroxysmal	*păr-ŏk-SĬZ-măl*	_____
nocturnal	*nŏk-TĔR-năl*	_____
dyspnea	*dĭsp-NĒ-ă*	_____
orthopnea	*or-THŎP-nē-ă*	_____
Coumadin	*KŪ-mă-dĭn*	_____
cardiovascular	*kăr-dē-ō-VĂS-kŭ-lăr*	_____

>>> MEDICAL RECORD 2-5: IMAGING REPORT

Term	**Pronunciation**	**Meaning**
coronal	*kŏ-RŌ-năl*	_____
sacrum	*SĀ-krŭm*	_____
herniation	*hĕr-nē-Ā-shŭn*	_____

>>> MEDICAL RECORD 2-6: LABORATORY REPORT

Term	**Pronunciation**	**Meaning**
sodium	*SŌ-dē-ŭm*	_____
glucose	*GLOO-kōs*	_____
leukocytes	*LOO-kō-sīts*	_____
nitrite	*NĪ-trīt*	_____

Critical Thinking: Analysis of Medical Records

This section provides experience in abstracting and analyzing information from medical records. Refer to Medical Records 2–2 through 2–6 as you answer the following questions.

>>> MEDICAL RECORD 2–2: PROGRESS NOTES

1. Does the patient have a history of hay fever or sore throat?

_____

2. What are the three medications prescribed to decrease inflammation and to open up the eustachian tubes?

_____

_____

>>> MEDICAL RECORD 2–3: HISTORY AND PHYSICAL EXAMINATION

3. What was the patient's CC?

_____

4. Does the patient suffer from nausea, diarrhea, or constipation?

_____

5. Did the physician note that there were increased breath sounds or any rales or wheezing?

_____

_____

6. Does the patient have any allergies?

_____

>>> MEDICAL RECORD 2–4: CONSULTATION

7. What was the patient's sharp pain associated with?

_____

8. What did the cardiovascular system examination reveal?

_____

_____

>>> MEDICAL RECORD 2-5: IMAGING REPORT

9. Why was the imaging study ordered for Timothy Anders?

_____

10. What abnormalities were found?

_____

>>> MEDICAL RECORD 2-6: LABORATORY REPORT

11. What laboratory tests were performed on Joleen Smythers?

_____

12. What type of sample(s) was used for the tests?

_____

Pathology Report

A pathology report, sometimes referred to as a *biopsy report*, contains the pathological findings in a tissue sample taken during surgery, biopsy, or autopsy. Although the wordings of the headers may vary between institutions, the central information contained within the report includes the name of the specimen submitted, the macroscopic or gross description (which is the appearance of the specimen before it is prepared for microscopic study), the microscopic findings, the cells and description of the tissue under the microscope, and the remarks and pathological diagnosis (diagnoses, plural). To become familiar with a pathology report, review Medical Record 2–7.

Operative Report

An operative report, also known as a *surgical report*, is a narrative description of a surgical procedure. An operative report is dictated by the physician and typed by a medical transcriptionist. The information contained in this report includes a detailed description of the operation performed, preoperative and postoperative diagnoses, anesthesia used, estimated blood loss, condition of the patient or complications encountered, and the names of the persons on the surgical team. Review Medical Record 2–8, which is the operative report for an elective surgical procedure to eliminate snoring that was performed on Carol Ottoman. The surgery performed on this patient is called laser-assisted uvulopalatoplasty.

Discharge Summary

The discharge summary is an important document in the patient's medical record. It contains a summary of the care rendered to a patient during the patient's stay in a hospital or any other health care facility. Information contained in this report includes admitting and discharge diagnoses, brief health history, physical examination findings, pertinent laboratory and diagnostic test results, any discharge medications, and a plan for follow-up care. To become familiar with the content of a discharge summary, review Medical Record 2–9 for John Tapper.

Medical Record 2–9. Discharge Summary

GENERAL HOSPITAL AND MEDICAL CENTER
2211 Fifth Avenue North • Healthy City, USA • (321) 123-4567

Discharge Summary

Patient Name: John Tapper   **Patient Number:** 34-55-90
Birth Date: 10/23/xx   **Room Number:** 342

DATE OF ADMISSION: 11/03/xx

DATE OF DISCHARGE: 11/09/xx

DISCHARGE SUMMARY: Mr. Tapper is a 78-year-old man who was transferred from Smith Hospital because of worsening shortness of breath and atrioventricular block. The patient was admitted and found to have congestive heart failure with severe left ventricular dysfunction, significant mitral regurgitation, and severe chronic obstructive pulmonary disease. The patient was aggressively diuresed using intravenous nitrates, diuretics, and dopamine. After several days of diuresis, the patient improved. In the meantime, the patient also underwent pacemaker implantation for atrioventricular block. He was put on Cordarone because of frequent atrial arrhythmias and was treated for his COPD with intravenous steroids.

At the time of discharge, the patient was doing reasonably well, ambulating in the hallways with oxygen, and had no symptoms.

His discharge medications include Micro-K 10 mEq t.i.d., aspirin 325 mg q.d., Isordil 20 mg t.i.d., Cordarone 200 mg q.d., digoxin 0.125 mg q.d., Lasix 20 mg q.d., Zestril 20 mg q.d., prednisone in tapering dose, and Combivent inhaler 2 puffs q.i.d.

The patient was given discharge arrangements including followup with Dr. Allay, his family physician, in one week and Dr. Bruno in 4-6 weeks.

BUN, creatinine, and electrolytes were ordered in one week.

CONDITION ON DISCHARGE: Fair.

Home oxygen therapy and home follow up for his congestive heart failure to include daily weights, fluid restrictions, etc., were all given to the patient and arrangements made.

_____
David Bruno, MD

cc: Michael Allay, MD
DB/bl
D&T: 11/09/xx

Medical Record 2–10. Emergency Department Report

GENERAL HOSPITAL AND MEDICAL CENTER
2211 Fifth Avenue North • Healthy City, USA • (321) 123-4567

Emergency Department Report

Patient Name: Nancy Frost **Patient Number:** 55-78-45
Birth Date: 02/14/xx **Room Number:** ER

CHIEF COMPLAINT: Fell, injured right leg.

HISTORY OF PRESENT ILLNESS: Patient fell four days ago onto some concrete when she tripped. She denies any other injuries. She has remained ecchymotic and swollen and subsequently presents for evaluation.

REVIEW OF SYSTEMS: She denies fever, chills, or any other injuries.

PHYSICAL EXAMINATION: She has ecchymosis across the entire lateral aspect of the distal right leg. She has no tenderness about the fibula or hip. She does have tenderness at the proximal fibula. She has no tenderness at the ankle or foot. Good dorsalis pedis pulses. Normal sensation of the foot. Capillary refill is normal. She has good sensation at the base of the web space between the great and second toe. Dorsiflexion at the ankle is strong. X-ray demonstrates a minimally displaced fracture at the proximal fibula.

I spoke with the orthopedic resident, and subsequently the patient was placed in Ace wrap, crutches, with no weight-bearing. Will follow up in ortho clinic.

DIAGNOSIS: Nondisplaced proximal fibula fracture, right leg.

_____

Franklin Dodge, MD

FD/bab
D: 05/01/xx
T: 05/01/xx

The Emergency Department Report

An emergency department report, also called an emergency room report, or emergency report, results when a patient is treated in an emergency department. A brief history, presenting complaint, physical examination results, diagnosis, and treatment plan are all contained within this type of medical report. Sometimes the condition is serious enough to warrant admission to the hospital (inpatient). Otherwise, treatment is administered and the patient is released from the hospital (outpatient). Review Medical Record 2–10, which is the emergency department report for Nancy Frost, who fell and injured her leg.

Reading and Dictionary Exercise

Check the box [✓] after you complete the exercise.

[   ] **1.** Underline the following words in the reports as you read the pathology report, the operative report, the discharge summary, and the emergency department report.

[   ] **2.** Use a medical dictionary and Appendix F to define the terms below.

[   ] **3.** Refer to Medical Records 2–7 through 2–10 as you complete this exercise.

Note: You are not expected to understand all the parts of the medical records. The important aspect of this exercise is to use all available resources to complete it. Eventually you will master the terminology, the pronunciation of words, and the format of these reports.

>>> MEDICAL RECORD 2–7: PATHOLOGY REPORT

Term	Pronunciation	Meaning
biopsy	BĪ-ŏp-sē	_____
endometrial	ĕn-dō-MĒ-trē-ăl	_____
hemorrhage	HĔM-ĕ-rĭj	_____
malignancy	mă-LĬG-năn-sē	_____
hyperplasia	hī-pĕr-PLĀ-zē-ă	_____
endometritis	ĕn-dō-mē-TRĪ-tĭs	_____
pathologist	pă-THŎL-ō-jĭst	_____

>>> MEDICAL RECORD 2–8: OPERATIVE REPORT

Term	Pronunciation	Meaning
apnea	ăp-NĒ-ă	_____

uvulopalatoplasty	*ū-vū-lō-păl-Ă-tō-plăs-tē*	_____
soft palate	*sŏft PĂL-ăt*	_____
oropharynx	*or-ō-FĂR-ĭnks*	_____
lidocaine	*LĪ-dō-kān*	_____
inferiorly	*ĭn-FĒ-rē-or-lē*	_____
posteriorly	*pŏs-TĒ-rē-or- lē*	_____
anteriorly	*ăn-TĬR-ē-or-lē*	_____

>>> MEDICAL RECORD 2-9: DISCHARGE SUMMARY

Term	Pronunciation	Meaning
atrioventricular	*ā-trē-ō-věn-TRĬK-ū-lăr*	_____
mitral	*MĪ-trăl*	_____
regurgitation	*rē-gŭr-jĭ-TĀ-shŭn*	_____
pulmonary	*PŬL-mō-ně-rē*	_____
diuresed	*dī-ū-RĒSD*	_____
intravenous	*ĭn-tră-VĒ-nŭs*	_____
diuretics	*dī-ū-RĚT-ĭks*	_____
dopamine	*DŌ-pă-mēn*	_____
Cordarone	*CŎRD-ă-rŏn*	_____
Micro-K	*MĪ-krō-kā*	_____
Isordil	*Ī-sŏr-dĭl*	_____
digoxin	*dĭ-JŎK-sĭn*	_____
Zestril	*ZĚS-trĭl*	_____
Combivent	*CŎM-bĭ-věnt*	_____

>>> MEDICAL RECORD 2-10: EMERGENCY DEPARTMENT REPORT

Term	Pronunciation	Meaning
ecchymotic	ĕk-ĭ-MŎT-ĭk	_____
ecchymosis	ĕk-ĭ-MŌ-sĭs	_____
lateral	LĂT-ĕr-ăl	_____
distal	DĬS-tăl	_____
dorsalis pedis	dor-SĀ-lĭs PĔ-dĭs	_____
capillary	KĂP-ĭ-lār-ē	_____
dorsiflexion	dor-sĭ-FLĔK-shūn	_____
proximal	PRŎK-sĭm-ăl	_____
fibula	FĬB-ū-lă	_____
ortho	ŏr-thō	_____

Critical Thinking: Analysis of Medical Records

This section provides experience in abstracting and analyzing information from various types of medical reports. Refer to Medical Records 2–7 through 2–10 as you answer the following questions.

>>> MEDICAL RECORD 2-7: PATHOLOGY REPORT

1. From what organ was the biopsy sample taken?

_____

2. Did the sample show evidence of carcinoma?

_____

_____

>>> **MEDICAL RECORD 2-8: OPERATIVE REPORT**

3. What procedure was performed on Carol Ottoman?

_____

4. Why was this procedure performed?

_____

>>> **MEDICAL RECORD 2-9: DISCHARGE SUMMARY**

5. Why was the patient transferred from Smith Hospital?

_____

6. What was done to improve the atrioventricular block?

_____

7. What was the patient's condition upon discharge?

_____

>>> **MEDICAL RECORD 2-10: EMERGENCY DEPARTMENT REPORT**

8. Why did Nancy Frost come to the emergency room?

_____

9. What type of fracture did the patient have?

_____

10. What treatment was she given for her injury?

_____

❖ ABBREVIATIONS

Abbreviations and symbols are frequently used to document patient care and are found in various medical reports. It is important to use standardized abbreviations in medical records so that they become familiar to all health-care practitioners.

ABBREVIATION	MEANING	ABBREVIATION	MEANING
BP	blood pressure	MD	medical doctor
BUN	blood urea nitrogen	mEq	milliequivalent
CBC	complete blood count	mg	milligram (1/1000 gram)
cc	cubic centimeter	mmol/L	millimole per liter
CC	chief complaint, craniocaudad (view, radiology)	MS	musculoskeletal, multiple sclerosis, mental status, morphine sulfate
cm	centimeter		
CO$_2$	carbon dioxide	OP	outpatient
COPD	chronic obstructive pulmonary disease	PERRLA	pupils equal, round, and reactive to light and accommodation
CPK	creatine phosphokinase	q	each, every
CV	cardiovascular	qd	every day
DO	doctor of osteopathy	qid	four times a day
EOMI	extraocular motion intact	RBC, rbc	red blood cell(s), red blood count
ER	emergency room, estrogen receptor	R/O	rule out
		S	sacral
GI	gastrointestinal	T	thoracic, temperature, time
GU	genitourinary	TIA	transient ischemic attack
h	hour	tid	three times a day
H&P	history and physical examination	UA	urinalysis
HEENT	head, eyes, ears, nose, and throat	WBC, wbc	white blood cell(s), white blood count
IP	inpatient		
L	liter, left, lumbar	y/o	years old

Activity 2–3: Clinical Application

Medical Reports

Consultation

Discharge Summary

Emergency Department Report

H&P

Imaging Report

Laboratory Report

Letter

Operative Report

Pathology Report

Progress Notes

Select the type of medical report from the list above that best describes each statement in the numbered list:

1. _____ enumeration of services rendered to a patient during the patient's stay in a hospital or other health-care facility.

2. _____ contains results of tests performed on tissue samples, blood, body fluids, etc.

3. _____ a narrative description of a surgical procedure.

4. _____ report that is initiated when a patient is treated in the ER.

5. _____ contains information by the health-care practitioner after examining, talking with, or meeting with a patient; also known as chart notes.

6. _____ report that contains the findings of x-ray procedures.

7. _____ business correspondence used to communicate patient information to other physicians, insurance companies, government offices, and the patient; often written in a business letter format.

8. _____ documents important data that focus on the medical history, social history, and the complaint or illness that prompted the patient to seek medical attention.

9. _____ contains the findings of a tissue sample taken during surgery, a biopsy, or an autopsy; also referred to as a biopsy report.

10. _____ examination of a patient by a specialist at the request of the primary care physician.

Correct Answers _____ × 10 = _____ % Score

The major surgical, diagnostic, and pathological suffixes and common prefixes are presented in this chapter. All of the word components introduced in this chapter are reinforced throughout the textbook.

In this chapter, suffixes that begin with a consonant are presented with a combining vowel (usually *o* followed by a slash (/) and then the suffix)—for example, *-o/scopy*, *-o/rrhaphy*, *-o/tomy*. The reason for the inclusion of the combining vowel *o* is to remind you to use a combining vowel to join the root to the suffix. Recall that the connecting vowel also helps with the ease of pronouncing medical words correctly.

Because the connecting *o* is merely a memory and constructive device and *not* part of the true suffix, you should look up such suffixes in the dictionary under the appropriate consonant and not under the connecting *o*. For example, you would look under *s* in the dictionary to find the definition of *o/scopy* rather than under *o*.

MEDICAL WORD COMPONENTS

Surgical Suffixes

A surgical suffix denotes an operative procedure. In operative terms, the root that is attached to the suffix indicates a body part upon which the surgical procedure is performed. For example, a *gastr/ectomy* is an excision (*-ectomy*) of the stomach (*gastr*). The suffix *-ectomy* denotes a surgical procedure; the root *gastr* denotes the body part. An *append/ectomy* is an excision (*-ectomy*) of the appendix (*append*). The suffix *-ectomy* denotes a surgical procedure; the root *append* denotes the body part.

Surgical suffixes indicate a type of treatment that a physician performs on a body part. Some surgical suffixes are also considered diagnostic suffixes because the surgical procedure is used to diagnose or confirm a patient's condition. The following are surgical suffixes denoting incisions.

Surgical Suffixes: Incisions

Suffix	Meaning	EXAMPLE	
		Term/Pronunciation	Definition
o/**centesis**	surgical puncture	arthr/o/**centesis*** ăr-thrō-sĕn-TĒ-sĭs	surgical puncture of a joint (*arthr/o*) space with a needle to remove accumulated fluid
-**ectomy**	excision, removal	mast/**ectomy** măs-TĔK-tŏ-mē	excision of the breast (*mast/o*)
-o/**stomy**	forming an opening (mouth)	col/o/**stomy** kō-LŎS-tō-mē	surgical opening of a portion of the colon (*col/o*) through the abdominal wall to its outside surface
-o/**tomy**	incision	phleb/o/**tomy** flē-BŎT-ō-mē	incision of a vein (*phleb/o*) to draw blood

*The suffix -centesis *can also be used to designate a diagnostic procedure. See also* amni/o/centesis *in the Diagnostic Suffixes section, which follows.*

Surgical Suffixes: Refracturing, Loosening, Crushing

Suffix	Meaning	EXAMPLE	
		Term/Pronunciation	Definition
-o/**clasis**	to break	oste/o/**clasis** ŏs-tē-ŎK-lă-sĭs	surgical fracture of a bone (*oste/o*) to correct a deformity
-o/**lysis**	separation, destruction, loosening	thromb/o/**lysis** thrŏm-BŎL-ĭ-sĭs	dissolution of a blood clot (*thromb/o*)
-o/**tripsy**	crushing	lith/o/**tripsy** LĬTH-ō-trĭp-sē	crushing of a stone or calculus (*lith/o*)

Surgical Suffixes: Plastic Operations

Suffix	Meaning	EXAMPLE	
		Term/Pronunciation	Definition
-o/**desis**	binding, fixation (of a bone or joint)	arthr/o/**desis** ăr-thrō-DĒ-sĭs	fixation of a joint (*arthr/o*) by a procedure that fuses the joint surfaces
-o/**pexy**	suspension, fixation (of an organ)	colp/o/**pexy** KŎL-pō-pĕk-sē	fixation of a relaxed and prolapsed vagina (*colp/o, vagin/o*) to the abdominal wall
-o/**plasty**	surgical repair	rhin/o/**plasty** RĪ-nō-plăs-tē	surgical repair of the nose (*rhin/o*) to change its structure; plastic surgery of the nose
-o/**rrhaphy**	suture	my/o/**rrhaphy** mī-OR-ă-fē	suture of a muscle (*my/o*)

Diagnostic Suffixes

Diagnostic suffixes are used to build words related to diagnostic procedures or tests. These tests may be ordered to establish or confirm a diagnosis. Some diagnostic suffixes are also used to describe a surgical procedure. The following are the major suffixes related to diagnostic procedures.

Diagnostic Suffixes

Suffix	Meaning	EXAMPLE	
		Term/Pronunciation	Definition
-o/**centesis**	surgical puncture	amni/o/**centesis*** ăm-nē-ō-sĕn-TĒ-sĭs	transabdominal puncture of the amniotic sac (*amni/o*) under ultrasound guidance using a needle and syringe to remove amniotic fluid *The sample fluid is studied to detect genetic disorders.*

*The suffix -centesis can also be used to designate a surgical procedure. See also arthr/o/centesis *in the Surgical Suffixes section above.*

Diagnostic Suffixes (Continued)

Suffix	Meaning	EXAMPLE	
		Term/Pronunciation	**Definition**
-o/**gram**	record, writing	angi/o/**gram** ĂN-jē-ō-grăm	a radiographic image of a blood vessel (*angi/o*) into which contrast medium has been injected *The term angiogram is also called arteriogram.*
-o/**graph**	instrument for recording	electr/o/cardi/o/**graph** ē-lĕk-trō-KĂR-dē-ō-grăf	instrument for recording electrical activity of the heart (cardi/o) *The CF electr/o means "electricity."*
-o/**graphy**	process of recording	angi/o/**graphy** ăn-jē-ŎG-ră-fē	a radiographic image of blood vessels (*angi/o*) and heart chambers after injecting a radiopaque contrast medium into a specific blood vessel or heart chamber *Examples of this radiographic procedure include cardiac angiography, cerebral angiography, and pulmonary angiography.*
-o/**meter**	instrument for measuring	crani/o/**meter** krā-nē-ŎM-ĕ-tĕr	instrument for measuring the skull (*crani/o*)
-o/**metry**	act of measuring	audi/o/**metry** aw-dē-ŎM-ĕ-trē	measurement of hearing (*audi/o*) acuity for various frequencies of sound waves
-o/**scope**	instrument to view or examine	endo/**scope** ĔN-dō-skōp	an instrument consisting of a tube and optical system for observing the inside (*endo-*) of a hollow organ or cavity *The prefix endo- means "in, within."*
-o/**scopy**	visual examination	endo/**scopy** ĕn-DŎS-kō-pē	visual examination or inspection of body organs or cavities with an endoscope *The prefix endo- means "in, within."*

Summary of Medical Word Building Rules

Rule 1: A word root is used to link a suffix that begins with a vowel.

Rule 2: A combining form (root + o) is used to link a suffix that begins with a consonant.

Rule 3: A combining form (root + o) is used to link multiple roots even if a root begins with a vowel.

Activity 3-1: Competency Verification

Surgical and Diagnostic Suffixes

Review the surgical and diagnostic suffixes and their examples in the previous section. Then pronounce each word listed in the example column aloud.

-o/clasis	-o/lysis	-o/rrhaphy
-o/desis	-o/meter	-o/stomy
-ectomy	-o/metry	-o/scopy
-o/gram	-o/pexy	-o/tomy
-o/graphy	-o/plasty	-o/tripsy

Use the components listed above to form medical words meaning:

1. the act of measuring hearing audi/_____

2. process of recording electrical activity of the heart electr/o/cardi/_____

3. forming an opening (mouth) into the colon col/_____

4. suture of muscle my/_____

5. incision of a vein (to draw blood) phleb/_____

6. record (radiographic image) of a blood vessel angi/_____

7. instrument for measuring the cranium or skull crani/_____

8. surgical repair of the nose rhin/_____

9. fixation of (to lift) a breast(s) mast/_____

10. binding or fixation of a joint arthr/_____

11. separation or loosening of a blood clot thromb/_____

12. surgical fracture of a bone oste/_____

13. excision (of all or part) of the colon col/_____

14. visual examination of the stomach gastr/_____

15. crushing a stone or calculus lith/_____

Correct Answers _____ × 6.67 = _____ **% Score**

Activity 3-2: Competency Verification
Surgical and Diagnostic Terms

Check the box [✓] as you complete each numbered section.

[ ] **1.** Review again the surgical and diagnostic suffixes and their examples in the previous section. Then pronounce each word listed in the example column aloud.

[ ] **2.** For the words below, first write the suffix and its meaning. Then translate the meaning of the remaining components starting with the first part of the word.

Note: You are not expected to know all of the word components at this time. They are reinforced throughout the other chapters in the textbook. If needed, refer to the previous sections or use Appendix B to complete this exercise.

Example: esophag/o/gastr/o/scopy
Answer: *scopy= visual examination; esophagus; stomach*

1. mast/ectomy _____

2. rhin/o/plasty _____

3. my/o/rrhapy _____

4. arthr/o/centesis _____

5. col/o/stomy _____

6. phleb/o/tomy _____

7. endo/scope _____

8. electr/o/cardi/o/graph _____

9. audi/o/metry _____

10. lith/o/tripsy _____

Correct Answers _____ × 10 = _____ % Score

Pathological Suffixes

A pathological suffix denotes a disease. The root that is attached to the suffix indicates a body part that is diseased. For example, *hepat/itis* is an inflammation of the liver. The pathological suffix is *-itis;* the root is *hepat.*

Pathological Suffixes

| Suffix | Meaning | EXAMPLE | |
		Term/Pronunciation	Definition
-algia	pain	neur/**algia** nū-RĂL-jē-ă	pain in a nerve (*neur/o*) or along the course of a nerve
-o/dynia		ot/o/**dynia** ō-tō-DĬN-ē-ă	pain in the ear (*ot/o*)
-o/cele	hernia, swelling	hepat/o/**cele** HĔP-ă-tō-sĕl	hernia of the liver (*hepat/o*)
-ectasis	dilation, expansion	bronchi/**ectasis** brŏng-kē-ĔK-tă-sĭs	chronic dilation of a bronchus (singular) or bronchi (plural)
-edema	swelling	lymph/**edema** lĭmf-ĕ-DĒ-mă	accumulation of lymph (*lymph/o*) in soft tissue and the resultant swelling caused by inflammation, obstruction, or removal of lymph channels
-emesis	vomiting	hemat/**emesis** hĕm-ă-TĔM-ĕ-sĭs	the vomiting of blood (*hemat/o, hem/o*)
-emia	blood condition	leuk/**emia** loo-KĒ-mē-ă	a malignancy of the blood (*-emia*) forming cells in the bone marrow
-iasis	abnormal condition (produced by something specified)	chol/e/lith/**iasis*** kō-lē-lĭ-THĪ-ă-sĭs	formation of bile (*chol/e*) stones (*-lith*) in the gallbladder or common bile duct *The CF* chol/e *refers to "bile," "gall";* -lith *refers to "stone, calculus."*
-itis	inflammation	gastr/**itis** găs-TRĪ-tĭs	inflammation of the stomach (*gastr/o*)
-o/lith	stone, calculus	chol/e/**lith*** KŌ-lĕ-lĭth	gallstone *The CF* chol/e *refers to "bile," "gall."*
-o/malacia	softening	oste/o/**malacia** ŏs-tē-ō-măl-Ā-shē-ă	an abnormal condition of softening and weakening of the bones (*oste/o*)
-o/megaly	enlargement	hepat/o/**megaly** hĕp-ă-tō-MĔG-ă-lē	enlargement of the liver (*hepat/o*)
-oma	tumor	carcin/**oma** kăr-sĭ-NŌ-mă	cancerous (*carcin/o*) tumor

* *In the words* chol/e/lith/iasis *and* chol/e/lith, *the connecting vowel is an* e. *Using an* e *is an exception to the rule of using the connecting vowel* o.

Pathological Suffixes (Continued)

Suffix	Meaning	EXAMPLE	
		Term/Pronunciation	Definition
-o/**pathy**	disease	neur/o/**pathy** *nū-RŎP-ă-thē*	any disease of the nerves (*neur/o*)
-o/**penia**	decrease, deficiency	leuk/o/**penia** *loo-kō-PĒ-nē-ă*	abnormal decrease of white blood cells (leukocytes)
-o/**plasia**	formation, growth	dys/**plasia** *dĭs-PLĀ-zē-ă*	abnormal formation or growth of tissue
-o/**plasm**		neo/**plasm** *NĒ-ō-plăzm*	a new (*neo-*) and abnormal formation of tissue, as a tumor or growth; usually used to denote a cancerous growth or tumor
-o/**rrhage**	bursting forth (of)	hem/o/**rrhage** *HĔM-ĕ-rĭj*	profuse discharge of blood (*hem/o*)
-o/**rrhagia**		men/o/**rrhagia** *mĕn-ō-RĀ-jē-ă*	profuse discharge of blood during menstruation (*men/o*)
-o/**rrhea**	discharge, flow	dia/**rrhea** *dī-ă-RĒ-ă*	frequent evacuation of watery stools *The prefix* dia- *means "through"* (*as in "running through"*).
-o/**rrhexis**	rupture	angi/o/**rrhexis** *ăn-jē-or-ĔK-sĭs*	rupture of a vessel (*angi/o*), especially a blood vessel
-**osis**	abnormal condition, increase (used only with blood cells)	cyan/**osis** *sī-ă-NŌ-sĭs*	an abnormal condition of blueness (*cyan/o*) of the skin, which indicates a decrease in oxygen
-o/**spasm**	involuntary contraction, twitching	blephar/o/**spasm** *BLĔF-ă-rō-spăsm*	twitching of the eyelid (*blephar/o*)
-o/**stenosis**	narrowing, stricture	arteri/o/**stenosis** *ăr-tē-rē-ō-stĕ-NŌ-sĭs*	abnormal narrowing of an artery (*arteri/o*)
-o/**toxic**	poison	thyr/o/**toxic** *thī-rō-TŎKS-ĭk*	pertaining to the toxic activity of the thyroid gland (*thyr/o*)
-o/**trophy**	development, nourishment	dys/**trophy** *DĬS-trō-fē*	tissue degeneration caused by poor (*dys-*) nourishment or prolonged disuse *The prefix* dys- *means "bad,"* *"painful," "difficult."*

Activity 3–3: Competency Verification

Pathological Suffixes

[   ] **1.** Review the suffixes denoting pathological conditions in the previous section. Then pronounce each word listed in the example column aloud.

-algia	-itis	-o/penia
-o/cele	-oma	-o/rrhage
-ectasis	-o/malacia	-osis
-emesis	-o/megaly	-o/spasm
-emia	-o/pathy	-o/stenosis

Use the word components listed above to form medical words meaning:

1. pain in a nerve   neur/_____

2. dilation or expansion of the bronchi   bronchi/_____

3. abnormal narrowing of an artery   arteri/_____

4. inflammation of the stomach   gastr/_____

5. cancerous tumor   carcin/_____

6. literally means "white blood"   leuk/_____

7. vomiting blood   hemat/_____

8. hernia of the liver   hepat/_____

9. disease of the nerves   neur/_____

10. twitching of an eyelid   blephar/_____

11. enlargement of the liver   hepat/_____

12. softening of bone   oste/_____

13. decrease or deficiency in white blood cells (leukocytes)   leuk/_____

14. bursting forth of blood   hem/_____

15. abnormal condition of blueness   cyan/_____

Correct Answers _____ × **6.67** = _____ **% Score**	

Activity 3–4: Competency Verification
Pathological Terms

Check the box [✓] as you complete each numbered section.

[   ] **1.** Review the components denoting pathological conditions and their examples in the previous section. Then pronounce each word listed in the example column aloud.

[   ] **2.** For the words below, first write the suffix and its meaning. Then translate the meaning of the remaining components starting with the first part of the word.

Note: You are not expected to know all of the word components at this time. They are reinforced throughout the other chapters in the textbook. If needed, refer to the previous sections or use Appendix B to complete this exercise.

> **Example:** oste/o/arthr/itis
> **Answer:** *itis*=inflammation; bone; joint(s)

1. gastr/itis   _____

2. hepat/o/megaly   _____

3. oste/o/malacia   _____

4. cyan/osis   _____

5. blephar/o/spasm   _____

6. thyr/o/toxic   _____

7. dia/rrhea   _____

8. neo/plasm   _____

9. neur/algia   _____

10. carcin/oma   _____

Correct Answers _____ × 10 = _____% Score

Adjective and Noun Suffixes

The following adjective and noun suffixes are commonly used to indicate whether a word is an adjective or noun. Many of these suffixes are used in everyday English.

Adjective Suffixes

In both medical and nonmedical terms, adjectives are used to modify nouns. The adjective suffixes meaning "pertaining to" or "relating to," or both, are summarized in the following section.

You will recognize many of these suffixes because they are the same ones used in everyday English.

Adjective Suffixes

Adjective Suffix	Meaning	EXAMPLE	
		Term/Pronunciation	Definition
-ac	pertaining to, relating to	cardi/**ac** KĂR-dē-ăk	relating to the heart (*cardi/o*)
-al		dent/**al** DĔN-tăl	relating to the teeth (*dent/o*)
-ar		ventricul/**ar** věn-TRĬK-ū-lăr	relating to a ventricle (*ventricul/o*) (of the heart or brain)
-ary		pulmon/**ary** PŬL-mō-nĕ-rē	relating to a lung (*pulmon/o*)
-eal		esophag/**eal** ē-sŏf-ă-JĒ-ăl	relating to the esophagus (*esophag/o*)
-ic		hepat/**ic** hĕ-PĂT-ĭk	relating to the liver (*hepat/o*)
-ical*		neur/o/log/**ical** nū-rō-LŎJ-ĭ-kăl	relating to the study of (*log/o*) nerves (*neur/o*)
-ile		pen/**ile** PĒ-nĭl	relating to the penis (*pen/o*)
-ory		audit/**ory** AW-dĭ-tō-rē	relating to hearing (*audit/o*)
-ose		gluc/**ose** GLŪ-kōs	relating to sugar, sweetness (*gluc/o*)
-ous†		cutane/**ous** kū-TĀ-nē-ŭs	relating to skin (*cutane/o*)
-tic		cyan/o/**tic** sī-ăn-ŎT-ĭk	relating to blue (*cyan/o*)

* -ical *is a combination of* -ic *and* -al.

† -ous *also means* "composed of," "producing."

Noun Suffixes

Nouns are names of persons, places, things, conditions, or states of being. Nouns added to word roots to create a noun are summarized in the following section. You will recognize many of these suffixes because they are the same ones used in everyday English.

Noun Suffixes

Noun Suffix	Meaning	EXAMPLE	
		Term/Pronunciation	**Definition**
-ia	condition	pneumon/**ia** *nū -MŌ-nē-ă*	a condition of inflamed lungs (*pneum/o*)
-ism		alcohol/**ism** *ĂL-kō-hŏl-ĭzm*	a chronic disease of dependence on alcoholic drinks
-y		neur/o/path/**y** *nū-RŎP-ă-thē*	any disease of the nerves (*neur/o*)
-iatry	medicine, treatment	psych/**iatry** *sī-KĪ-ă-trē*	the branch of medicine concerned with the diagnosis, treatment, and prevention of mental illness *The combining form psych/o refers to "the mind"; the noun suffix -iatry, means "medicine" or "treatment."*
-ician	specialist	obstetr/**ician** *ŏb-stĕ-TRĬSH-ăn*	a specialist in the branch of medicine concerned with pregnancy and childbirth *The combining form obstetr/o means "midwife"; the noun suffix -ician means "specialist."*
-ist		dermat/o/log/**ist** *dĕr-mă-TŎL-ō-jĭst*	a specialist in the study of the skin (*dermat/o*) *The combining form log/o means "study of"; the noun suffix -ist means "specialist."*

Activity 3–5: Competency Verification

Nouns and Adjectives

Determine whether the underlined words are nouns or adjectives. Remember, an adjective modifies a noun. In the space provided, write either *adj* **for adjective or** *noun***.**

1. He was diagnosed with pulmon/ary edema. _____

2. The patient was treated for pneumon/ia. _____

3. A dent/ist is a specialist in the treatment of teeth. _____

4. He has a lesion over the left nas/al tip, which was biopsied. _____

5. Neur/o/log/ical studies were recommended to evaluate the numbness in his left leg. _____

6. Audit/ory acuity testing is a physical assessment of hearing. _____

7. The urolog/ist specializes in urinary tract disorders _____

8. The dermat/o/log/ist treats skin diseases. _____

9. She was diagnosed with cardi/ac arrhythmia. _____

10. Neur/o/path/y is a disease affecting the nervous system. _____

Correct Answers _____ × 10 = _____ **% Score**

Prefixes

Prefixes are word parts placed at the beginning of a word. Substituting one prefix for another changes the meaning of a medical word. Not all, but many medical words contain prefixes. You will recognize many of them because they are the same ones that are used in everyday English.

Prefixes

		EXAMPLE	
Prefix	**Meaning**	**Term/Pronunciation**	**Definition**
a-	without, not	**a**/mast/ia ă-MĂS-tē-ă	absence of breasts (*mast/o*) in women caused by a congenital defect *The noun suffix* -ia *means "condition (of)."*
an-		**an**/orexia ăn-ō-RĔK-sē-ă	loss of appetite (-*orexia*)
brady-	slow	**brady**/pnea brăd-ĭp-NĒ-ă	abnormally slow breathing (-*pnea*)
dia-	through, across	**dia**/rrhea dī-ă-RĒ-ă	frequent passage of watery bowel movements *The suffix* -rrhea *means "discharge," "flow."*
dipl-	double	**dipl**/opia dĭp-LŌ-pē-ă	double vision (-*opia*)
dys-	bad, painful, difficult	**dys**/pepsia dĭs-PĔP-sē-ă	difficult or painful digestion (-*pepsia*) *Dyspepsia is not a disease in itself but is symptomatic of other diseases or disorders.*
endo-	in, within	**endo**/scopy ĕn-DŎS-kō-pē	visual examination (-*scopy*) or inspection of body organs or cavities by use of an endoscope

Prefixes (Continued)

Prefix	Meaning	EXAMPLE	
		Term/Pronunciation	**Definition**
hyper-	excessive, above normal	**hyper**/glyc/emia *hī-pĕr-glī-SĒ-mē-ă*	excessive amount of sugar (*glyc/o*) in the blood (*-emia*), as in diabetes
hypo-	under, below	**hypo**/glyc/emia *hī-pō-glī-SĒ-mē-ă*	abnormally low level of sugar (*glyc/o*) in the blood (*-emia*)
im-	not	**im**/potence *ĬM-pō-tĕns*	inability of a man to achieve or maintain an erection (*-potence*) The suffix *-potence literally means "power."*
in-	in, not	**in**/somn/ia *in-SŎM-nē-ă*	condition (*-ia*) of not being able to sleep (*somn/o*) The suffix *-ia means "condition."*
macro-	large	**macro**/cephal/y *măk-rō-SĔF-ă-lē*	abnormally large size of the head (*cephal/o*) *The noun ending* -y *denotes a condition.*
micro-	small	**micro**/cephal/y *mī-krō-SĔF-ă-lē*	abnormally small size of the head (*cephal/o*) *The noun ending* -y *denotes a condition.*
neo-	new	**neo**/plasm *NĒ-ō-plăzm*	a new and abnormal formation (*-plasm*) of tissue, as a tumor or growth; usually used to denote a cancerous growth or tumor *The suffix* -plasm *means "formation," "growth."*
pseudo-	false	**pseudo**/cyesis *soo-dō-sī-Ē-sĭs*	a false pregnancy (*-cyesis*); condition in which all of the usual signs and symptoms of pregnancy occur in a person who is not pregnant
syn-*	union, together, joined	**syn**/dactyl/ism *sĭn-DĂK-tĭl-ĭzm*	congenital anomaly characterized by the fusion of the fingers or toes (*dactyl/o*) *The suffix* -ism *is a noun ending denoting a condition.*
tachy-	rapid	**tachy**/pnea *tăk-ĭp-NĒ-ă*	an abnormally rapid rate of breathing (*-pnea*)

* Appears as sym- *before* b, p, ph, *or* m.

Activity 3-6: Competency Verification
Prefixes

Review the prefixes and their examples in the previous section. Then pronounce each word in the example column aloud.

a-	dipl-
brady-	dys-
hypo-	neo-
im-	pseudo-
micro-	tachy-

Use the word components listed above to form medical words meaning:

1. double vision   _____/opia

2. a false pregnancy   _____/cyesis

3. absence of breasts   _____/mast/ia

4. a deficiency of blood sugar   _____/glyc/emia

5. an abnormally small size of head   _____/cephal/y

6. rapid breathing   _____/pnea

7. a new formation or growth of tissue _____/plasm

8. inability of a man to achieve an erection; the   _____/potence
   condition of being not potent

9. bad, painful, or difficult digestion   _____/pepsia

10. slow breathing   _____/pnea

Correct Answers _____ × 10 = _____ % Score

Activity 3–7: Competency Verification
Suffixes and Prefixes

-centesis	-oma	dipl-
-dynia	-osis	dys-
-ectomy	-pathy	endo-
-edema	-plasty	hypo-
-emesis	-rrhexis	macro-
-gram	-scope	neo-
-lith	-stenosis	tachy-
-malacia	-tomy	
-megaly	-tripsy	

Match the word components listed above with the definitions given in the numbered list:

1. _____ under, below

2. _____ excision, removal

3. _____ large

4. _____ instrument to view

5. _____ softening

6. _____ double

7. _____ puncture

8. _____ tumor

9. _____ disease

10. _____ new

11. _____ stone, calculus

12. _____ rupture

13. _____ rapid

14. _____ swelling

15. _____ bad, painful, difficult

16. _____ record, a writing

17. _____ enlargement

18. _____ vomiting

19. _____ abnormal condition

20. _____ within

21. _____ narrowing, stricture

22. _____ incision (of)

23. _____ crushing

24. _____ surgical repair

25. _____ pain

Correct Answers _____ × 4 = _____% **Score**

Activity 3-8: Competency Verification
Medical Terms

amni/o/centesis	col/o/stomy	hepat/o/cele	pseudo/cyesis
an/orexia	dia/rrhea	hyper/glyc/emia	rhin/o/plasty
audi/o/metry	dys/pepsia	leuk/emia	tachy/pnea
blephar/o/spasm	electr/o/cardi/o/graph	mast/ectomy	thromb/o/lysis
bronchi/ectasis	gastr/o/scopy	macro/cephal/y	
carcin/oma	hem/o/rrhage	oste/o/clasis	
chol/e/lith/iasis	hemat/emesis	oste/o/malacia	

Match the words listed above with the definitions given in the numbered list:

1. _____ abnormally large size of a head

2. _____ difficult or painful digestion

3. _____ puncture of the amniotic sac

4. _____ visual examination of the stomach

5. _____ rapid breathing

6. _____ profuse discharge of blood

7. _____ hernia of the liver

8. _____ loss of appetite

9. _____ softening of the bones

10. _____ cancerous tumor

11. _____ vomiting blood

12. _____ excision of a breast

13. _____ frequent evacuation of watery stools

14. _____ surgical opening (mouth) of a portion of the colon through the abdominal wall to its outside surface

15. _____ surgical repair of the nose

16. _____ a false pregnancy

17. _____ surgical fracture of a bone

18. _____ separation, destruction, or loosening of a blood clot

19. _____ a malignancy of the blood-forming cells in the bone marrow; literally means "white blood"

PLANES OF REFERENCE

To visualize and study the structural arrangements of various organs, the body may be sectioned (cut) and diagrammed according to planes of reference. A plane is an imaginary flat surface that separates two portions of the body or an organ. Thinking in terms of body planes helps you understand the anatomic relationship of one part to another.

Four fundamental planes (midsagittal, sagittal, coronal, and transverse) are frequently used to depict structural arrangement. Locate these planes in Figure 4–3, which offers an illustration of the planes in the anatomic position.

- **Midsagittal (median) plane.** A vertical plane that passes through the midline of the body and divides the body or organ into equal right and left sides.

- **Sagittal plane.** A plane that is parallel to a midsagittal plane that divides the body or organ into unequal right and left sides.

- **Frontal (coronal) plane.** A plane from side to side that separates the body into anterior (front) and posterior (back) portions

- **Transverse (horizontal) plane.** A plane that separates the body into superior (upper) and inferior (lower) portions.

Body planes are also used to describe the view in which radiographic images are taken. For example, an anteroposterior chest radiograph is taken in the coronal or frontal plane. Prior to the development of the computed tomographic (CT) radiographic scan (which displays an image along a transverse plane), conventional radiographic images were on a vertical plane, and the dimensions of body irregularities were difficult, if not impossible, to ascertain.

MEDICAL WORD COMPONENTS

Combining Forms

Basic Structural Units

The basic structural units of the body consist of cells and tissues. These structures make up the upper levels of anatomic structures. The combining forms representing these structures are summarized in the following chart.

Combining Forms: Cells and Tissues

Combining Form	Meaning	EXAMPLE	
		Term/Pronunciation	**Definition**
adip/o	fat	**adip**/oid ĂD-ĭ-poyd	resembling (-*oid*) fat
lip/o		**lip**/ectomy lĭ-PĔK-tō-mē	excision of (-*ectomy*) of fatty tissue
cyt/o	cell	**cyt**/o/logy* sī-TŎL-ō-jē	study of (-*logy*) cells *Cytology includes the study of formation, structure, and function of cells.*
chondr/o	cartilage	**chondr**/oma kŏn-DRŌ-mă	tumor (-*oma*) composed of cartilage
fibr/o	fiber, fibrous tissue	**fibr**/o/blast FĪ-brō-blăst	any cell from which connective tissue develop *The suffix* -blast *means "embryonic cell."*

* The combining form log/o *means study of. Combine* log/o *and* y *to form a new suffix meaning study of. Recall from Chapter 1, the* y *is a noun ending. In this book, the suffix meaning study of will be listed as* –logy.

Combining Forms: Cells and Tissues (Continued)

Combining Form	Meaning	EXAMPLE	
		Term/Pronunciation	**Definition**
hist/o	tissue	**hist**/o/logist† hĭs-TŎL-ō-jĭst	specialist in the study of (-*logist*) tissues
my/o	muscle	**my**/o/pathy mī-ŎP-ă-thē	diseased (-*pathy*) muscle or muscle tissue
sarc/o	flesh (connective tissue)	**sarc**/oma săr-KŌ-mă	a cancer arising from connective tissue such as muscle or bone *The word root* sarc *indicates a malignant (cancerous) growth.* *The suffix* -oma *means "tumor."*

†*The combining form* log/o *means "study of." Combine* log/o *and* -ist *to form a new suffix meaning "specialist in the study of." Recall from Chapter 1 that the suffix* -ist *means "specialist." In this book, the suffix meaning "specialist in the study of" will be listed as* –logist.

Parts of the Body

The following combining forms refer to such body parts or regions as the skull, chest, and vertebrae.

Combining Forms: Parts of the Body

Combining Form	Meaning	EXAMPLE	
		Term/Pronunciation	**Definition**
abdomin/o	abdomen	**abdomin**/al ăb-DŎM-ĭ-năl	pertaining to (-*al*) the abdomen
cervic/o	neck, cervix uteri (neck of the uterus)	**cervic**/al SĔR-vĭ-kăl	pertaining to (-*al*) the neck of the body or the neck of the uterus
coccyg/o	coccyx (tailbone)	**coccyg**/eal kŏk-SĬJ-ē-ăl	pertaining to (-*eal*) the coccyx or tailbone
crani/o	cranium, skull	**crani**/o/tomy krā-nē-ŎT-ō-mē	incision (-*tomy*) of the skull *This procedure is performed to remove tumors or to control cranial bleeding.*
ili/o	ilium (lateral flaring portion of hip bone)	**ili**/ac IL-ē-ăk	pertaining to (-*ac*) the ilium
inguin/o	groin	**inguin**/al ĬN-gwĭ-năl	pertaining to (-*al*) the groin
lumb/o	loins (lower back)	**lumb**/ar LŬM-băr	pertaining to (-*ar*) the loin area or lower back
pelv/i	pelvis	**pelv**/ic PĔL-vĭk	pertaining to (-*ic*) the pelvis

Combining Forms: Parts of the Body (Continued)

Combining Form	Meaning	EXAMPLE	
		Term/Pronunciation	Definition
sacr/o	sacrum	**sacr**/al SĀ-krăl	pertaining to (-*al*) the sacrum *The sacrum is the region of the lower back.*
spin/o	spine	**spin**/al SPĪ-năl	relating to (-*al*) the spine or spinal column
thorac/o	chest	**thorac**/ic thō-RĂS-ĭk	pertaining to (-*ic*) the chest
umbilic/o	umbilicus, navel	**umbilic**/al ūm-BĬL-ĭ-kăl	pertaining to (-*al*) the umbilicus
viscer/o	internal organs	**viscer**/al VĬS-ĕr-ăl	pertaining to the viscera *The viscera are the internal organs enclosed within a body cavity, especially the abdominal organs.*
vertebr/o	vertebrae (backbone)	inter/**vertebr**/al ĭn-tĕr-VĔRT-ĕ-brĕl	pertaining to (-*al*) the area between (inter-) two adjacent vertebrae

Activity 4–2: Competency Verification
Word Components: Parts of the Body

Check the box [✓] as you complete each numbered section.

[ ] **1.** Review the word components for the basic structural units, regions, and parts of the body in the previous sections. Then pronounce each word aloud.

[ ] **2.** For the words below, first write the suffix and its meaning. Then translate the meaning of the remaining components starting with the first part of the word.

Note: You are not expected to know all of the word components at this time. They are reinforced throughout the other chapters in the textbook. If needed, refer to the previous sections or use Appendix B to complete the exercise.

Example: epi/gastr/ic
Answer: *ic*=pertaining to; above, upon; stomach

1. lip/ectomy _____

2. spin/al _____

3. chondr/oma _____

4. lumb/ar _____

5. umbilic/al _____

6. fibr/o/blast _____

7. inguin/al _____

8. hist/o/logist _____

9. crani/o/tomy _____

10. thorac/ic _____

Correct Answers _____ × 10 = _____% **Score**

Position and Direction

The following combining forms are used most frequently to describe the relationship of one body part to another in reference to the anatomic position, but they may also be used to denote a body structure.

Combining Forms: Position and Direction

Combining Form	Meaning	EXAMPLE	
		Term/Pronunciation	**Definition**
anter/o	anterior, front	**anter**/o/later/al AN-tĕr-ō-lăt-ĕr-ăl	pertaining to (-*al*) the front and to one side (*later/o*)
caud/o	tail	**caud**/ad KAW-dăd	with reference to movement in a posterior direction or toward (-*ad*) the tailbone
cephal/o	head	**cephal**/ic sĕ-FĂL-ĭk	pertaining to (-*ic*) the head
dist/o	far, farthest	**dist**/al DĬS-tăl	farthest from the center, midline of the body or trunk *The suffix* -al *means* "pertaining to."
dors/o	back (of the body)	**dors**/al DŌR-săl	pertaining to (-*al*) the back side of the body
later/o	side, to one side	**later**/al LĂT-ĕr-ăl	pertaining to (-*al*) one side of the body
medi/o	middle	**medi**/al MĒ-dē-ăl	pertaining to (-*al*) the middle
poster/o	back (of the body), behind, posterior	**poster**/o/medi/al pŏs-tĕr-ō-MĒ-dē-ăl	situated posteriorly and in the median plane (*medi/al*)

Combining Forms: Position and Direction (Continued)

Combining Form	Meaning	EXAMPLE	
		Term/Pronunciation	Definition
proxim/o	near, nearest	**proxim**/al PRŎK-sĭm-ăl	pertaining (-al) to a position nearest to the trunk of the body *For example, the ankle is proximal to the foot.*
ventr/o	belly, belly side	**ventr**/al VĔN-trăl	pertaining to (-al) the belly side of the body

Prefixes and Suffixes

In this section, prefixes are listed alphabetically and highlighted whereas suffixes are defined in the right-hand column on an as-needed basis.

Prefixes: Position and Direction

Prefix	Meaning	EXAMPLE	
		Term/Pronunciation	Definition
ab-	from, away from	**ab**/duct/ion ăb-DŬK-shŭn	movement away from the midline of the body *The combining form* duct/o *means "to lead", "to carry"; the suffix* -ion *means "the act of."*
ad-*	toward	**ad**/duct/ion ă-DŬK-shŭn	movement toward the midline of the body *The combining form* duct/o *means "to lead," "to carry;" the suffix* -ion *means "the act of."*
epi-	above, upon	**epi**/gastr/ic ĕp-ĭ-GĂS-trĭk	pertaining to (-ic) the area above the stomach (gastr/o)
hypo-	under, below	**hypo**/derm/ic hī-pō-DĔR-mĭk	pertaining to (-ic) under the skin (derm/o)
infra-		**infra**/cost/al ĭn-fră-KŎS-tăl	pertaining to (-al) the area below the ribs (cost/o)
inter-	between	**inter**/cost/al ĭn-tĕr-KŎS-tăl	pertaining to (-al) the area between the ribs (cost/o)

* The prefix ad- *can also be used as a suffix as illustrated in the term* caud/ad *(toward the tail or tailbone).*

Activity 4–3: Competency Verification

Word Components: Position and Direction

Check the box [✓] as you complete each numbered section.

[   ] **1.** Review the terms of position and direction in the previous sections. Then pronounce each term aloud.

[   ] **2.** In the words below, first write the suffix and its meaning. Then translate the meaning of the remaining components starting with the first part of the word.

> *Note: You are not expected to know all of the word components at this time. They are reinforced throughout the other chapters in the textbook. If needed, refer to the previous sections or use Appendix B to complete the exercise.*

> **Example:** epi/gastr/ic
> **Answer:** *ic* = pertaining to; above, upon; stomach

1. proxim/al _____

2. dors/al _____

3. cephal/ic _____

4. caud/ad _____

5. ventr/al _____

6. anter/o/later/al _____

7. infra/cost/al _____

8. hypo/derm/ic _____

9. dist/al _____

10. poster/o/medi/al _____

Correct Answers _____ × 10 = _____ **% Score**

BODY CAVITIES

A body cavity is a hollow space within the body that contains internal organs, also known as viscera. The body consists of two ventral (anterior) cavities and two dorsal (posterior) cavities (see Fig. 4–5).

Ventral Cavity

Label Figure 4–5 as you read the following material.

Two ventral cavities, called the (1) **thoracic** and (2) **abdominopelvic,** are located in the front or anterior side of the body. A thick muscular wall, called the (3) **diaphragm,** separates the two cavities. The thoracic cavity contains the lungs and heart. The abdominopelvic cavity is further divided into two subdivisions—the (4) **abdominal** and (5) **pelvic** cavities. The abdominal cavity contains the stomach, intestines, spleen, liver, and other organs. The pelvic cavity contains the urinary bladder and reproductive organs such as the uterus in women and the prostate gland in men.

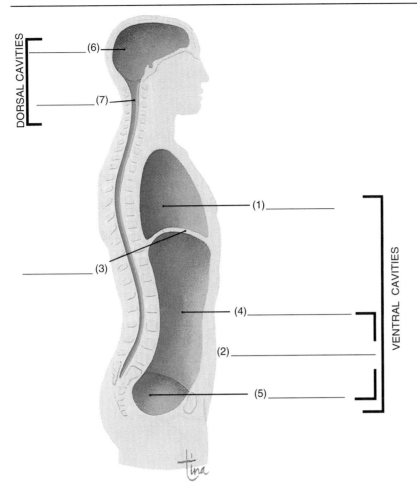

Figure 4–5. Body cavities. (Lateral view from the right side.) (Adapted from Scanlon, VC, and Sanders, TS: Essentials of Anatomy and Physiology, ed 3. FA Davis, Philadelphia, 1999, p 14, with permission.)

When the body is subjected to physical trauma (as often happens in an automobile accident), the most vulnerable abdominopelvic organs are those within the abdominal cavity. This is because the walls are formed only by trunk muscles and are not reinforced by bone. The pelvic organs receive a somewhat greater degree of protection from the bony pelvis.

Dorsal Cavity

Two dorsal cavities, the (6) **cranial** and the (7) **spinal** cavities are located in the back or dorsal side of the body. The cranial cavity is formed by the skull and contains the brain. The spinal cavity is formed by the spine (backbone) and contains the spinal cord.

Activity 4–4: Competency Verification

Body Cavities

Check your labeling of body cavities in Appendix C.

DIVISIONS OF THE ABDOMINOPELVIC CAVITY

Because the abdominopelvic cavity contains more organs than any other body cavity, it is useful to describe the location of organs within the abdominopelvic cavity. To do so, the abdominal pelvic cavity is divided into quadrants and regions.

Four Quadrants

Four quadrants identify the placement of internal organs in the abdominopelvic cavity. Generally, the quadrants are used for clinical examination and reporting. For example, a physician might describe a patient's abdominal pain in the LUQ (left upper quadrant), indicating different clinical possibilities than if the pain was in the RLQ (right lower quadrant). The quadrants are also used to describe the location of surgical procedures and to denote incision sites or location of tumors. Therefore, you will find quadrant references in operative reports as well as physical examinations. A variety of medical reports are included in the medical records sections of various chapters. Refer to Figure 4–6A as you read the following information about the quadrants and the organs contained within each of them, as shown in Table 4–2.

Nine Regions

Whereas the quadrant designation is better suited for clinical examination and reporting, the region designation (Fig. 4–6B) is used mainly to identify the location of internal organs. For example, the liver is located in the epigastric and right hypochondriac regions.

The abdominopelvic cavity can be divided into nine regions. Refer to Figure 4–6B to locate the nine regions as you read the following information.

- **Hypochondriac:** The upper right region and the upper left region located under the cartilage of the ribs.

- **Epigastric:** The middle region located above the stomach.

- **Lumbar:** the middle right region and the middle left region located near the waist

- **Umbilical:** The middle region located in the area of the navel or umbilicus.

- **Inguinal:** The lower right region and the lower left region located near the groin. These regions are also called *iliac regions* because they are located near the ilium (the upper portion of the hip bone located on both sides of the body).

- **Hypogastric:** The lower middle region located below the stomach or umbilical region

Spinal Column

The spinal column, or vertebral column, is separated into five divisions: cervical, thoracic, lumbar, sacral, and coccygeal. It is important to point out that the spinal column and spinal cord are two different structures. Whereas the spinal column is composed of the bones (vertebrae) that extend from the neck (cervical) downward to the tailbone (coccygeal), the spinal cord is composed of nervous tissue. The bony spinal column protects the delicate tissue of the spinal cord. The names, numbers, and abbreviations of the vertebrae are illustrated in Figure 4–7 and listed below.

There are 7 cervical, 12 thoracic, 5 lumbar, and 5 sacral vertebrae. There are 4 to 5 small coccygeal vertebrae fused into 1 coccyx, as illustrated in Figure 4–7. Abbreviations are used in medical records to denote the exact names and positions of vertebrae as listed here:

- The 7 cervical vertebrae, C1 through C7, are located in the neck region.

- The 12 thoracic vertebrae, T1 through T12, are located in the chest region.

- The 5 lumbar vertebrae, L1 through L5, are located in the lower back region.

- The 5 sacral vertebrae, S1 through S5, are located above the tail region.

- The 4 coccygeal vertebrae, 4 fused vertebrae, are not individually designated are located in the tail region.

TABLE 4–2:	Quadrants
QUADRANT	**ORGANS**
Right upper quadrant (RUQ)	Right lobe of the liver, gallbladder, part of the pancreas, and part of the small and large intestines.
Right lower quadrant (RLQ)	Part of the small and large intestines, appendix, right ovary, right fallopian tubes and right ureter.
Left upper quadrant (LUQ)	Left lobe of the liver, stomach, spleen, part of the pancreas, part of the small and large intestines.
Left lower quadrant (LLQ)	Part of the small and large intestines, left ovary, left fallopian tubes and left ureter.

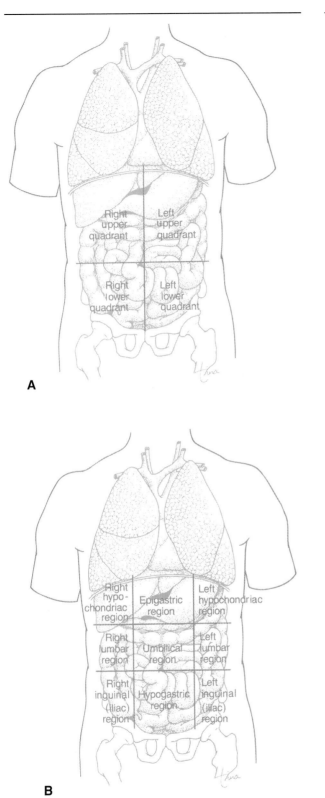

A

B

Figure 4–6. *Divisions of the abdominopelvic cavity. (A) Four quadrants. (B) Nine regions. (Adapted from Scanlon, VC, and Sanders, TS: Essentials of Anatomy and Physiology, ed 3. FA Davis, Philadelphia, 1999, p 16, with permission.)*

Right upper quadrant

Left upper quadrant

Right lower quadrant

Left lower quadrant

Right hypo-chondriac region

Epigastric region

Left hypochondriac region

Right lumbar region

Umbilical region

Left lumbar region

Right inguinal (iliac) region

Hypogastric region

Left inguinal (iliac) region

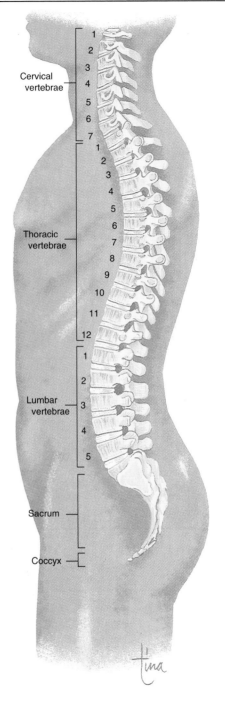

Cervical vertebrae

Thoracic vertebrae

Lumbar vertebrae

Sacrum

Coccyx

Figure 4–7. *The spinal (vertebral) column. (From Scanlon, VC, and Sanders, TS: Essentials of Anatomy and Physiology, ed 3. FA Davis, Philadelphia, 1999, p 112, with permission.)*

❖ ABBREVIATIONS

ABBREVIATION	MEANING	ABBREVIATION	MEANING
AP	anteroposterior	LUQ	left upper quadrant
C1, C2, etc.	first cervical vertebra, second cervical vertebra, etc.	MS	musculoskeletal, multiple sclerosis, mental status, morphine sulfate
CV	cardiovascular		
GI	gastrointestinal	RLQ	right lower quadrant
GU	genitourinary	RUQ	right upper quadrant
lat	lateral	S1, S2, etc.	first sacral vertebra, second sacral vertebra, etc.
L1, L2, etc.	first lumbar vertebra, second lumbar vertebra, etc.		
		T1, T2, etc.	first thoracic vertebra, second thoracic vertebra, etc.
LLQ	left lower quadrant		

Activity 4–5: Competency Verification
Planes of Reference, Position, and Direction

Select the word that best describes the statements that follow:

anterior
deep
distal
dorsal recumbent
external
(frontal) coronal
Fowler

inferior
internal
lateral
medial
midsagittal
posterior
prone

proximal
sagittal
superficial
superior
supine
transverse

Refer to Figure 4–3 and Table 4–1 to complete the following exercise items:

1. _____ pertaining to the midline or near the middle of the body

2. _____ near the point of attachment to the trunk or a structure

3. _____ the opposite of superior

4. _____ the front of the body

5. _____ toward the side

6. _____ the opposite of internal

7. _____ away from the surface

8. _____ within, interior to

9. _____ toward the surface

10. _____ below; toward the tail

11. _____ farther from the point of attachment to the trunk or a structure

12. _____ above; toward the head

Refer to Figure 4–4 to complete the following items:

13. _____ lying flat on the abdomen with the head slightly turned to the side

14. _____ lying flat on the back with arms at the sides or above the head

15. _____ semi-sitting position with the head of the examination table tilted at a 45- to 60-degree angle

16. _____ supine position with the legs sharply flexed at the knees and the feet on the examination table

Refer to Figure 4–3 to complete the following items:

17. _____ a plane that separates the body into anterior and posterior portions

18. _____ a plane that separates the body into superior and inferior portions

19. _____ a vertical plane that divides the body into equal right and left sides

20. _____ a plane parallel to the midsagittal plane that divides the body into unequal right and left sides

Correct Answers _____ **× 5 =** _____% **Score**

Activity 4-6: Competency Verification
Areas of the Abdomen, Body Cavities, and Spinal Column

Supply the word(s) that best describe(s) the statements that follow.
Refer to Figure 4–6 and Table 4–2 to complete the following items:

1. _____ quadrant that contains the left lobe of the liver, stomach, spleen, part of the pancreas, and part of the small and large intestine

2. _____ quadrant that contains the right lobe of the liver, gallbladder, part of the pancreas, and part of the small and large intestine

3. _____ quadrant that contains part of the small and large intestine, left ovary, left fallopian tube, and left ureter

4. _____ region of the navel

5. _____ region above the stomach

6. _____ lower middle region below the umbilical region

7. _____ upper region located below the right rib

8. _____ upper region located below the left rib

Refer to Figure 4–5 to complete the following items:

9. _____ the cavity that houses the cranial and spinal cavities

10. _____ another name for the anterior cavity

11. _____ muscular organ that separates the thoracic and abdominal cavities

12. _____ lower portion (cavity) of the abdominopelvic cavity

Refer to Figure 4–7 to complete the following items:

13. _____ the first seven vertebrae of the spinal column located in the neck area

14. _____ the number of vertebrae contained in the lumbar region

15. _____ the terminal portion of the vertebral column, also called the tailbone

Correct Answers _____ × 6.7 = _____ **% Score**

Activity 4–7: Competency Verification
Build Medical Words

anter/o	hist/o	neur/o	epi-
cephal/o	inguin/o	pelv/i	hypo-
chondr/o	later/o	poster/o	inter-
cyt/o	medi/o	umbilic/o	-ic
derm/o	my/o	vertebr/o	-tomy
dist/o		viscer/o	

Use the word components listed above to form medical words meaning:

1. pertaining to the middle   _____/al

2. (pertaining to) farthest from the center   _____/al

3. pertaining to the region above the stomach   _____/gastr/_____

4. enlargement of the internal organs   _____/megaly

5. pertaining to the area between the ribs   _____/cost/al

6. pertaining to the navel region   _____/al

7. pertaining to the abdomen and pelvis   abdomin/o/_____/ic

8. study of tissues   _____/o/logy

9. (pertaining to) under the skin   _____/_____/ic

10. incision of the skull   crani/o/_____

11. pertaining to both sides   bi/_____/al

12. pertaining to the groin   _____/al

13. specialist in the study of nerves   _____/logist

14. pertaining to the side and middle   _____/o/_____/al

15. pertaining to the front and back   _____/o/_____/ior

16. tumor composed of cartilage   _____/oma

17. specialist in the study of cells   _____/logist

18. pertaining to the area between vertebrae   _____/_____/al

19. pertaining to the head   _____/ic

20. diseased muscle   _____/pathy

Correct Answers _____ × **5** = _____ **% Score**

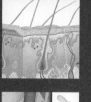
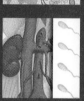
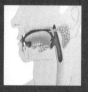
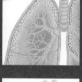

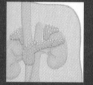

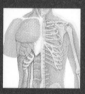

chapter

5 Dermatology

Chapter Outline

STUDYING THE INTEGUMENTARY SYSTEM

INTEGUMENTARY SYSTEM AT A GLANCE

STRUCTURE AND FUNCTION

Skin

Accessory Structures of the Skin

STUDYING DERMATOLOGY TERMINOLOGY

MEDICAL WORD COMPONENTS

Combining Forms

Prefixes

Suffixes

PATHOLOGICAL CONDITIONS

CUTANEOUS LESIONS

BURNS

DIAGNOSTIC PROCEDURES

SURGICAL AND THERAPEUTIC PROCEDURES

OTHER PROCEDURES

PHARMACOLOGY

MEDICAL RECORDS

Medical Record 5–1: History and Physical Examination

Medical Record 5–2: Consultation

Medical Record 5–3: Operative Report

Medical Record 5–4: Dermatology Report

Objectives

Upon completion of this chapter, you will be able to:

- Describe the type of medical treatment a dermatologist provides.
- Name the layers of the skin and the accessory structures of the skin.
- Recognize, pronounce, build, and spell terms related to the integumentary system.
- Describe pathological conditions, diagnostic tests, surgical procedures, and other treatments related to the integumentary system.
- Demonstrate your knowledge of this chapter by successfully completing the activities and the analysis of medical records.

About the Medical Specialty of Dermatology

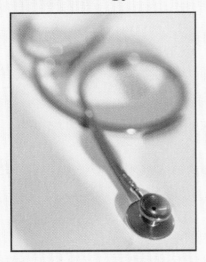

Dermatology is the branch of medicine concerned with the study of the skin, diseases of the skin, and the relationship of cutaneous lesions to systemic disease. The physician who specializes in the diagnosis and treatment of skin diseases is called a **dermatologist.** Many diagnostic procedures, such as microscopic and microbiologic examination of the skin and its secretions, are used to determine the cause of pathological conditions. Once a diagnosis is confirmed, several methods may be used to treat skin disorders.

Besides medications (topical and injected) and therapeutic treatments, such as ultraviolet light therapy, numerous surgical procedures are available for treatment. Surgical procedures may involve the use of a scalpel, a surgical curette (a device for scraping and removing tissue or debris), an electrosurgical unit, a freezing surgical device, or a laser beam.

Another important part of the dermatologist's practice is the treatment of skin manifestations (signs, symptoms) caused by internal diseases of the body, such as skin lesions that result from a sexually transmitted disease. The dermatologist's scope of practice includes the management of skin cancers, moles, and other skin tumors. This specialist also uses various techniques for the enhancement and correction of cosmetic skin defects and prescribes measures to maintain the skin in a state of health.

To understand the role of health-care practitioners in the field of dermatology, it is essential to understand the structure and function of the integumentary system as well as the medical specialty of dermatology.

Selected Key Terms

albinism ĂL-bĭn-ĭzm *albin=white* *ism=condition*	A group of inherited disorders that produce a deficiency or absence of pigment in the skin, hair, and eyes, or eyes only, related to an abnormality in the production of melanin.
androgen ĂN-drō-jĕn	Generic term for an agent, usually a hormone (testosterone, androsterone), that stimulates the activity of the accessory male sex organs or encourages the development of male characteristics (masculinization). Hormonal secretions are discussed in Chapter 10.
avascular ă-VĂS-kū-lăr *a=without, not* *vascul=vessel* *ar=pertaining to*	Referring to a kind of tissue that does not have blood vessels; not receiving a sufficient supply of blood in tissues. The reduced flow may be the result of blockage by a blood clot or the deliberate stoppage of flow during surgery, or of measures taken to control a hemorrhage. Synonymous with *nonvascular*.
collagen KŎL-ă-jĕn	Dense connective tissue strands, or fibers, of the tendons, the ligaments, and the fascia.
dissipated dĭ-sĭ-PĂT-ĕd	Scattered in various directions; dispersed.
ductule DŬK-tūl *duct= to lead, carry* *ule=small, minute*	A very small duct.

melanin MĔL-ă-nĭn	The pigment produced by melanocytes that gives color to hair, skin, and the choroid of the eye.
melanocyte MĔL-ăn-ō-sīt *melano=black* *cyte=cell*	A melanin-forming cell. Those of the skin are found in the lower epidermis.
pathogens PĂTH-ō-jĕnz	Any microorganisms capable of producing disease.
pore PŌR	Minute opening, especially on an epithelial surface; the opening of the secretory duct of a sweat gland.
sebum SĒ-bŭm	An oily, fatty secretion of the sebaceous glands of the skin.
sebaceous sē-BĀ-shŭs	Containing, or pertaining to, sebum. Sebum is an oily, fatty matter secreted by the sebaceous glands of the skin.
squamous SKWĀ-mŭs	Platelike, scaly, or covered with scales.
stratified STRĂT-ĭ-fīd	Arranged in layers.
subcutaneous sŭb-kū-TĀ-nē-ŭs *sub=under, below* *cutane=skin* *ous=pertaining to*	Beneath the skin. Synonymous with *hypodermis*.
sudoriferous sū-dor-ĬF-ĕr-ŭs	Sweat-secreting. Refers to glands of the skin.

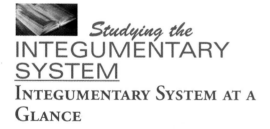

Studying the
INTEGUMENTARY SYSTEM

INTEGUMENTARY SYSTEM AT A GLANCE

The skin, the largest organ of the body, and its accessory structures (glands, hair, and nails) form the **integumentary system.** Not only does the skin work together with other body systems to control body temperature, but it also influences the functions of other organs as illustrated in Figure 5–1. The specialized functions of the skin are as follows:

Thermoregulation: The skin has a complex structure of impulse carrying nerves and blood vessels that play an important role in the maintenance of body temperature. The brain's thermoregulatory centers, located in the hypothalamus, regulate heat production and heat loss. To maintain a normal body temperature, the centers respond to changes in body temperature and send signals to the skin's nerve fibers. When the body experiences excessive heat, reflex signals trigger the dilation of blood vessels and stimulate the sweat glands to excrete a moisture secretion, which in turn, carries the heat away and, thus, cools off the body.

Bacterial protection: Acid secretions produced in minute amounts by the skin protect the body from bacterial invasion and against excessive loss of heat, salts, and water. Generally, secretions from the skin are slightly acidic in nature.

Sensory functions: An elaborate network of nerve fibers under the skin's surface records sensations of pain, temperature, and pressure. These sensory mes-

Body System Connections
Integumentary System

THE CARDIOVASCULAR SYSTEM
◆ To a great extent, body temperature is controlled by changes in the skin's blood flow.

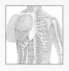

THE MUSCULOSKELETAL SYSTEM
◆ The skin protects muscles and bones. ◆ Body temperature is regulated by involuntary muscle contractions (shivering). ◆ The skin's ability to absorb vitamin D helps to provide calcium for bones.

THE DIGESTIVE SYSTEM
◆ Dietary calcium assimilation is activated when the skin absorbs vitamin D from exposure to the sun.
◆ Surplus calorie consumption may be stored as subcutaneous fat.

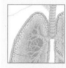

THE NERVOUS SYSTEM
◆ The nervous system reacts to information provided by the skin's sensory receptors. ◆ The activity of sweat glands and blood vessels of the skin is regulated by the nervous system.

THE ENDOCRINE SYSTEM
◆ Hormones activate either the decomposition or the synthesis of subcutaneous fat.

THE RESPIRATORY SYSTEM
◆ The skin protects the respiratory organs. ◆ Changes in respiratory rate may be due to stimulation of the skin's receptors.

THE FEMALE REPRODUCTIVE SYSTEM
◆ The skin's sensory receptors influence the suckling reflex and erotic stimuli. ◆ The skin's ability to stretch during pregnancy accommodates the growing fetus.

THE URINARY AND MALE REPRODUCTIVE SYSTEMS
◆ The kidneys partially compensate for water and electrolyte loss caused by sweating. ◆ Erotic stimuli are greatly influenced by the skin's sensory receptors.

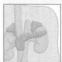

THE LYMPHATIC AND IMMUNE SYSTEMS
◆ Lymphatic vessels prevent edema by draining excess tissue fluid. ◆ The immune system depends on the skin as a first line of defense against pathogenic invasion.

Figure 5–1 *The interrelationship of the integumentary system with other body systems.*

sages are transmitted to the spinal cord and brain by the nerve endings located in the skin.

Sweat and sebum production: Two important glands, the sweat (sudoriferous) glands and the sebaceous (oil) glands, are located under the skin's surface. Sweat glands produce a watery secretion, or sweat, which cools the body through evaporation. Sebaceous glands produce **sebum,** an oily secretion that functions as a lubricant on the skin's surface. Secretions of both glands rise to the skin's outer layers through its ducts and are deposited on the surface of the skin by skin pores.

STRUCTURE AND FUNCTION

The integumentary system consists of the skin and its associated structures (hair, glands, and nails). Included in this system are the millions of sensory receptors and a vascular network. As such, the skin is a dynamic interface between the body and the external environment. It is the largest organ of the body, consisting of several kinds of tissues that are structurally arranged to function together. The skin protects the body from the environment and prevents the entry of harmful substances.

Skin

Structurally, the skin consists of two parts: an outer layer called the **epidermis** and an inner layer called the dermis. Beneath the dermis is a **subcutaneous layer.** Label the structures in Figure 5–2 as you read the following material.

Epidermis

The (1) **epidermis** is the protective layer of the skin composed of **stratified squamous** epithelium that varies in thickness. The stratified squamous epithelium consists of flattened, scale-like cells that are arranged in several layers (**strata).** Unlike the dermis and subcutaneous tissue, the epidermis is **avascular** and does not contain blood vessels, lymphatic vessels, or nerve endings. It depends on the rich supply of blood vessels in the dermis for nourishment and skin tone.

Depending on its location in the body, the epidermis is organized into four or five cellular layers. For example, the epidermis of the palms and soles is the thickest and has five layers because these areas are exposed to greater friction. Although the epidermis can be subdivided into four or five layers, the two most important are the outermost layer, the (2) **stratum corneum,** and the innermost layer, the (3) **stratum germinativum,** also called the *basal layer.*

Stratum Corneum

The stratum corneum, the horny layer of the epidermis, consists of many layers of dead cells filled with a hard, horny protein called *keratin,* which continuously flakes away. The horny cells serve as a protective covering and are an effective barrier against **pathogens** and most chemicals, although microscopic breaks in the epidermis are sufficient to permit pathogen entry. Because keratin is relatively waterproof, it minimizes the loss of water and prevents dehydration. At the same time, it prevents the entry of excess water by way of the body surface.

Stratum Germinativum

Continuous cell division takes place in the basal layer. As new basal cells multiply, they are pushed up a hard protein called toward the stratum corneum. As these cells are being pushed up toward the surface, they flatten, shrink, and become filled with keratin. Eventually, the keratinized cells are worn off and replaced by underlying new cells that, in turn, become keratinized and die. The entire process, in which a cell forms in the basal layers, rises to the surface, becomes keratinized, and sloughs off, takes about 1 month.

Another type of specialized epithelial cells, known as **melanocytes,** is found primarily in the epidermis. These specialized epithelial cells synthesize the pigment **melanin,** providing a protective barrier to the ultraviolet radiation in sunlight. Exposure to ultraviolet radiation leads to increased melanin production. When the skin is exposed to ultraviolet radiation, both the amount and the darkness of melanin increase. This process causes the skin to tan, further protecting the body against radiation. Inability of melanin to absorb excessive amounts of ultraviolet rays results in inflamed, sunburned skin. If exposure to the sun is prolonged over a period of several years, wrinkling of the skin or even skin cancer may result. Because dark-skinned people have more melanin, they generally have fewer wrinkles and a lower incidence of skin cancer. Thus melanin serves a vital protective function.

Because the number of melanocytes is about the same in all races, differences in skin color are attributed to the amount of pigment the melanocytes produce. When the pigment is absent in the hair and eyes as well as the skin, the individual most likely has an inherited inability to produce melanin. This results in the condition known as **albinism,** and the person is called an *albino.*

Continue to label Figure 5–2 as you read the following material.

Dermis

Also known as the *corium,* the (4) **dermis** lies under the epidermis. It consists of dense connective tissue that is rich with blood and lymph vessels, nerve endings, oil and sweat glands, and hair follicles. All of the latter structures are embedded in the deep connective tissue containing collagenous and elastic fibers.

Collagenous fibers are very tough and resistant to a pulling force, yet are somewhat flexible. Because they often occur in bundles, these fibers have a great deal of strength. In addition to strength, the combination of elastic and collagenous fibers provides the skin with extensibility and elasticity. *Extensibility* is the ability to stretch; *elasticity* is the ability to return to its original shape after extension or contraction. The skin's ability to stretch can readily be seen during pregnancy, obesity, and edema. In such cases of extreme stretching, small tears occur that are initially red. Although they do not disappear, they eventually turn from red to silvery white streaks called *striae.*

Subcutaneous Tissue

The hypodermis or (5) **subcutaneous tissue,** located beneath the dermis, is another connective tissue layer that binds the dermis to the underlying structures. Collagenous and elastic fibers reinforce the hypodermis—particularly on the palms and soles, where the skin is firmly attached to the underlying structures. The underlying structures are composed of (6) **adipose tissue,** which contains

lipocytes (fat cells). The amount of adipose tissue in the hypodermis varies with the sex, age, region of the body, and nutritional state of the individual. The subcutaneous layer, or hypodermis, also functions to store lipids, insulate and cushion the body, and regulate temperature. In addition, the hypodermis stores excess nutrients as a potential energy source, and generally supports and protects various organs in the body, such as the subcutaneous layer of adipose tissue around the kidneys and the fatty padding around bones and joints.

Because the subcutaneous tissue is rich in adipose tissue, many fat-soluble drugs and medications are injected into this tissue. A subcutaneous injection is often used when a patient is unable to take medicine orally. A hypodermic needle is so named because it is used to inject the drug below the dermis into the tissue of the hypodermis.

Accessory Structures of the Skin

The integumentary system is composed not only of the skin but also its accessory structures: the glands, hair, and nails. These are discussed in the following sections.

Glands

All of the skin's glands are located in the dermis and are formed from epithelial tissue. Two important glands of the skin, the sweat (sudoriferous) glands and the sebaceous (oil) glands, are referred to as *exocrine glands* because they excrete substances through ducts.

Continue to label Figure 5–2 as you read the following material.

The (7) **sudoriferous glands** secrete perspiration or sweat onto the surface of the skin through (8) **pores.** Its main function is to help maintain body temperature and excrete certain wastes. Sweat glands are located primarily on the palms, soles, forehead, and armpits (axillae). Modified sudoriferous glands known as *ceruminous glands* are found only in the external auditory canal (ear canal). They secrete cerumen (earwax), which is a combined secretion of the ceruminous and sebaceous glands. Not only does cerumen provide protection because it is a water and insect repellent, but it also keeps the tympanum (eardrum) from drying out. Excessive secretions of cerumen can interfere with hearing. This is discussed in greater detail in Chapter 17.

The (9) **sebaceous glands,** located in the dermis, produce an oily substance known as **sebum.** They secrete their sebum through ducts (exocrine glands) into the hair follicle. The sebum is then **dissipated** to the surface of the skin, where it protects, lubricates, and helps to waterproof the skin. If the drainage **ductule** for the sebaceous glands becomes blocked, the glands may become infected resulting in acne. Congested sebum in the sebaceous glands causes the formation of pimples or whiteheads, and if the sebum is dark, it forms blackheads. Sex hormones, particularly **androgens,** regulate the production and secretion of sebum. During adolescence the secretions increase, but they

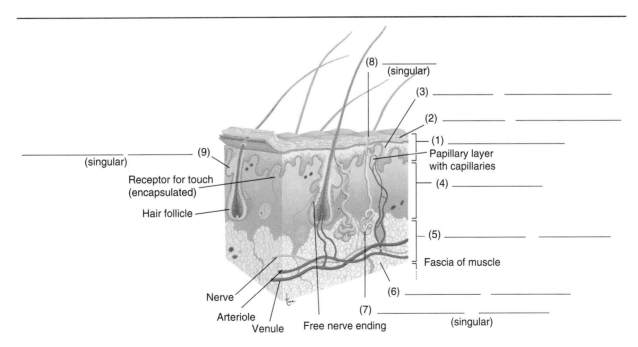

Figure 5–2   *The structure of the skin and subcutaneous tissue. (Adapted from Scanlon, VC, and Sanders, TS: Essentials of Anatomy and Physiology, ed 3. FA Davis, Philadelphia, 1999, p 85, with permission.)*

diminish as a person gets older. The loss of sebum, which lubricates the skin, may be the reason for wrinkles that form as a person ages.

Sebaceous glands are present over the entire body except on the soles of the feet and the palms of the hands. They are especially prevalent on the scalp and face, around openings such as the nose, mouth, external ear, and anus, as well as on the upper back.

Hair

Hair is found on nearly all parts of the body. Certain parts, such as the palms of the hands, soles of the feet, dorsal surfaces of the fingers and toes, lips, nipples, and parts of the external reproductive organs (the penis in men; the clitoris, labia minora, and labia majora in women) are the exceptional hairless parts of the body. The main purpose of hair is protection, even though its effectiveness is limited. Hair of the scalp provides insulation from cold for the head and protects the scalp from injury and the sun's rays. Hair in the nostrils and external ear canal protects these structures against airborne particles and dust. Some secondary functions of hair are to distinguish individuals and to serve as an ornament and source for sexual attraction.

Label Figure 5–3 as you read about the hair follicle.

Hair fibers contain a hard protein substance called keratin. The growth of hair is very similar to the growth of the epidermal layer of skin. Each individual hair evolves from a group of epidermal cells at the base of a tubelike depression known as a *hair follicle.* The (1) **follicle,** which starts at the dermis, contains the (2) **hair root.** Epidermal cells are nourished by dermal blood vessels at the deep end of the follicle. As these epidermal cells divide and grow, older cells are pushed toward the surface. The cells that move upward and away from their nutrient supply become keratinized and die. The cellular remains form a developing hair, whose (3) **hair shaft** extends away from the skin's surface. This explains why a hair is composed of dead epidermal cells. The deep-lying cells at its base are nourished by dermal blood vessels.

Like skin color, hair color is determined by the amount of pigment the epidermal melanocytes produce. Melanocytes lie at the deep end of a follicle, and if they produce large quantities of melanin, the hair is dark. If small quantities of pigment are produced, the hair is blond, and if no pigment is produced, the hair is white. As people age, they slowly stop producing melanin, and that is why the hair color changes to gray.

Nails

As you read the following material, label Figure 5–4.

Both the fingernails and the toenails serve as protection from injury. The fingernails also aid the fingers

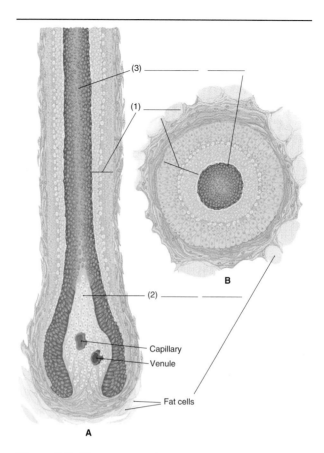

Figure 5–3 *The structure of a hair follicle. (A) Longitudinal section. (B) Cross-section (Adapted from Scanlon, VC, and Sanders, TS: Essentials of Anatomy and Physiology, ed 3. FA Davis, Philadelphia, 1999, p 89, with permission.)*

in grasping and picking up small objects. The nail is made up of hard keratin, consisting of keratinized stratified squamous epithelial cells. These cells form by cell division in the (1) **nail root** and produce keratin.

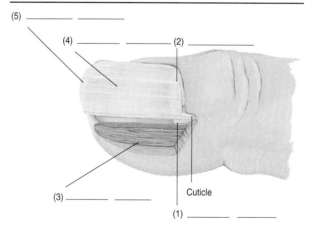

Figure 5–4 *The structure of a fingernail shown in longitudinal section. (Adapted from Scanlon, VC, and Sanders, TS: Essentials of Anatomy and Physiology, ed 3. FA Davis, Philadelphia, 1999, p 89, with permission.)*

The keratin produced in the nail is a stronger form of protein than the keratin produced in the hair. The (2) **lunula,** the half-moon–shaped area at the base of the nail, is the growing region. As the nail grows, it stays attached and slides forward over the layer of epithelium called the (3) **nail bed.** This epithelial layer is continuous with the epithelium of the skin. Most of the (4) **nail body** is pink living tissue, with the exception of the whitish lunula, because of the underlying vascular tissue, but the (5) **free edge** of the nail itself consists of keratinized dead cells. Thus, cutting a nail is not painful unless you cut it too short by cutting the living tissue.

Activity 5–1: Competency Verification
Structures Related to the Skin, Hair, and Nails

Review Figures 5–2, 5–3, and 5–4 and check your labeling in Appendix C.

Activity 5–2: Competency Verification
Layers of the Skin

androgen	glands	sebaceous
basal layer	hair	stratum corneum
dermis	melanocytes	subcutaneous tissue
epidermis	nails	sudoriferous
follicle	pores	

Match the terms listed above with the definitions given in the numbered list.

1. _____ Protective outer layer of skin that is avascular.

2. _____ Innermost layer of epidermis where continuous cell division takes place.

3. _____ Specialized epithelial cells that synthesize the pigment melanin, providing a barrier from ultraviolet sun rays.

4. _____ Inner vascular layer that is rich in blood vessels, nerves, and glands.

5. _____ Layer located beneath the dermis; contains adipose tissue and binds the dermis to underlying structures.

6. _____ A gland that secretes perspiration into the skin through pores.

7. _____ A gland that produces an oily substance known as sebum.

8. _____ Opening(s) on the skin's surface.

9. _____, _____, _____ The three accessory organs of the integumentary system.

10. _____ Hormone that regulates the secretion of sebum.

Correct Answers _____ × 10 = _____ **% Score**

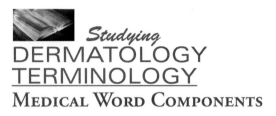

Studying
DERMATOLOGY TERMINOLOGY
MEDICAL WORD COMPONENTS

The major word components related to dermatology consist of various types of skin cells and structures and accessory structures of the skin. They also include word components that denote skin color and pathological conditions.

Combining Forms

The following chart outlines combining forms pertinent to the integumentary system.

Combining Forms: Integumentary System

Combining Form	Meaning	EXAMPLE	
		Term/Pronunciation	**Definition**
adip/o	fat	**adip**/o/cyte AD-ĭ-pō-sīt	a fat (*adipose*) cell
lip/o		**lip**/oma lĭ-PŌ-mă	a benign fatty tumor Lipoma *is synonymous with* adipoma.
cutane/o	skin	sub/**cutane**/ous sŭb-kū-TĀ-nē-ŭs	under (*sub-*) the skin The suffix -ous *means "pertaining to."*
derm/o		hypo/**derm**/ic hī-pō-DĔR-mĭk	under (*hypo-*) the skin Hypodermic *is synonymous with* subcutaneous.
dermat/o		**dermat**/itis dĕr-mă-TĪ-tĭs	inflammation of the skin
hidr/o	sweat	**hidr**/osis hī-DRŌ-sĭs	abnormal condition of (-*osis*) sweat Do not confuse hidr/o (*sweat*) with hydr/o (*water*).
sudor/o		**sudor**/esis sū-dō-RĒ-sĭs	profuse sweating The suffix -esis *means "condition."*
histi/o	tissue	**histi**/o/blast HĬS-tē-ō-blăst	a tissue-forming cell The suffix -blast *refers to an embryonic cell.*
hist/o		**hist**/o/logy hĭs-TŎL-ō-jē	study of (-*logy*) the microscopic structure of tissue
ichthy/o	dry, scaly (fishlike)	**ichthy**/osis ĭk-thē-Ō-sĭs	abnormal condition (-*osis*) of dry, scaly skin, resembling fish skin Congenital disorder of keratinization (*hard tissue*) characterized by non-inflammatory dryness and scaling of the skin. It can also be acquired and is often associated with other defects and with abnormalities of lipid (*fat*) metabolism.

Activity 5–4: Competency Verification
Combining Forms, Prefixes, and Suffixes

Check the box [✓] as you complete each numbered section.

[　] **1.** Review the word components related to color and the prefixes and suffixes related to the integumentary system. Then pronounce each word aloud.

[　] **2.** In the spaces below, first write the suffix and its meaning. Then translate the meaning of the remaining word components, starting with the first part of the word.

> **Example:** leuk/o/cyte
> **Answer:** *cyte*=**cell; white**

1. erythr/o/cyte   _____

2. cirrh/osis   _____

3. xanth/o/derma   _____

4. jaund/ice   _____

5. cyan/o/derma   _____

6. melan/oma   _____

7. an/hidr/osis   _____

8. scler/o/derma   _____

9. dermat/o/logy   _____

10. sub/ungu/al   _____

Correct Answers _____ **× 10 =** _____ **% Score**

PATHOLOGICAL CONDITIONS

PATHOLOGICAL CONDITION	DESCRIPTION
abscess ĂB-sĕs	A localized collection of pus in any body part, resulting from the invasion of a pyogenic (pus-forming) bacterium.
acne ĂK-nē	An inflammatory papular and pustular eruption of the skin.
acne vulgaris ĂK-nē vŭl-GĀ-rĭs	An eruption, predominantly on the face, upper back, and chest, made up of comedones (blackheads), cysts, papules, and pustules on an inflammatory base. The condition occurs in most people during puberty and adolescence because of increased secretion of androgens.

PATHOLOGICAL CONDITIONS (CONTINUED)

PATHOLOGICAL CONDITION	DESCRIPTION
alopecia *ăl-ō-PĒ-shē-ă*	Partial or complete absence or loss of hair, especially of the head; baldness. The condition may be due to the aging process, disease, injury, or treatment (chemotherapy).
basal cell carcinoma *BĀ-săl sĕl kăr-sĭ-NŌ-mă*	Malignant tumor of the basal cell layer of the epidermis that is locally invasive but rarely metastasizes. The condition occurs most frequently on areas of the skin exposed to the sun.
carbuncle *KĂR-bŭng-kl*	Pyogenic infection of the skin, or abscess. This infection is made up of several furuncles developing in adjoining hair follicles with multiple drainage sinuses. The most common sites of these lesions are hairy parts of the body exposed to irritation, pressure, friction, or moisture (Fig. 5–5). See also *furuncle*. ***Figure 5–5*** *Carbuncle-furuncle—two distinct abcesses. Erythematous, tender, deeply indurated, 1-cm or larger lesions that surround one or several pustular hair follicles. Lesions drain creamy pus when incised and may heal with scarring. (From Goldsmith, LA, et al. Adult and Pediatric Dermatology: A Color Guide to Diagnosis and Treatment. FA Davis, Philadelphia, 1997, p 364, with permission.)*
cellulitis *sĕl-ū-LĪ-tĭs*	Inflammation of cellular or connective tissue.
cicatrix *SĬK-ă-trĭks*	Firm scar tissue that forms in the healing of a sore or wound.
comedo *KŎM-ē-dō*	Blackhead; discolored dried sebum plugging an excretory duct of the skin.
contusion *kŏn-TOO-zhŭn*	An injury in which the skin is not broken, caused by a blow to the body and characterized by swelling, discoloration, and pain. The immediate application of cold may limit the development of a contusion. Also called a *bruise*.
cyst *sĭst*	Closed sac or pouch in or under the skin, with a definite wall, that contains fluid, semifluid, or solid material.
sebaceous *sē-BĀ-shŭs*	A cyst filled with sebum (fatty material) from a sebaceous gland. The cyst may enlarge as sebum collects and may become infected.
dermatitis *dĕr-mă-TĪ-tĭs* *dermat=skin* *itis=inflammation*	Inflammation of the skin.
seborrheic *sĕb-ō-RĒ-ĭk*	An acute or subacute form of dermatitis characterized by dry or moist greasy scales. Common sites are the scalp, eyelids, face, external surfaces of the ears, axillae, breasts, groin, and gluteal folds.

Pathological Conditions (Continued)

PATHOLOGICAL CONDITION	DESCRIPTION
dermatomycosis *dĕr-mă-tō-mī-KŌ-sĭs* *dermato=skin* *myc=fungus* *osis=abnormal condition*	Fungal infection of the skin.
discoid lupus erythematosus (DLE) *DIS-koyd LŪ-pŭs ĕr-ĭ-thĕ-mă-TŌ-sŭs*	A chronic skin disease characterized by remissions and exacerbations of a scaling, red, macular rash. These lesions contain plugged follicles and are atrophic. In one form the lesions are above the chin; in the second form, on the rest of the body. The disease is limited to the skin in 90% of patients, but may eventually develop into systemic lupus erythematosus. Thought to be an autoimmune disorder, it is approximately five times more common in women than in men. Also called *cutaneous lupus erythematosus*.
ecchymosis *ĕk-ĭ-MŌ-sĭs*	Black-and-blue mark on the skin caused by hemorrhages into the skin from injury or by leakage of blood from blood vessels underneath the skin. Commonly called a bruise. Ecchymosis differs from petechiae only in size (larger than 3 mm in diameter).
eczema *ĔK-zĕ-mă*	Generic term for inflammatory condition of the skin; a superficial dermatitis of unknown cause. In the early stage eczema may be pruritic, erythematous, papulovesicular, edematous, and weeping. Later it becomes crusted, scaly, thickened, and hardened. Exacerbating factors include sudden temperature changes, humidity, psychologic stress, fibers, detergents, and perfumes. Eczema is not a distinct disease entity (Fig. 5–6). 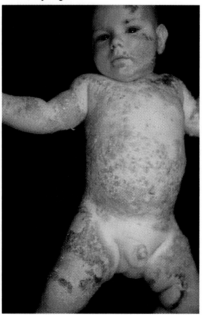 ***Figure 5–6*** *Scattered eczema of the trunk of an infant. (From Goldsmith, LA, et al: Adult and Pediatric Dermatology: A Color Guide to Diagnosis and Treatment. FA Davis, Philadelphia, 1997, p 243, with permission.)*
erythema *ĕr-ĭ-THĔ-mă*	Redness or inflammation of the skin or mucous membranes resulting from dilation and congestion of superficial capillaries. Examples of erythema are nervous blushes and mild sunburn.

Pathological Conditions (Continued)

PATHOLOGICAL CONDITION	DESCRIPTION
erythroderma *ĕ-rĭth-rō-DĔR-mă* *erythro=red* *derma=skin*	Abnormal redness of the skin, usually related to widespread areas of erythema.
exanthematous viral disease *ĕks-ăn-THĔM-ă-tŭs VĪ-răl dĭ-ZĒZ*	Viral infection characterized by a rash. Examples are scarlet fever, measles, and chickenpox.
furuncle *FŪ-rŭng-kl*	An abscess involving the entire hair follicle and adjacent subcutaneous tissue (see Fig. 5–5). Also known as a *boil*.
gangrene *GĂNG-grēn*	Necrosis or death of tissue, usually the result of ischemia (loss of blood supply), bacterial invasion, and subsequent putrefaction (decomposition of proteins by bacteria). The extremities are most often affected, but gangrene can occur anywhere in the body. Occurs as a result of certain diseases such as diabetes, or degenerative changes such as arteriosclerosis. The dead matter must be removed before healing can take place.
granuloma *gran-yū-LŌ-mă*	One of a variety of inflamed, granular-appearing tissues; a benign mass of granulation tissue.
herpes *HĔR-pēz*	A word used to indicate vesicular eruption caused by a virus, especially herpes simplex or herpes zoster, and the condition commonly called *cold sore* or *fever blister*. When used as a single word, "herpes" usually refers to herpes simplex (Fig. 5–7). *Figure 5–7 Herpes simplex. (From Goldsmith, LA, et al: Adult and Pediatric Dermatology: A Color Guide to Diagnosis and Treatment. FA Davis, Philadelphia, 1997, p 306, with permission.)*
zoster *HĔR-pēz ZŎS-tĕr*	An acute inflammatory eruption of highly painful vesicles on the trunk of the body or occasionally on the face, which mainly affects adults. Characterized by the development of painful vesicular skin eruptions that follow the underlying route of cranial or spinal nerves inflamed by the virus; also called *shingles* (Fig. 5–8). *Figure 5–8 Herpes zoster (shingles). (From Goldsmith, LA, et al: Adult and Pediatric Dermatology: A Color Guide to Diagnosis and Treatment. FA Davis, Philadelphia, 1997, p 86, with permission.)*

PATHOLOGICAL CONDITIONS (CONTINUED)

PATHOLOGICAL CONDITION	DESCRIPTION
hirsutism HŬR-sūt-ĭzm	Condition characterized by excessive growth of hair or presence of hair in unusual places, especially in women.
hyperhidrosis hī-pĕr-hī-DRŌ-sĭs *hyper=excessive, above normal* *hidr=sweat* *osis=abnormal condition*	Excessive perspiration often caused by heat, hyperthyroidism, strong emotion, menopause, or infection.
ichthyosis ĭk-thē-Ō-sĭs	A condition in which the skin is dry and scaly, resembling fish skin. Because ichthyosis is so easily recognized, a variety of diseases have been called by this name.
vulgaris vŭl-GĂ-rĭs	A hereditary form of ichthyosis with two genetically distinct types—dominant and sex-linked:
dominant DŎM-ĭ-nănt	Dominant ichthyosis vulgaris is produced by an autosomal dominant gene. It is characterized by dry, rough, scaly skin; it is not present at birth and is usually noticed between the ages of 1 and 4 years. Many cases improve in later life.
sex-linked SĔKS-linkt	A form of ichtyosis present only in men and transmitted by a woman as a recessive gene. Onset of scattered large brown scales is seen in early infancy. The scalp may be involved, but the face is spared except for the sides and in front of the ears. There is little tendency for this condition to improve with age.
impetigo ĭm-pĕ-TĪ-gō	Inflammatory skin disease characterized by isolated pustules that become crusted and rupture (Fig. 5–9). ***Figure 5–9*** *Impetigo. (From Goldsmith, LA, et al: Adult and Pediatric Dermatology: A Color Guide to Diagnosis and Treatment. FA Davis, Philadelphia, 1997, p 331, with permission.)*
Kaposi sarcoma KĂP-ō-sē săr-KŌ-mă	A vascular malignancy that is often first apparent in the skin or mucous membranes but may involve the viscera. Characterized by cutaneous purplish-blue nodules, usually on the lower extremities. It is the most common AIDS-related tumor and causes structural and functional damage. When associated with AIDS, it progresses aggressively, involving the lymph nodes, the viscera, and sometimes the gastrointestinal tract.
keloid KĒ-lŏyd	An overgrowth of scar tissue at the site of a wound of the skin.

PATHOLOGICAL CONDITIONS (CONTINUED)

PATHOLOGICAL CONDITION	DESCRIPTION
keratosis kĕr-ă-TŌ-sĭs *kerat=horny tissue, hard* *osis=abnormal condition*	Any horny growth on the skin (e.g., a callus or wart).
actinic ăk-TĬN-ĭk	A horny, premalignant lesion of the skin caused by excessive exposure to sunlight. The regular use of sunscreen prevents the development of solar keratoses and will most probably reduce the risk of skin cancer; synonymous with *solar keratosis*.
seborrheic sĕb-ō-RĒ-ĭk	A benign skin tumor that may be pigmented, made up of immature epithelial cells. Common in elderly people. Its etiology is unknown.
laceration lăs-ĕ-RĀ-shŭn	Wound or irregular tear of the flesh.
lesion LĒ-zhŭn	A wound, injury, or pathological change in body tissue. A lesion may be described as benign, cancerous, gross, occult, or primary.
lipoma lĭ-PŌ-mă *lip=fat* *oma=tumor*	A benign growth made up of fatty tissue; synonymous with adipoma.
melanoma mĕl-ă-NŌ-mă *melan=black* *oma=tumor*	Any of a group of malignant, darkly pigmented neoplasms that originate in the skin and are made up of melanocytes.
nevus (nevi, plural) NĒ-vŭs (NĒ-vī)	A pigmented skin blemish that is usually benign but may become cancerous. Many nevi are congenital, but some are acquired. Any change in color, size, or texture or any bleeding or itching of a nevus merits investigation. Also known as a *mole* or *birthmark*.
onychia ō-NĬK-ē-ă *onych=nail* *ia=condition*	Inflammation of the nailbed. Also called *onychitis*.
pediculosis pē-dĭk-ū-LŌ-sĭs *pedicul=a louse* *osis=abnormal condition*	Infestation with lice. Transmitted by personal contact or common use of brushes, combs, or headgear.
petechia (petechiae, plural) pē-TĒ-kē-ă (pē-TĒ-kē-ē)	Minute or small hemorrhagic spot on the skin. Petechia is a smaller version of ecchymosis.
pruritus proo-RĪ-tŭs	Itching, which may be a symptom of a process such as an allergic response.

PATHOLOGICAL CONDITIONS (CONTINUED)

PATHOLOGICAL CONDITION	DESCRIPTION
psoriasis *sō-RĪ-ă-sĭs*	Chronic skin disease characterized by itchy red patches covered with silvery scales.
purpura *PŬR-pū-ră*	Any of several bleeding disorders characterized by bleeding into the skin. Minute hemorrhagic spots of pinhead size are known as petechiae and larger hemorrhagic areas are known as *ecchymoses* or *bruises*.
pustule *PŬS-tūl*	Small elevation of skin filled with lymph or pus.
scabies *SKĀ-bēz*	Contagious skin disease transmitted by the itch mite.
seborrhea *sĕb-or-Ē-ă* *sebo=sebum* *rrhea=discharge, flow*	Any of several common skin conditions in which an overproduction of sebum by the sebaceous glands results in excessive oiliness or dry scales.
shingles *SHĬNG-lz*	See *herpes zoster*.
squamous cell carcinoma *SKWĀ-mŭs sĕl kăr-sĭ-NŌ-mă*	A slow-growing malignant tumor of squamous epithelium. May grow not only in the skin but also wherever squamous epithelium exists (nose, mouth, esophagus, lungs, bladder, and so forth); also called epidermoid carcinoma.
suppuration *sŭp-ū-RĀ-shŭn*	The formation of pus. Synonymous with *pyogenesis* and *pyosis*.
systemic lupus erythematosus (SLE) *sĭs-TĔM-ĭk LŪ-pŭs ĕr-ĭ-thē-mă-TŌ-sŭs*	A chronic autoimmune inflammatory disease involving multiple organ systems and marked by periods of exacerbation and remission. This condition is characterized by a butterfly rash over the nose. The disease is most prevalent in nonwhite women of childbearing age. Sometimes confused with *discoid lupus erythematosus* (DLE).
tinea *TĬN-ē-ăh*	Any fungal skin disease, frequently caused by ringworm. Names of various forms indicate the body part affected (e.g., tinea barbae [beard], tinea corporis [body], tinea pedis [athlete's foot]).
ulcer *ŬL-sĕr*	An open sore or lesion of the skin or mucous membrane accompanied by sloughing of inflamed necrotic tissue. If the sore becomes infected, pus forms.
decubitus *dē-KŪ-bĭ-tŭs*	An inflammation, sore, or ulcer in the skin over a bony prominence caused by impaired circulation in a portion of the body surface from lying in one position over a prolonged period of time. A decubitus (lying down) ulcer is also known as a *pressure sore* or *bedsore*.
urticaria *ŭr-tĭ-KĀ-rē-ă*	Allergic reaction of the skin characterized by eruption of pale-red elevated patches called *wheals* (hives).
vitiligo *vĭt-ĭl-Ī-gō*	Localized loss of skin pigmentation characterized by milk-white patches.

PATHOLOGICAL CONDITIONS (CONTINUED)

PATHOLOGICAL CONDITION	DESCRIPTION
xerosis zē-RŌ-sĭs *xer=dry* *osis=abnormal condition*	Dry skin; also called xeroderma (Fig. 5–10).

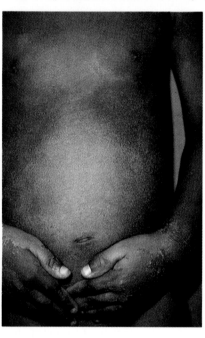

Figure 5–10 Xerosis. (From Goldsmith, LA, et al: Adult and Pediatric Dermatology: A Color Guide to Diagnosis and Treatment. FA Davis, Philadelphia, 1997, p 132, with permission.)

Activity 5-5: Clinical Application
Pathological Conditions

alopecia	granuloma	pediculosis
cicatrix	hirsutism	pruritus
comedo	hyperhidrosis	pustule
dermatomycosis	ichthyosis	scabies
ecchymosis	keratosis	sebaceous cyst
erythroderma	laceration	ulcer
furuncle	melanoma	vitiligo
gangrene	onychia	xeroderma

Match the diagnoses listed above with the definitions given in the numbered list:

1. _____ A condition in which the skin is dry and scaly, resembling fish skin.

2. _____ Any horny growth of the skin, such as a callus or wart.

3. _____ Fungal infection of the skin.

4. _____ Absence or loss of hair.

5. _____ Collection of discolored dried sebum plugging an excretory duct of the skin; a blackhead.

6. _____Excessive perspiration.

7. _____Irregular tear of the flesh; a wound.

8. _____Dry skin.

9. _____Small elevation of skin filled with lymph or pus.

10. _____Contagious skin disease transmitted by the itch mite.

11. _____Inflammation of the nail bed.

12. _____Firm scar tissue that forms in the healing of a sore or wound.

13. _____Discoloration on the skin consisting of large, irregularly formed hemorrhagic areas. The color is blue-black, changing in time to greenish-brown or yellow; commonly caused by a bruise.

14. _____An abscess involving the entire hair follicle and adjacent subcutaneous tissue. Also called a *boil*.

15. _____Loss of skin pigmentation characterized by milk-white patches.

16. _____An open sore or lesion of the skin or mucous membrane accompanied by sloughing of inflamed necrotic tissue. If the sore becomes infected, pus forms.

17. _____Infestation with lice, transmitted by personal contact or common use of combs or headgear.

18. _____A cyst filled with sebum (fatty material).

19. _____Excessive growth of hair in unusual places, especially in women.

20. _____Abnormal redness of the skin, usually related to widespread areas of erythema.

Correct Answers _____ × 5 = _____ **% Score**

CUTANEOUS LESIONS

Evaluation of skin lesions, injuries, or changes to tissue helps establish skin disorders. Lesions are described as primary or secondary lesions. Primary skin lesions are the initial reaction to pathologically altered tissue. Secondary skin lesions are the changes that take place in the primary lesion due to infection, scratching, trauma, or various stages of a disease. Lesions are also described according to type and appearance. Some of the major primary and secondary skin lesions are described and illustrated on the next page.

BURNS

Three basic types of burns are thermal, chemical, and electrical. Thermal burns are the most common and are caused by contact with hot substances, fire, steam, or scalds. Chemical burns are caused by alkalies or acids. Electrical burns are caused by either low- or high-voltage currents.

The surface appearance of the wound determines the burn classification. Burns can be either partial thickness or full thickness (Fig. 5–11).

PRIMARY LESIONS

FLAT LESIONS
Flat, discolored, circumscribed lesions of any size

Macule
Flat, pigmented, circumscribed area less than 1 cm in diameter. **Examples**: freckle, flat mole, or rash that occurs in rubella.

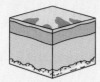

--- ELEVATED LESIONS ---

Solid   *Fluid filled*

Papule
Solid raised lesion less than 1 cm in diameter that may be the same color as the skin or pigmented. **Examples**: nevus, warts, pimples, ringworm, psoriasis, eczema.

Vesicle
Elevated, circumscribed, fluid-filled lesion, less than 0.5 cm in diameter. **Examples**: poison ivy, shingles, chickenpox.

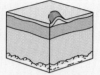

Nodule
Palpable, circumscribed lesion, larger and deeper than a papule (0.6 to 2 cm in diameter), extends into the dermal area. **Examples**: intradermal nevus, benign or malignant tumor.

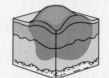

Bulla
A vesicle or blister larger than 1 cm in diameter. **Examples**: second degree burns, severe poison oak, ivy dermatitis.

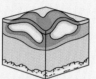

Tumor
Solid, elevated lesion larger than 2 cm in diameter that extends into the dermal and subcutaneous layers. **Examples**: lipoma, steatoma, dermatofibroma, hemangioma.

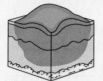

Pustule
Small, raised, circumscribed lesion that contains pus; usually less than 1 cm in diameter. **Examples**: acne, furuncle, pustular psoriasis, scabies.

Wheal
Elevated, firm, rounded lesion with localized skin edema (swelling) that varies in size, shape, and color; white in the center with a pale-red periphery, accompanied by itching. **Examples:** hives, insect bites, urticaria.

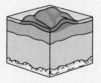

SECONDARY LESIONS

DEPRESSED LESIONS
Depressed lesions caused by loss of skin surface

Excoriations
Linear scratch marks or traumatized abrasions of the epidermis. **Examples**: scratches, abrasions, chemical or thermal burns.

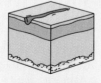

Ulcer
An open sore or lesion that extends to the dermis and usually heals with scarring. **Examples**: pressure sore, basal cell carcinoma.

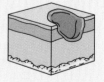

Fissure
Small slit or cracklike sore that extends into the dermal layer; could be caused by continuous inflammation and drying.

Adapted from Williams, LS, and Hopper, PD: Understanding Medical-Surgical Nursing. FA Davis, Philadelphia, 1999, p 1084, with permission.

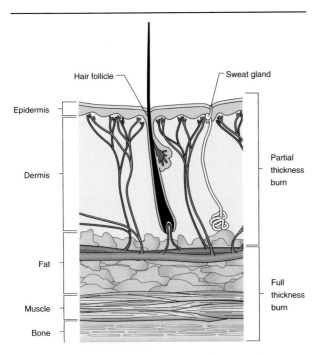

Figure 5–11 *Partial- and full-thickness burns, and structures affected. (From Williams, LS, and Hopper, PD: Understanding Medical-Surgical Nursing. FA Davis, Philadelphia, 1999, p 1182, with permission.)*

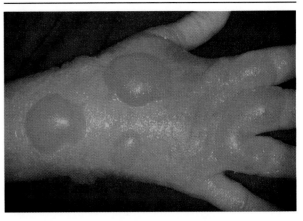

Figure 5–12 *A blistered partial-thickness thermal burn. (From Goldsmith, LA, Lazarus, GS, and Tharp, MD: Adult and Pediatric Dermatology: A Color Guide to Diagnosis and Treatment. FA Davis, Philadelphia, 1997, p 318, with permission.)*

The method used most frequently of estimating the burn area is known as the *rule of nines*. This methodology divides the total body surface into areas consisting of 9% or multiples of 9% as illustrated in Figure 5–13.

Partial-thickness burns are further categorized as superficial partial-thickness burns and deep partial-thickness burns. *Superficial partial-thickness* burns damage only two or three layers of the epidermis and generally tend to heal in 2 to 7 days. Sunburns or steam burns are good examples of this type of burn. *Deep partial-thickness burns* are more painful and involve the entire epidermal layer and even part of the dermis. The epidermis is blistered or broken as shown in Figure 5–12. If deep partial-thickness burns become infected or there is a greater degree of trauma to the area involved, they can develop into full-thickness burns.

Full-thickness burns affect all skin layers, including the subcutaneous tissue. The center of the burned area may feel painless due to destruction of nerve endings, whereas the surrounding areas may become extremely painful.

The extent of the burn is calculated by the percentage of total body surface area (TBSA) burned.

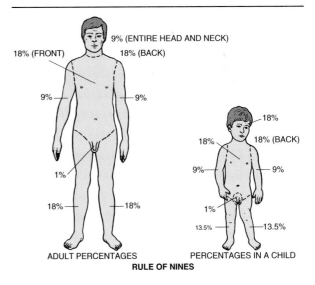

Figure 5–13 *The rule of nines. (From Venes, D [ed]: Taber's Cyclopedic Dictionary, ed 19. FA Davis, Philadelphia, 2001, p 1907, with permission.)*

Activity 5–6: Clinical Application

Skin Lesions and Burns

bulla	furuncle	thermal burn
chemical burn	keratosis	tumor
deep partial-thickness burn	macule	ulcer
fissure	superficial partial-thickness burn	wheal

Match the diagnoses listed above with the definitions given in the numbered list:

1.＿＿＿＿＿＿＿＿＿＿An open sore or lesion that extends to the dermis and usually heals with scarring, such as a pressure sore.

2.＿＿＿＿＿＿＿＿＿＿A vesicle or blister larger than 1 cm in diameter. Examples are poison ivy and dermatitis.

3.＿＿＿＿＿＿＿＿＿＿A flat, pigmented circumscribed area less than 1 cm in diameter. Examples are freckles and flat moles.

4.＿＿＿＿＿＿＿＿＿＿Small slit or cracklike sore that extends into the dermal layer.

5.＿＿＿＿＿＿＿＿＿＿Caused by contact with hot substances, fire, or steam.

6.＿＿＿＿＿＿＿＿＿＿Elevated, firm, rounded lesion with localized swelling that varies in size, shape, and color; it is white in the center with a pale red periphery, accompanied by itching. Examples are hives and insect bites.

7.＿＿＿＿＿＿＿＿＿＿Characterized by damage to only two or three layers of the epidermis; tending to heal in 2 to 7 days.

8.＿＿＿＿＿＿＿＿＿＿Caused by alkalies or acids.

9.＿＿＿＿＿＿＿＿＿＿Solid, elevated lesion larger than 2 cm in diameter that extends into subcutaneous layers. Examples are lipoma and steatoma.

10.＿＿＿＿＿＿＿＿＿＿Characterized by damage to all of the skin layers, including the subcutaneous tissue.

Correct Answers ＿＿＿＿ × 10 = ＿＿＿＿% **Score**

DIAGNOSTIC PROCEDURES

PROCEDURE	DESCRIPTION
biopsy (bx) BĪ-ŏp-sē	Excision of a small piece of living tissue from an organ or other part of the body for microscopic examination to confirm or establish a diagnosis, estimate prognosis, or follow the course of a disease.
aspiration ăs-pĭ-RĀ-shŭn	Removal of tissue for microscopic examination by suction through a fine needle attached to a syringe. The procedure is used primarily to obtain cells from a lesion containing fluid or when fluid is formed in a serous cavity.
needle NĒ-dl	Removal of tissue by inserting a hollow needle through the skin or external surface of an organ or tumor to draw off a sample of diseased tissue for histological study.
punch pŭnch	Method that removes a small cylindrical specimen for biopsy by means of a special instrument that pierces the organ directly or through the skin or a small incision in the skin. Used to obtain tissue when complete excision of the diseased area is not feasible.
shave shāv	Technique performed with a surgical blade or a razor blade. Used for lesions that are elevated above the skin level or confined to the epidermis and upper dermis, or to protrusions of lesions from internal sites.
frozen section (FS) FRŌ-zĕn SĔK-shŭn	A surgical procedure to cut a thin piece of tissue from a frozen specimen for immediate pathological examination. Commonly used for rapid diagnosis of malignancy, while patient awaits surgery, to determine conservative or radical approach.
skin test skĭn tĕst	A test to determine the reaction of the body to a substance by observing the results of injecting the substance intradermally or of applying it topically to the skin. Used to detect allergens, to determine immunity, and to diagnose disease.
intradermal ĭn-tră-DĔR-măl *intra =in, within* *derm =skin* *al =pertaining to*	A procedure used to identify suspected allergens by subcutaneously injecting the patient with small amounts of extracts of the suspected allergens and observation of the skin for a subsequent reaction. Performed to detect immunity to diphtheria (Schick test) and sensitivity to tuberculosis (Mantoux test).
patch păch	The simplest type of skin test, in which a small piece of gauze or filter paper is impregnated with a minute quantity of the suspected allergy-causing substance (food, pollen, animal fur, and so on), and is applied to the skin, usually on the forearm. After a certain length of time, the patch is removed and the reaction observed. If the skin is reddened or swollen, the result is positive. If there is no reaction, the test result is negative.
scratch skrăch	Type of skin test in which a small quantity of a solution containing a suspected allergen is placed on a lightly scratched area of the skin. If redness or swelling occurs at the scratch sites within 15 to 20 minutes, allergy to the substance is indicated and the test result is considered positive. If no reaction has occurred after 30 minutes, the substance is removed and the result is considered negative.

SURGICAL AND THERAPEUTIC PROCEDURES

PROCEDURE	DESCRIPTION
curettage *kū-rĕ-TAZH*	Scraping of a cavity, wound, or other surface using a spoonlike cutting instrument called a *curette*. Can be performed with a blunt or a sharp curette or by suction.
cryosurgery *krī-ō-SĔR-jĕr-ē* *cryo=cold*	A procedure using subfreezing temperature (achieved by liquid nitrogen or carbon dioxide) to destroy tissue. Used to treat malignant tumors and to control pain and bleeding.
débridement *dā-brēd-MŎN*	Removal of dead or damaged tissue from a wound or burn site to prevent infection and to facilitate healing.
electrosurgery *ē-lĕk-trō-SŬR-jĕr-ē*	Electrosurgical procedures performed with various electric instruments that operate on high-frequency electric current. Kinds of electrosurgery include electrocautery, electrocoagulation, electrodesiccation, and fulguration.
electrocautery *ē-lĕk-trō-KAW-tĕr-ē*	The application of a needle or snare heated by electric current for the destruction of tissue. Used in procedures such as removing warts or polyps and cauterizing small blood vessels to limit blood loss during surgery.
electrocoagulation *ē-lĕk-trō-kō-ăg-ū-LĀ-shŭn*	Hardening (coagulation) of tissue by means of a high-frequency electric current from an electrocautery device. The heat producing the coagulation is generated within the tissue to be destroyed.
electrodesiccation *ē-lĕk-trō-dĕs-ĭ-KĀ-shŭn*	Destruction of tissue by burning with an electric spark. Used primarily for eliminating small superficial growths but may be also used with curettage for eradicating abnormal tissue deeper in the skin. In the latter case, layers of skin may be burned and then successively scraped away. The procedure is performed under local anesthesia.
fulguration *fŭl-gŭ-RĀ-shŭn*	Destruction of tissue by means of long high-frequency electric sparks. See *electrodesiccation*.
escharotomy *ĕs-kăr-ŎT-ō-mē* *escharo=scab (caused by burning)* *tomy=incision*	A surgical incision in an eschar (scab) to lessen constriction, as might be done following a burn; used to prevent wound infection of the burn site.
irrigation *ĭr-ĭ-GĀ-shŭn*	The process of washing out a body cavity or wounded area with a stream of water or other fluid. It is also used to cleanse a tube or drain inserted into the body, such as an indwelling catheter. The solutions used for cleansing should be sterile and have an approximate temperature slightly warmer than body temperature.

Surgical and Therapeutic Procedures (Continued)

PROCEDURE	DESCRIPTION
laser surgery LĀ-zĕr SŬR-jĕr-ē	Surgery using a laser device. Lasers are used in surgery to divide or cause adhesions, or to destroy or fix tissue in place. Lasers have multiple treatment applications. In dermatology, they are used for obliteration of blood vessels, superficial removal of warts and skin cancers, removal of excess tissue in enlarged noses, superficial removal of pigmented conditions (brown spots) and port-wine nevi, and removal of tattoos and superficial wrinkles.
lipectomy lĭ-PĔK-tō-mē *lip=fat* *ectomy=excision, removal*	Surgical excision of subcutaneous fat. If suction is used, the procedure is called *liposuction* or *suction lipectomy*.
liposuction līp-ō-SŬK-shŭn	A technique for removing subcutaneous fat tissue with a suction pump device. Used primarily to remove or reduce localized areas of fat around the abdomen, breasts, legs, face, and upper arms where the skin is contractile enough to redrape in a normal manner. Also called *suction lipectomy*.
rhytidoplasty, **rhytidectomy** RĬT-ĭ-dō-plăs-tē, rĭt-ĭ-DĔK-tō-mē *rhytido=wrinkle* *plasty=surgical repair* *ectomy=excision, removal*	A procedure in reconstructive plastic surgery in which the skin of the face is tightened, wrinkles are removed, and the skin is made to appear firm and smooth. An incision is made at the hairline, and excess skin is separated from the supporting tissue and excised. The edges of the remaining skin are pulled up and back and sutured at the hairline. The sutures are removed several days after discharge in an outpatient facility or in the surgeon's office.
skin graft skĭn grăft	Skin obtained from another part of the body, or from a donor, and used to repair a defect or trauma of the skin.
autograft, **homograft** AW-tō-grăft, HŌ-mō-grăft *auto=self, own* *homo=same*	Any tissue obtained from one part of the body and implanted at another location in the same individual. Used in several kinds of plastic surgery, most commonly to replace skin lost in severe burns.
heterograft, **xenograft** HĔT-ĕ-rō-grăft, ZĔN-ō-grăft *hetero = different* *xeno = foreign, strange*	Tissue obtained from an individual of one species for transplantation to an individual of a different species.

OTHER PROCEDURES

PROCEDURE	DESCRPTION
abrasion *ă-BRĀ-zhŭn*	A scraping away of a diseased or scarred area.
chemabrasion *kēm-ă-BRĀ-shŭn*	Application of chemicals to remove the surface layer of skin cells. May be used to treat scars, tattoos, abnormal pigmentation, or diseased skin cells.
dermabrasion *DĔRM-ă-brā-zhŭn*	Use of rotating brushes, sandpaper, or other abrasive materials to remove scars, lesions, and fine wrinkles from the skin.
cautery *KAW-tĕr-ē*	A technique used to destroy tissue by electricity, freezing, heat, or corrosive chemicals. Used in potentially infected wounds and to destroy excess granulation tissue.
chemical peel *KĔM-ĭ-kăl pēl*	Application of an acid solution to peel the top skin layers, allowing new, smoother skin with tighter cells to occupy the surface. Immediately after the peel, there may be considerable swelling, which subsides after 7 to 10 days as new skin begins to form. This procedure eliminates wrinkles, blemishes, pigment spots, and sun-damaged areas of the skin.

PHARMACOLOGY

DRUG CLASSIFICATION	THERAPEUTIC ACTION
anesthetics *ăn-ĕs-THĔT-ĭks*	Agents or drugs that reduce or eliminate sensation with or without loss of consciousness.
general	Anesthetics that affect the whole body and are accompanied by loss of consciousness.
local	Anesthetics that affect a particular region of the body.
topical	Substances used to relieve pain on the skin's surfaces caused by wounds, hemorrhoids, sunburn, and itching. Topical anesthetics, which numb the skin layers and mucous membranes, are administered directly by means of sprays, creams, gargles, suppositories, and other preparations.
anti-infectives, antibacterials *ăn-tĭ-ĭn-FĔK-tĭvs,* *ăn-tĭ-băk-TĒ-rē-ăls*	Agents that eliminate epidermal infections. Can be administered either topically or systemically. Topical medications create a skin environment that is lethal to microbes. Generally, a specific fungicide must be prescribed for a given fungus strain, whereas one antibiotic effectively eliminates several type of bacteria.
antifungals, antimycotics *ăn-tĭ-FŬNG-găls,* *ăn-tĭ-mī-KŌT-ĭks*	Substances that kill fungi or inhibit their growth or reproduction Can be administered either topically or systemically. In general, a specific fungicide is prescribed for a given fungus strain, whereas one antibiotic effectively eliminates several types of bacteria. Antifungals produce a skin condition that is lethal to microbes.

PHARMACOLOGY (CONTINUED)

DRUG CLASSIFICATION	THERAPEUTIC ACTION
antipruritics *ăn-tĭ-proo-RĬT-ĭks*	Substances commonly used as ointments, creams, or lotions to prevent or relieve itching. Topical anesthetics, corticosteroids, and antihistamines are used as antipruritic agents.
antiseptics *ăn-tĭ-SĔP-tĭks*	Topically applied agents that inhibit the growth and reproduction of microorganisms and destroy bacteria, thus preventing the development of infections in cuts, scratches, and surgical incisions.
astringents *ă-STRĬN-jĕnts*	Topical agents that cause contraction of tissue, arrest of secretions, or control of bleeding. Astringents shrink the blood vessels locally, dry up secretions from seeping lesions, decrease sweating, and lessen skin sensitivity.
corticosteroids *kor-tĭ-kō-STĒR-oyds*	Hormonelike preparations used as anti-inflammatory agents; topical agents that are administered for their immunosuppressive and anti-inflammatory properties. Produce vasoconstriction and are often used to relieve pruritus (itching). Corticosteroids are a mainstay of therapy for conditions that include eczema, psoriasis, insect bites, and contact dermatitis. Oral corticosteroids may be given to act systemically in severe or widespread cases of inflammation and pruritus.
keratolytics *kĕr-ă-tō-LĬT-ĭks*	Substances that promote dissolution or peeling of the horny layer of the epidermis. Potent keratolytic preparations are effective for removing warts and corns. Milder preparations are effective in promoting the shedding of scales and crusts in eczema, psoriasis, seborrheic dermatitis, and other dry, scaly conditions. Very weak keratolytics irritate inflamed skin, acting as tonics to promote healing.
parasiticides *păr-ă-SĬT-ĭ-sīds*	Drugs applied topically to kill insect parasites that infest the skin. Scabicides, potentially toxic and irritating to the skin, kill mites and their eggs. They must be used with caution in treating children. Pediculicides destroy lice and their eggs.
protectives *prō-TĔK-tĭvs*	Substances that function by covering, cooling, drying, or soothing inflamed skin. Protectives provide a long-lasting film, which protects the skin from air, water, and clothing during the natural healing process. Unlike other cooling agents, they do not penetrate or soften the skin.
retinoids *RĔT-ĭ-noyds*	Natural compounds and synthetic derivatives of retinol that exhibit vitamin A activity. Retinoids may be used in the treatment of conditions that include acne, keratinization disorders, skin cancer, psoriasis, and cutaneous aging.

❖ ABBREVIATIONS

The following abbreviations are primarily related to dermatology, but they also include abbreviations used in this chapter's medical records.

ABBREVIATION	MEANING	ABBREVIATION	MEANING
Bx, bx	biopsy	**oint, ung**	ointment
BCC	basal cell carcinoma	**po**	by mouth (per os)
cm	centimeter	**PERRLA**	pupils equal, round, and reactive
decub	decubitus (ulcer); bedsore		to light and accommodation
derm	dermatology	**postop**	postoperative
DLE	discoid lupus erythematosus	**PSS**	progressive systemic
EAHF	eczema, asthma, and hay fever;		scleroderma
	eczema, allergy, hay fever	**qh**	every hour (This abbreviation
EKG, ECG	electrocardiogram		may also contain any number to
FS	frozen section		indicate the number of hours
ID	intradermal		between administration of
IM	intramuscular; infectious		medication or therapy, e.g., q8h.)
	mononucleosis	**R/O**	rule out
IMP	impression; synonymous with	**SC, sc, subcu,**	subcutaneous
	diagnosis (Dx)	**sub q**	
I&D	incision and drainage	**SLE**	systemic lupus erythematosus
IV	intravenous	**SMAS**	superficial musculoaponeurotic
JVD	jugular venous distention		system [flap] (plastic surgery)
mg	milligram (1/1000 gram)	**XP, XDP**	xeroderma pigmentosum
mm	millimeter		

Activity 5–7: Clinical Application

Diagnostic, Surgical, and Therapeutic Procedures

antibacterials	débridement
antimycotics	dermabrasion
aspiration	irrigation
autograft	keratolytics
cryosurgery	lipectomy
curettage	topical anesthetics

Match the terms listed above with the statements given in the numbered list:

1. _____ Surgical transplantation of any tissue from one part of the body to another location in the same individual.

2. _____ Substances that promote dissolution or peeling of the horny layer of the epidermis.

3. _____ Process of washing out a body cavity or wound area with a stream of water or other fluid.

4. _____ Agents that kill fungi or inhibit their growth or reproduction.

5. _____ Using subfreezing temperatures, usually liquid nitrogen or carbon dioxide, to destroy tissue.

6. _____ Scraping of a cavity, wound, or other surface using a spoonlike instrument.

7. _____ Agents used on the skin to relieve pain caused by wounds or sunburn.

8. _____ Surgical excision of fatty tissue.

9. _____ Use of rotating brushes, sandpaper, or other abrasive materials to remove the epidermis; may be used to remove scars or lesions from the skin.

10. _____ Agents that destroy bacteria or inhibit their growth.

Correct Answers _____ × 10 = _____% **Score**

Activity 5–8: Build Medical Words
Diagnostic, Symptomatic, and Surgical Terms

Use *dermat/o* (skin) to build medical words meaning:

1. inflammation of the skin _____

2. specialist in skin (diseases) _____

Use *adip/o* or *lip/o* (fat) to build medical words meaning:

3. tumor consisting of fat _____

4. cell consisting of fat _____

Use *onych/o* (nail) to build medical words meaning:

5. inflammation of the nail _____

6. tumor of the nail _____

7. disease of the nails _____

8. softening of the nails _____

Use *trich/o* (hair) to build medical words meaning:

9. disease of the hair _____

10. abnormal condition of the hair _____

Use *xer/o* (dry) to build medical words meaning:

11. skin that is dry _____

12. abnormal condition of dryness _____

Use the suffix *-derma* (skin) to build medical words meaning:

13. white skin _____

14. blue skin _____

15. yellow skin _____

Use the suffix *-cyte* (cell) to build medical words meaning:

16. red cell _____

17. white cell _____

18. black cell _____

Use the prefixes *an-* (without, not) or *hyper-* (excessive, above normal) to build medical words meaning:

19. abnormal condition without sweat _____

20. abnormal condition of excessive sweat _____

Correct Answers _____ **× 5 =** _____ **% Score**

MEDICAL RECORDS

Authentic medical records, including a history and physical examination, a consultation, an operative report, and a dermatopathology report, are presented in this section.

The following dictionary exercise and medical record analysis will help you develop skills to abstract information and master the terminology in the reports. Accurate interpretation is important because information of this type is used in numerous areas of the medical practice, such as initiation of treatments, evaluation of patient's progress, and completion of insurance claims.

Reading and Dictionary Exercise

Place a check mark [✓] after you complete the exercise.

[   ] **1.** Underline the following words in the records as you read the history and physical examination, consultation, operative report, and dermatopathology report. These medical records can be found at the end of the chapter.

[   ] **2.** Use a medical dictionary and Appendix F, Part 2 to define the following terms. The words are listed below in sequential order, as they appear in the reports.

Note: You are not expected to fully understand all the parts of the medical records. The important aspect of this exercise is to use all resources that are available to complete it. Eventually you will master the terminology and format of these reports.

> > > MEDICAL RECORD 5-1: HISTORY AND PHYSICAL EXAMINATION

Term	Pronunciation	Meaning
erythromycin	ĕ-rĭth-rō-MĪ-sĭn	_____
Benadryl	BĔN-ă-drĭl	_____
impetigo	ĭm-pĕ-TĪ-gō	_____
dysphagia	dĭs-FĀ-jē-ă	_____
edema	ĕ-DĒ-mă	_____
cyanosis	sī-ă-NŌ-sĭs	_____
hemoptysis	hē-MŎP-tĭ-sĭs	_____
hepatitis	hĕp-ă-TĪ-tĭs	_____
jaundice	JAWN-dĭs	_____
diarrhea	dī-ă-RĒ-ă	_____
hematuria	hē-mă-TŪ-rē-ă	_____
anemia	ă-NĒ-mē-ă	_____
paresthesia	păr-ĕs-THĒ-zē-ă	_____
hyperemia	hī-pĕr-Ē-mē-ă	_____
supple	SŬ-pl	_____
thyromegaly	thī-rō-MĔG-ă-lē	_____
rhonchi	RŎNG-kī	_____
organomegaly	or-gă-nō-MĔG-ă-lē	_____
clubbing	KLŬB-ĭng	_____
Homans' sign	HŌ-mănz sīn	_____

> > > MEDICAL RECORD 5-2: CONSULTATION

Term	Pronunciation	Meaning
lesions	LĒ-zhŭns	_____

edematous	ĕ-DĒM-ă-tŭs	_____
weeping	WĒ-pĭng	_____
pustular	PŬS-tū-lĕr	_____
Duricef	DŪ-rĭ-sĕf	_____
Ancef	ĂN-sĕf	_____
Unasyn	ŪN-ă-sĭn	_____
pruritus	proo-RĪ-tŭs	_____
Cleocin	klē-ō-SĬN	_____
ciprofloxacin	sĭp-rō-FLŎCKS-ă-sĭn	_____
impetigo	ĭm-pĕ-TĪ-gō	_____
Staphylococcus	stăf-ĭl-ō-KŎK-ŭs	_____
Streptococcus	strĕp-tō-KŎK-ŭs	_____
vancomycin	VĂN-kō-mī-sĭn	_____
mupirocin	mū-PĒR-rō-sĭn	_____

> > > MEDICAL RECORD 5-3: OPERATIVE REPORT

Term	Pronunciation	Meaning
lipectomy	lĭ-PĔK-tō-mē	_____
analgesia	ăn-ăl-JĒ-zē-ă	_____
Betadine	BĔ-tă-dīn	_____
bilaterally	bī-LĂT-ĕr-ăl-ē	_____
Marcaine	MĂR-kān	_____
temporal scalp	TĔM-por-ăl skălp	_____
inferiorly	ĭn-FĒ-rē-or-lē	_____
preauricular region	prē-aw-RĬK-ū-lăr RĒ-jŭn	_____
posteriorly	pŏs-TĒ-rē-or-lē	_____
zygoma	zī-GŌ-mă	_____
postauricular	pōst-aw-RĬK-ū-lăr	_____

> > > MEDICAL RECORD 5-4: DERMATOPATHOLOGY REPORT

Term	Pronunciation	Meaning
Nofavil	NŎ-fă-vĭl	_____
plaque	plăk	_____
punch	pŭnch	_____
lentigo	lĕn-TĪ-gō	_____
malignancy	mă-LĬG-năn-sē	_____
basal cell	BĀ-săl sĕl	_____
carcinoma	kăr-sĭ-NŌ-mă	_____
atypical	ā-TĬP-ĭ-kăl	_____
melanocytic	mĕl-ă-nō-SĬT-ĭk	_____
squamous	SKWĀ-mŭs	_____
melanocytes	MĔL-ăn-ō-sīts	_____
papillary	PĂP-ĭ-lăr-ē	_____

Critical Thinking: Analysis of Medical Records

This section provides experience in abstracting and analyzing information from medical records. At the same time, it reinforces the material presented in this chapter.

> > > MEDICAL RECORD 5-1: HISTORY AND PHYSICAL EXAMINATION

1. What was Ms. Anderline's chief complaint, and what was her previous diagnosis?

_____

_____

2. Place a "+" in the space provided for positive findings and a "−" for negative findings. A positive finding indicates the patient had a history (Hx) of this condition; a negative finding indicates the patient did not have a history of this condition.

_____ high blood pressure   _____ edema

_____ ringing in the ears   _____ thyroid disease or diabetes

_____ dysphagia   _____ blood clots, anemia

_____ chest pain   _____ varicose veins

3. What does the dermatologist mean when he states in the physical examination section that there is "no discharge or ulcers"?

_____

4. What was Dr. Smith's diagnosis?

_____

> > > MEDICAL RECORD 5-2: CONSULTATION

5. Why was the patient admitted to the hospital, and what type of treatment did she receive?

_____

_____

6. Was the patient allergic to any medication? If so, explain.

_____

_____

_____

7. What was the physician's diagnosis or impression and what type of therapy was continued?

_____

_____

8. What body structure is the physician talking about when he suggests adding mupirocin ointment to the *nares* to get rid of the putative (commonly considered) staph carriage?

_____

_____

> > > MEDICAL RECORD 5-3: OPERATIVE REPORT

9. a. What type of operation was performed, and why and where was it was performed?

_____

_____

b. Why and where was a small stab incision made and how was the excess fat removed?

_____

_____

> > > MEDICAL RECORD 5-4: DERMATOPATHOLOGY REPORT

10. What did the clinical data indicate for several months and for many years?

_____

11. What were the diagnoses for the left upper back and the left ear?

_____

_____

12. What was the purpose of examining the 0.2 × 0.2 cm punch specimen?

_____

_____

Audio Practice

Listen to the audio CD-ROM to practice the pronunciation of selected medical terms from this chapter.

Medical Record 5–1. History and Physical Examination

GENERAL HOSPITAL AND MEDICAL CENTER
2211 Fifth Avenue North • Healthy City, USA 12345 • (321) 123-4567

History and Physical Examination

Patient Name: Amy Anderline   **Patient Number:** 48-34-33
Birth Date: 06/01/xx   **Room Number:** 183

HISTORY

CHIEF COMPLAINT: Rash over the face.

PRESENT ILLNESS: The patient is a 31-year-old black female. She stated that last week she started having some itching in the forehead, and she went to the doctor, and he prescribed an antibiotic (erythromycin) and Benadryl, and one to two days after, the rash was covering all over the face. The patient was diagnosed with impetigo, and she was admitted to the hospital for more investigation and treatment.

PAST HISTORY: High blood pressure.

ALLERGIES: Sulfa.

CURRENT MEDICATIONS: Benadryl and erythromycin.

REVIEW OF SYSTEMS:
Integument: No other dermatological complaints or lesions previously except for the one she has at the present time.
HEENT & Oral: No history of dizziness, ringing in the ears, blurred vision, or loss of consciousness. No bloody nose or dysphagia.
Cardiovascular: No history of chest pain, shortness of breath, edema, or cyanosis.
Respiratory: No history of chronic obstructive pulmonary disease, shortness of breath, tuberculosis, hemoptysis, or chronic cough.
Gastrointestinal: No history of ulcers, melena, hematemesis, hepatitis, jaundice, or marked alteration in weight or appetite. No history of chronic vomiting, diarrhea, or constipation.
Genitourinary: Denies any urgency, hesitancy, dysuria or hematuria.
Reproductive: Noncontributory.
Metabolic & Endocrine: No history of thyroid disease or diabetes.
Breasts: The patient denies any masses or nipple discharge.
Blood, Lymphatic: No history of blood clots, anemia, or bleeding disorder.
Skeletal: There is no pain, tenderness, swelling, or joint limitation of motion.
Neuromuscular: No history of paresthesias, numbness, or gait problems.

Continued

History and Physical Examination, page 2
Patient Name: Amy Anderline   **Patient Number:** 48-34-33

Mental: No history of mental disease.
Vascular, Peripheral: No history of lower limb edema or varicose veins.

PERSONAL & SOCIAL HISTORY: The patient does not smoke or drink.

FAMILY HISTORY: Unremarkable for any medical problems.

PHYSICAL EXAMINATION

VITAL SIGNS: Per nursing notes.
GENERAL APPEARANCE & MENTAL STATUS: The patient is an alert and oriented, well-developed, well-nourished 31-year-old black female.
INTEGUMENT: There is a rash all over the face. No discharge or ulcers.
HEENT & ORAL: Normocephalic. PERRLA. Sclerae nonicteric. Nose and throat showed no hyperemia, congestion, or discharge. Mucous membranes appeared to be adequately moistened.
NECK: Supple. No rigidity or painful motion. No thyromegaly, JVD, or carotid bruits.
NODES: No lymphadenopathy.
BREASTS: No masses or nipple discharge.
LUNGS: Essentially clear. No rhonchi or wheezes.
CARDIOVASCULAR: Regular rate and rhythm. No murmurs, gallops, or extra sounds.
ABDOMEN: Soft, nontender. No organomegaly or mass. Active bowel sounds.
GENITAL & RECTAL: Deferred.
SKELETAL: Full range of motion of articulation. No pain or joint swelling.
NEUROMUSCULAR: Deep tendon reflexes are present. Cranial nerves are intact. No focal deficits.
VASCULAR, PERIPHERAL: No cyanosis, clubbing, or edema. Pulses intact. No Homans sign.

IMPRESSION: Impetigo, under investigation and treatment.

_____
J. B. Smith, MD

JBS/ab

D: 06/13/xx
T: 06/14/xx

Medical Record 5–2. Consultation

GENERAL HOSPITAL AND MEDICAL CENTER
2211 Fifth Avenue North • Healthy City, USA 12345 • (321) 123-4567

Consultation

Patient Name: Amy Anderline   **Patient Number:** 48-34-33
Birth Date: 06/01/xx   **Room Number:** 131

DATE: 02/08/xx

CONSULTATION

CONSULTING PHYSICIAN: Elmer Haig, M.D.

REASON FOR CONSULTATION: The chart was reviewed, the patient was examined. The history is well outlined in the chart. In brief, the patient is a 31-year-old black female. She has two children. Neither of the children have had any facial lesions or any other infections. She has no pets at home. She apparently developed some infection of the forehead about 2 weeks ago, and this spread to her nose, and then subsequently to her whole face. This became progressively more edematous with weeping of apparent pustular material from the whole face diffusely. Indeed the patient was seen by Dr. X as well as Dr. Y, and she was placed on Duricef and then subsequently erythromycin in view of the fact that it did not seem to respond to the Duricef. She was also seen in the emergency room at one point and given a gram of Ancef, I believe. Certainly she is a fairly good historian and actually named the medication.

The patient was admitted for IV antibiotics, and indeed on admission her face was so swollen that she was almost unable to open her eyes. She was placed on Unasyn, and this appeared to be working over the course of 2 days. However, she developed some pruritus of her feet which was thought to be perhaps an allergy of some sort, and this was changed to Cleocin. I was called yesterday and changed the dose to 900 mg IV q.8h. as well as added ciprofloxacin at 750 mg p.o. q.12h. in view of the lack of knowledge as to the nature of the culprit. All cultures thus far have been negative, including those that were done on an outpatient basis at Dr. S's office as well as the cultures done here. Indeed no bacteria were even seen on the Gram stain of the facial drainage. This, of course, could be because she had been on antibiotics.

On physical examination, she is slightly obese. Her whole face is covered with essentially a cellulitis which is weeping of yellowish material which looks purulent. Apparently there was a lot of edema earlier. There is very little now. There are submandibular nodes which are palpable as well as submental nodes which are also palpable. The balance of the exam is essentially as documented.

Continued

Medical Record 5–4. Dermatopathology Report
___

GENERAL HOSPITAL AND MEDICAL CENTER
2211 Fifth Avenue North • Healthy City, USA 12345 • (321) 123-4567

Pathology Report
___

Patient Name: George Franks   **Patient Number:** 33-43-12
Birth Date: 04/12/xx   **Room Number:** OP

CLINICAL DATA: A: Scaly slightly pearly plaque for several months; biopsy only, 2 mm punch closed with 5–0 Novafil.

B: Brown pink plaque for many years; biopsy only, 2 mm punch closed with 5–0 Novafil.

A: Lentigo, R/O lentigo malignancy
B: Basal cell carcinoma.

DIAGNOSIS: A: LEFT UPPER BACK:
ATYPICAL MELANOCYTIC PROLIFERATION, MOST COMPATIBLE WITH MALIGNANT MELANOMA, MEASURING APPROXIMATELY 0.25 MM IN THICKNESS (PUNCH BIOPSY) (172.9).

B: EAR, LEFT:
SUPERFICIAL SQUAMOUS CELL CARCINOMA (173.2).
___

SPECIMEN A:

GROSS DESCRIPTION: 0.2 × 0.2 cm punch.

MICROSCOPIC DESCRIPTION: Initial and deeper sections examined. Within the epidermis, extending to peripheral margins, there is an increased number of plump, variably atypical melanocytes present singly and in collections. In areas, single melanocytes predominate and are scattered at all levels of the epidermis. In only one of multiple levels of sectioning, there is a small collection of melanocytes within the papillary dermis.

Pathologist: _____
                        Nora Roff, M.D.

NR/bab

d&t: 05/25/xx

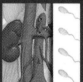

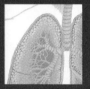

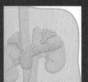

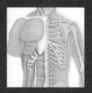

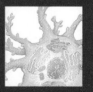

chapter

6 Urology

Chapter Outline

Objectives

Upon completion of this chapter, you will be able to:

- Describe the type of medical treatment a urologist provides.
- Name the organs of the urinary system and discuss their primary function.
- Recognize, pronounce, build, and spell terms related to the genitourinary system.
- Describe pathological conditions, diagnostic tests, surgical procedures, and other treatments related to the genitourinary system.
- Demonstrate your knowledge of this chapter by successfully completing the activities and the analysis of medical records.

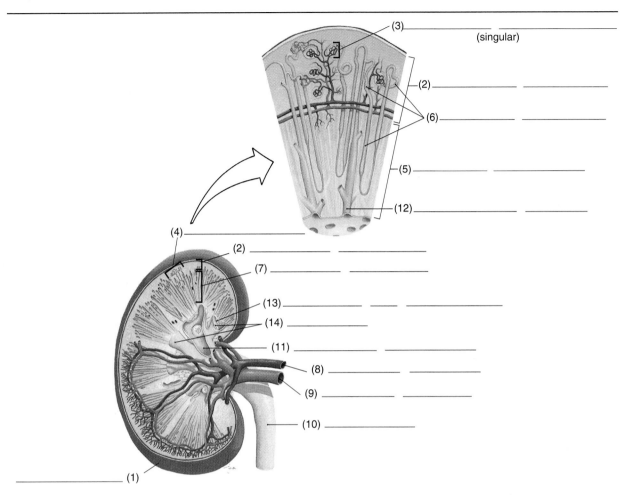

(3)_____ _____
(singular)

(2)_____ _____ _____

(6)_____ _____ _____

(5)_____ _____

(12)_____ _____

(4)_____

(2)_____ _____

(7)_____ _____

(13)_____ _____ _____

(14)_____

(11)_____ _____

(8)_____ _____

(9)_____ _____

(10)_____

(1)_____

Figure 6–3 *Frontal section of the right kidney showing internal structure and blood vessels. The magnified section of the kidney shows several nephrons. (Adapted from Scanlon, VC, and Sanders, T: Understanding Human Structure and Function. FA Davis, Philadelphia, 1997, p 405, with permission.)*

porarily stored until it is expelled from the body through the urethra.

As you read the following material, label Figure 6–4.

Nephron

Each kidney contains over 1 million tiny blood-processing units known as nephrons, which carry out the processes that form urine. The tubular portion of the nephron is divided into three parts: a (1) **proximal convoluted tubule,** the (2) **loop of Henle,** and a (3) **distal convoluted tubule.** The capsule that surrounds and encloses the (4) **glomerulus** is the (5) **Bowman capsule.** Glomerular filtrate, the fluid that transports filtered products and toxins, is collected in the Bowman capsule and eliminated through urine. To maintain **homeostasis,** electrolytes, nutrients, and water are returned to the blood.

The distal convoluted tubules of several nephrons drain into a collecting tubule. Fluid is then drained by the collecting tubule from the (6) **renal cortex** into the (7) **renal medulla.** This fluid, now called *urine,* passes through the renal pelvis and out of the kidney into the ureter (see Fig. 6–3). The muscular walls of the ureter propel the urine into the bladder. A flaplike fold of mucous membrane covers the opening through which urine enters the bladder. This fold acts as a valve, allowing urine to enter the bladder from the ureter but preventing it from backing up. The urinary bladder stores the urine until it is **voided.** Sustained contraction of the internal urethral sphincter (circular muscle) prevents the bladder from emptying until pressure within the bladder increases to a certain level. Once the pressure level is reached, there is an urge to urinate. The process that expels urine from the urinary bladder is called *micturition* or *urination.*

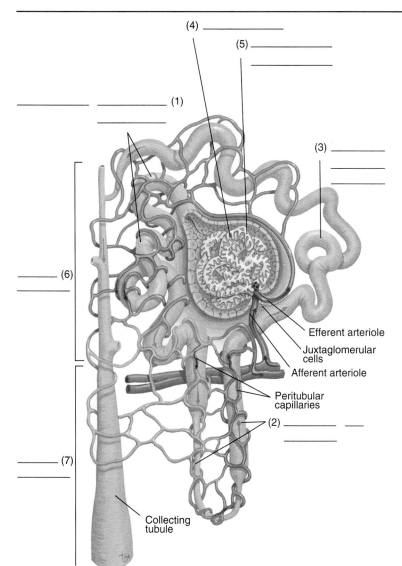

(4) _____

(5) _____
_____

_____ _____ (1)
_____

(3) _____
_____
_____

Efferent arteriole

Juxtaglomerular cells

Afferent arteriole

Peritubular capillaries

(6)

(2) _____ __

(7)

Collecting tubule

Figure 6–4 *A nephron with associated blood vessels. The arrows indicate the direction of the blood flow and the flow of renal filtrate. (Adapted from Scanlon, VC, and Sanders, T: Understanding Human Structure and Function. FA Davis, Philadelphia, 1997, p 406, with permission.)*

Activity 6-1: Competency Verification
Frontal Section of Right Kidney, and Nephron with Associated Blood Vessels

Review Figures 6–3 and 6–4, and check your labeling in Appendix C.

Urine Formation

Urine formation begins by filtration of blood through capillary pores known as glomeruli (singular, *glomerulus*) as illustrated in Figure 6–4, structure (4). Three major processes are involved in the formation of urine: glomerular filtration, which takes place in the renal corpuscles; tubular reabsorption, which takes place in the renal tubules; and tubular secretion, which also takes place in the renal tubules.

Glomerular filtration requires blood pressure that forces plasma, dissolved substances, and proteins out of the glomeruli. The newly formed fluid is called renal **filtrate** and ends up in the Bowman capsule (see Fig. 6–4, structure (5)).

Tubular reabsorption consists of the recovery of useful substances from the renal filtrate, which is returned to the blood in the peritubular capillaries. Approximately 99% of the renal filtrate is reabsorbed. In a healthy person, all proteins found in the renal filtrate are reabsorbed. Healthy urine has no protein.

Tubular secretion adds unwanted substances or waste products from the blood to the renal filtrate, which is then excreted as urine. Examples of waste products are ammonia or metabolic products of medications. In summary, tubular reabsorption conserves useful substances; tubular secretion involves filtering waste products, which are voided in urine.

Blood Pressure

Besides producing urine and excreting waste products, the kidneys play an important role in regulating blood pressure because blood volume, which is controlled by the kidneys, has a direct effect on blood pressure. When blood pressure decreases, so that blood flow is diminished, the juxtaglomerular cells (see Fig. 6–4) in the kidney secrete the enzyme renin and discharge it in the blood. The enzyme renin then initiates a mechanism that activates the contraction of arterioles to raise the blood pressure and blood flow in the kidneys and restore it to normal levels. Keep in mind that normal blood pressure is essential to healthy body functioning. Normal blood pressure is only one of the many factors the urologist uses to identify predisposing causes, symptoms, and eventually treatment of urinary tract disorders.

STRUCTURE AND FUNCTION OF THE MALE REPRODUCTIVE SYSTEM

Several organs in the man serve as parts of both the urinary tract and the reproductive system. Diseases of these organs may produce disorders of either or both systems. For this reason, diseases of the male reproductive system are usually treated by the urologist and are covered in this chapter.

The organs of the male reproductive system include the testes and several ducts and glands. In both men and women, the organs of the reproductive system are adapted to produce and unite **gametes** that contain specific genes. In men, the reproductive role is to produce and deliver sperm to the female reproductive organs.

Label Figure 6–5 as you learn about the organs of the male reproductive system.

Structures of the male reproductive system can be divided into two categories based on function: primary sex organs and secondary sex organs.

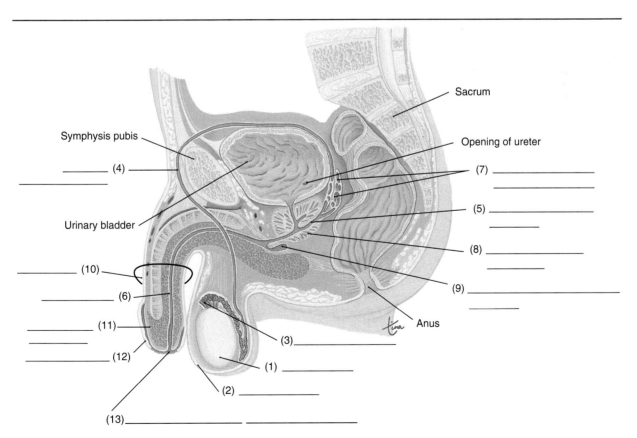

Figure 6–5 *The male reproductive system. (Adapted from Scanlon, VC, and Sanders, T: Understanding Human Structure and Function. FA Davis, Philadelphia, 1997, p 442, with permission.)*

Primary Sex Organs

The primary sex organs for both men and women are called **gonads.** In men, the (1) **testes** (singular, **testis**), also called *testicles* (singular, *testicle*), are paired oval glands that descend into the (2) **scrotum.** The testes contain specialized structures that are responsible for producing the gametes, or sperm. The testes also produce and secrete sex hormones. At the onset of puberty the testes produce the hormone **testosterone.** The appropriate amounts and timing of the production and secretion of male sex hormones cause the development of secondary sex organs and the expression of secondary sex characteristics.

Secondary Sex Organs

Secondary sex organs are structures that are essential in caring for and transporting sperm through the network of tubules within the male reproductive system. There are three categories of secondary sex organs: the sperm-transporting ducts, the accessory glands, and the copulatory organ.

The sperm-transporting ducts include the (3) **epididymis,** a comma-shaped organ; the (4) **vas deferens,** also called the ductus deferens; two (5) **ejaculatory ducts;** and the (6) **urethra.**

The accessory glands are the (7) **seminal vesicles,** which lie on the posterior wall of the bladder; the single (8) **prostate gland;** and two small glands located on each side of the prostate, the (9) **bulbourethral glands.** The bulbourethral glands, also known as **Cowper glands,** secrete a thick, clear mucus that drains into the urethra. This alkaline secretion, which is released before ejaculation, neutralizes any acidic urine that might be present in the urethra.

The copulatory organ, the (10) **penis,** an external genital organ, contains **erectile tissue.** It has the dual function of being the organ of copulation and of urination. Semen travels through the urethral duct, which is enclosed within the penis. The distal end of the penis is called the (11) **glans penis** and is covered with a fold of skin called the (12) **prepuce** or **foreskin** and encloses the (13) **urethral orifice.**

The penis is used to introduce semen and spermatozoa (sperm) into the vagina. Within the penis are three cylindrical masses of tissue. All three masses are enclosed by fascia and loose-fitting skin and consist of erectile tissue permeated by blood sinuses. Under the influence of sexual stimulation, the arteries supplying the penis dilate, and large quantities of blood enter the blood sinuses. Expansion of these spaces compresses the veins, draining the penis so that most entering blood is retained. These **vascular** changes result in an erection. The erect penis is capable of penetrating the female vagina to deposit sperm. During ejaculation, the smooth muscle at the base of the urinary bladder is closed because of the higher pressure in the urethra caused by expansion of the penis. Thus urine is not expelled during ejaculation and semen does not enter the urinary bladder. The penis returns to its flaccid state when the arteries constrict and pressure on the veins is relieved.

Activity 6–2: Competency Verification
Organs of the Male Reproductive System

Review Figure 6–5, and check your labeling in Appendix C.

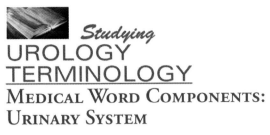

Studying
UROLOGY TERMINOLOGY
MEDICAL WORD COMPONENTS: URINARY SYSTEM
Combining Forms

Combining Forms: Kidney

Combining Form	Meaning	EXAMPLE	
		Term/Pronunciation	Definition
glomerul/o	glomerulus	**glomerul**/o/scler/osis *glō-měr-ū-lō-sklě-RŌ-sĭs*	a severe kidney disease in which glomerular function of blood filtration is lost as fibrous scar tissue replaces the glomeruli (plural). *The combining form* scler/o *means "hardening"; sclera refers to the outer layer of the eyeball; the suffix* -osis *means "an abnormal condition" or "increase" (used primarily with blood cells). In this case, the abnormal condition is a kidney disease.*
nephr/o	kidney	**nephr**/oma *ně-FRŌ-mǎ*	tumor (-*oma*) of the kidney
ren/o		**ren**/al *RĒ-nǎl*	pertaining to (-*al*) the kidney
pyel/o	renal pelvis	**pyel**/o/lith/o/tomy *pī-ě-lō-lĭth-ŎT-ō-mē*	incision (-*tomy*) to remove renal calculi (*lith/o*) from the pelvis of the kidney

Combining Forms: Urinary Tract

Combining Form	Meaning	EXAMPLE	
		Term/Pronunciation	Definition
cyst/o	bladder	**cyst**/o/scope *SĬST-ō-skōp*	an instrument for examining (-*scope*) and treating lesions of the urinary bladder, ureter, and kidney *The suffix* -scope *can be broken down further into its root* scop/o *and noun ending* e.
vesic/o		**vesic**/o/vagin/al *věs-ĭ-kō-VĂJ-ĭ-nǎl*	pertaining to the urinary bladder and vagina (*vagin/o*)

Combining Forms: The Urinary Tract (Continued)

Combining Form	Meaning	EXAMPLE	
		Term/Pronunciation	**Definition**
meat/o	opening, meatus	**meat**/o/tomy mē-ă-TŎT-ō-mē	incision (-*tomy*) to enlarge a meatus *A meatotomy of the urethra or ureter is performed to enlarge the passage.*
trigon/o	trigone (triangular region at base of the bladder)	**trigon**/itis trĭg-ō-NĪ-tĭs	inflammation (-*itis*) of the trigone *The trigone, a triangular region at the bladder base, is outlined between two ureteral openings and one urethral opening. It is of clinical importance because infections tend to persist in this region.*
ureter/o	ureter	**ureter**/o/cele ū-RĒ-tĕr-ō-sēl	cystlike dilation or swelling of the ureter near its opening into the bladder *A ureterocele may lead to obstruction of the flow of urine, hydronephrosis, and loss of renal function. The suffix -cele means "hernia," "swelling."*
urethr/o	urethra	**urethr**/o/dynia ū-rē-thrō-DĬN-ē-ă	pain (-*dynia*) in the urethra
ur/o	urinary tract, urine	**ur**/o/graphy ū-RŎG-ră-fē	process of recording (-*graphy*) x-ray images of the urinary tract (kidneys, ureter, or bladder) after introduction of a contrast medium

Activity 6–3: Competency Verification
Medical Word Components: Urinary System

Check the box [✓] as you complete each numbered section.

[   ] **1.** Review the word components for the kidneys and the urinary tract in the previous section. Then pronounce each term listed below aloud.

[   ] **2.** For the words below, first write the suffix and its meaning. Then translate the meaning of the remaining components starting with the first part of the word.

> **Example:** glomerul/o/scler/osis
> **Answer:** *osis* = abnormal condition; increase (used primarily with blood cells) glomerulus; hardening, sclera

1. nephr/oma   _____

2. cyst/o/scope   _____

3. ureter/o/cele   _____

4. pyel/o/lith   _____

5. cyst/itis   _____

6. urethr/o/dynia   _____

7. ureter/itis   _____

8. glomerul/o/scler/osis   _____

9. trigon/itis   _____

10. pyel/o/lith/o/tomy   _____

Correct Answers _____ × 10 = _____% **Score**

Combining Forms: Urine

Combining Form	Meaning	EXAMPLE	
		Term/Pronunciation	**Definition**
albumin/o	albumin (protein)	**albumin**/oid ăl-BŪ-mĭ-noyd	resembling (-_oid_) albumin
azot/o	nitrogenous	**azot**/uria ăz-ō-TŪ-rē-ă	an increase in nitrogenous compounds in the urine (-_uria_), especially urea in the urine
kal/i*	potassium (an electrolyte)	hypo/**kal**/emia hī-pō-kă-LĒ-mē-ă	an abnormally low concentration of potassium in the blood (-_emia_). _The prefix_ hypo- _means_ "under," "below."
ket/o	ketone bodies (acids and acetones)	**ket**/osis kē-TŌ-sĭs	abnormal accumulation of ketone bodies; this condition is also known as _ket/o/acid/osis_ because of the accumulation of acids in the tissues and blood _The suffix_ -osis _means_ "abnormal condition, increase" (used primarily with blood cells).
keton/o		**keton**/uria kē-tō-NŪ-rē-ă	ketone bodies in the urine (-_uria_)

*_The combining vowel for the root_ kal _(potassium) is an_ i. _Examples:_ kal/i/meter, kal/i/um.

Combining Forms: Urine (Continued)

Combining Form	Meaning	EXAMPLE	
		Term/Pronunciation	**Definition**
ur/o	urine, urinary tract	**ur**/emia *ū-RĒ-mē-ă*	excessive amounts of urea and other nitrogenous waste products in the blood (-*emia*)
urin/o		**urin**/o/meter *ū-rĭ-NŎM-ĕ-tĕr*	a device for determining the specific gravity of urine *The suffix* -meter *refers to an instrument for measuring.*

Prefixes and Suffixes

In this section, prefixes are listed alphabetically and highlighted whereas suffixes are defined in the right-hand column on an as-needed basis.

Prefixes: Urinary System

Prefix	Meaning	EXAMPLE	
		Term/Pronunciation	**Definition**
an-	without, not	**an**/uria *ăn-Ū-rē-ă*	absence of urine (-*uria*) formation
dia-	through, across	**dia**/lysis *dī-ĂL-ĭ-sĭs*	the process of removing toxic materials from the blood when the kidneys are unable to do so *The suffix* -lysis *means* "separation," "destruction," "loosening."
dys-	bad, painful, difficult	**dys**/uria *dĭs-Ū-rē-ă*	difficult or painful urination, symptomatic of numerous conditions *The suffix* -uria *refers to* urine.
hyper-	excessive, above normal	**hyper**/kal/emia *hī-pĕr-kă-LĒ-mē-ă*	excessive amount of potassium (*kal/i*)* in the blood (-*emia*)
hypo-	under, below	**hypo**/azot/uria *hī-pō-ăz-ō-TŪ-rē-ă*	excretion of abnormally small quantities of nitrogenous compounds (*azot/o*) in the urine (-*uria*)
poly-	many, much	**poly**/uria *pŏl-ē-Ū-rē-ă*	excessive secretion and discharge of urine (-*uria*)
supra-	above, excessive	**supra**/ren/al *soo-pră-RĒ-năl*	*Located above the kidneys (ren/o)* *The suffix* -al *means* "pertaining to."

The combining vowel for the root kal *(potassium) is an* i. *Examples:* kal/i/meter, kal/i/um.

Activity 6–4: Competency Verification
Medical Word Components: Urine

Check the box [✓] as you complete each numbered section.

[ ] **1.** Review the word components related to urine and the urinary system in the previous two sections. Then pronounce each word aloud.

[ ] **2.** For the words below, first write the suffix and its meaning. Then translate the meaning of the remaining components, starting with the first part of the word.

> **Example:** albumin/oid
> **Answer:** *oid* = resembling; albumin (protein)

1. ket/osis _____

2. ur/emia _____

3. an/uria _____

4. supra/ren/al _____

5. dia/lysis _____

6. keton/uria _____

7. hypo/azot/uria _____

8. urin/o/meter _____

9. poly/uria _____

10. hyper/kal/emia _____

Correct Answers _____ × 10 = _____% **Score**

MEDICAL WORD COMPONENTS: MALE REPRODUCTIVE SYSTEM

Combining Forms: Male Reproductive System

Combining Form	Meaning	EXAMPLE	
		Term/Pronunciation	**Definition**
andr/o	male	**andr**/o/gen ĂN-drō-jĕn	producing (*-gen*) a male *A substance producing or stimulating the development of male characteristics (masculinization) such as the hormones testosterone and androsterone.*

Combining Forms: Male Reproductive System (Continued)

Combining Form	Meaning	EXAMPLE	
		Term/Pronunciation	Definition
balan/o	glans penis	**balan**/o/plasty BĂL-ă-nō-plăs-tē	plastic surgery of the glans penis to correct a congenital defect or to serve an aesthetic purpose *The suffix* -plasty *means "surgical repair."*
gonad/o	gonads, sex glands	**gonad**/o/pathy gŏn-ă-DŎP-ă-thē	any disease of the sexual glands *Gonad is a generic term referring to both the female sex glands, or ovaries, and the male sex glands, or testes. Each forms the cells necessary for human reproduction, spermatozoa from the testes and ova from the ovaries.*
orch/o	testes	**orch**/itis or-KĪ-tĭs	inflammation (*-itis*) of one or both of the testes
orchi/o		**orchi**/o/pexy or-kē-ō-PĔX-ē	surgical fixation (*-pexy*) of an undescended testicle by implanting it into the scrotum
orchid/o		**orchid**/ectomy or-kĭ-DĔK-tō-mē	excision (*-ectomy*) of one or more testicles.
test/o		**test**/is TĔS-tĭs	one of the pair of male gonads that produce sperm and testosterone *The suffix* -is *designates the singular form of* test/es *(plural).*
prostat/o	prostate gland	**prostat**/o/megaly prŏs-tă-tō-MĔG-ă-lē	enlargement (*-megaly*) of the prostate
spermat/o	sperm	**spermat**/o/lysis spĕr-măt-ŎL-ĭ-sĭs	destruction (*-lysis*) of sperm
sperm/o		oligo/**sperm**/ia ŏl-ĭ-gō-SPĔR-mē-ă	a temporary or permanent deficiency in the number of spermatozoa in the semen *The combining form* olig/o *means "scanty."*
vas/o	vessel, vas deferens, duct	**vas**/ectomy văs-ĔK-tō-mē	a procedure for male sterilization involving the bilateral surgical removal (*-ectomy*) of a part of the vas deferens

Prefixes and Suffixes

In this section, prefixes are listed alphabetically and highlighted whereas suffixes are defined in the right-hand column on an as-needed basis.

Prefixes: Male Reproductive System

Prefix	Meaning	EXAMPLE	
		Term/Pronunciation	**Definition**
a-	without, not	**a**/sperm/ia ă-SPĔR-mē-ă	failure to form semen or ejaculate *The suffix -ia means "condition"; the combining form sperm/o refers to spermatozoa, sperm cells.*
an-		**an**/orch/ism ăn-OR-kĭzm	congenital absence of one or both testicles *The suffix -ism means "condition."*
circum-	around	**circum**/cision sĕr-kŭm-SĬ-zhŭn	removal of the end of the prepuce of the penis *The suffix -cision refers to cutting.*
para-	near, beside, beyond	**para**/phim/osis păr-ă-fĭ-MŌ-sĭs	an abnormal condition (-*osis*) characterized by an inability to replace the foreskin in its normal position after it has been retracted behind the glans penis *Phim/o means "muzzle"; a muzzle restrains and has a tightening effect. The tightness of the prepuce of the penis prevents the retraction of the foreskin over the glans.*

Activity 6–5: Competency Verification

Medical Word Components: Male Reproductive System

Check the box [✓] as you complete each numbered section.

[   ] **1.** Review the word components related to the male reproductive organs in the previous two sections and their examples. Then pronounce each word aloud.

[   ] **2.** For the words below, first write the suffix and its meaning. Then translate the meaning of the remaining components, starting with the first part of the word.

> **Example:** para/phym/osis
> **Answer:** *osis* = abnormal condition; near, beside beyond; muzzle

1. orch/itis   _____

2. pyel/o/lith/o/tomy_____

3. balan/o/plasty   _____

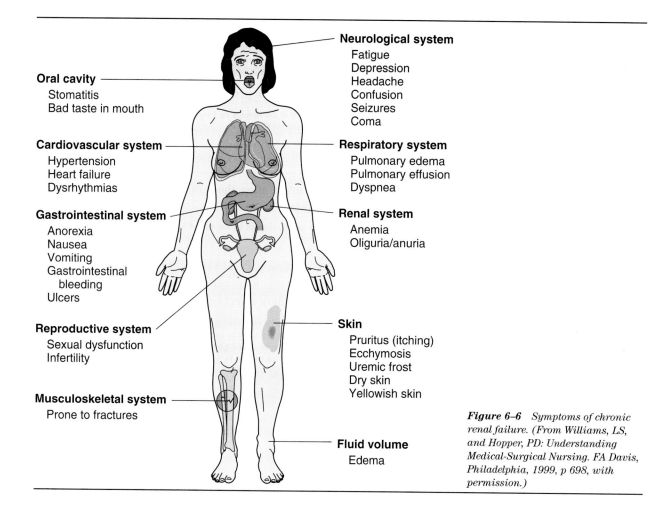

Neurological system
Fatigue
Depression
Headache
Confusion
Seizures
Coma

Oral cavity
Stomatitis
Bad taste in mouth

Cardiovascular system
Hypertension
Heart failure
Dysrhythmias

Respiratory system
Pulmonary edema
Pulmonary effusion
Dyspnea

Gastrointestinal system
Anorexia
Nausea
Vomiting
Gastrointestinal
  bleeding
Ulcers

Renal system
Anemia
Oliguria/anuria

Reproductive system
Sexual dysfunction
Infertility

Skin
Pruritus (itching)
Ecchymosis
Uremic frost
Dry skin
Yellowish skin

Musculoskeletal system
Prone to fractures

Fluid volume
Edema

Figure 6–6 Symptoms of chronic renal failure. (From Williams, LS, and Hopper, PD: Understanding Medical-Surgical Nursing. FA Davis, Philadelphia, 1999, p 698, with permission.)

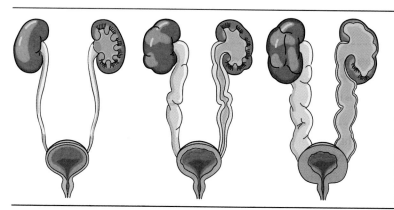

Figure 6–7 Hydronephrosis. Progressive thickening of the bladder wall and dilatation of ureters and kidneys results from obstruction of urine flow. (From Williams, LS, and Hopper, PD: Understanding Medical-Surgical Nursing. FA Davis, Philadelphia, 1999, p 694, with permission.)

Disorders of the Male Reproductive System (Continued)

PATHOLOGICAL CONDITION	DESCRIPTION
phimosis *fĭ-MŌ-sĭs* *phimo=muzzle* *osis=abnormal condition*	Stenosis of preputial orifice in which the foresl over the glans penis. The tightness (muzzling) of the prepuce of the penis prevents t glans.
prostatic cancer *prŏs-TĂT-ĭk KĂN-sĕr*	A malignant neoplasm of the prostate tissue, cr per part of the urethra. Prostate cancer tends to metastasize, often spreading to the bo detected. it is the second leading cause of cancer deaths in men (af *of the prostate.*
prostatism *PRŎS-tă-tĭzm* *prostat=prostate gland* *ism=condition*	Any condition of the prostate gland that interfe from the bladder. The condition is characterized by frequent uncomfortable urina may occur with development of uremia. Causes include benign hy nodular hyperplasia.
sexually transmitted disease (STD, venereal disease) *SĔKS-ŭ-al-ē trăns-mĭt-ĕd dĭ-zēz*	A contagious disease acquired by sexual interco These diseases are among the most common communicable di recent years despite improved methods of diagnosis and treatmen herpes genitalis, syphilis, and a complex array of other infections a
chlamydial infection *klă-MĬD-ē-ă*	An infection caused by the bacterium *Chlamyd* In men, chlamydial infections cause urethritis with a whitish chlamydial infections cause an inflammation of the cervix (cerviciti an increased risk of pelvic infections. Antibiotics are used to treat cl refrain from sexual intercourse until the treatment is completed.
genital wart *JĔN-ĭ-tăl wŏrt*	A wart of the genitalia caused by human papillo Genital warts are transmitted through sexual intercourse. In wor cer of the cervix. Treatment is not particularly effective because recu may include the application of a topical medication to destroy the condoms may reduce the transmission of genital warts, but individ tact with anyone who has the lesion.
gonorrhea *gŏn-ō-RĒ-ă*	An infection caused by the bacterium *Neisseria* Most often affects the genitourinary tract with symptoms of dys vaginal discharge. It can also affect the eyes, oral mucosa, rectum, a gonorrhea.
herpes genitalis *hĕr-pēz jĕn-ĭ-TĂL-ĭs*	An infection of the genital and anorectal skin a herpes simplex virus (HSV). Usually spread by sexual contact with infected body secretions ual intercourse (Fig. 6–8).

Figure 6–8
primary in
[ed]: Taber
FA Davis, I
permission

Disorders of the Urinary System (Continued)

PATHOLOGICAL CONDITION	DESCRIPTION
polycystic kidney *pŏl-ē-SĬS-tĭk KĬD-nē* *poly=many, much* *cyst=bladder* *ic=pertaining to*	A hereditary condition in which the kidneys are enlarged and contain many cysts. Congenital cysts gradually enlarge and may cause high blood pressure and loss of kidney function.
polydipsia *pŏl-ē-DĬP-sē-ă* *poly=many, much* *dips=thirst* *ia=condition*	Excessive thirst. A sign of diabetes mellitus or diabetes insipidus (see Chapter 10).
pyelonephritis *pī-ĕ-lō-nĕ-FRĪ-tĭs*	A bacterial infection of the renal pelvis and renal medulla of one or both kidneys. Bacteria may gain access to the bladder via the urethra and ascend to the kidney or may reach the kidney through the bloodstream. In acute pyelonephritis, pus forms in the renal pelvis and adjacent renal medulla. Chronic pyelonephritis results from reinfection causing some form of obstruction and leads to destruction of renal tissue and scar formation. Urinalysis reveals pyuria.
pyuria *pī-Ū-rē-ă* *py=pus* *uria=urine*	The presence of white blood cells in the urine. Usually a sign of an infection in the urinary tract. Excessive leukocytes suggest an infection or inflammation of the kidney or bladder. Freshly passed urine may be cloudy in appearance.
renal hypertension *RĒ-năl hī-pĕr-TĔN-shŭn* *ren=kidney* *al=pertaining to* *hyper=above normal* *tension=tension*	High blood pressure resulting from a kidney disease.
urgency *ŬR-jĕn-sē*	A sudden compelling urge to urinate.
urinary incontinence *Ū-rĭ-năr-ē ĭn-KŎNT-ĭn-ĕns* *urin=urine* *ary=pertaining to* *in=in, not* *continence=to hold back*	Intermittent or complete absence of ability to control the release of urine from the bladder.
Wilms tumor *vĭlmz TŪ-mor*	Rapidly developing, malignant kidney tumor that usually occurs in children.

Disorders of the Male Reproductive System

PATHOLOGICAL CONDITION	DESCRIPTION
anorchism ăn-OR-kĭzm *an=without* *orch=testes* *ism=condition (of)*	Congenital absence of one or both testes.
balanitis băl-ă-NĪ-tĭs	Inflammation of the skin covering the glans penis.
benign prostatic hyperplasia (BPH) bē-NĪN prŏs-TĂT-ĭk hī-pĕr-PLĀ-zē-ă *hyper=excessive, above normal* *plasia=formation, growth*	A nonmalignant enlargement of the prostate due to e prostatic tissue. The most common benign neoplasm in men over 60 years of age. An in completely and urinary obstructions are symptoms. Also called *benign prosta hyperplasia*.
cryptorchidism krĭpt-OR-kĭd-ĭzm *crypt=hidden* *orchid=testes* *ism=condition (of)*	Failure of testicles to descend into the scrotum.
epididymitis ĕp-ĭ-dĭd-ĭ-MĪ-tĭs *epididym=epididymis* *itis=inflammation*	Acute or chronic inflammation of the epididymis. May result from venereal disease, urinary tract infection, prostatitis, prost of indwelling catheters.
epispadias ĕp-ĭ-SPĀ-dē-ăs *epi=above, upon* *spadias=a rent (a slit, a fissure)*	A congenital (birth) defect in which the urethra opens the penis, near the glans penis, instead of at the tip. Treatment is surgical redirection of the opening of the urethra to its norm penis.
hydrocele HĪ-drō-sēl *hydro=water* *cele=hernia, swelling*	An accumulation of fluid in any saclike cavity or duct, p; tal sac or along the spermatic cord. Usually the result of inflammation of the epididymis or testis or by venous for hydrocele is surgical removal of the sac through an incision in the scrotu
hypospadias hī-pō-SPĀ-dē-ăs *hypo=under, below* *spadias=a rent (a slit; a fissure)*	A congenital defect in which the male urethra opens on the penis instead of at the tip. Treatment consists of surgical redirection of the opening of the urethra to end of the penis.
impotence ĬM-pō-těns *im=not* *potence=power*	The inability of a man to achieve or maintain an erectio

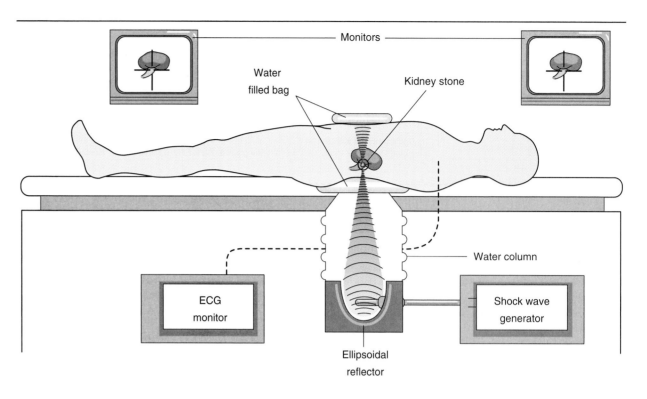

Figure 6–10 *Extracorporeal shock-wave lithotripsy. (From Williams, LS, and Hopper, PD: Understanding Medical-Surgical Nursing. FA Davis, Philadelphia, 1999, p 693, with permission.)*

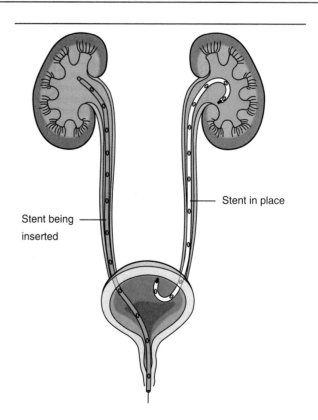

Figure 6–11 *Ureteral stents. (From Williams, LS, and Hopper, PD: Understanding Medical-Surgical Nursing. FA Davis, Philadelphia, 1999, p 695, with permission.)*

Disorders of the Urinary System (Continued)

PATHOLOGICAL CONDITION	DESCRIPTION
polycystic kidney pŏl-ē-SĬS-tĭk KĬD-nē *poly=many, much* *cyst=bladder* *ic=pertaining to*	A hereditary condition in which the kidneys are enlarged and contain many cysts. Congenital cysts gradually enlarge and may cause high blood pressure and loss of kidney function.
polydipsia pŏl-ē-DĬP-sē-ă *poly=many, much* *dips=thirst* *ia=condition*	Excessive thirst. A sign of diabetes mellitus or diabetes insipidus (see Chapter 10).
pyelonephritis pī-ĕ-lō-nĕ-FRĪ-tĭs	A bacterial infection of the renal pelvis and renal medulla of one or both kidneys. Bacteria may gain access to the bladder via the urethra and ascend to the kidney or may reach the kidney through the bloodstream. In acute pyelonephritis, pus forms in the renal pelvis and adjacent renal medulla. Chronic pyelonephritis results from reinfection causing some form of obstruction and leads to destruction of renal tissue and scar formation. Urinalysis reveals pyuria.
pyuria pī-Ū-rē-ă *py=pus* *uria=urine*	The presence of white blood cells in the urine. Usually a sign of an infection in the urinary tract. Excessive leukocytes suggest an infection or inflammation of the kidney or bladder. Freshly passed urine may be cloudy in appearance.
renal hypertension RĒ-năl hī-pĕr-TĔN-shŭn *ren=kidney* *al=pertaining to* *hyper=above normal* *tension=tension*	High blood pressure resulting from a kidney disease.
urgency ŬR-jĕn-sē	A sudden compelling urge to urinate.
urinary incontinence Ū-rĭ-nār-ē ĭn-KŎNT-ĭn-ĕns *urin=urine* *ary=pertaining to* *in=in, not* *continence=to hold back*	Intermittent or complete absence of ability to control the release of urine from the bladder.
Wilms tumor vĭlmz TŪ-mor	Rapidly developing, malignant kidney tumor that usually occurs in children.

Disorders of the Male Reproductive System

PATHOLOGICAL CONDITION	DESCRIPTION
anorchism ăn-OR-kĭzm *an=without* *orch=testes* *ism=condition (of)*	Congenital absence of one or both testes.
balanitis băl-ă-NĪ-tĭs	Inflammation of the skin covering the glans penis.
benign prostatic hyperplasia (BPH) bē-NĬN prŏs-TĂT-ĭk hī-pĕr-PLĀ-zē-ă *hyper=excessive, above normal* *plasia=formation, growth*	A nonmalignant enlargement of the prostate due to excessive growth of prostatic tissue. The most common benign neoplasm in men over 60 years of age. An inability to empty the bladder completely and urinary obstructions are symptoms. Also called *benign prostatic hypertrophy* and *prostatic hyperplasia.*
cryptorchidism krĭpt-OR-kĭd-ĭzm *crypt=hidden* *orchid=testes* *ism=condition (of)*	Failure of testicles to descend into the scrotum.
epididymitis ĕp-ĭ-dĭd-ĭ-MĪ-tĭs *epididym=epididymis* *itis=inflammation*	Acute or chronic inflammation of the epididymis. May result from venereal disease, urinary tract infection, prostatitis, prostatectomy, or prolonged use of indwelling catheters.
epispadias ĕp-ĭ-SPĀ-dē-ăs *epi=above, upon* *spadias=a rent (a slit, a fissure)*	A congenital (birth) defect in which the urethra opens on the upper side of the penis, near the glans penis, instead of at the tip. Treatment is surgical redirection of the opening of the urethra to its normal position at the end of the penis.
hydrocele HĪ-drō-sēl *hydro=water* *cele=hernia, swelling*	An accumulation of fluid in any saclike cavity or duct, particularly the scrotal sac or along the spermatic cord. Usually the result of inflammation of the epididymis or testis or by venous obstruction. The treatment for hydrocele is surgical removal of the sac through an incision in the scrotum.
hypospadias hī-pō-SPĀ-dē-ăs *hypo=under, below* *spadias=a rent (a slit; a fissure)*	A congenital defect in which the male urethra opens on the undersurface of the penis instead of at the tip. Treatment consists of surgical redirection of the opening of the urethra to its normal position at the end of the penis.
impotence ĬM-pō-tĕns *im=not* *potence=power*	The inability of a man to achieve or maintain an erection.

Disorders of the Male Reproductive System (Continued)

PATHOLOGICAL CONDITION	DESCRIPTION
phimosis fī-MŌ-sĭs *phimo=muzzle* *osis=abnormal condition*	Stenosis of preputial orifice in which the foreskin cannot be pushed back over the glans penis. The tightness (muzzling) of the prepuce of the penis prevents the retraction of the foreskin over the glans.
prostatic cancer prŏs-TĂT-ĭk KĂN-sĕr	A malignant neoplasm of the prostate tissue, creating pressure on the upper part of the urethra. Prostate cancer tends to metastasize, often spreading to the bones of the spine or pelvis before it is detected. it is the second leading cause of cancer deaths in men (after lung cancer); also called *carcinoma of the prostate*.
prostatism PRŎS-tă-tĭzm *prostat=prostate gland* *ism=condition*	Any condition of the prostate gland that interferes with the flow of urine from the bladder. The condition is characterized by frequent uncomfortable urination and nocturia. Retention of urine may occur with development of uremia. Causes include benign hypertrophy, carcinoma, prostatitis, and nodular hyperplasia.
sexually transmitted disease (STD, venereal disease) SĔKS-ŭ-al-ē trăns-mĭt-ĕd dĭ-zēz	A contagious disease acquired by sexual intercourse or genital contact. These diseases are among the most common communicable diseases, and the incidence has risen in recent years despite improved methods of diagnosis and treatment. They include chlamydia, gonorrhea, herpes genitalis, syphilis, and a complex array of other infections and clinical syndromes.
chlamydial infection klă-MĬD-ē-ă	An infection caused by the bacterium *Chlamydia trachomatis*. In men, chlamydial infections cause urethritis with a whitish discharge from the penis. In women, chlamydial infections cause an inflammation of the cervix (cervicitis) with a mucopurulent discharge and an increased risk of pelvic infections. Antibiotics are used to treat chlamydial infection. The patient should refrain from sexual intercourse until the treatment is completed.
genital wart JĔN-ĭ-tăl wōrt	A wart of the genitalia caused by human papillomavirus (HPV). Genital warts are transmitted through sexual intercourse. In women, they may be associated with cancer of the cervix. Treatment is not particularly effective because recurrence of warts is common. Treatment may include the application of a topical medication to destroy the wart or surgical excision. Using latex condoms may reduce the transmission of genital warts, but individuals are advised to avoid sexual contact with anyone who has the lesion.
gonorrhea gŏn-ō-RĒ-ă	An infection caused by the bacterium *Neisseria gonorrhoeae*. Most often affects the genitourinary tract with symptoms of dysuria and a greenish-yellow urethral or vaginal discharge. It can also affect the eyes, oral mucosa, rectum, and joints. Antibiotics are used to treat gonorrhea.
herpes genitalis hĕr-pēz jĕn-ĭ-TĂL-ĭs	An infection of the genital and anorectal skin and mucosa caused by the herpes simplex virus (HSV). Usually spread by sexual contact with infected body secretions and can be transmitted through sexual intercourse (Fig. 6–8).

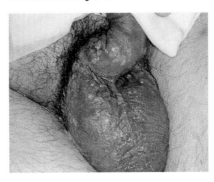

Figure 6–8 *Herpes genitalis. Widespread primary infection. (From Thomas, CL [ed]: Taber's Cyclopedic Dictionary, ed 18. FA Davis, Philadelphia, 1997, p 894, with permission.)*

Disorders of the Male Reproductive System (Continued)

PATHOLOGICAL CONDITION	DESCRIPTION
syphilis SĬF-ĭ-lĭs	An infection caused by the bacterium *Treponema pallidum* and characterized by lesions that may involve any organ or tissue. The disease is spread by sexual contact with an infected partner, and can also be passed through the placenta from an infected mother to her unborn infant. If left untreated, the end result is blindness, insanity, and eventual death. Penicillin is an effective treatment for primary syphilis.
trichomoniasis trĭk-ō-mō-NĪ-ă-sĭs	An infection of the vagina, urethra, or prostate caused by the bacterium *Trichomonas vaginalis*. In men, the infection is usually asymptomatic, but may be evidenced by a persistent or recurrent urethritis, dysuria, or urinary frequency. In women, it is characterized by itching; burning; and frothy, pale yellow to green, malodorous (strong-smelling) vaginal discharge. Treatment includes an anti-infective drug called Flagyl (metronidazole). Reinfection is common if sexual partners are not treated simultaneously.
varicocele VĂR-ĭ-kō-sēl *varico=dilated vein* *cele=hernia, swelling*	Swollen, enlarged, herniated veins near the testis.

Activity 6–6: Clinical Application
Pathological Conditions

anorchism	epispadias	nocturia
aspermia	glomerulosclerosis	orchitis
azotemia	gonorrhea	phimosis
balanitis	hydrocele	pyelonephritis
cryptorchidism	hyperkalemia	ureterocele
dysuria	hypospadias	ureterolithiasis
enuresis	nephroma	urinary incontinence

Match the terms listed above with the definitions given in the numbered list:

1. _____ inflammation of the testes.

2. _____ presence of calculi in the ureter.

3. _____ inflammation of the skin that covers the glans penis.

4. _____ infection of the renal pelvis, tubules, and interstitial tissue.

5. _____ accumulation of fluid in the space around the testis.

6. _____ excessive urination at night.

7. _____ retention of excessive amounts of nitrogenous compounds in the blood.

8. _____ involuntary discharge of urine that occurs after the age by which bladder control should have been established; also called *nocturnal bedwetting*.

9. _____ inability to control urine from the bladder.

10. _____ failure of testicles to descend into the scrotum.

11. _____ congenital defect in which the male urethra opens on the upper side of penis instead of at the end.

12. _____ sexually transmitted disease that affects the genitourinary tract.

13. _____ congenital defect in which the male urethra opens on the underside of the penis instead of at the end.

14. _____ stenosis of preputial orifice so that the foreskin cannot be pushed back over the glans penis.

15. _____ fibrous scar tissue that has replaced the glomeruli causing loss of blood filtration.

16. _____ kidney tumor.

17. _____ swelling of the ureter.

18. _____ excessive amount of potassium in the blood.

19. _____ failure to form semen or to ejaculate.

20. _____ absence of one or more testicles.

Correct Answers _____ × 5 = _____ **% Score**

DIAGNOSTIC PROCEDURES AND TESTS

Selected diagnostic tests are performed to confirm a disease or condition a person may have or to determine a change in the body or its functions; they are also used to determine a diagnosis. Keep in mind the various pathological conditions to help you understand the reasons behind these procedures and tests.

Imaging Procedures

PROCEDURE	DESCRIPTION
intravenous pyelogram (IVP) *ĭn-tră-VĒ-nŭs PĪ-ĕ-lō-grăm* *intra=within* *ven=vein* *ous=pertaining to* *uro=urinary tract, urine* *gram=writing, record*	Procedure in which a contrast medium is injected intravenously and serial x-ray films are taken to provide visualization and important information of the entire urinary tract: kidneys, ureters, bladder, and urethra. **Also known as intravenous urography (IVU) or excretory urogram.**
KUB (kidneys, ureters, bladder) *KĬD-nēz, Ū-rĕ-ters, BLĂD-dĕr*	A radiograph obtained without the use of a contrast medium that illustrates the size, shape, and location of the kidneys in relationship to other organs in the abdominopelvic region.

Imaging Procedures (Continued)

PROCEDURE	DESCRIPTION
radiography rā-dē-ŎG-ră-fē *radio=radiation, x-ray* *graphy=process of recording*	Examination of any part of the body for diagnostic purposes, using x-rays, with the record of the findings usually impressed upon a photographic film.
renal scan RĒ-năl skăn *ren=kidney* *al=pertaining to*	An imaging procedure that determines renal function and shape. A radioactive substance or radiopharmaceutical that concentrates in the kidney is injected intravenously. The radioactivity is measured as it accumulates in the kidneys and is recorded as an image. This is a nuclear medicine procedure.
retrograde pyelogram (RP) PĪ-ĕ-lō-grăm *pyelo=renal pelvis* *gram=a writing, record*	Procedure in which a contrast medium is introduced through a cystoscope directly into the bladder and ureters, using small-caliber catheters. This radiographic procedure provides detailed visualization of the urinary collecting system and is useful in locating obstructions in the urinary tract. It may also be used as a substitute for an IVP when a patient is allergic to the contrast medium.
ultrasonography, ultrasonogram ŭl-tră-sŏn-ŎG-ră-fē, ŭl-tră-SŎN-ō-grăm *ultra=excess, beyond* *sono=sound* *graphy=process of recording* *sono=sound* *gram= record, writing*	A method of producing an image or photograph of an organ or tissue using sound waves. Ultrasonic echoes are recorded as they strike tissues of different densities. Ultrasound tests are used to diagnose diseases of the kidneys, heart, gallbladder, and so on.
voiding cystourethrography (VCUG) voyd-ĭng sĭs-tō-ū-rē-THRŎG-ră-fē *cysto=bladder* *urethro=urethra* *graphy=process of recording*	Radiography of the bladder and urethra after the introduction of a contrast medium and during the process of voiding urine. The bladder is filled with an opaque contrast medium before the procedure.

Clinical Procedures

PROCEDURE	DESCRIPTION
catheterization kăth-ĕ-tĕr-ĭ-ZĀ-shŭn *catheter=something inserted* *ization=process (of)*	Insertion of a catheter (a hollow flexible tube) into a body cavity or organ to instill a substance or remove a fluid. The most common type of catheterization is to insert a catheter through the urethra and into the bladder to withdraw urine. Catheterization is also used as a method of treatment, as illustrated in the Therapeutic Procedures section of this chapter.
cystoscopy sĭs-TŎS-kō-pē *cysto=bladder* *scopy=visual examination*	Visual examination of the urinary bladder by inserting a cystoscope into the urethra. In addition to visualization, cystoscopy is used to obtain biopsies of tumors or other growths and to remove polyps.

Clinical Procedures (Continued)

PROCEDURE	DESCRIPTION
digital rectal examination (DRE) *DĬJ-ĭ-tăl RĔK-tăl ĕg-zăm-ĭ-NĀ-shŭn*	Insertion of a finger into the male rectum to palpate (use fingers to examine) the rectum and prostate.
renal biopsy, percutaneous *RĒ-năl BĪ-ŏp-sē, pĕr-kū-TĀ-nē-ŭs* *ren=kidney* *al=pertaining to* *bi=life* *opsy=view (of)* *per=through* *cutane=skin* *ous=pertaining to*	Obtaining renal tissue for analysis by use of a needle inserted through the skin. Used to establish a diagnosis of renal dysfunction to determine prognosis in patients with renal disease and to establish an appropriate therapy.

Laboratory Tests

TEST	DESCRIPTION
blood urea nitrogen (BUN) *blŭd ū-RĒ-ă NĪ-trō-jĕn*	A test that measures the amount of urea (nitrogenous waste product) normally excreted by the kidneys into the blood. An increase in the BUN level usually indicates decreased renal function.
creatinine clearance test *krē-ĂT-ĭn-ĭn KLĒR-ăns tĕst*	Test that measures the level of creatinine (a waste product) in the blood. Used to determine the rate at which creatinine is removed from the blood by the kidneys. An increase of serum creatinine levels is an indication of impaired glomerular function.
prostate-specific antigen (PSA) test *PRŎS-tăt-spĕ-SĬF-ĭk ĂN-tĭ-jĕn tĕst*	Blood test to screen for prostate cancer. An elevated level of a protein produced by the prostate indicates the possibility of a tumor or other disease of the prostate.
urinalysis (UA) *ū-rĭ-NĂL-ĭ-sĭs* *urin=urine* *a=connecting vowel* *lysis=separation, destruction, loosening* *Note: The root* urin *uses the connecting vowel* a. *This is an exception to the rule of using an* o *as the connecting vowel.*	A physical, chemical, and microscopic analysis of the urine. Refer to the following section for a comprehensive discussion of this diagnostic procedure.

Urinalysis

Although its value is often underestimated, urinalysis (urine analysis), as its name implies, contributes a wealth of important clinical information, not only about renal function but also about the state of health and functioning of many body systems. Urinalysis is a simple but important aspect of a physical examination. The voided urine specimen is tested for color, clarity, specific gravity, chemical composition, and for the presence of microscopic bacteria, crystals, and casts.

The normal characteristics and pathological significance of urine are summarized in Table 6–1. Review the table to obtain a more comprehensive understanding of pathologies related to the urinary system.

TABLE 6–1: Normal Characteristics and Pathological Significance of Urine

CHARACTERISTIC	DESCRIPTION AND NORMAL FINDINGS	PATHOLOGICAL SIGNIFICANCE
Color	A fresh specimen is generally pale yellow, straw-colored, or amber, depending on its concentration.	Dark amber suggests dehydration. Yellow-brown to green urine indicates excessive bilirubin. Cloudiness of freshly voided urine indicates infection. Nearly colorless urine is seen with a large fluid intake or diabetes insipidus.
Odor	Normal urine odor is aromatic. Urine that has been standing for a while develops a strong ammonia smell.	With infection, urine becomes foul smelling. In diabetic ketoacidosis, urine has a fruity odor.
pH	This measures the degree of acid or alkaline solution that is present in urine. Normal urine is slightly acid (6.5) with a normal range of 4.6–8.0. The pH is greatly affected by the food eaten. On standing, urine becomes alkaline due to the diffusion of carbon dioxide into the air.	A pH below 4.6 is seen with metabolic and respiratory acidosis. A pH above 8.0 is seen when urine has been standing or with infection because bacteria decompose urea to form ammonia.
Specific gravity	This reflects the amount of dissolved wastes, minerals, and solids in the urine. The normal range is 1.010–1.025.	Low specific gravity indicates excessive fluid intake or diabetes insipidus. High specific gravity is seen with dehydration; a low specific gravity indicates overhydration.
Protein	The normal range of protein in urine is 0–8 mg/dL. Urine normally has small amounts of protein, but not in sufficient quantity to produce a positive result by ordinary means of testing. Elevated albumin levels are usually responsible for positive urinary test results.	Persistent proteinuria is seen with renal disease from damage to the glomerulus. Intermittent protein in the urine can result from strenuous exercise, dehydration, or fever. As a general rule, protein in the urine is a significant sign of renal problems.
Glucose	Sugar is not normally found in urine.	The presence of glucose in the urine indicates diabetes mellitus, excessive glucose intake, or low renal threshold for glucose reabsorption.
Ketone bodies	Ketones (also referred to as *acetones,* which are a type of ketone body) are breakdown products from fat catabolism in cells. Normally there are none in the urine.	The presence of ketones in the urine indicates diabetes mellitus with ketonuria or starvation from breakdown of body fats into ketones.
Bilirubin	Bilirubin is a pigment substance from hemoglobin breakdown that may appear in the urine, darkening it, as a manifestation of liver or gallbladder disease. Normally it is not present in the urine.	Bilirubin in the urine indicates liver disorders causing jaundice. Bilirubin may appear in the urine before jaundice is visible.
Casts	Casts are accumulations of proteins that have leaked through the glomeruli and have been pushed through the tubules like toothpaste through a tube. They may contain inclusions of red blood cells (RBC), white blood cells (WBC), bacteria, and other substances.	The presence of casts usually indicates renal infection or renal damage.
Pus	Pyuria produces a cloudy (turbid) appearance to urine.	Large numbers of leukocytes (WBCs) are present because of infection or inflammation in the kidney or bladder.

Surgical and Therapeutic Procedures

Surgical Procedures

PROCEDURE	DESCRIPTION
circumcision *sĕr-kŭm-SĬ-zhŭn* *circum=around* *cision=to cut*	Surgical removal of the foreskin or the prepuce of the penis. Uncircumcised men exhibit a higher incidence of syphilis, gonorrhea, and penile malignancies. The remaining foreskin is easily retracted and the glans penis is fully exposed after circumcision.
cystolitholapaxy *SĬS-tō-lĭth-ŏl-ā-pĕk-sē*	Removal of a kidney stone from the bladder by crushing it and then extracting the particles via irrigation.
kidney transplantation, renal transplantation *KĬD-nē trăns-plăn-TĀ-shŭn,* *RĒ-năl trăns-plăn-TĀ-shŭn* *ren=kidney* *al=pertaining to* *trans=through, across*	Surgical implantation of a kidney from a compatible donor into a recipient. This is the most successful of any organ transplant procedure, and is often performed using a kidney donated by a close relative. A computer search can also find a tissue match, often with a person who has just suffered accidental death. Transplantation is used to treat end-stage renal disease (Fig. 6–9).

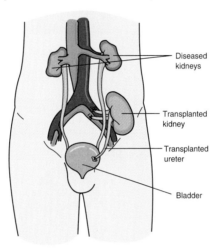

Diseased kidneys

Transplanted kidney

Transplanted ureter

Bladder

Figure 6–9 *A transplanted kidney is placed in the abdomen. The kidneys are usually left in place. (From Williams, LS, and Hopper, PD: Understanding Medical-Surgical Nursing. FA Davis, Philadelphia, 1999, p 708, with permission.)*

PROCEDURE	DESCRIPTION
lithotripsy *LĬTH-ō-trĭp-sē* *litho=stone, calculus* *tripsy=crushing*	A procedure for eliminating a calculus in the renal pelvis, ureter, bladder, or gallbladder. The calculus may be crushed surgically or by using a noninvasive method such as high-energy, shock-wave lithotripsy, or pulsed-dye laser. The fragments may then be expelled or washed out.
extracorporeal shock-wave lithotripsy *ĕks-tră-kor-POR-ē-ăl* *shŏk-wāv LĬTH-ō-trĭp-sē* *extra=outside* *orpor=body* *al=pertaining to*	A noninvasive procedure to break up kidney stones. The shock waves are focused on the stones, disintegrating them and permitting their passage in the urine. Also called *extracorporeal lithotripsy* (see Fig. 6–10).
stent placement *stĕnt PLĀS-mĕnt*	Use of a device to hold open vessels, tubes, or an obstructed ureter (Fig. 6–11).
vasectomy *văs-ĔK-tō-mē* *vas=vessel, vas deferens* *ectomy=excision, removal*	Removal of all or a segment of the vas deferens, also called *ductus deferens*. Bilateral vasectomy is the most successful method of male contraception or sterilization, preventing the release of sperm in the semen. A vasectomy can also be reversed (Fig. 6–12).

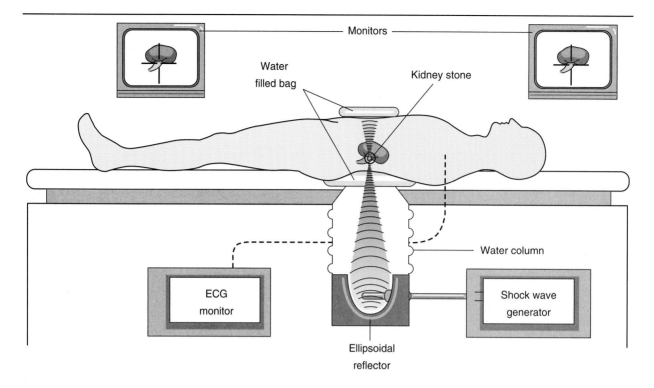

Figure 6–10 *Extracorporeal shock-wave lithotripsy. (From Williams, LS, and Hopper, PD: Understanding Medical-Surgical Nursing. FA Davis, Philadelphia, 1999, p 693, with permission.)*

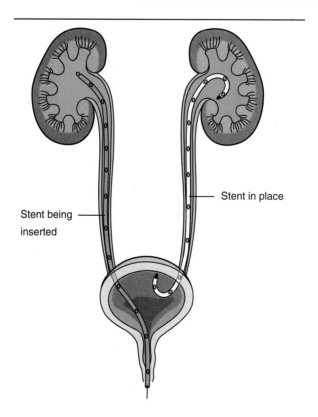

Figure 6–11 *Ureteral stents. (From Williams, LS, and Hopper, PD: Understanding Medical-Surgical Nursing. FA Davis, Philadelphia, 1999, p 695, with permission.)*

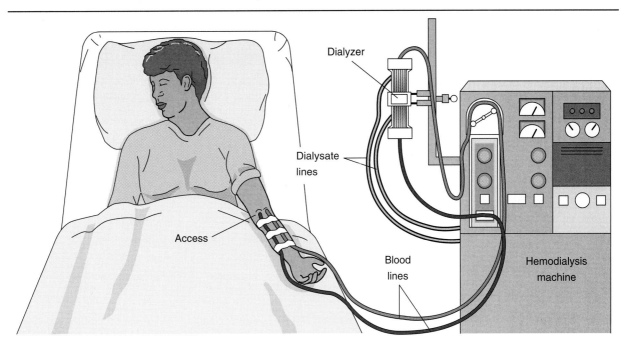

Dialyzer

Dialysate lines

Access

Blood lines

Hemodialysis machine

Figure 6–14 *Hemodialysis. (From Williams, LS, and Hopper, PD: Understanding Medical-Surgical Nursing. FA Davis, Philadelphia, 1999, p 705, with permission.)*

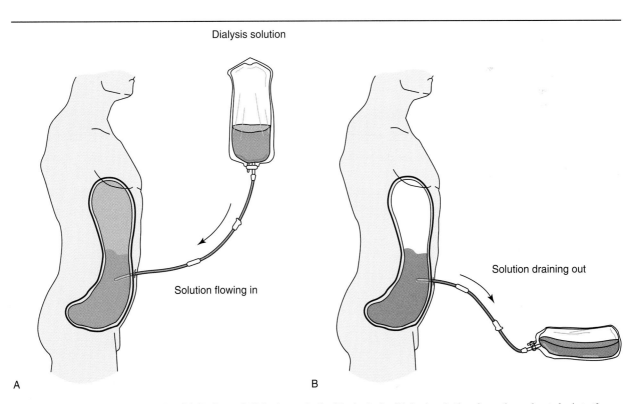

Dialysis solution

Solution flowing in

Solution draining out

A

B

Figure 6–15 *Peritoneal dialysis. (A) Peritoneal dialysis works inside the body. Dialysis solution flows through a tube into the abdominal cavity, where it collects waste products from the blood. (B) Periodically the used dialysis solution is drained from the abdominal cavity, carrying away waste products and excess water from the blood. (From Williams, LS, and Hopper, PD: Understanding Medical-Surgical Nursing. FA Davis, Philadelphia, 1999, p 707, with permission.)*

The Urinary Tract (Continued)

DRUG CLASSIFICATION	THERAPEUTIC ACTION
antispasmodics *ăn-tĭ-spăz-MŎD-ĭks*	Drugs that relieve spasms and act to relax the smooth muscle in the wall of the urethra, bladder, and intestine, allowing normal urination. Catheterization, UTI irritations, or renal calculi can cause ureteral spasms, renal colic, spasms of the bladder sphincter, and urinary retention.
diuretics *dī-ū-RĔT-ĭks*	Substances that increase the rate of secretion. Diuretics cause extra sodium and water to be excreted from the circulating blood volume and are useful in the treatment of hypertension. There are several categories of diuretics, depending on the basis of the site of their action within the kidney.
potassium supplements *pō-TĂS-ē-ŭm SŬP-lě-měnts*	Supplements used concurrently with many diuretics to counteract the potassium-depletion effect. Even though foods, such as bananas and broccoli, are rich in potassium, dietary sources alone are usually not sufficient to replenish potassium loss caused by diuretics.
sulfonamides *sŭl-FŎN-ă-mīdz*	Substances used to treat UTIs. Inhibit the growth of bacteria, but do not kill them as antibiotics do. Therefore they are not true antibiotics. Sulfonamides are also called *sulfa drugs*.
urinary alkalinizers *Ū-rĭ-nār-ē ĂL-kă-lĭn-īz-ĕrz*	Substances that inhibit stone formation by reducing urine acidity.
uricosurics *ū-rĭ-kō-SŪ-rĭks*	Substances used to treat gout because they increase urinary excretion of uric acid.

Reproductive System

DRUG CLASSIFICATION	THERAPEUTIC ACTION
estrogen hormones *ĔS-trō-jěn HOR-mōnz*	Substances that suppress gonadotropic and testicular androgenic hormones in men. Used to treat some prostatic cancers.
gonadotropins *gŏn-ă-dō-TRŌ-pĭnz*	Hormonal preparations used to raise sperm count in infertility cases.
spermicidals *spěr-mĭ-SĪ-dălz*	Substances that destroy sperm and are often used within the woman's vagina for contraception. Can also be found in lubricants and spermicidal condoms.

❖ ABBREVIATIONS

ABBREVIATION	MEANING	ABBREVIATION	MEANING
AGN	acute glomerular nephritis	IVU	intravenous urography
ARF	acute renal failure	K	potassium (an electrolyte)
BNO	bladder neck obstruction	KUB	kidneys, ureters, bladder
BPH	benign prostatic hyperplasia, benign prostatic hypertrophy	Na	sodium (an electrolyte)
		PKU	phenylketonuria
BUN	blood urea nitrogen	pH	symbol for degree of acidity or alkalinity
CAPD	continuous ambulatory peritoneal dialysis	prn	as needed, as required
cath	catheterization, catheter	PSA	prostate-specific antigen
CRF	chronic renal failure	RP	retrograde pyelogram
cysto	cystoscopy	sp.gr.	specific gravity
DRE	digital rectal examination	STD	sexually transmitted disease
ED	erectile dysfunction, emergency department	TURP	transurethral resection of prostate (for prostatectomy)
ESRD	end-stage renal disease	UA	urinalysis
ESWL	extracorporeal shock-wave lithotripsy	US	ultrasound
		UTI	urinary tract infection
EU	excretory urogram; same as IVP	VCUG	voiding cystourethrogram; voiding cystourography
GU	genitourinary		
GFR	glomerular filtration rate	VDRL	Venereal Disease Research Laboratories
HD	hemodialysis		
IVP	intravenous pyelogram; same as EU		

Activity 6–7: Clinical Application
Diagnostic Tests, Treatments, and Abbreviations

catheterization	KUB (kidneys, ureters, bladder)
circumcision	spermicidals
cystoscopy	stent placement
dialysis	ultrasonography
DRE	uricosurics
gonadotropins	voiding cystourethrography

Match the terms listed above with the definitions given in the numbered list:

1. _____ agents that increase urinary secretion of uric acid; used to treat gout.

2. _____ insertion of a catheter into a body cavity or organ to instill a substance or remove a fluid; used to withdraw urine from the bladder.

3. _____ x-ray of the bladder and urethra done before, during, and after voiding urine.

4. _____ agents that destroy sperm; used within the woman's vagina for contraception.

5. _____ agents used to raise sperm count in infertility cases.

6. _____ procedure used to produce an image or photograph of an organ or tissue via sound waves.

7. _____ use of a device to hold open vessels or tubes, that is, an obstructed ureter.

8. _____ process of diffusing blood across a semipermeable membrane to remove toxic materials and to maintain fluid balance.

9. _____ removal of the end of the prepuce of the penis; usually done at birth.

10. _____ an x-ray study obtained without a contrast medium that illustrates the size, shape, and location of the kidneys in relationship to other organs in the abdominopelvic region.

Correct Answers _____ × 10 = _____% **Score**

Activity 6–8: Build Medical Words
Diagnostic, Symptomatic, and Surgical Terms

Use *nephr/o* (kidney) to build medical words meaning:

1. tumor of the kidney _____

2. calculus in the kidney _____

3. study of the kidney _____

Use *pyel/o* (renal pelvis) to build medical words meaning:

4. writing, record of the renal pelvis _____

5. dilation of the renal pelvis _____

Use *ureter/o* (ureter) to build medical words meaning:

6. hernia, swelling of the ureter _____

7. surgical repair of a ureter _____

Use *urethr/o* (urethra) to build medical words meaning:

8. narrowing or stricture of the urethra _____

9. pain in the urethra _____

10. inflammation of the urethra _____

Use *azot/o* (nitrogenous compounds) to build medical words meaning:

11. nitrogenous compounds in the urine _____

12. nitrogenous compounds in the blood _____

Use *orchid/o* (testes) to build medical words meaning:

13. excision of a testicle _____

14. incision of a testicle _____

Use *poly-* (many, much) to build medical words meaning

15. much urine _____

16. condition of excessive thirst _____

Use *prostat/o* (prostate gland) to form medical words meaning:

17. enlargement of the prostate gland _____

18. inflammation of the prostate gland _____

Use *vas/o* (vessel, vas deferens, duct) to form medical words meaning:

19. pertaining to the vas deferens _____

20. excision of a part of the vas deferens _____

Correct Answers _____ **× 5 =** _____ **% Score**

MEDICAL RECORDS

Pete Hernandez was treated for a urinary disorder. Authentic medical records, including a urology consultation, a discharge summary, and a pathology report, are presented in this section.

The following reading and dictionary exercise and medical record analysis will help you develop skills to abstract information and master the terminology in the reports. Accurate interpretation is important because information of this type is used in numerous areas of the medical practice, such as initiation of treatments, evaluation of the patient's progress, and completion of insurance claims.

 Reading and Dictionary Exercise

Place check mark in the box [✓] after you complete the exercise.

[ ] **1.** Underline the following words in the reports as you read the urology consultation, discharge summary, and pathology report. These medical records can be found at the end of the chapter.

[ ] **2.** Use a medical dictionary and Appendix F, Part 2 to define the following terms.

Note: You are not expected to fully understand all the parts of the medical records. The important aspect of this exercise is to use all available resources to complete it. Eventually you will master the terminology and format of these reports.

> > > MEDICAL RECORD 6-1: UROLOGY CONSULTATION

Term	Pronunciation	Meaning
voiding	*voyd-ĭng*	_____
catheter	*KĂTH-ĕ-tĕr*	_____
prostatism	*PRŎS-tă-tĭzm*	_____
nocturia	*nŏk-TŪ-rē-ă*	_____
hematuria	*hē-mă-TŪ-rē-ă*	_____
dysuria	*dĭs-Ū-rē-ă*	_____
Triaminic	*trī-ă-MĬ-nĭk*	_____
benign	*bē-NĪN*	_____
prostatic hypertrophy	*prŏs-TĂT-ĭk* *hī-PĔR-trŏ-fē*	_____
Septra	*SĔP-tră*	_____

> > > MEDICAL RECORD 6-2: DISCHARGE SUMMARY

Term	Pronunciation	Meaning
adenocarcinoma	*ăd-ĕ-nō-kăr-sĭn-Ō-mă*	_____
cystoscopy	*sĭs-TŎS-kō-pē*	_____
dilatation	*dĭl-ă-TĀ-shŭn*	_____
cystolitholapaxy	*SĬS-tō-lĭth-ŏl-ā-păk-sē*	_____
Foley catheter	*FŌ-lē KĂTH-ĕ-tĕr*	_____
electrocardiogram	*ē-lĕk-trō-KĂR-dē-ō-grăm*	_____
hyperplasia	*hī-pĕr-PLĀ-zē-ă*	_____
transurethral resection	*trăns-ū-RĒ-thrăl* *rē-SĔK-shŭn*	_____
postoperative	*pōst-ŎP-ĕr-ă-tĭv*	_____
Cipro	*sĭp-RŌ*	_____

> > > MEDICAL RECORD 6-3: PATHOLOGY REPORT

Term	Pronunciation	Meaning
pathology	pă-THŎL-ō-jē	_____
atypical	ā-TĬP-ĭ-kăl	_____
histiocytic	hĭs-tē-ō-SĬ-tĭk	_____
involution	ĭn-vō-LŪ-shŭn	_____
comorbidities	kō-mŏr-BĬD-ĭ-tēz	_____

Critical Thinking: Analysis of Medical Records

This section provides experience in abstracting and analyzing information from medical records. At the same time, it reinforces the material presented in this chapter.

> > > MEDICAL RECORD 6-1: UROLOGY CONSULTATION

1. What brought Mr. Hernandez to the emergency room?

   _____

2. Place a "+" in the space provided for positive findings and a "−" for negative findings. This information is documented in the consultation report. A positive finding indicates the patient had a history (Hx) of this condition; a negative finding indicates the patient did not have a history of this condition.

   _____hematuria   _____normal urinary flow

   _____hesitancy   _____enlarged prostate

   _____nocturia   _____dysuria

   _____urinary tract infections

3. What is the purpose of a urinary catheter?

   _____

   _____

4. Why was the patient put on the antibiotic Septra?

   _____

   _____

5. What type of surgery was advised?

   _____

> > > MEDICAL RECORD 6-2: DISCHARGE SUMMARY

6. What type of operation and special procedures did the surgeon perform?

_____

7. What medication was Mr. Hernandez prescribed upon discharge from the hospital, and why was it prescribed?

_____

8. What laboratory reports are pending?

_____

9. What was his final diagnosis?

_____

> > > MEDICAL RECORD 6-3: PATHOLOGY REPORT

10. How were the specimens labeled in the gross description, parts A and B, of the pathology report?

_____

11. Were there any signs of malignancy in the biopsy performed on the prostate tissue?

_____

12. What abnormalities were found in the bladder?

_____

 Audio Practice

Listen to the audio CD-ROM to practice the pronunciation of selected medical terms from this chapter.

Medical Record 6–1. Urology Consultation

GENERAL HOSPITAL AND MEDICAL CENTER
2211 Fifth Avenue North • Healthy City, USA 12345 • (321) 123-4567

Urology Consultation

Patient Name: Pete Hernandez
Date: 12/14/xx

Referring Physician: E. Roberts, MD, UMC Emergency Room

REASON FOR CONSULTATION:
Pete Hernandez is a 70-year-old Caucasian male who had increasing difficulty in voiding the last several days. Finally he came to the emergency room on 11/27/xx. A Foley catheter was inserted and 1,600 cc. of residual urine was obtained. Our office was contacted and he was given an appointment on 12/17/xx. However, over the weekend he removed the catheter and again was unable to void. He was seen in our office on an emergency basis this morning, and a catheter was reinserted because of acute retention and 1,500 cc. was recorded. Patient does have some symptoms of prostatism and recent nocturia x4. He has some hesitancy and slowing of the stream. He has no hematuria or dysuria. No urinary tract infections.

PAST MEDICAL HISTORY:

Occupation:	He is a retired office worker and security guard.
Habits:	Alcohol: Socially. Nothing heavy. None significantly recently.
Smoking:	None
Surgeries:	None
Medications:	Triaminic which has been intermittent and this has been discontinued; aspirin prn.
Family History:	No heart disease or diabetes

PHYSICAL EXAMINATION:

Height:	6'0" Weight: 173 pounds
Vital Signs:	Blood pressure 140/70, pulse 88, respirations 18, temperature 98 degrees.
HEENT:	Unremarkable, Neck was supple.
Chest:	Clear
Heart:	Irregular sinus rhythm. No murmurs
Abdomen:	Benign and obese. No CVA tenderness.
Genitalia:	Penis and testicles are normal
Prostate:	2-3+ enlarged, smooth, symmetric and benign in quality.
Urine:	Clear.
Culture obtained:	Foley was draining clear amber urine.

Continued

Urology Consultation, page 2
Patient Name: Pete Hernandez

IMPRESSION: 1. Benign prostatic hypertrophy with bladder outlet obstruction and recurrent urinary retention with a large residual urine volume

ADVISED:
1. IVP
2. Septra, 1 DS tablet q12h for 14 days
3. Probable TURP. He has a very high residual. Probably represents a decompensated bladder
4. Prostate obstruction surgery

_____

Joan Summerlin, M.D

JS:urs

D: 12-14xx
T: 12/14/xx

Body System Connections
Digestive System

THE CARDIOVASCULAR SYSTEM
◆ The digestive system provides nutrients for absorption by the blood; the blood transports these nutrients to all body cells.

THE ENDOCRINE SYSTEM
◆ Local hormones influence digestive activity; cholecystokinin stimulates contraction of the gallbladder and secretion of pancreatic enzymes. ◆ The pancreas contains hormone-producing cells that play a role in the digestive process. ◆ The digestive system provides vital nutrients to endocrine organs.

THE FEMALE REPRODUCTIVE SYSTEM
◆ The reproductive system depends on the digestive system to provide adequate nutrients, including fats, and to make conception and normal fetal development possible.

THE INTEGUMENTARY SYSTEM
◆ Dietary calcium assimilation is activated when the skin absorbs vitamin D from the sun. ◆ Surplus calorie consumption may be stored as subcutaneous fat.

THE LYMPHATIC AND IMMUNE SYSTEMS
◆ Lymphoid nodules in the intestinal walls prevent invasion of pathogens. ◆ Immune cells protect digestive tract organs against infection.

THE MUSCULOSKELETAL SYSTEM
◆ Muscles play an important role in the digestive system. They facilitate mastication, swallowing, and movement of digestive ingredients throughout the entire gastrointestinal tract. ◆ Dietary calcium is absorbed by the digestive system to help normal bone development.

THE NERVOUS SYSTEM
◆ The nervous system affects the rate of digestive functioning. ◆ The digestive system provides nutrients needed for normal neural functioning.

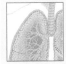

THE RESPIRATORY SYSTEM
◆ A common anatomical structure is shared by the respiratory and digestive systems. ◆ The respiratory system provides oxygen and removes carbon dioxide produced by the organs in the digestive system.

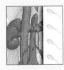

THE URINARY AND MALE REPRODUCTIVE SYSTEMS
◆ Fluids lost during digestion are partially restored by the kidneys. ◆ Both the liver and kidneys activate the release of vitamin D. ◆ The male reproductive system depends on the digestive system to provide adequate nutrients in order to produce viable sperm.

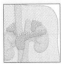

Figure 7–1 *The interrelationship of the digestive system with other body systems.*

food into smaller particles while mixing it with saliva—a fluid that contains important digestive enzymes. The teeth are surrounded by pink fleshy tissue known as (1) **gingiva** (gums). Each tooth consists of three main parts: the (2) **crown,** the (3) **neck,** and the (4) **root.**

The crown is covered with (5) **enamel,** which gives the teeth a white appearance. Enamel is the hardest substance in the body and protects the teeth from friction. Beneath the enamel is the main structure of the tooth, the (6) **dentin.** It is yellowish, bony tissue that is considerably softer than enamel. Under the dentin, the innermost part of the tooth, the (7) **pulp cavity,** contains (8) **nerve** endings and (9) **blood vessels.** The (10) **cementum** is a protective layer that covers

the root. Holding the tooth in place is the (11) **periodontal membrane.**

Salivary Glands

Label the salivary glands in Figure 7–4 as you read the following material.

The oral cavity contains three pairs of salivary glands that produce saliva: the (1) **sublingual glands,** the (2) **submandibular glands,** also called submaxillary glands, and the (3) **parotid glands.** The ducts of these three glands carry saliva to the mouth. Even though the secretion of saliva is continuous, the amount of saliva at any given time differs. The amount of saliva in the mouth increases whenever there is an object in the mouth, regardless of whether or not it is

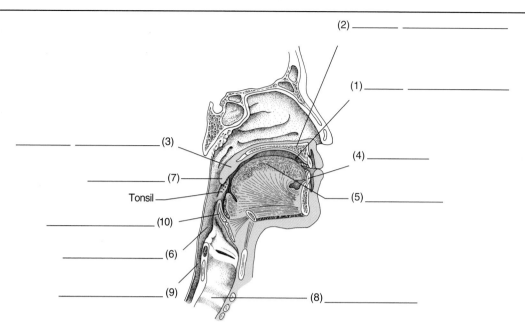

Figure 7–2 *Sagittal view of the head showing oral, nasal, and pharyngeal components of the digestive system. (Adapted from Gylys, BA, and Wedding, ME: Medical Terminology: A Systems Approach, ed 4. FA Davis, Philadelphia, 1999, p 86, with permission.)*

edible. The amount of saliva present in the mouth also increases at the sight or smell of food.

Pharynx and Esophagus

Finish labeling the structures in Figure 7–2 as you read the following material. Once food is chewed, it is formed into a round, sticky mass called a *bolus*, which is pushed by the tongue from the mouth into the (6) **pharynx,** or throat. Its downward movement is guided into the pharynx by the soft, fleshy V-shaped tissue called the (7) **uvula.** The lowest portion of the pharynx divides into two tubes: one that leads to the lungs, called the (8) **trachea,** and one that leads to the stomach, called the (9) **esophagus.**

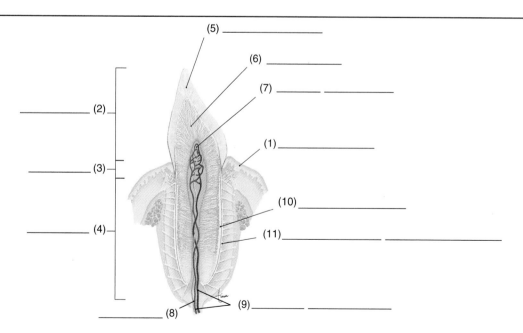

Figure 7–3 *Longitudinal section of a tooth, showing the internal structure. (Adapted from Scanlon, VC, and Sanders, TS: Essentials of Anatomy and Physiology, ed 3. FA Davis, Philadelphia, 1999, p 354, with permission.)*

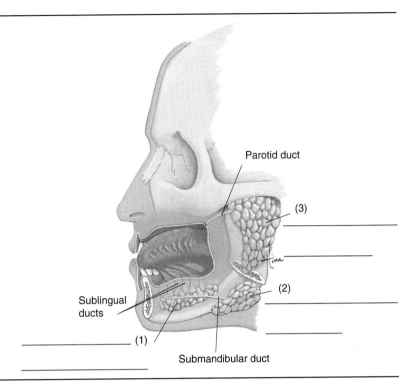

Parotid duct

(3)

(2)

Sublingual
ducts

(1)

Submandibular duct

Figure 7–4 *The salivary glands shown in left lateral view. (Adapted from Scanlon, VC, and Sanders, TS: Essentials of Anatomy and Physiology, ed 3. FA Davis, Philadelphia, 1999, p 354, with permission.)*

The pharynx serves a dual role because it is a passageway for both air and food and has both respiratory and digestive functions. During the process of swallowing, a small flap of tissue, called the (10) **epiglottis,** covers the trachea. Its purpose is to prevent food from entering the trachea and going into the lungs.

The esophagus (see Fig. 7–2), the third organ involved in the process of swallowing (deglutition), is a muscular tube that is about 10 inches long. It goes through an opening in the diaphragm, called the esophageal hiatus, and terminates in the superior portion of the stomach. The esophagus propels food, which is in the form of a bolus, to the stomach by rhythmic, wavelike contractions of muscles that line its walls. This process, known as **peristalsis,** is also how food is moved through the stomach and small intestines.

Activity 7–1: Competency Verification
Digestive Process

Review Figures 7–2 and 7–3, and check your labeling in Appendix C.

Stomach

Label Figure 7–5 as you read about the structures and function of the stomach.

The stomach, located in the left upper quadrant (LUQ) of the abdominal cavity, is a food reservoir and the first major site of digestion. A muscular ring, known as the (1) **lower esophageal sphincter (LES)** or cardiac sphincter, controls the passage of food from the esophagus into the stomach. When the LES relaxes, the muscular ring opens to allow food to enter the stomach and then contracts to prevent the backup of stomach contents into the esophagus. If the LES does not contract completely, gastric juice may back up into the esophagus causing a painful condition known as *heartburn.*

The stomach comprises an upper portion called the (2) **fundus,** the large central portion called the (3) **body,** and the lower portion, known as the (4) **pylorus** or **antrum.** When empty, the stomach collapses inward, and forms longitudinal folds called (5) **rugae** (wrinkles). The rugae allow the stomach to distend, or greatly increase in size, when it is full. The rugae also contain the digestive glands that produce the enzyme **pepsin** and **hydrochloric acid.** These enzyme secretions, coupled with the mechanical

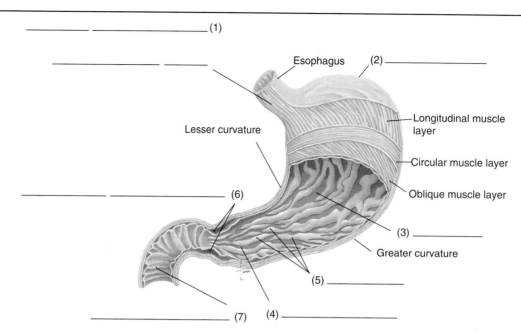

_____ _____ (1)

Esophagus (2) _____

Longitudinal muscle
layer

Circular muscle layer

Oblique muscle layer

Lesser curvature

_____ _____ _____ (6)

(3) _____

Greater curvature

(5) _____

_____ (7) (4) _____

Figure 7–5 *The stomach in anterior view. The stomach wall has been sectioned to show the muscle layers and the rugae of the mucosa. (Adapted from Scanlon, VC, and Sanders, TS: Essentials of Anatomy and Physiology, ed 3. FA Davis, Philadelphia, 1999, p 359, with permission.)*

mixing and churning, turn foodstuffs into a semiliquid form called **chyme.** Food slowly leaves the stomach through the (6) **pyloric sphincter** into the first part of the small intestine called the (7) **duodenum.**

Activity 7–2: Competency Verification
Salivary Glands and Stomach

Review Figures 7–4 and Figure 7–5, and check your labeling in Appendix C.

Small Intestine

The small intestine is a continuation of the GI tract that extends from the pyloric sphincter to the first part of the large intestine. Digestion continues in the small intestine as enzymes are added to the chyme and absorption of nutrients into the bloodstream occurs.

Label Figure 7–6 as you continue to read about the GI tract.

The small intestine, a coiled 20-foot-long tube, winds from the pyloric sphincter of the stomach to the beginning of the large intestine, filling much of the abdominal cavity. The small intestine comprises three parts: the (1) **duodenum,** the uppermost division, the (2) **jejunum,** and the (3) **ileum.** Approximately 90 percent of the absorption of nutrients occurs in the small intestine. The remaining 10 percent

of absorption takes place in the (4) **stomach** and large intestine. Secretions from the accessory organs, the (5) **liver,** (6) **gallbladder,** and (7) **pancreas,** as well as enzymes secreted by glands in the small intestine, aid in the digestion of food (chyme).

Throughout the length of the small intestine (Fig. 7–7*A*) food absorption takes place in microscopic fingerlike projections called villi (Fig. 7–7*B*). Inside the villi are tiny capillary networks that permit digested nutrients to be absorbed into the bloodstream and lymph vessels. A microscopic view of three villi (singular, villus) showing the internal structure is illustrated in Figure 7–7*C*. Review the figure to visualize the small intestine and its microscopic vessels that promote digestion. Any undigested or unabsorbed material from the small intestine is passed on to the large intestine to be excreted from the body. For a graphic illustration of the pathway of food through the digestive system, see Flowchart 7–1.

Large Intestine

The large intestine, also known as the large bowel, is about 5-feet long and extends from the ileum to the anus. It is named "the large intestine" because its diameter is larger than that of the small intestine. The large intestine is structurally divided into the cecum, colon, rectum, and anal canal.

Label Figure 7–8 as you read the following material.

The first part of the large intestine, the (1) **cecum,** is a dilated pouch that hangs inferiorly to the

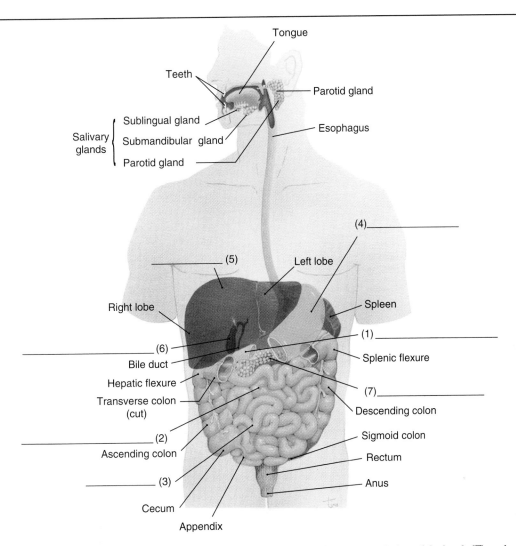

Tongue

Teeth

Parotid gland

Sublingual gland

Salivary
glands

Submandibular gland

Esophagus

Parotid gland

(4)_____

(5)

Left lobe

Right lobe

Spleen

(1)_____

(6)

Splenic flexure

Bile duct

Hepatic flexure

(7)_____

Transverse colon
(cut)

Descending colon

(2)

Sigmoid colon

Ascending colon

Rectum

(3)

Anus

Cecum

Appendix

Figure 7–6   *The digestive organs shown in anterior view of the trunk and left lateral view of the head. (The spleen is not a digestive organ but is included to show its location relative to the stomach, pancreas, and colon.) (Adapted from Scanlon, VC, and Sanders, TS: Essentials of Anatomy and Physiology, ed 3. FA Davis, Philadelphia, 1999, p 353, with permission.)*

(2) **ileocecal valve.** The purpose of the ileocecal valve is to prevent backup of colon materials into the small intestine. Attached to the cecum is a wormlike, dead-end projection, the (3) **appendix.** The appendix serves no purpose in the digestive process, but problems arise if it becomes inflamed or infected. The open, superior portion of the cecum is continuous with the colon. The cecum merges with the colon, which is divided into ascending, transverse, descending, and sigmoid portions. The (4) **ascending colon** extends superiorly from the cecum along the right abdominal wall to the inferior surface of the liver. Here the colon bends abruptly to the left at the (5) **hepatic flexure** and transversely crosses the upper abdominal cavity as the (6) **transverse colon.** At the left abdominal wall, another right-angle bend

known as the (7) **splenic flexure** turns the transverse colon downward to become the (8) **descending colon.** The descending colon continues downward to the brim of the pelvis to form the S-shaped bend called the (9) **sigmoid colon** and extends to the (10) **rectum.** The last 2 to 3 centimeters of the rectum are called the (11) **anal canal.** The (12) **anus,** the external opening of the anal canal, is where waste products or feces are eliminated from the body.

Activity 7-3: Competency Verification
Small Intestine and Large Intestine

Review Figures 7–6 and Figure 7–8, and check your labeling in Appendix C.

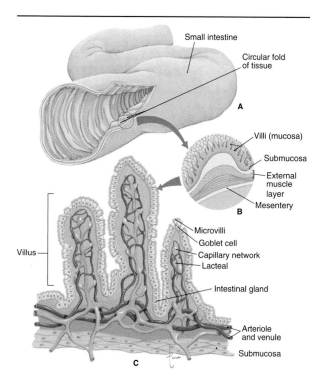

Figure 7–7 *The small intestine. (A) Section through the small intestine. (B) Magnified view of a section of the intestinal wall showing the villi and the four layers. (C) Microscopic view of three villi showing the internal structure. (Adapted from Scanlon, VC, and Sanders, TS: Essentials of Anatomy and Physiology, ed 3. FA Davis, Philadelphia, 1999, p 366, with permission.)*

Accessory Organs of Digestion: Liver, Gallbladder, and Pancreas

Chemical digestion in the small intestines is not only facilitated by its own secretions but it is also greatly dependent on the activities of the three accessory organs of digestion: the liver, the gallbladder, and the pancreas.

Although food does not pass through these organs, they play a vital role in the proper digestion and absorption of nutrients. The liver, gallbladder, and pancreas are not located directly in the alimentary canal.

Label Figure 7–9 as you learn about the structures and functions of the liver, the gallbladder, and the pancreas.

Liver

The (1) **liver,** the largest glandular organ in the body, comprises two major lobes and two minor lobes. The liver is located beneath the diaphragm in the right upper quadrant (RUQ) of the abdominal cavity and weighs approximately 3 to 4 pounds. The functions of the liver are vital to life. An important digestive

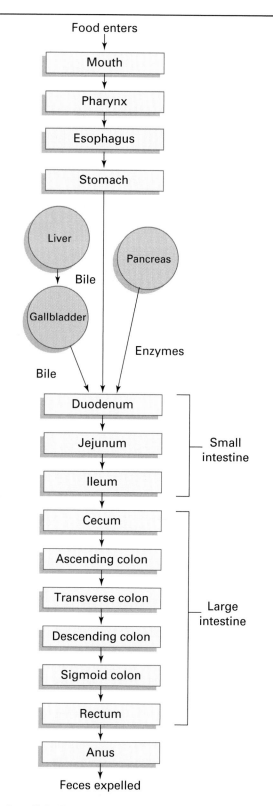

Flowchart 7–1 *Pathway of food through the digestive system.*

function of the liver is the production of bile for the **emulsification** of fats in the small intestine. Bile mainly comprises bile salts, bile pigments, and cho-

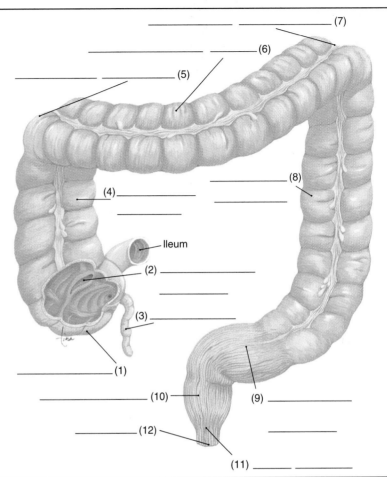

_____ _____ (7)

_____ _____ (6)

_____ (5)

(4) _____

(8)

_____

Ileum

(2) _____

_____

(3) _____

(1) _____

_____ (10)

(9) _____

(12) _____

(11) _____ _____

Figure 7–8 _The large intestine shown in anterior view. (Adapted from Scanlon, VC, and Sanders, TS: Essentials of Anatomy and Physiology, ed 3. FA Davis, Philadelphia, 1999, p 368, with permission.)_

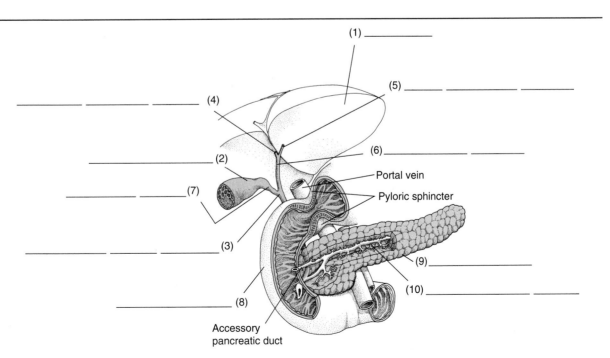

(1) _____

(5) _____ _____

(4)

_____ _____ _____

(6) _____

Portal vein

(2) _____

Pyloric sphincter

_____ _____

(7)

_____ _____ _____ _____

(3)

(9) _____

(10) _____ _____

(8) _____

Accessory pancreatic duct

Figure 7–9 _The liver, gallbladder, pancreas, and duodenum with associated ducts and blood vessels. (Adapted from Gylys, BA, and Wedding, ME: Medical Terminology: A Systems Approach, ed 4. FA Davis, Philadelphia, 1999, p 90, with permission.)_

lesterol. The main component of bile pigment is **bilirubin,** which is an orange-brown or even greenish pigment that is evident in serum and urine. If bilirubin is present in high concentrations in serum or urine, it causes jaundice and may be an indication of a liver disease, bile duct obstruction, or an anemia that results in excessive destruction of RBCs.

Besides its digestive function of producing bile, the liver performs several other important functions:

- Produces blood proteins such as prothrombin and fibrinogen, which aid in blood clotting.
- Performs an excretory function in that it carries bilirubin and excess cholesterol to the intestines for elimination in feces.
- Destroys old erythrocytes and releases bilirubin.
- Removes or transforms toxic substances (detoxification) into less harmful components. Potentially harmful substances, such as DDT may be present in the liver of humans who eat sprayed fruits and vegetables. In addition, alcohol and medications are transformed into less toxic substances.
- Stores glycogen, copper, iron, and vitamins A, B_{12}, D, E, and K.
- Helps regulate the blood glucose concentration by either removing glucose (sugar) from or adding glucose to the blood, according to the needs of the body. After a carbohydrate-rich meal, the liver can remove some glucose and convert it into glycogen (starch), which is then stored in the liver cells. This process is known as *glycogenesis.* The liver also has the ability to reverse this process and transform glycogen (starch) to glucose when the sugar level in the blood is too low. This is known as *glycogenolysis.* Additionally, whenever the body needs sugar, the liver has the ability to transform proteins and fats into glucose. This process is known as *gluconeogenesis.*

Gallbladder

The (2) **gallbladder** serves as a storage area for bile. When bile is needed for digestion, the gallbladder releases it into the duodenum through the (3) **common**

bile duct. Bile is also drained from the liver through the (4) **right hepatic duct** and the (5) **left hepatic duct.** These two ducts eventually form the (6) **hepatic duct.** The (7) **cystic duct** of the gallbladder merges with the hepatic duct to form the common bile duct, which leads into the (8) **duodenum.**

As bile squirts into the duodenum from the common bile duct, it mixes with pancreatic juices. Here, the bile aids in emulsification, the breaking down of large fat globules into smaller ones. Without bile, most ingested fat could not be digested. Bile production is stimulated by hormone secretions, which are produced in the duodenum as soon as food enters the small intestine.

Pancreas

Continue labeling the pancreas in Figure 7–9 as you read the following material.

The (9) **pancreas** is an elongated, somewhat flattened organ that lies posterior and slightly inferior to the stomach and is connected to the duodenum. It performs both endocrine and exocrine functions. As an endocrine gland, the pancreas secretes insulin directly into the bloodstream. This process helps maintain normal blood sugar levels. For a comprehensive discussion of the endocrine function of the pancreas, review Chapter 10.

As an exocrine gland, the pancreas produces digestive enzymes that pass into the duodenum through the (10) **pancreatic duct.** The digestive enzymes contain trypsin, which breaks down proteins; amylase, which breaks down carbohydrates; and lipase, which breaks down fats.

Activity 7–4: Competency Verification
Accessory Digestive Organs

Review Figure 7–9, and check your labeling in Appendix C.

Activity 7–5: Competency Verification
Tracing the Route of Digestion

anus	ileum	pylorus
ascending colon	jejunum	rectum
descending colon	LES	stomach
duodenum	oral cavity	teeth
epiglottis	pharynx	transverse colon
esophagus		

Place the terms listed above in sequential order, using the numbered list below.

1. _____ beginning of the GI tract; receptacle for food.

2. _____ organs of mastication.

3. _____ structure that serves as a passageway for both air and food.

4. _____ structure that covers the trachea to prevent food from entering the lungs.

5. _____ the tube that leads to the stomach.

6. _____ structure that controls passage of food from the esophagus to the stomach; also called the cardiac sphincter.

7. _____ a reservoir for food enabling gradual digestion.

8. _____ lower portion of the stomach; also called the antrum.

9. _____ first part of the small intestine.

10. _____ second part of the small intestine.

11. _____ third part of the small intestine.

12. _____ structure that extends superiorly from the cecum along the right abdominal wall to the inferior surface of the liver.

13. _____ structure that extends across the abdominal cavity.

14. _____ structure that descends to the sigmoid colon.

15. _____ external opening for the elimination of feces from the body.

Correct Answers _____ × 6.67 = _____% Score

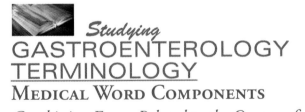

Studying
GASTROENTEROLOGY TERMINOLOGY
MEDICAL WORD COMPONENTS
Combining Forms Related to the Organs of Ingestion

Combining Forms: Organs of Ingestion

Combining Form	Meaning	EXAMPLE	
		Term/Pronunciation	Definition
MOUTH			
or/o	mouth	**or**/al ŌR-ăl	pertaining to (-*al*) the mouth

Combining Forms: Organs of Ingestion (Continued)

Combining Form	Meaning	EXAMPLE	
		Term/Pronunciation	**Definition**
stomat/o *stō-mă-TŎP-ă-thē*	mouth	**stomat**/o/pathy	any disease (-*pathy*) of the mouth. Stomatopathy *is synonymous with stomatosis.*
gloss/o	tongue	**gloss**/itis *glŏs-SĪ-tĭs*	inflammation (-*itis*) of the tongue
lingu/o		**lingu**/al *LĬNG-gwăl*	pertaining to (-*al*) the tongue
bucc/o	cheek	**bucc**/al *BŬK-ăl*	pertaining to (-*al*) the cheek
cheil/o	lip	**cheil**/osis *kī-LŌ-sĭs*	abnormal condition (-*osis*) of the lips *This disorder is characterized by scales and fissures caused by a deficiency of vitamin B complex, especially riboflavin, in the diet.*
labi/o		**labi**/al *LĀ-bē-ăl*	pertaining to (-*al*) the lip
dent/o	teeth	**dent**/ist *DĔN-tĭst*	specialist (-*ist*) in the treatment of teeth
odont/o		orth/**odont**/ist *ŏr-thō-DŎN-tĭst*	a specialist (-*ist*) in dentistry who is concerned with the diagnosis, prevention, and correction of malpositions and imperfect contacts of the teeth *The combining form orth/o means "straight." The term orthodontist literally means "specialist in straight teeth."*
gingiv/o	gum(s)	**gingiv**/it is *jĭn-jĭ-VĪ-tĭs*	inflammation of the gums
sial/o	saliva, salivary gland	**sial**/o/lith *sī-ĂL-ō-lĭth*	a calculus or stone (-*lith*) formed in a salivary gland or duct *The salivary glands are the exocrine glands in the mouth that secrete saliva.*

Combining Forms: Organs of Ingestion (Continued)

Combining Form	Meaning	EXAMPLE	
		Term/Pronunciation	Definition
ESOPHAGUS AND PHARYNX **esophag/o**	esophagus	**esophag/o/cele** *ē-SŎF-ă-gō-sēl*	A hernia (-*cele*) of the esophagus *The mucous membrane herniates through a weakened area in the wall of the esophagus.*
pharyng/o	pharynx (throat)	**pharyng/itis** *făr-ĭn-JĪ-tĭs*	inflammation (-*itis*) of the pharynx (throat)

Activity 7–6: Competency Verification
Medical Word Components: Mouth, Esophagus, and Pharynx

Check the box [✓] as you complete each numbered section.

[   ] **1.** Review the components related to the mouth, esophagus, and pharynx in the previous section. Then pronounce each term aloud.

[   ] **2.** For the following words, first write the suffix and its meaning. Then translate the meaning of the remaining components starting with the first part of the word.

> **Example:** esophag/o/gastr/o/scopy
> **Answer:** *scopy*=visual examination; esophagus; stomach

1. dent/ist   _____

2. gingiv/itis   _____

3. esophag/itis   _____

4. stomat/o/pathy   _____

5. gloss/itis   _____

6. orth/odont/ist   _____

7. esophag/o/cele   _____

8. cheil/osis   _____

9. labi/al   _____

10. sial/o/lith   _____

Correct Answers _____ **× 10 =** _____ **% Score**

Combining Forms Related to the Organs of Digestion

Combining Forms: Organs of Digestion

Combining Form	Meaning	EXAMPLE	
		Term/Pronunciation	Definition
STOMACH			
gastr/o	stomach	**gastr**/ectomy *găs-TRĔK-tō-mē*	partial or total removal (-*ectomy*) of the stomach (Fig. 7–10)
pylor/o	pylorus, pyloric sphincter	**pylor**/o/plasty *pī-LOR-ō-plăs-tē*	surgical repair (-*plasty*) of the pyloric sphincter
SMALL INTESTINE			
duoden/o	duodenum	**duoden**/o/scopy *dū-ŏd-ĕ-NŎS-kō-pē*	visual examination (-*scopy*) of the duodenum *The duodenum is the first part of the small intestine.*
enter/o	intestine (usually small intestine)	**enter**/o/pathy *ĕn-tĕr-ŎP-ă-thē*	an intestinal disease (-*pathy*)
jejun/o	jejunum	**jejun**/o/rrhaphy *jĕ-joo-NOR-ă-fē*	suture (-*rrhaphy*) of the jejunum *The jejunum is the second part of the small intestine.*
ile/o	ileum	**ile**/itis *ĭl-ē-Ī-tĭs*	inflammation (-*itis*) of the ileum *The ileum is the third part of the small intestine.*

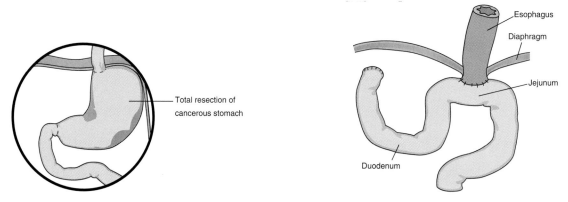

Figure 7–10 *Total gastrectomy. (From Williams, LS, and Hopper, PD: Understanding Medical-Surgical Nursing. FA Davis, Philadelphia, 1999, p 587, with permission.)*

Combining Forms: Organs of Digestion (Continued)

Combining Form	Meaning	EXAMPLE	
		Term/Pronunciation	Definition
LARGE INTESTINE			
append/o	appendix	**append**/ectomy ăp-ĕn-DĔK-tō-mē	excision (-*ectomy*) of the appendix *Recall that the appendix is the wormlike projection that hangs from the cecum.*
appendic/o		**appendic**/itis ă-pĕn-dĭ-SĪ-tĭs	inflammation (-*itis*) of the appendix (Fig. 7–11)
col/o	colon	**col**/o/stomy kō-LŎS-tō-mē	surgical creation of an artificial opening (-*stomy*) on the abdominal wall by incising the colon and drawing it out to the surface *When* -stomy *is used with a combining form for an organ, it refers to a surgical opening to the outside of the body. A colostomy is performed for colon cancer, obstructive tumors, and severe abdominal wounds.*
colon/o		**colon**/o/scopy kō-lŏn-ŎS-kō-pē	visual examination (-*scopy*) of the inner surface of the colon using a colonoscope.
sigmoid/o	sigmoid colon	**sigmoid**/o/tomy sĭg-moyd-ŎT-ō-mē	incision (-*tomy*) of the sigmoid colon
rect/o	rectum	**rect**/o/cele RĔK-tō-sēl	herniation (-*cele*) or protrusion of the rectum *Rectocele is synonymous with proctocele.*
proct/o	anus, rectum	**proct**/o/dynia prŏk-tō-DĬN-ē-ă	pain (-*dynia*) in the rectum or around the anus

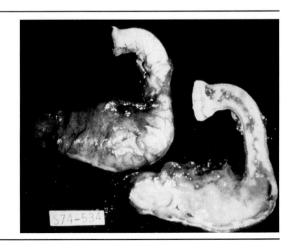

Figure 7–11 *Inflamed appendix, following its removal. (With permission from the late Dr. W. R. Spence.)*

Activity 7–7: Competency Verification

Medical Word Components: Stomach, Small Intestine, and Colon

Check the box [✓] as you complete each numbered section.

[ ] **1.** Review the word components related to the stomach, small intestine, and colon in the previous section. Then pronounce each word aloud.

[ ] **2.** For the words below, first write the suffix and its meaning. Then translate the meaning of the remaining components starting with the first part of the word.

> **Example:** jejun/itis
> **Answer:** *itis* = inflammation; jejunum (first part of the small intestine)

1. gastr/ectomy   _____

2. append/ectomy   _____

3. jejun/o/rrhaphy   _____

4. enter/o/pathy   _____

5. colon/o/scopy   _____

6. pylor/o/plasty   _____

7. rect/o/cele   _____

8. proct/o/dynia   _____

9. col/o/stomy   _____

10. sigmoid/o/scopy   _____

Correct Answers _____ **× 10 =** _____ **% Score**

Combining Forms: Accessory Organs of Digestion

Combining Form	Meaning	EXAMPLE	
		Term/Pronunciation	**Definition**
LIVER **hepat**/o	liver	**hepat**/o/megaly hĕp-ă-tō-MĔG-ă-lē	enlargement (-*megaly*) of the liver
GALLBLADDER **cholangi**/o	bile vessel	**cholangi**/o/gram kō-LĂN-jē-ō-grăm	radiographic record (-*gram*) of the bile ducts obtained by cholangiography

Combining Forms: Accessory Organs of Digestion (Continued)

Combining Form	Meaning	EXAMPLE Term/Pronunciation	Definition
chol/e*	bile, gall	**chol**/e/lith/iasis kō-lē-lĭ-THĪ-ă-sĭs	formation or presence of calculi, or bile stones (-*lith*), in the gallbladder or common duct *The suffix* -iasis *means " abnormal condition (produced by something specified)."*
cholecyst/o	gallbladder	**cholecyst**/ectomy kō-lē-sĭs-TĔK-tō-mē	excision of the gallbladder
choledoch/o	bile duct	**choledoch**/o/stomy kō-lĕd-ō-KŎS-tō-mē	forming an opening (-*stomy*) into the common bile duct
PANCREAS **pancreat**/o	pancreas	**pancreat**/oma păn-krē-ă-TŌ-mă	pancreatic tumor (-*oma*)

The combining vowel e *is used instead of* o. *This is an exception to the rule.*

Prefixes and Suffixes

In this section, prefixes are listed alphabetically and highlighted whereas suffixes are defined in the right-hand column as necessary.

Prefixes

Prefix	Meaning	EXAMPLE Term/Pronunciation	Definition
an-	without, not	**an**/orexia ăn-ō-RĔK-sē-ă	loss of appetite (-*orexia*); aversion to food
dia-	through, across	**dia**/rrhea dī-ă-RĒ-ă	abnormally frequent discharge or flow (-*rrhea*) of fluid fecal matter from the bowel
dys-	bad, painful, difficult	**dys**/pepsia dĭs-PĔP-sē-ă	difficult digestion (-*pepsia*)
hyper-	excessive, above normal	**hyper**/emesis hī-pĕr-ĔM-ĕ-sĭs	excessive vomiting (-*emesis*)
peri-	around	**peri**/odont/ist pĕr-ē-ō-DŎN-tĭst	a specialist (-*ist*) in periodontics *Periodontics is the branch of dentistry concerned with the treatment of abnormal conditions of the tissues around the teeth.*

Prefixes (Continued)

Prefix	Meaning	EXAMPLE	
		Term/Pronunciation	**Definition**
post-	after, behind	**post**/prandial *pōst-PRĂN-dē-ăl*	after a meal (-*prandial*)
sub-	under, below	**sub**/lingu/al *sŭb-LĬNG-gwăl*	pertaining to (-*al*) the area under the tongue

Activity 7–8: Competency Verification

Medical Word Components: Accessory Digestive Organs
Prefixes and Suffixes: Gastroenterology

Check the box [✓] as you complete each numbered section

[   ] **1.** Review the components of the accessory digestive organs, and the prefixes and suffixes related to gastroenterology in the previous sections. Then pronounce each word aloud.

[   ] **2.** For the words below, first write the suffix and its meaning. Then translate the meaning of the remaining components starting with the first part of the word.

> **Example:** cholecyst/itis
> **Answer:** *itis*= inflammation, gallbladder

1. hepat/o/megaly   _____

2. chol/e/lith/iasis   _____

3. cholecyst/ectomy   _____

4. cholangi/o/gram   _____

5. dys/pepsia   _____

6. post/prandial   _____

7. sub/ling/ual   _____

8. hyper/emesis   _____

9. an/orexia   _____

10. hepat/oma   _____

Correct Answers _____ × 10 = _____ **% Score**

PATHOLOGICAL CONDITIONS
Disorders Related to the Organs of Ingestion
Mouth, Esophagus, and Pharynx

PATHOLOGICAL CONDITION	DESCRIPTION
MOUTH	
cheilitis *kī-LĪ-tĭs* *cheil=lip* *itis=inflammation*	Inflammation of the lip.
dental caries *DĔN-tăl KĀR-ēz*	A plaque disease caused by the complex interaction of food, especially starches and sugars, with bacteria that form dental plaque; tooth decay.
leukoplakia *loo-kō-PLĀ-kē-ă* *leuko=white* *plakia= plaque*	A precancerous, slowly developing change in the mucous membrane characterized by thickened, white, firmly attached patches that are slightly raised and sharply circumscribed. They may appear on the lips, the mucosa of the mouth, as well on the penis or vulva. Malignant potential is evaluated by microscopic study of biopsied tissue. Those that occur on the lips and in the mouth are usually associated with pipe or cigarette smoking.
periodontal disease *pĕr-ē-ō-DŎN-tăl dĭ-ZĒZ* *peri=around* *odont=teeth* *al=pertaining to*	A disease of the supporting structures of the teeth (the periodontium) including the gums and bone structure to which the teeth are anchored. The most common symptom is bleeding gums but loosening of the teeth, receding gums, abscesses in pockets between the gums and the teeth, and necrotizing ulcerative gingivitis may be present as the disease process continues. Proper dental hygiene, including proper brushing of the teeth, use of dental floss, and periodic removal of plaque help to prevent periodontal disease.
sialoadenitis *sī-ă-lō-ăd-ě-NI-tĭs* *sialo=saliva, salivary gland* *aden=gland* *itis=inflammation*	Inflammation of a salivary gland.
stomatitis *stō-mă-TĪ-tĭs* *stomat=mouth* *itis=inflammation*	Any inflammatory condition of the mouth. It may result from infection by bacteria, viruses, or fungi; from exposure to certain chemicals or drugs; from vitamin deficiency; or from a systemic inflammatory disease.
aphthous *ĂF-thŭs*	A recurring condition characterized by the eruption of painful ulcers (commonly called *canker sores*) on the mucous membranes of the mouth. The cause is unknown, but an autoimmune basis is suspected. Fever, mental stress, or exposure to some foods may precede these lesions.
herpetic *hĕr-PĚT-ĭk*	A form of stomatitis caused by a herpes virus infection. Commonly known as *cold sores* or *fever blisters*.

Disorders Related to the Organs of Ingestion
Mouth, Esophagus, and Pharynx (Continued)

PATHOLOGICAL CONDITION	DESCRIPTION
thrush *thrŭsh*	An infection of the mouth or throat, especially in infants and young children, caused by *Candida albicans.* It is characterized by formation of white patches and ulcers and frequently by fever and gastrointestinal inflammation.
ESOPHAGUS	
esophageal varices *ē-sŏf-ă-JĒ-ăl VĂR-ĭ-sēz* *esophag=esophagus* *eal=pertaining to*	Tortuous (twisted) dilatation of esophageal veins situated at the distal end of the esophagus, especially susceptible to ulceration and hemorrhage.
PHARYNX	
pharyngitis *făr-ĭn-JĪ-tĭs* *pharyng=pharynx (throat)* *itis=inflammation*	This most common throat disorder is an acute or chronic inflammation of the pharynx. It is widespread among adults who live or work in dusty or dry environments, use their voices excessively, habitually use tobacco or alcohol, or suffer from chronic sinusitis, persistent coughs, or allergies. Uncomplicated pharyngitis usually subsides in 3 to 10 days.

Disorders Related to the Organs of Digestion
Stomach, Small Intestine, Large Intestine, Rectum, and Anus

PATHOLOGICAL CONDITION	DESCRIPTION
STOMACH	
achalasia *ăk-ă-LĀ-zē-ă*	An abnormal condition characterized by inability of a muscle to relax, particularly the cardiac sphincter of the stomach.
gastroenteritis *găs-trō-ĕn-tĕr-Ī-tĭs* *gastro=stomach* *enter=intestine* *itis=inflammation*	Inflammation of the stomach and small intestine, accompanying numerous gastrointestinal disorders. The condition may be attributed to bacterial enterotoxins, bacterial or viral invasion, chemical toxins, or miscellaneous conditions such as lactose intolerance.
gastroesophageal reflux *găs-trō-ĕ-sŏf-ă-JĒ-ăl RĒ-flŭks* *gastro=stomach* *esophag=esophagus* *eal=pertaining to*	A backflow of contents of the stomach into the esophagus; often the result of incompetence of the lower esophageal sphincter. Gastric juices are acid and therefore produce burning pain in the esophagus.
pyloric stenosis *pī-LŌR-ĭk stĕ-NŌ-sĭs* *pylor=pylorus* *ic=pertaining to, relating to*	A narrowing of the pyloric sphincter at the outlet of the stomach, causing an obstruction that blocks the flow of food into the small intestine. The condition occurs as a congenital defect in 1 of 200 newborns and occasionally in older adults secondary to an ulcer or fibrosis at the outlet. Treatment involves surgical section of the thickened muscle around the pyloric orifice.

Disorders Related to the Organs of Digestion
Stomach, Small Intestine, Large Intestine, Rectum, and Anus (Continued)

PATHOLOGICAL CONDITION	DESCRIPTION
dysentery DĬS-ĕn-tĕr-ē	Inflammation of the intestine, especially of the colon, which may be caused by chemical irritants, bacteria, protozoa, or parasites. Dysentery is common in underdeveloped areas of the world and in times of disaster and social disorganization when sanitary living conditions, clean food, and safe water are not available. It is characterized by diarrhea, colitis, and abdominal cramps.
Hirschsprung disease HĬRSH-sprŭngz dĭ-ZĒZ	Congenital absence of autonomic ganglia (groups of nerve cells) in the smooth muscle wall of the colon, which causes poor or absent peristalsis in the involved segment of the colon, accumulation of feces, and dilation of the bowel (megacolon). Symptoms include intermittent vomiting, diarrhea, and constipation. The abdomen may become distended to several times its normal size. During youth, impairments of autonomic nervous function are usually from injuries to the spinal cord or autonomic nerves. In older adults, the efficiency of the autonomic nervous system declines. The condition is corrected surgically by removing the inactive bowel. Also known as *congenital aganglionic megacolon*.
intestinal obstruction ĭn-TĔS-tĭ-năl ŏb-STRŬK-shŭn	Partial or complete obstruction of the small or large bowel lumen. Complete obstruction in any part of the bowel, if untreated, can cause death within hours from shock and vascular collapse. Intestinal obstruction is most likely after abdominal surgery or in persons with congenital bowel deformities. Intestinal obstruction results from mechanical or nonmechanical (neurogenic) blockage of the lumen.
mechanical mĕ-KĂN-ĭ-kăl	An obstruction that occurs when there is a blockage within the intestine from pressure on the intestinal walls. The obstructions may be caused by adhesions and strangulated hernias (usually associated with small-bowel obstruction); carcinomas (usually associated with large-bowel obstruction); foreign bodies, such as fruit pits, gallstones, or worms; compression of the bowel wall from stenosis; intussusception; volvulus of the sigmoid or cecum; tumors; or atresia (Fig. 7–14).
nonmechanical NŎN-mĕ-kăn-ĭ-kăl	An obstruction that occurs when the intestinal peristalsis decreases or stops because of vascular or neuromuscular pathology. The obstruction usually results from paralytic ileus, the most common of all intestinal obstructions. Paralytic ileus is a physiological form of intestinal obstruction that usually develops in the small bowel after abdominal surgery. Other nonmechanical causes of obstruction include electrolyte imbalances; toxicity, such as that associated with uremia or generalized infection; neurogenic abnormalities, such as spinal cord lesions; and thrombosis or embolism of mesenteric vessels.
intussusception ĭn-tŭ-sŭ-SĔP-shŭn	The sliding of the inner segment of intestine into another segment. This kind of intestinal obstruction may involve segments of the small intestine, the colon, or the terminal ileum and cecum. Intussusception occurs most often in infants and small children and is characterized by abdominal pain, vomiting, and presence of bloody mucus in the stool. Barium enema is used to confirm the diagnosis, and surgery is usually necessary to correct the obstruction (see Fig 7–14A).
irritable bowel syndrome (IBS) Ĭ-rĭ-tă-bĕl BŎW-ĕl SĬN-drōm	Chronic or periodic diarrhea alternating with constipation. It is accompanied by straining and abdominal cramps. Although the cause is unknown, contributing or aggravating factors include anxiety and stress with initial symptoms occurring early in life. Also called *spastic colon*.
polyposis coli pŏl-ē-PŌ-sĭs KŌ-lī *polyp=small growth* *osis=abnormal condition*	A condition of multiple polyps in the large intestine.

Disorders Related to the Organs of Digestion
Stomach, Small Intestine, Large Intestine, Rectum, and Anus (Continued)

PATHOLOGICAL CONDITION	DESCRIPTION

Figure 7–14   *Mechanical bowel obstructions. (A) Intussusception. (B) Volvulus (From Williams, LS, and Hopper, PD: Understanding Medical-Surgical Nursing. FA Davis, Philadelphia, 1999, p 609, with permission.)*

volvulus *VŎL-vū-lŭs*	A twisting of the bowel on itself, causing intestinal obstruction (see Fig. 7–14*B*).

RECTUM AND ANUS

fistula *FĬS-tū-lă*	An abnormal tubelike passage from a normal cavity or tube to a free surface or to another cavity.
anal *Ā-năl*	A fistula near the anus that may open into the rectum.
hemorrhoids *HĔM-ō-roydz*	Dilated, tortuous (twisted) veins in the mucous membrane. Constipation, straining at stool, prolonged sitting, and anorectal infections are factors that contribute to the development of hemorrhoids. Other factors may be loss of muscle tone due to old age, pregnancy, and receptive anal intercourse.
external *ĕks-TĔR-năl*	Hemorrhoids that involve veins outside the anal sphincter. They are usually not painful, and bleeding does not occur unless a hemorrhoidal vein ruptures or thromboses.
internal *ĭn-TĔR-năl*	Hemorrhoids that involve veins above the internal sphincter of the anus. If they become large enough to protrude from the anus, they become constricted and painful. Small internal hemorrhoids may bleed with defecation.

Activity 7-9: Clinical Application

Pathological Conditions: Organs of Ingestion and Digestion

achalasia	leukoplakia
cheilitis	pharyngitis
Crohn disease	pyloric stenosis
hemorrhoids	stomatitis
Hirschsprung disease	thrush
intussusception	volvulus

Match the terms listed above with the definitions given in the numbered list:

1. _____a chronic inflammation that is distinguished from closely related bowel disorders by its inflammatory pattern; usually of the ileum.

2. _____infection of the mouth or throat caused by *Candida albicans.*

3. _____inflammation of the lip.

4. _____inflammation of the mouth.

5. _____a precancerous, slowly developing change in a mucous membrane characterized by white patches.

6. _____an abnormal condition characterized by inability of a muscle to relax, particularly the cardiac sphincter of the stomach.

7. _____congenital absence of autonomic ganglia in the smooth muscular wall of the colon.

8. _____intestinal obstruction caused by a twisting of the bowel on itself.

9. _____the inner segment of intestine that has been pushed into another segment.

10. _____dilated, tortuous veins in the mucous membrane.

Correct Answers _____ × 10 = _____% **Score**

Disorders Related to the Accessory Organs of Digestion: Liver, Pancreas, and Gallbladder

PATHOLOGICAL CONDITION	DESCRIPTION
LIVER	
cirrhosis *sĭr-RŌ-sĭs* *cirrh=yellow* *osis=abnormal condition*	Chronic liver disease characterized by the destruction of liver cells; eventually leads to impaired liver function and jaundice. The most common cause of cirrhosis is chronic alcoholism.
hepatitis *hĕp-ă-TĪ-tĭs* *hepat=liver* *itis=inflammation*	Inflammatory condition of the liver, characterized by jaundice, hepatomegaly, anorexia, abdominal and gastric discomfort, abnormal liver function, clay-colored stools, and tea-colored urine.
viral hepatitis (VH) *VĪ-răl hĕp-ă-TĪ-tĭs* *hepat=liver* *itis=inflammation*	Inflammation of the liver caused by a virus; marked by hepatic cell destruction, necrosis, and autolysis, leading to anorexia, jaundice, and hepatomegaly. In most patients, hepatic cells eventually regenerate with little or no residual damage, allowing ready recovery. However, old age and serious underlying disorders make complications more likely. The prognosis is poor if edema and hepatic encephalopathy develop. Five types of viral hepatitis are recognized: A, B,C, D, and E.
hepatitis A (HAV) *hĕp-ă-TĪ-tĭs ā*	Hepatitis caused by hepatitis A virus. This form of hepatitis is characterized by the slow onset of signs and symptoms. The virus may be spread by direct contact through feces-contaminated food or water. The infection most often occurs in young adults and is usually followed by complete recovery. Prophylaxis with immune globulin (immunization) is effective in household and sexual contacts. A vaccine for immunization is available. Also called *acute infectious hepatitis*.
hepatitis B (HBV) *hĕp-ă-TĪ-tĭs bē*	Hepatitis caused by hepatitis B virus. The virus is transmitted in contaminated serum in blood transfusion, by sexual contact with an infected person, or by the use of contaminated hypodermic needles and dental and surgical instruments. It can also be transmitted by body fluids, such as saliva, semen, and tears. Severe infection may cause prolonged illness, destruction of liver cells, cirrhosis, or death. A vaccine that provides immunity is available for infants, teenagers, and adults at risk for exposure. The vaccine is also recommended for dentists, hospital personnel, laboratory technicians, and patients who require frequent transfusions. Also called *serum hepatitis*.
hepatitis C (HCV) *hĕp-ă-TĪ-tĭs sē*	Also known as non-A, non-B hepatitis because is not caused by the A or B virus. A type of hepatitis transmitted largely by blood transfusion or percutaneous inoculation, as when intravenous drug users share needles. The disease progresses to chronic hepatitis in up to 50% of patients acutely infected. HCV increases the risk of hepatocellular carcinoma.
hepatitis D (HDV) *hĕp-ă-TĪ-tĭs dē*	Also known as delta hepatitis, a form of hepatitis that occurs only in patients infected with hepatitis B. HDV relies on HBV replication and cannot replicate independently. The disease usually develops into a chronic state. It is transmitted sexually and through needle sharing. The only intervention is prevention of HBV.

Disorders Related to the Accessory Organs of Digestion: Liver, Pancreas, and Gallbladder (Continued)

PATHOLOGICAL CONDITION	DESCRIPTION
hepatitis E (HEV) *hĕp-ă-TĪ-tĭs ē*	Also known as *epidemic non-A, non-B hepatitis*, a self-limited type of hepatitis, which is common in developing countries and which may occur after natural disasters because of fecally contaminated water or food. There is currently no serological test available.

■ PANCREAS

pancreatitis *păn-krē-ă-TĪ-tĭs* *pancreat=pancreas* *itis=inflammation*	An inflammatory condition of the pancreas that may be acute or chronic.
acute *ă-KŪT*	Pancreatitis of sudden onset. Generally the result of damage to the biliary tract, as by infectious disease or from certain drugs. It is characterized by severe abdominal pain (generally epigastric or upper left) radiating to the back, fever, anorexia, nausea, and vomiting. There may be jaundice if the common bile duct is obstructed.
chronic *KRŎ-nĭk*	Pancreatitis of slow progression or frequent recurrence. Symptoms are similar to those of the acute form. When the cause is alcohol abuse, there may be calcification, atrophy, fatty degeneration, and scarring of the smaller pancreatic ducts. Abdominal pain, nausea, and vomiting occur, as well as steatorrhea and creatorrhea, caused by the diminished output of pancreatic enzymes. Pancreatic insulin production may be diminished, and diabetes mellitus develops in some patients, which leads to the malfunction of the pancreas; causes are similar to those of the acute form.

■ GALLBLADDER

cholelithiasis *kō-lē-lĭ-THĪ-ă-sĭs* *chole=bile, gall* *lith=stone, calculus* *iasis=abnormal condition (produced by something specified)*	The presence or formation of stones in the gallbladder, also known as gallstones. The gallbladder can be a site of blockage that prevents bile from leaving the gallbladder. If stones cannot pass spontaneously into the duodenum, cholangiography or similar procedures will reveal their location, and they can be removed or a cholecystectomy may be performed. Cholelithiasis may cause jaundice, right upper quadrant pain, obstruction, and inflammation of the gallbladder.

OTHER DISORDERS

DISORDER	DESCRIPTION
achlorhydria *ă-klor-HĪ-drē-ă* *a=without* *chlor=green* *hydr=water* *ia=condition*	Absence of hydrochloric acid in the gastric juice. May be associated with gastric carcinoma, gastric ulcer, pernicious anemia, adrenal insufficiency, or chronic gastritis.
anorexia *ăn-ō-RĔK-sē-ă* *an=without, not* *orexia=appetite*	Lack or loss of appetite, resulting in the inability to eat. Anorexia should not be confused with *anorexia nervosa*, which is a complex psychogenic eating disorder characterized by an all-consuming desire to remain thin. Anorexia nervosa and a similar eating disorder called *bulimia nervosa* are discussed in Chapter 20.

OTHER DISORDERS (CONTINUED)

DISORDER	DESCRIPTION
ascites ă-SĪ-tēz	Abnormal accumulation of fluid in the peritoneal cavity. General abdominal swelling, hemodilution, edema, or a decrease in urinary output may accompany the condition. Ascites may be a complication of cirrhosis, congestive heart failure, nephrosis, malignant neoplastic disease, peritonitis, or various fungal and parasitic diseases.
borborygmus bŏr-bō-RĬG-mŭs	An audible abdominal sound produced by hyperactive intestinal peristalsis. Borborygmi (singular, *borborygmus*) are rumbling, gurgling, and tinkling noises heard in abdominal auscultation. It is caused by passage of gas through the liquid contents of the intestine.
cachexia kă-KĔKS-ē-ă	A state of ill health, malnutrition, and wasting. It may occur in many chronic diseases, malignancies, and infections.
constipation kŏn-stĭ-PĀ-shŭn	A change in normal bowel habits characterized by decreased infrequent, difficult defecation or passage of hard, dry stools; sluggish action of the bowels.
diarrhea dī-ă-RĒ-ă *dia=through, across* *rrhea=discharge, flow*	A change in bowel habits characterized by the frequent passage of loose, fluid, unformed stools. It is a common symptom of gastrointestinal disturbances.
dyspepsia dĭs-PĔP-sē-ă *dys=bad, painful, difficult* *pepsia=digestion*	A vague feeling of epigastric discomfort, felt after eating. There is an uncomfortable feeling of fullness, heartburn, bloating, and nausea. Dyspepsia is not a disease in itself but symptomatic of other diseases or disorders.
flatus FLĀ-tŭs	Air or gas in the intestine that is passed through the rectum.
hernia HĔR-nē-ă	A protrusion or projection of an organ or a part of an organ through the wall of the cavity that normally contains it (Fig. 7–15).
femoral FĔM-or-ăl	A loop of intestine descends through the femoral canal into the groin. Surgical repair, or herniorrhaphy, is the usual treatment (see Fig. 7–15).

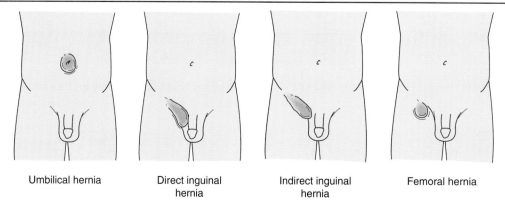

Umbilical hernia   Direct inguinal hernia   Indirect inguinal hernia   Femoral hernia

Figure 7–15 *Types of hernias. (From Williams, LS, and Hopper, PD: Understanding Medical-Surgical Nursing. FA Davis, Philadelphia, 1999, p 609, with permission.)*

OTHER DISORDERS (CONTINUED)

DISORDER	DESCRIPTION
hiatal hī-Ā-tăl	Protrusion of a portion of the stomach upward through the diaphragm, commonly producing no symptoms. The major difficulty in symptomatic patients is gastroesophageal reflux, the backflow of the acid contents of the stomach into the esophagus. Diagnosis is made easily on x-ray films, and the hernia may be an incidental finding on a chest radiograph. Surgical treatment is usually unnecessary, and efforts should be directed to alleviating the discomfort associated with reflux (Fig. 7–16).
inguinal ĬNG-gwĭ-năl	A type of hernia in which a loop of intestine enters the inguinal canal; in a man it sometimes fills the entire scrotal sac. An inguinal hernia is usually repaired surgically to prevent the herniated segment from becoming strangulated, gangrenous, or obstructive, thereby blocking passage of waste through the bowel. Of all hernias, 75% to 80% are inguinal hernias (see Fig. 7–15).
umbilical ŭm-BĬL-ĭ-kăl	A soft, skin-covered protrusion of intestine and omentum through a weakness in the abdominal wall around the umbilicus. It usually closes spontaneously within 1 to 2 years, although large hernias may require surgical closure (see Fig. 7–15).

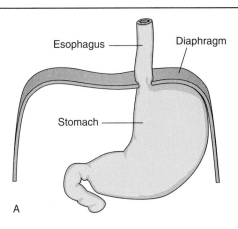

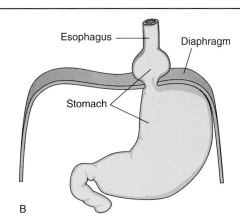

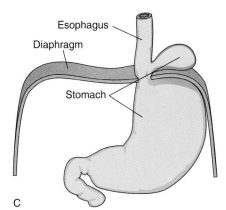

Figure 7–16   *Types of hiatal hernias. (A) Normal esophagus and stomach. (B) Sliding hiatal hernia. (C) Rolling hiatal hernia. (From Williams, LS, and Hopper, PD: Understanding Medical-Surgical Nursing. FA Davis, Philadelphia, 1999, p 579, with permission.)*

OTHER DISORDERS (CONTINUED)

DISORDER	DESCRIPTION
jaundice JAWN-dĭs	A yellow discoloration of the skin, mucous membranes, and sclerae of the eyes, caused by higher than normal amounts of bilirubin in the blood. Jaundice is a symptom of many disorders, including liver diseases, biliary obstruction, and hemolytic anemias. Also called *icterus*.
melena MĔL-ĕ-nă	Abnormal black tarry stool that has a distinctive odor and contains digested blood. It usually results from bleeding in the upper gastrointestinal tract and is often a sign of peptic ulcer or small intestinal disease.
nausea NAW-sē-ă	Unpleasant wave-like sensation in the throat or abdomen, usually preceding vomiting. Motion sickness, early pregnancy, diseases of the central nervous system, chemotherapy, and certain gallbladder disturbances may precipitate nausea. Sight or odor of obnoxious matter, or conditions or mental images of the same may result in nausea.
pruritus ani proo-RĪ-tŭs Ā-nē	Itching of varying intensity of the skin around the anus.
steatorrhea stē-ă-tō-RĒ-ă *steato=fat* *rrhea=discharge, flow*	Higher than normal amounts of fat in the feces; any condition in which fats are poorly absorbed by the small intestine.

Activity 7-10: Clinical Application

Pathologic Conditions: Accessory Digestive Organs and Related Terms

anorexia   hepatitis
ascites   hernia
borborygmus   jaundice
cachexia   melena
cholelithiasis   steatorrhea
flatus   volvolus

Match the terms listed above with the definitions given in the numbered list:

1. _____ abnormal amount of fat in the feces.

2. _____ intestinal gas that is passed through the rectum.

3. _____ black tarry stools that contain digested blood.

4. _____ protrusion of an organ or a part of an organ through the wall of the cavity that normally contains it.

5. _____ an audible abdominal sound produced by hyperactive intestinal peristalsis.

6. _____state of ill health and wasting that may occur in many chronic diseases, malignancies, and infections.

7. _____inflammation of the liver.

8. _____another word for gallstones.

9. _____a yellow discoloration of the skin caused by excessive bilirubin in the serum.

10. _____lack of appetite, resulting in inability to eat.

Correct Answers _____ × 10 = _____% Score

Diagnostic Procedures and Tests

Imaging Procedures

PROCEDURE	DESCRIPTION
barium enema (lower GI series) *BĂ-rē-ŭm ĔN-ĕ-mă*	Radiographic examination of the rectum and colon following administration of barium sulfate (radiopaque contrast medium) into the rectum. This procedure is used for diagnosis of obstructions, tumors, or other abnormalities, such as ulcerative colitis (Fig. 7–17). 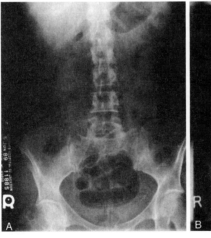 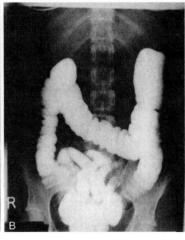 ***Figure 7–17*** *(A) An image of a patient who was poorly prepared for a barium enema. (B) An image of a patient who was adequately prepared for a barium enema. (From Williams, LS, and Hopper, PD: Understanding Medical-Surgical Nursing. FA Davis, Philadelphia, 1999, p 630, with permission.)*
barium swallow (upper GI series) *BĀ-rē-ŭm SWĂ-lō*	Radiographic examination of the esophagus, stomach, and small intestine following oral administration of barium sulfate (radiopaque contrast medium). Structural abnormalities of the esophagus and vessels, such as esophageal varices, may be diagnosed by use of this technique. Also used to locate swallowed objects.

Imaging Procedures (Continued)

PROCEDURE	DESCRIPTION
cholangiography kō-lăn-jē-ŎG-ră-fē	Radiographic examination for outlining the major bile ducts by intravenous injection or direct instillation of a radiopaque contrast material. This procedure has been virtually replaced by ultrasound and nuclear medicine procedures.
intravenous ĭn-tră-VĒ-nŭs	In intravenous cholangiography (IVC), a contrast agent is injected slowly into the vein, and radiographs are taken of the region of the gallbladder. Operative and postoperative cholangiography use the injection of contrast material into the common bile duct via a drainage T-tube inserted during surgery to reveal any small, residual gallstones that are still present. These procedures have been virtually replaced by ultrasound examinations.
percutaneous transhepatic pĕr-kū-TĀ-nē-ŭs trăns-hĕ-PĂT-ĭk *per=through* *cutane=skin* *ous=pertaining to* *trans=through, across* *hepat=liver* *ic=pertaining to*	A radiographic examination of the structure of the bile ducts. In percutaneous transhepatic cholangiography (PTC), a needle is passed directly into the hepatic duct, after which an opaque contrast medium is injected.
oral cholecystography (OCG) OR-ăl kō-lē-sĭs-TŎG-ră-fē *cholecysto=gallbladder* *graphy=process of recording*	A radiographic examination of the gallbladder after the ingestion of a contrast medium. At least 12 hours before the study, the patient has a fat-free meal and ingests a contrast material containing iodine, usually in the form of tablets. The iodine, which is opaque to x-rays, is excreted by the liver into the bile which is stored in the gallbladder. After the procedure, the patient consumes a fatty meal or **cholecystokinin,** which stimulates the gallbladder to contract, expelling bile and contrast material into the bile duct. Additional radiographs are taken 1 hour later. The test is useful in the diagnosis of cholecystitis, cholelithiasis, and tumors. This procedure is being replaced by ultrasound and nuclear medicine procedures.
computed tomography (CT) cŏm-pū-tĭd tō-MŎG-ră- fē	A radiographic imaging modality that is more sensitive than a conventional x-ray examination. A scanner and detector circle the patient's body, sending images to a computer, which allows the radiographer and physician to view any part of the body. The image produced represents a detailed cross section of tissue structure. CT is most frequently used to visualize the brain, abdomen, and chest. This procedure is painless and noninvasive and requires no special preparation. It was once called a computerized axial tomography (CAT) scan.
abdominal CT	Provides visualization of the internal organs of the abdomen, such as the gallbladder, liver, bile ducts, pancreas, kidneys, ureters, and bladder. Used in the diagnosis of tumors, cysts, inflammation, abscesses, obstructions, perforation, bleeding, aneurysms, and obstruction.

Imaging Procedures (Continued)

PROCEDURE	DESCRIPTION
endoscopic retrograde cholangiopancreatog- raphy (ERCP) *ĕn-dō-SKŎP-ĭk RĚT-rō-grād kō-LĂN-jē-ō-păn-krē-ă-TŎG- ră-fē*	Direct radiographic visualization with a fiberoptic endoscope, including radiographic fluoroscopy, to examine the size and the filling of the pancreatic and biliary ducts.

Used to detect strictures (narrowing) of the common bile duct, gallstones, cysts, tumors, and anatomical variations of the pancreatic and biliary ducts (Fig. 7–18).

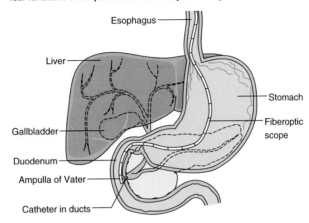

Figure 7–18 *Endoscopic retrograde cholangio- pancreatography (ERCP). (From Williams, LS, and Hopper, PD: Understanding Medical-Surgical Nursing. FA Davis, Philadelphia, 1999, p 632, with permission.)*

PROCEDURE	DESCRIPTION
fluoroscopy *floo-RŎS-kō-pē* *fluoro=luminous, fluorescence* *scopy=visual examination*	A radiographic technique for visually examining a part of the body or the function of an organ with a fluoroscope. An important advantage of fluoroscopy over conventional radiography is that the technique offers moving or dynamic images of internal organs, such as the heart and digestive tract organs.
magnetic resonance imaging (MRI) *măg-NĚT-ĭk RĚZ-ō-năns Ĭ-mă-jĭng*	Imaging procedure that uses radiofrequency radiation as its source of energy. Among its advantages are superior soft tissue contrast resolution, ability to image in multiple planes, and lack of ionizing radiation hazards. MRI is regarded as superior to computed tomography for most central nervous system abnormalities, particularly those of the posterior fossa, brainstem, and spinal cord. It has become an important tool in musculoskeletal and pelvic imaging; used to identify disease or deformity in the gastrointestinal tract.
ultrasonography *ŭl-tră-sŏn-ŎG-ră-fē* *ultra=excess, beyond* *son=sound* *graphy=process of recording*	Use of sound waves (ultrasound) to produce an image of an organ or tissue. Ultrasonic echoes are recorded as they strike tissues of different densities. Ultrasound diagnosis differs from radiologic diagnosis in that there is no ionizing radiation involved; synonymous with *sonography*.
abdominal	Ultrasonographic visualization of the internal organs of the abdomen, such as the liver gallbladder, bile ducts, pancreas, kidneys, bladder, and ureters.

Clinical Procedures

PROCEDURE	DESCRIPTION
endoscopy ĕn-DŎS-kō-pē *endo=in, within* *scopy=visual examination*	Visualization of the interior of organs and cavities of the body with an endoscope. The organ being examined dictates the name of the endoscopic procedure. Besides direct visualization, this procedure also is used to aspirate fluid, perform a biopsy, and coagulate areas of bleeding. A laser can also be passed through the endoscope, which permits endoscopic surgery. It is an important tool in establishing or confirming a diagnosis or of detecting a pathological condition.
upper GI	Visual examination of the esophagus (esophagoscopy), stomach (gastroscopy), and duodenum (duodenoscopy), using a lighted, fiberoptic endoscope (Fig. 7–19). Used to identify tumors, esophagitis, gastroesophageal varices, peptic ulcers, the source of upper GI bleeding, and the establishment of the presence and extent of varices in the lower esophagus and stomach in patients with liver disease. 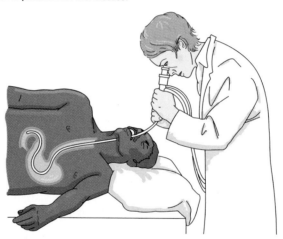 ***Figure 7–19*** *Gastroscopy. (From Williams, LS, and Hopper, PD: Understanding Medical-Surgical Nursing. FA Davis. Philadelphia, 1999, p 565, with permission.)*
lower GI	Visual examination of the colon (colonoscopy), sigmoid colon (sigmoidoscopy), rectum, and anal canal (proctoscopy) using a lighted, fiberoptic endoscope. Used to identify pathological conditions in the colon.

Laboratory Tests

TEST	DESCRIPTION
stool culture stool KŪL-tūr	The plating of feces to one or more culture media to grow colonies of microorganisms for the purpose of identifying specific pathogen(s).
stool guaiac **(hemoccult)** GWĪ-ăk	Test performed on feces using the reagent gum guaiac to detect the presence of blood in the feces that is not apparent on visual inspection (obscure, hidden, or occult blood). Hemoccult is the trade name of a modified guaiac test.

Laboratory Tests (Continued)

TEST	DESCRIPTION
liver function tests (LFTs)	A battery of tests used to determine liver cell dysfunction and liver disease.
alanine aminotransferase (ALT) *ĂL-ă-nēn* *ă-mē-nō-TRĂNZ-fĕr-āz*	Blood test to measure the concentration of the enzyme ALT in the blood. This test is considered a sensitive index of liver damage caused by a variety of disorders and numerous drugs, including alcohol. Elevations may also be seen in nonhepatic disorders.
alkaline phosphatase (ALP) *ĂL-kă-lĭn FŎS-fă-tās*	Test to measure the concentration of the enzyme ALP in the blood. Increased levels of ALP are found in liver disease.
aspartate aminotransferase (AST) *ă-SPĂR-tāt* *ă-mē-nō-TRĂNZ-fĕr-āz*	Test to measure the concentration of the enzyme AST in the blood, which is released following damage to cells, particularly cardiac muscle and liver cells.
gamma glutamyltransferase (GGT) *GĂM-ă glū-tă-mĭl-TRĂNZ-fĕr-āz*	Blood test to determine liver cell dysfunction and to detect alcohol-induced liver disease. It is also used to monitor the cessation or reduction of alcohol consumption.
bilirubin *bĭl-ĭ-ROO-bĭn*	Test to measure the bilirubin concentration in the blood. Patients with high levels of bilirubin have impaired liver function and appear jaundiced. Serum bilirubin levels are measured as total bilirubin, indirect bilirubin, and direct bilirubin.

OTHER DIAGNOSTIC PROCEDURES

PROCEDURE	DESCRIPTION
biopsy *BĪ-ŏp-sē* *bi=life* *opsy=view of*	Removal of a small piece of living tissue for microscopic examination, usually to establish or confirm a diagnosis, estimate prognosis, or follow the course of a disease.
aspiration *ăs-pĭ-RĀ-shŭn*	Removal of living tissue, for microscopic examination, by suction through a fine needle attached to a syringe.
liver	A special needle is introduced into the liver under local anesthesia to obtain a specimen for pathological examination.
needle	Removal of tissue for microscopic examination by use of a needle, usually attached to a syringe.

Surgical and Therapeutic Procedures
Surgical Procedures

PROCEDURE	DESCRIPTION
anastomosis *ă-năs-tō-MŌ-sĭs*	Surgical connection between two vessels; surgical joining of two ducts, blood vessels, or bowel segments to allow flow from one to another.
ileorectal *ĭl-ē-ō-RĔK-tăl* *ileo=ileum* *rect=rectum* *al=pertaining to, relating to*	Connection between the ileum and rectum after total colectomy, as is sometimes performed in the treatment of ulcerative colitis.
intestinal *ĭn-TĔS-tĭ-năl*	Connection of two portions of the intestines, also called *enteroenterostomy*.
cheilorrhaphy *kī-LOR-ă-fē* *cheilo=lip* *rrhaphy=suture*	Surgical procedure that sutures the lip, such as in the repair of a congenitally cleft lip or a lacerated lip.
colostomy *kō-LŎS-tō-mē* *colo=colon* *stomy=forming an opening (a mouth)*	Surgical creation of an artificial anus on the abdominal wall by incising the colon and drawing it out to the surface through which feces will be expelled into a disposable bag. It is performed for cancer of the colon, benign obstructive tumors, and severe abdominal wounds. Colostomy may be permanent or temporary. A temporary colostomy may be done to divert feces after surgery, as in the repair of the bowel in Hirschsprung disease, or from an inflamed area; it is repaired when the colon has healed or the inflammation subsides.
hemorrhoidectomy *hĕm-ō-royd-ĔK-tō-mē*	Excision of one or more hemorrhoids.
lithotripsy *LĬTH-ō-trĭp-sē* *litho=stone, calculus* *tripsy=crushing*	A procedure for eliminating a calculus in the renal pelvis, ureter, bladder, or gallbladder. It may be crushed surgically or by using a noninvasive method such as a hydraulic, or high-energy, shock-wave or a pulsed-dye laser. The fragments may then be expelled or washed out.
extracorporeal shock-wave *ĕks-tră-kor-POR-ē-ăl*	Extracorporeal shock-wave lithotripsy (ESWL) uses shock waves as a noninvasive method to destroy stones in the gallbladder or biliary ducts. Patients who are considered poor surgical risks and who have few cholesterol stones that are not calcified are the most likely candidates for ESWL. Ultrasound is used to locate the stone(s) and to monitor the destruction of the stones. After ESWL, the patient is usually placed on a course of oral dissolution drugs to ensure complete removal of all stones and stone fragments (Fig. 7–20).

Surgical Procedures (Continued)

PROCEDURE	DESCRIPTION

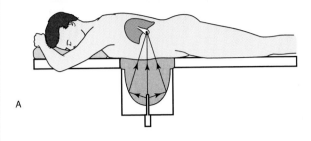

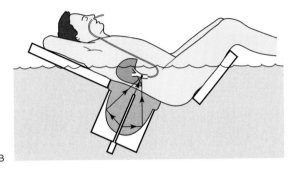

Figure 7–20 *Extracorporeal shock-wave lithotripsy. Shock waves are transmitted through water to break up gallstones. (A) Position for stones in gallbladder. Client is lying on a fluid-filled bag. (B) Position for stones in common bile duct. Client is in a water bath. (From Williams, LS, and Hopper, PD: Understanding Medical-Surgical Nursing. FA Davis, Philadelphia, 1999, p 665, with permission.)*

paracentesis
păr-ă-sĕn-TĒ-sĭs

para = near, beside, beyond

centesis = puncture

Surgical puncture of the peritoneal cavity (abdomen) to withdraw fluid.

An incision is made in the skin, and a hollow cannula or catheter is passed through the incision into the cavity to allow outflow of fluid into a collecting device. This procedure is most commonly performed to remove excessive accumulations of fluid.

Therapeutic Procedures

PROCEDURE	DESCRIPTION

gastric lavage
GĂS-trĭk lă-VĂZH

Washing out of the stomach; used to empty the stomach when the contents are irritating, as in prolonged postanesthetic vomiting and some cases of regurgitant vomiting in acute intestinal obstruction.

nasogastric intubation
nā-zō-GĂS-trĭk ĭn-too-BĀ-shŭn

naso = nose

gastr = stomach

ic = pertaining to, relating to

Insertion of a nasogastric tube through the nose into the stomach to relieve gastric distension by removing gas, gastric secretions, or food; to instill medication, food, or fluids; or to obtain a specimen for laboratory analysis (Fig. 7–21).

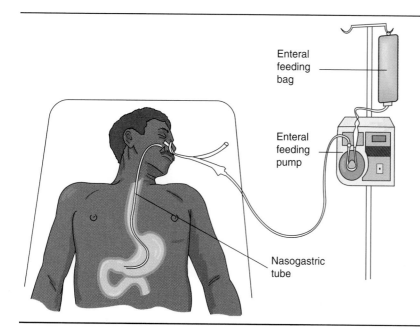

Enteral
feeding
bag

Enteral
feeding
pump

Nasogastric
tube

Figure 7–21 *Nasogastric tube connected to tube feeding pump. (Adapted from Williams, LS, and Hopper, PD: Understanding Medical-Surgical Nursing. FA Davis, Philadelphia, 1999, p 567, with permission.)*

PHARMACOLOGY

Over-the-counter or prescribed gastrointestinal drugs are used to treat disease conditions of the stomach and intestines. These conditions include diarrhea, constipation, peptic ulcers, ulcerative colitis, irritable bowel syndrome (IBS), or gallstones.

DRUG CLASSIFICATION	THERAPEUTIC ACTION
antacids ănt-ĂS-ĭdz	Drugs that exert a therapeutic effect by neutralizing acid, especially in the stomach and duodenum. Used to relieve gastritis, ulcer pain, indigestion, and reflux esophagitis (heartburn). Some antacids are combined with other ingredients, such as calcium. This is an additional benefit in women to supplement dietary calcium intake. Another combination antacid contains an additional ingredient, simethicone, to relieve flatulence. Most antacids are available without prescription.
antidiarrheals ăn-tī-dī-ă-RĒ-ălz	Drugs that relieve diarrhea either by absorbing the excess fluids that cause diarrhea or by lessening intestinal motility (slowing the movement of fecal material through the intestine), allowing more time for absorption of water.
antiemetics, **antinauseants** ăn-tī-ĕ-MĚT-ĭks, ăn-tī-NĂW-sē-ănts	Drugs that prevent or relieve nausea and vomiting, mainly by acting on brain control centers to stop nerve impulses. Also used to control motion sickness and dizziness associated with inner ear infections. Drugs that inhibit serotonin receptors are especially effective for the prevention of chemotherapy-induced nausea and vomiting. Some antihistamines and tranquilizers have antiemetic properties.
antiflatulents ăn-tī-FLĂT-ū-lĕnts	Drugs that reduce the feeling of gaseousness and flatulence accompanying indigestion. These agents facilitate the passing of gas by breaking down gas bubbles to a smaller size and by mildly stimulating intestinal motility. Cathartics, laxatives, and purgatives promote bowel movement or defecation or both. In smaller doses, they relieve constipation and are called *laxatives*; in larger doses, they evacuate the entire GI tract and are called *purgatives* (used before surgery or intestinal radiological examinations).

Pharmacology (Continued)

DRUG CLASSIFICATION	THERAPEUTIC ACTION
bismuth compounds *BĬZ-mŭth CŎM-poundz*	Agents that may be used for protective effects in ulcer disease and for mild to moderate diarrhea. These drugs are part of combination therapy for ulcers that are related to *Helicobacter pylori* infection.
emetics *ĕ-MĔT-ĭks*	Agents that induce vomiting, especially in cases of poisoning.
H₂ blockers (H₂ receptor antagonists)	Drugs used to treat ulcers and gastroesophageal reflux disease (GERD) by blocking the release of acid in the gastric parietal cells, which line the stomach.
mucosal protective agents *mū-KŌ-săl*	Agents that act topically on the ulcer surface and bind directly to necrotic areas, forming a protective layer over the ulcer, allowing it to heal.
prostaglandins *PRŎS-tă-glănd-ĭnz*	Substances that inhibit acid secretion and stimulate the production of protective mucus bicarbonate. These drugs may be especially useful in patients on long-term aspirin or nonsteroidal anti-inflammatory drug (NSAID) therapy to prevent the common side effect of gastric ulcers.
proton pump inhibitors *PRŌ-tŏn pŭmp in-HĬB-ĭ-tŏrz*	Specifically inhibit acid production; used in the treatment of peptic ulcers and gastroesophageal reflux disease (GERD).

❖ ABBREVIATIONS

COMMON ABBREVIATION	MEANING	COMMON ABBREVIATION	MEANING
BM	bowel movement	NG	nasogastric
Dx	diagnosis	PE	physical examination, pulmonary embolism
GB	gallbladder		
GER	gastroesophageal reflux	PMH	past medical history
GERD	gastroesophageal reflux disease	RLQ	right lower quadrant
GI	gastrointestinal	RUQ	right upper quadrant
HAV	hepatitis A virus		
HBV	hepatitis B virus		
HCV	hepatitis C virus	**DIAGNOSTIC TEST**	**MEANING**
HDV	hepatitis D virus		
HEV	hepatitis E virus	ABC	aspiration biopsy cytology
IBS	irritable bowel syndrome	ALT	alanine aminotransferase (elevated in liver and heart disease); new name for SGPT; enzyme tests of liver function
IV	intravenous		
LLQ	left lower quadrant		
LUQ	left upper quadrant		

DIAGNOSTIC TEST	MEANING
AST	angiotensin sensitivity test, aspartate aminotranferase (new name for SGOT)
alk phos	alkaline phosphatase
Ba	barium
BaE, BE	barium enema
BAO	basal acid output
BUN	blood urea nitrogen
cm	centimeter
CT	computed tomography
CT scan,	computed tomography scan
CAT scan	(x-ray images in a cross-sectional view)
Dx	diagnosis
EGD	esophagogastroduodenoscopy
ERCP	endoscopic retrograde cholangiopancreatography
ERS	endoscopic retrograde sphincterectomy
ESWL	extracorporeal shock-wave lithotripsy
FBS	fasting blood sugar
GBS	gallbladder series
GGT	gamma glutamyltransferase
GTT	glucose tolerance test
IVC	intravenous cholangiography
LFT	liver function test(s)
MAO	maximal acid output
OCG	oral cholecystography
PO	postoperative, period of onset

DIAGNOSTIC TEST	MEANING
PUD	peptic ulcer disease
UGI	upper gastrointestinal tract (x-ray)
MRI	magnetic resonance imaging
US	ultrasound

MEDICATION TIME SCHEDULE	MEANING
ac	before meals (ante cibum)
bid	twice a day
hs	at bedtime
npo	nothing by mouth
pc, pp	after meals (postprandial)
po	by mouth (per os)
prn	as required
qam, qm	every morning
qd	every day
qh	every hour (This abbreviation may also contain a number to indicate the number of hours between administration of medication or therapy, e.g., q8h.)
q2h	every 2 hours
qid	four times a day
qod	every other day
qpm, qn	every night
stat	immediately
tid	three times a day

Activity 7-11: Clinical Application

Diagnostic Tests, Treatments, Abbreviations, and Pharmacology

anastomosis
antacids
antidiarrheals
antiemetics
barium enema (lower GI series)
barium swallow (upper GI series)
biopsy
BUN
cathartics, laxatives, purgatives
computed tomography (CT)
emetics
endoscopic retrograde cholangiopancreatography (ERCP)

endoscopy
lithotripsy
magnetic resonance imaging (MRI)
nasogastric intubation
paracentesis
qam
qd
qid
stat
stool culture
tid

Match the terms listed above with the definitions given in the numbered list:

1. _____ radiographic examination of rectum and colon following administration of barium sulfate into the rectum.

2. _____ imaging procedure that uses radiofrequency radiation as its source of energy. Among its advantages are superior soft tissue contrast resolution, ability to image in multiple planes, and lack of ionizing radiation hazards; regarded as a superior procedure to CT.

3. _____ a surgical connection between two vessels, such as joining two bowel segments to allow flow from one to another.

4. _____ radiographic visualization with a fiberoptic endoscope including x-ray fluoroscopy to examine the size of and the filling of the pancreatic and biliary ducts.

5. _____ visualization of the interior of organs and cavities of the body with an endoscope.

6. _____ the plating of feces to one or more culture media to grow colonies of microorganisms for the purpose of identifying specific pathogen(s).

7. _____ a radiographic technique that is more sensitive than a conventional x-ray examination. It produces a film that represents a detailed cross section of tissue structure.

8. _____ excision of a small piece of living tissue for microscopic examination, usually to confirm or establish a diagnosis.

9. _____ radiographic examination of the esophagus, stomach, and small intestine following oral administration of a contrast medium.

10. _____surgical crushing of a calculus.

11. _____insertion of a tube through the mouth into the stomach to relieve gastric distension, to instill medications, food, or fluids, or to obtain a specimen for laboratory analysis.

12. _____agents that neutralize acid; used to relieve gastritis, indigestion, ulcer pain, and reflux esophagitis.

13. _____agents used to suppress nausea and vomiting; also used to control motion sickness and dizziness associated with inner ear infections.

14. _____agents that promote bowel movement or defecation or both.

15. _____agents that induce vomiting, especially in cases of poisoning.

16. _____every morning.

17. _____every day.

18. _____four times a day.

19. _____immediately.

20. _____three times a day.

Correct Answers _____ × 5 = _____ **Score**

Activity 7-12: Build Medical Words
Diagnostic, Symptomatic, and Surgical Terms

Use *esophag/o* (esophagus) to build words meaning:

1. inflammation of the esophagus _____

2. instrument to view or examine the esophagus _____

3. visual examination of the esophagus (with an endoscope) _____

Use *gastr/o* (stomach) to build words meaning:

4. inflammation of the stomach _____

5. disease of the stomach _____

6. enlargement of the stomach _____

Use *duoden/o* (duodenum), *jejun/o* (jejunum), or *ile/o* (ileum) to build words meaning:

7. visual examination of the duodenum (with an endoscope) _____

8. incision of the duodenum _____

9. suture of the jejunum _____

10. incision of the ileum _____

Use *enter/o* (small intestine) to build words meaning:

11. inflammation of the small intestine _____

12. disease of the small intestine _____

Use *col/o* (colon) to build words meaning:

13. visual examination of the colon (with an endoscope) _____

14. suture of the colon _____

Use *proct/o* (anus, rectum) or *rect/o* (rectum) to build words meaning:

15. herniation of the rectum _____

16. narrowing or constriction of the rectum _____

Use *cholecyst/o* (gallbladder) to build words meaning:

17. inflammation of the gallbladder _____

18. abnormal condition of gallstones _____

Use *hepat/o* (liver) or *pancreat/o* (pancreas) to build words meaning:

19. enlargement of the liver _____

20. inflammation of the pancreas _____

Correct Answers _____ × 5 = _____ % Score

MEDICAL RECORDS

This section covers medical records of a patient diagnosed with acute cholecystitis with cholelithiasis. Included are a consultation, an operative report, a pathology report, and a discharge summary.

The following reading and dictionary exercise and medical record analysis will help you develop skills to abstract information and master the terminology in the reports. In turn, you will be able to understand the importance of accurately interpreting information from a medical record. Accurate interpretation is important because this information is used to initiate treatments, evaluate the patient's progress, and complete insurance claims for third-party reimbursements.

Reading and Dictionary Exercise

Place a check mark in the box [✓] after you complete the exercise.

[   ] **1.** Underline the following words in the records as you read aloud the consultation, the operative report, the pathology report, and the discharge summary. These medical records can be found at the end of the chapter.

[   ] **2.** Use a medical dictionary and Appendix F, Part 2 to define the following terms.

Note: You are not expected to fully understand all the parts of the medical records. The important aspect of this exercise is to use all resources that are available to complete it. Eventually you will master the terminology and format of these reports.

> > > MEDICAL RECORD 7-1: CONSULTATION

Term	Pronunciation	Meaning
jaundice	JAWN-dĭs	_____
hysterectomy	hĭs-tĕr-ĔK-tō-mē	_____
appendectomy	ă-pĕn-DĔK-tō-mē	_____
hypertension	hī-pĕr-TĔN-shŭn	_____
afebrile	ă-FĔB-rĭl	_____
edentulous	ē-DĔNT-ū-lŭs	_____
organomegaly	or-gă-nō-MĔG-ă-lē	_____
bruits	brwē	_____
guaiac	GWĪ-ăk	_____
varicosities	văr-ĭ-KŌS-ĭ-tēz	_____
cholecystitis	kō-lē-sĭs-TĪ-tĭs	_____
cholelithiasis	kō-lē-lĭ-THĪ-ă-sĭs	_____
exogenous	ĕks-ŎJ-ĕ-nŭs	_____
obesity	ō-BĒ-sĭ-tē	_____
hypercholesterolemia	hī-pĕr-kō-lĕs-tĕr-ōl-Ē-mē-ă	_____
cholangiograms	kō-LĂN-jĕ-ō-grămz	_____

> > > MEDICAL RECORD 7-2: OPERATIVE REPORT

Term	Pronunciation	Meaning
purulent	PŪR-ū-lĕnt	_____
gangrenous	GĂNG-grĕ-nŭs	_____
peritonitis	pĕr-ĭ-tō-NĪ-tĭs	_____
cholecystectomy	kō-lē-sĭs-TĔK-tō-mē	_____
cholangiography	kō-lăn-jē-ŎG-ră-fē	_____
endotracheal	ĕn-dō-TRĀ-kē-ăl	_____
anesthetic	ăn-ĕs-THĔT-ĭk	_____
peritoneal cavity	pĕr-ĭ-tō-NĒ-ăl	_____
exudate	ĔKS-ū-dāt	_____
omentum	ō-MĔN-tŭm	_____
perforation	pĕr-fō-RĀ-shŭn	_____
anaerobic	ăn-ĕr-Ō-bĭk	_____
fossa	FŎS-ă	_____
fundus	FŬN-dŭs	_____
duodenum	dū-ō-DĒ-nŭm	_____
electrocoagulation	ē-lĕk-trō-kō-ăg-ū-LĂ-shŭn	_____
lavaged	lă-VĂZHD	_____
saline	SĀ-lēn	_____
infrahepatic	ĭn-fră-hĕ-PĂT-ĭk	_____

> > > MEDICAL RECORD 7-3: PATHOLOGY REPORT

Term	Pronunciation	Meaning
gangrene	GĂNG-grēn	_____
serosal	sĕ-RŌ-săl	_____
hemorrhagic	hĕm-ō-RĂJ-ĭk	_____
edematous	ĕ-DĒ-mă-tŭs	_____
mucosa	mū-KŌ-să	_____

purulence   *PŪR-ū-lĕns*   _____

polyps   *PŎL-ĭps*   _____

induration   *ĭn-dū-RĀ-shŭn*   _____

ulceration   *ŭl-sĕr-Ā-shŭn*   _____

necrosis   *nĕ-KRŌ-sĭs*   _____

epithelium   *ĕp-ĭ-THĒ-lē-ŭm*   _____

lithiasis   *lĭth-Ī-ă-sĭs*   _____

> > > MEDICAL RECORD 7-4: DISCHARGE SUMMARY

Term	Pronunciation	Meaning
Cipro	*SĪ-prō*	_____
Flagyl	*FLĂ-jĭl*	_____
Darvocet	*DĂR-vō-sĕt*	_____
Nitro-Bid	*NĪ-trō-bĭd*	_____
Synthroid	*SĬN-throyd*	_____
Aldactone	*ăl-DĂK-tōn*	_____
hemoglobin	*HĒ-mō-glō-bĭn*	_____
hematocrit	*hē-MĂT-ō-krĭt*	_____
anemia	*ă-NĒ-mē-ă*	_____
electrolytes	*ē-LĔK-trō-līts*	_____
creatinine	*krē-ĂT-ĭn-ēn*	_____
sodium	*SŌ-dē-ŭm*	_____
potassium	*pō-TĂS-ē-ŭm*	_____
enterococcus	*ĕn-tĕr-ō-KŎK-ŭs*	_____
bronchospasm	*BRŎNG-kō-spăzm*	_____
paroxysm	*PĂR-ŏk-sĭzm*	_____
tachycardia	*tăk-ē-KĂR-dē-ă*	_____
dehydration	*dē-hī-DRĀ-shŭn*	_____

Critical Thinking: Analysis of Medical Records

This section provides experience in abstracting and analyzing information from medical records. At the same time, it reinforces the material presented in this chapter.

> > > MEDICAL RECORD 7-1: CONSULTATION

1. What type of surgeries did this patient have in the past?

_____

_____

2. What is Dr. Lee's diagnosis of this patient?

_____

_____

3. What findings in the physical examination led the doctor to suspect a gallbladder problem?

_____

_____

_____

_____

4. Does the physician think the patient can tolerate surgery at this time?

_____

_____

> > > MEDICAL RECORD 7-2: OPERATIVE REPORT

5. What did the surgeon observe immediately upon opening the peritoneal cavity?

_____

6. What else did he observe on the medial portion of the wall?

_____

_____

7. What complication arose with the coagulating mechanism during surgery? Was the surgeon able to rectify the problem?

_____

_____

> > > MEDICAL RECORD 7-3: PATHOLOGY REPORT

8. What type and size of calculi did the pathologist find when he examined the excised gallbladder?

_____

_____

9. What made the pathologist conclude there was purulence present in the mucosa?

_____

_____

> > > MEDICAL RECORD 7-4: DISCHARGE SUMMARY

10. Upon discharge, what antibiotics did the patient have to take? Why were these prescribed?

_____

11. Did the patient have an uneventful recovery?

_____

12. Why was the patient sent home with a short prescription of iron tablets? How will the doctor know that the iron tablets were effective?

_____

_____

_____

Audio Practice

Listen to the audio CD-ROM to practice the pronunciation of selected medical terms from this chapter.

Medical Record 7–1. Consultation

GENERAL HOSPITAL AND MEDICAL CENTER
2211 Fifth Avenue North • Healthy City, USA 12345 • (321) 123-4567

Consultation

Patient Name: Jeanne Waters
Date of Birth: 04/23/1936

Patient Number: 67-53-22
Room Number: 323

DATE OF CONSULTATION: 05-01-20xx

REASON FOR CONSULTATION:
Dr. Stillwater has asked me to see Jeanne Waters, a 64-year-old widowed Caucasian female, a convalescent home resident in surgical consultation on the afternoon of May 1, 20xx, for evaluation of acute gallbladder disease. She was seen at approximately 1630 hours on that date.

This lovely elderly patient related that she became ill suddenly on the morning of April 27, 20xx, following a very small meal of cereal and juice. The pain and discomfort started in the upper abdomen and progressed to the right side of the abdomen. She tried some soup at noon but vomited about three times. She has really eaten very little since and had only ginger ale on the present date. On the next day, because of the abdominal pain, it happened that she was visiting her cardiologist, Dr. Joseph, and he modified her pacemaker. He also noted the abdominal discomfort and suggested an echo scan of the gallbladder and made arrangements. Nevertheless, with her progressive discomfort, the nurse at her convalescent home suggested that she be seen earlier, and this was done by Dr. Richardson, taking calls for Dr. Stillwater, who admitted her on 04/30/xx. Questioning for other previous similar symptoms is unrewarding and there is nothing to suggest jaundice, chills or fever. I refer you to the laboratory data obtained to date. She has had a previous lower abdominal surgery in the distant past including total hysterectomy and appendectomy. She carries the disease processes of coronary artery disease with a bypass in 19xx as well as a total hip replacement surgery. She had hypertension and hypothyroidism treated by Dr. Stillwater. She described an allergy to penicillin.

PHYSICAL EXAMINATION:
General: Pleasant, alert, elderly female who is quite obese but appearing her approximate chronological age.
Vital Signs: As noted in the nursing record, essentially afebrile to date.
Skin: Clear.
Lymphatics: Unremarkable.
HEENT: Ears, nose and throat are clear.
Chest: Clear.
Heart: A pacemaker is present in the left upper chest.

Continued

Consultation, page 2
Patient Name: Jeanne Waters   **Patient Number:** 67-53-22

Breasts: Modest size, no masses.
Abdomen: Moderately obese with very tender globular mass in the right upper quadrant. No other organomegaly or masses. Bowel sounds are normal, no bruits.
Pelvic/Rectal: Within normal limits except the noted soft, yellow-brown stool on the rectal glove. Guaiac negative.
Extremities: Evidence of previous hip surgery, no edema. There are fair distal pulses. No venous varicosities.

IMPRESSION:
1. Acute cholecystitis with cholelithiasis.
2. Exogenous obesity.
3. Chronic coronary artery disease.
4. Hypercholesterolemia, all by history and previously treated.
5. Status post total hip replacement surgery.

COMMENT:
I believe she has acute gallbladder disease until proven otherwise. I recommended that she have open gallbladder surgery with cholangiograms and explained this procedure to her at length including further care and possible postoperative complications. I believe she understands and agrees. I have also discussed the matter with Dr. Stillwater who feels that she is in the best shape possible at this point, and the surgery will be arranged as soon as the operating schedule permits.

I appreciate the opportunity to see this patient in consultation.

_____
Robert E. Lee, M.D.

REL/gmi
D: 05/01/xx
T: 05/04/xx

Medical Record 7–2. Operative Report

GENERAL HOSPITAL AND MEDICAL CENTER
2211 Fifth Avenue North • Healthy City, USA 12345 • (321) 123-4567

Operative Report

Patient Name: Jeanne Waters
Birth Date: 04/23/1936

Patient Number: 67-53-22
Room Number: 323

DATE OF PROCEDURE: 05/04/xx

PREOPERATIVE DIAGNOSIS: Acute cholecystitis with cholelithiasis.

POSTOPERATIVE DIAGNOSIS: Acute purulent cholecystitis with gangrenous change in wall and early perforation and localized peritonitis.

PROCEDURE PERFORMED: Cholecystectomy with operative cholangiography.

SURGEON: Robert E. Lee, MD.

ASSISTANT: E. M. Grant, M.D.

PROCEDURE: The patient was placed supine on an operating table and a general endotracheal anesthetic was administered uneventfully by Dr. Morse. The abdomen was prepared with heavy cleansing alcohol. The operating field was draped in sterile towels and sheets. A primary right subcostal incision was used in this very large (about 250 pounds) patient with an extremely generous abdomen.

Upon opening the peritoneal cavity, it was noted immediately that the gallbladder was quite inflamed and the omentum was packed around it. There was a fibrinous exudate overlying parts of the omentum but this could gradually be released revealing a markedly thickened and reddened gallbladder consistent with acute cholecystitis. In addition, on its medial portion of the wall, there was a gangrenous area that showed evidence of perforation and a purulent collection of about 25 cc of material as well as the fibrinous exudate. This was cultured for aerobic and anaerobic organisms. The gallbladder was released from the gallbladder fossa starting at the fundus and working to the neck, and because of the intense inflammation, this patient had marked vascular changes in the liver bed. These were packed away as dissection proceeded which could be done essentially with a finger until reaching a thickened area at the neck of the gallbladder. In this portion, very careful and gradual blunt dissection was performed identifying the cystic artery which was clamped divided and doubly ligated with 2-0 Tevdek and then clipped with a metallic staple.

Continued

Operative Report, page 2
Patient Name: Jeanne Waters   **Patient Number:** 67-53-22

The cystic duct was identified. In this patient, it was quite short measuring not more than 10 mm in length and extending into the common duct which could be visualized below and the common hepatic duct above. The neck of the gallbladder was tied with 2-0 Tevdek. The cystic duct was opened. Common clear bile escaped. Two operative cholangiograms using half strength radiopaque dye of about 10 cc each injection were obtained showing no evidence of filling defects and ready entrance of dye into the duodenum. The cystic duct was then clamped and doubly tied with the 2-0 Tevdek adjacent to the common duct but no impinging on it. As the films were being developed, the rest of the gallbladder was being released by blunt dissection and totally removed intact.

Not mentioned previously was that it was first decompressed before dissection was performed placing a purse string suture at the fundus and releasing all the purulent bile with a trocar and this bile was also cultured for aerobic and anaerobic organisms.

Now going on, the operative areas were inspected gradually and slowly, and hemostasis obtained with electrocoagulation. Unfortunately, our coagulating mechanisms sent off alarms apparently from her pacemaker or the right hip prosthesis so that several of these were tried. Fortunately, a satisfactory connection could be obtained and electrocoagulation proceeded to a satisfactory level.

In this patient, the liver was quite friable throughout. In all areas where there were raw surfaces, either Gelfoam or Surgicel packs were placed and hemostasis appeared secure when all of this was completed.

The operative areas were lavaged with copious physiologic saline, returns were clear. Two one inch Penrose drains were placed in the infrahepatic space and brought out through a separate inferior stab wound. The intestinal contents were replaced.

In view of the findings described, a general exploration was not performed in this patient except to note there was no evidence of acute disease within the duodenum or distal stomach which was decompressed with a nasogastric tube during the procedure.

The abdomen was closed in layers using running #0 Vicryl and the peritoneum and fascia supplementing the anterior fascia with interrupted #0 Vicryl, interrupted 3-0 Vicryl in the subcuticular tissues, and metallic staples in the skin. Lavage of all layers was performed with physiologic saline as closure was accomplished. Appropriate dressings were applied. Sponge, needle, and instrument counts were correct.

Continued

Operative Report, page 3
Patient Name: Jeanne Waters   **Patient Number:** 67-53-22

ESTIMATED BLOOD LOSS: Blood loss was abdominal about 700 cc because of the inflammatory findings described.

The patient's vital signs remained quite stable throughout and she was transferred to the Recovery Room in satisfactory condition.

_____

Robert E. Lee, M.D.

REL/sl
D: 05/01/xx
T: 05/04/xx

Medical Record 7–3. Pathology Report

GENERAL HOSPITAL AND MEDICAL CENTER
2211 Fifth Avenue North • Healthy City, USA 12345 • (321) 123-4567

Pathology Report

Patient Name: Jeanne Waters   **Patient Number:** 67-53-22
Birth Date: 04/23/19xx   **Room Number:**   323

SPECIMEN: Gallbladder.

CLINICAL DATA: None provided
                     PREOP DX: Acute cholecystitis.
                     POSTOP DX: Acute cholecystitis with gangrene and perforation.

GROSS DESCRIPTION: Received is a large collapsed gallbladder which measures up to approximately 14.3 cm in length and between 4.0 and 7.0 cm in diameter. The gallbladder is partly opened. The gallbladder shows an area of perforation through a mottled, red-brown-tan dull serosa. Exudate focally covers the serosal surface. There is an area of marked thinning and the perforation including the area of thinning varies up to 2.5 x 1.5 cm in greatest dimension. Three black spherical calculi are present within the lumen of the gallbladder varying up to approximately 1.7 cm in greatest diameter. The wall is irregularly hemorrhagic, edematous and varies up to 1.0 cm in greatest thickness. The mucosa shows a patchy appearance alternating between red-brown and greenish with obvious areas of purulence present. No plaques, polyps, or areas of significant induration are encountered. Representative sections submitted.

MICROSCOPIC DESCRIPTION: Sections of gallbladder show multiple areas of mucosal ulceration with transmural necrosis and marked acute and chronic inflammation. There is also extensive edema in the wall of the gallbladder with fresh mural hemorrhage. Areas containing an intact mucosa show mucous cell metaplasia of the epithelium with a patchy slight chronic inflammatory cell infiltrate. No Rokitansky-Aschoff sinuses are identified.

DIAGNOSIS: 1. GALLBLADDER, CHOLECYSTECTOMY – ACUTE
                         GANGRENOUS CHOLECYSTITIS.
                     2. LITHIASIS.
                     3. MILD CHRONIC CHOLECYSTITIS.

———————————————————
Richard W. Gisson, MD

RWG/bab
D&T: 05/04/xx

Medical Record 7–4. Discharge Summary

GENERAL HOSPITAL AND MEDICAL CENTER
2211 Fifth Avenue North • Healthy City, USA 12345 • (321) 123-4567

Discharge Summary

Patient Name: Jeanne Waters   **Patient Number:** 67-53-22
Birth Date: 04/23/1936   **Room Number:** 323

DATE OF ADMISSION: April 30, 20xx

DATE OF DISCHARGE: May 7, 20xx

DISCHARGE MEDICATIONS:
1. Cipro 500 mg b.i.d.
2. Flagyl 500 mg t.i.d. for 5 days.
3. Darvocet-N 100 q.4h. p.r.n.
4. Nitro-Bid ½ inch q.6h.
5. Synthroid 0.25 mg q.d.
6. Aldactone 25 mg q.d.

HISTORY OF PRESENT ILLNESS: The patient presented with abdominal pain on the right side with vomiting. The patient was seen by Dr. Joseph for possible pacemaker problem, and ultrasound of the abdomen was done in view of this patient's problem. The patient presented to the emergency room with these complaints in my absence and was found to have acute cholecystitis secondary to cholelithiasis. The patient was admitted, was given Rocephin intravenously. Dr. Lee was consulted relative to surgery. The patient's admission hemoglobin was 12.1, hematocrit 37, WBC 15.7. At the time of discharge, hemoglobin is 9, hematocrit 27, WBC 7.4. This anemia is secondary to blood loss at the time of surgery. The patient's iron level is 10. Electrolytes show BUN 49, creatinine 2.5 at the time of admission. At the time of discharge, BUN is 25, creatinine 1.6, sodium 141, potassium 3.8, chloride 112. Anaerobic and aerobic cultures from core blood show group D strep, not enterococcus, and the patient was being sent home with Cipro and Flagyl. Acute cholecystitis was seen on the pathology report.

In recovery, the patient had problem with bronchospasm, and a small paroxysm of atrial tachycardia was seen. The patient was seen by Dr. Joseph for cardiology consultation.

The patient overall remained stable, hemoglobin remained stable during the hospitalization. She is being sent home with a short prescription of multi-vitamins and iron tablets. A CBC will be checked on an outpatient basis. The patient will be followed by Home Health nurse.

Continued

Discharge Summary, page 2
Patient Name: Jeanne Waters   **Patient Number:** 67-53-22

DISCHARGE DIAGNOSES:
1. Acute cholecystitis secondary to acute cholelithiasis.
2. Anemia secondary to blood loss.
3. Hypertension.
4. Dehydration.

_____
Andrew Stillwater, MD

AS/jg
D: 05/07/xx
T: 05/09/xx

cc: Robert E. Lee, MD

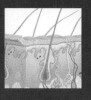

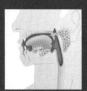
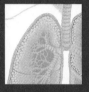

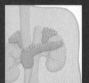

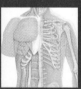

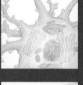

chapter

8 Pulmonology

Chapter Outline

Objectives

Upon completion of this chapter, you will be able to:

- Describe the type of treatment a pulmonologist provides.
- Name the organs of the respiratory system and discuss their functions.
- Recognize, pronounce, build, and spell terms related to the respiratory system.
- Describe pathological conditions, diagnostic tests, surgical procedures, and other treatments related to the respiratory system.
- Demonstrate your knowledge of this chapter by successfully completing the activities and analysis of medical records.

About Pulmonology

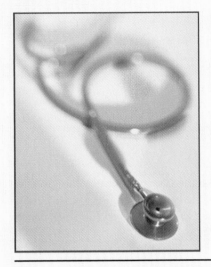

The medical specialty of **pulmonology** focuses on the diagnosis and treatment of diseases involving the lower respiratory tract: the lungs, its airways and blood vessels, and the chest wall (thoracic cage). Physicians who treat respiratory disorders are called **pulmonologists.** Some of the disorders pulmonologists treat include asthma, emphysema, chronic bronchitis, occupational and industrial lung disease, and pulmonary vascular disease. Pulmonologists also work with patients who require specialized ventilator support or lung transplantation. In general, pulmonologists are specialized to diagnose and manage pulmonary disorders as well as acute and chronic respiratory failure. Diagnosis and management of pulmonary disorders require a patient history and physical examination. They may also require pulmonary function testing, arterial blood gas analysis, chest x-rays, and chemical or microbiological tests. When needed, special tests and procedures, such as endoscopy and biopsy, are performed.

To grasp the scope of practice and the role of health-care practitioners in the medical specialty of pulmonology, it is important to understand the structure and function of the respiratory system as well as the language of medicine that is related to this medical specialty.

Selected Key Terms

alveoli (singular, **alveolus**) *ăl-VĒ-ō-lī*	Thin-walled microscopic air sacs in the lungs that exchange gases.
apex *Ā-pěks*	The top, the end, or the tip of a structure, such as the apex of the lungs or the apex of the heart.
bifurcate *BĪ-fŭr-kāt*	Divide in two branches or divisions; become forked.
bronchial tree *BRŎNG-kē-ăl* *bronchi=bronchus* *al=pertaining to*	Branched airways of the bronchi (singular, **bronchus**) and bronchioles that lead from the trachea to the microscopic airways in the lungs.
ciliated epithelium *SĬL-ē-ā-tĕd ĕp-ĭ-THĒ-lē-ŭm*	Epithelial tissue with hairlike processes (**cilia**) on the surface.
erythrocytes *ĕ-RĬTH-rō-sīts* *erythro=red* *cytes=cells*	Red blood cells (RBCs); erythrocytes transport oxygen and carbon dioxide (CO_2).
eustachian tubes *ū-STĀ-kē-ăn*	The tubes that connect the middle ear and the nasopharynx. These tubes are normally closed but open during yawning, chewing, and swallowing to allow equalization of the air pressure in the middle ear with atmospheric pressure; also called *auditory tubes.*
glottis *GLŎT-ĭs*	A slitlike opening through which air passes between the vocal cords.
hemoglobin *hē-mō-GLŌ-bĭn*	Component of RBCs that transports oxygen to the cells of the body.

homeostasis *hō-mē-ō-STĀ-sĭs* *homeo=same* *stasis=standing still*	A relative constancy or equilibrium in the internal environment of the body. This balance is naturally maintained by adaptive responses that promote a healthy survival.
olfactory nerves *ŏl-FĂK-tō-rē*	Nerves that transmit signals controlling the sense of smell.
patent *PĀ-tĕnt*	Wide open and unblocked, such as a patent airway.
phrenic nerve *frĕn-ĭk*	Nerve that extends through the thorax and provides innervation of the diaphragm.
pleural membranes *PLOO-răl*	Double-folded membranes that enclose the lungs; comprise the visceral and parietal pleura.
uvula *Ū-vū-lă*	Small, soft structure suspended from the soft palate.

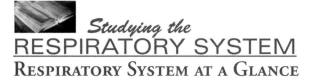

Studying the RESPIRATORY SYSTEM

Respiratory System at a Glance

Even though the human body requires oxygen continuously, it is incapable of storing it. Consequently, we need to move air into and out of the lungs 24 hours a day. Yet we rarely think of our vital need to breathe until we develop a breathing disorder. We usually breathe 12 to 20 times per minute and faster if there is physical exertion involved or the need arises. The underlying need to breathe is controlled by involuntary centers in the brain, mainly the medulla oblongata.

Besides the involuntary centers in the brain, the breathing process is dependent on the anatomic structures and the physical functions of organs in the respiratory system. The primary function of the respiratory system is the exchange of gases between the environmental air and the blood. This function involves three processes:

1. Ventilation, or breathing, the inspiration (inflow) and expiration (outflow) of air into and out of the lungs

2. External respiration, the exchange of gases between the air in the lungs and the bloodstream

3. Internal respiration, the exchange of gases between the bloodstream and the cells.

The first two functions are carried out by the respiratory system, and the third is carried out by the cardiovascular system. Nevertheless, the respiratory system, in conjunction with the cardiovascular system, transports a continuous supply of oxygen necessary to sustain the life of all body cells. It is essential that the circulatory system function properly for the transportation of these gases in the bloodstream. Failure of either system has the same effect on the body: disruption of **homeostasis** and rapid death of cells from oxygen starvation.

The interrelationship of the respiratory system with other body systems is illustrated in Figure 8–1.

Structure and Function

The respiratory system is divided into the upper respiratory tract and the lower respiratory tract. The upper respiratory tract comprises structures located outside the chest cavity: the air passages of the nose, nasal cavities, pharynx, larynx, and upper trachea. The lower respiratory tract comprises structures located within the chest cavity: the lower trachea and the lungs, as well as the bronchial tubes and alveoli. Pleural membranes and the respiratory muscles are also part of the respiratory system.

Label Figure 8–2 as you read the following material.

Air enters and exits the respiratory system through the (1) **nose,** which consists of bone and cartilage. The (2) **nostrils** (nares) are lined with a mucous membrane and hairs (**cilia**), which filter, moisten, and warm incoming air. The mucous membrane is composed of **ciliated epithelial** tissue and is highly vascular. A bony, cartilaginous plate called the *nasal septum* separates the two nasal cavities. The (3) **olfactory recep-**

Body System Connections
Respiratory System

THE CARDIOVASCULAR SYSTEM

◆ The heart pumps oxygen-deficient blood to the lungs, where the blood exchanges carbon dioxide for oxygen-rich blood.

THE DIGESTIVE SYSTEM

◆ A common anatomic structure is shared by the digestive and respiratory systems. ◆ The respiratory system provides oxygen and removes carbon dioxide produced by the organs in the digestive system.

THE ENDOCRINE SYSTEM

◆ The release of certain hormones increases the rate of cellular respiration and dilates the bronchial tubes.

THE FEMALE REPRODUCTIVE SYSTEM

◆ Respiration rate increases during sexual activity. ◆ Fetal respiration starts before birth.

THE INTEGUMENTARY SYSTEM

◆ The skin protects the respiratory organs. ◆ Changes in respiratory rate may be due to stimulation of the skin's receptors.

THE LYMPHATIC AND IMMUNE SYSTEMS
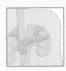
◆ A collection of lymphatic tissue around the tonsils protects the opening to the respiratory tract from pathogenic invasion. ◆ Immune cells patrol the lungs and defend against infection.

THE MUSCULOSKELETAL SYSTEM
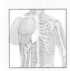
◆ Muscles related to breathing help the respiratory system expel carbon dioxide and inhale oxygen-rich air. ◆ The rib cage protects the lungs from injury, and provides attachments for muscles involved in breathing.

THE NERVOUS SYSTEM

◆ The nervous system regulates the rate and depth of breathing.

THE URINARY AND MALE REPRODUCTIVE SYSTEMS
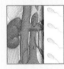
◆ Both the kidneys and the lungs control the pH (acid/base balance) of the body's internal environment. ◆ Water lost through breathing is restored by the kidneys. ◆ Respiration rate increases during sexual activity.

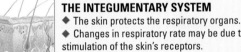

Figure 8–1 *The interrelationship of the respiratory system with other body systems.*

tors, located in the upper nasal cavities, are the receptors of the sense of smell. They also detect vaporized chemicals and other odors that may be harmful if one continues to breathe them. The **olfactory nerves** pass through the (4) **ethmoid bone** to the brain.

Pharynx

The throat, or **pharynx,** is located posteriorly to the nasal and oral cavities and functions as an air passage. It is divided into three parts: the nasopharynx, oropharynx, and laryngopharynx. The (5) **nasopharynx** is located behind the nasal cavities and is above the level of the (6) **soft palate.** Recall from Chapter 7 that the pharynx serves a dual role because it is a passageway for both air and food and has both respiratory and digestive functions.

The (7) **uvula** is part of the soft palate located at the back of the throat. During swallowing, the soft palate and its pendulous uvula close off the nasopharynx and prevent food from entering the nasal cavity. The (8) **pharyngeal tonsils** (adenoids) are masses of lymphoid tissue found on the posterior wall of the nasopharynx. Two (9) **eustachian tubes** join the nasopharynx and middle ear cavity. The eustachian tubes are normally closed but open during yawning, swallowing, or chewing to allow equalization of the air pressure in the middle ear with atmospheric pressure.

Although the nasopharynx is for air passage only, the (10) **oropharynx,** which lies behind the oral cavity, is both a food and an air passage. The (11) **palatine tonsils,** commonly known as the tonsils, are located in the oropharynx. Together with the (12) **lingual ton-**

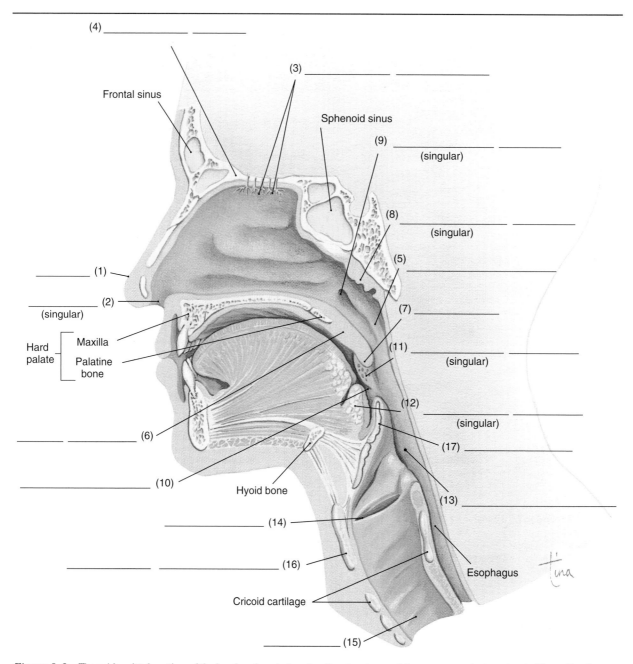

(4) _____ _____

Frontal sinus

(3) _____ _____

Sphenoid sinus

(9) _____ _____
(singular)

(8) _____ _____
(singular)

(5) _____

(1) _____

(2) _____
(singular)

(7) _____

Hard palate — Maxilla

Palatine bone

(11) _____
(singular)

(6) _____

(12) _____
(singular)

(17) _____

(10) _____

Hyoid bone

(13) _____

(14) _____

(16) _____

Esophagus

Cricoid cartilage

(15) _____

Figure 8–2 *The midsagittal section of the head and neck showing the structures of the upper respiratory tract. (From Scanlon, VC, and Sanders, TS: Essentials of Anatomy and Physiology, ed 3. FA Davis, Philadelphia, 1999, p 327, with permission.)*

sils, the palatine tonsils and the adenoids form a ring of lymphatic tissue around the pharynx designed to destroy **pathogens** that penetrate the mucosa.

As discussed previously, the (13) **laryngopharynx** is both a food and an air passageway. It opens anteriorly into the larynx and posteriorly into the esophagus. Muscular wall contraction of the oropharynx and laryngopharynx is part of the swallowing reflex.

Larynx

The (14) **larynx,** also known as the *voice box,* is responsible for sound production. It also functions as an air passageway between the pharynx and the (15) **trachea.** It comprises nine pieces of cartilage connected with ligaments. The larynx is made of firm, flexible tissue, which is **patent** at all times, unlike the esophagus, which is a collapsible muscular tube.

The (16) **thyroid cartilage,** commonly called the *Adam's apple,* is the largest of the individual cartilages. The (17) **epiglottis** is the uppermost cartilage and it closes over the top of the larynx during swallowing to prevent food entry into the airway.

Activity 8-1: Competency Verification
Upper Respiratory Tract and Larynx

Review Figure 8–2, and check your labeling in Appendix C.

Trachea

Label the structures of the respiratory system in Figure 8–3 as you continue to learn about the structure and function of the respiratory system.

The (1) **trachea,** or windpipe, is a passageway for air to the bronchi. It comprises smooth muscle embedded with 16 to 20 C-shaped cartilage rings that provide rigidity to keep the air passage patent. The trachea is about 4½ inches in length. It extends from the larynx and **bifurcates** into the right and left bronchi. One branch of the trachea leads to the (2) **left primary bronchus** (plural, bronchi) and the other to the

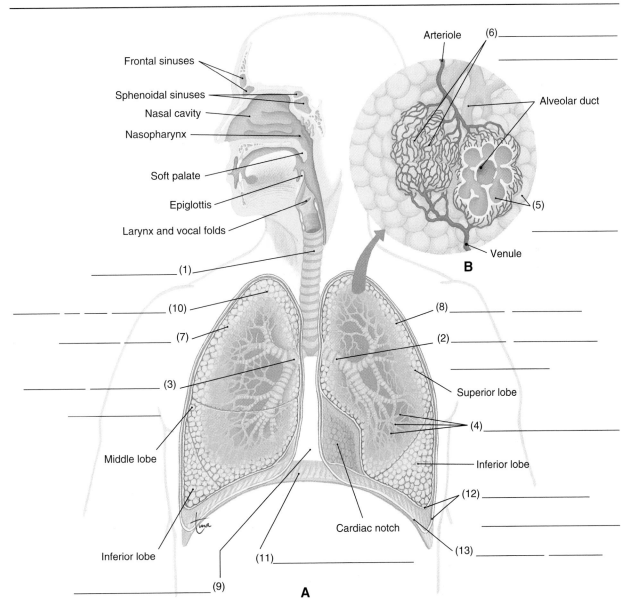

Figure 8–3 *The respiratory system. (A) Anterior view of the upper and lower respiratory tracts. (B) Microscopic view of alveoli and pulmonary capillaries. (The colors represent the vessels, not the oxygen content of the blood within the vessels.) (From Scanlon, VC, and Sanders, TS: Essentials of Anatomy and Physiology, ed 3. FA Davis, Philadelphia, 1999, p 330, with permission.)*

(3) **right primary bronchus.** The bronchi, like the trachea, contain C-shaped cartilage rings.

Once the primary bronchi enter the lungs, they subdivide into smaller bronchi, eventually forming (4) **bronchioles.** The continuous branching of the bronchi and bronchioles from the trachea resembles an inverted tree trunk with branches and is commonly referred to as the **bronchial tree.** Several structural changes take place as the branching becomes more extensive in the bronchial tree. The branches become smaller and smaller and no cartilage is present in the walls of the bronchioles. Absence of cartilage in the walls of the bronchioles becomes clinically significant in asthma when constriction of the bronchi occurs. The smallest bronchioles eventually terminate in clusters of (5) **alveoli** (singular, alveolus), also known as the *air sacs of the lungs.* They are like tiny balloons that expand and contract with inflow and outflow of air.

The inner surface of the alveoli is covered with a lipid material known as *surfactant,* which helps prevent the alveoli from collapsing. Because gases must dissolve in a liquid in order to enter or leave a cell, the alveoli are lined with a very thin layer of tissue fluid the function of which is to diffuse the gases.

Each lung has millions of alveoli that are encased by an extensive network of (6) **pulmonary capillaries.** It is through the moist walls of both the alveoli and the pulmonary capillaries that the blood picks up inhaled oxygen and deposits carbon dioxide, which is to be exhaled. The oxygen is transported in the blood by bonding to **hemoglobin,** a protein on the surface of RBCs, or **erythrocytes.** The pathway of inhaled air (oxygenated) and exhaled air containing carbon dioxide is illustrated in Flowchart 8–1. (Red represents oxygenated air; blue represents deoxygenated air.)

Lungs

The lungs are located on either side of the heart and are encircled by the rib cage. The (7) **right lung** has three lobes and the (8) **left lung** has two lobes. The (9) **mediastinum** is the space between the right and left lungs and contains the heart, aorta, trachea, esophagus, and bronchi. The (10) **apex of the lung** is at the level of the clavicle and the base rests on the (11) **diaphragm** below. The middle portion located in the midline region has an indentation called the *hilus.* That is where the primary bronchus and the pulmonary artery and veins enter the lungs.

A double-folded membrane known as the (12) **pleural membranes** or **pleura** surrounds the lungs. The outer layer of the pleura, which lines the thoracic cavity, is called the *parietal layer.* The inner layer of the pleura, which covers the lung, is known

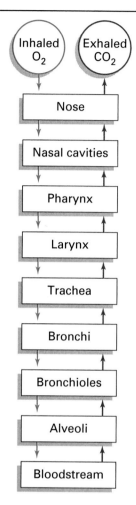

Flowchart 8–1 *Pathway of inhaled air (oxygenated) and exhaled air containing carbon dioxide. Red represents oxygenated air; blue represents deoxygenated air.*

as the *visceral pleura.* The (13) **pleural space,** a small space between these membranes, is filled with a serous fluid that prevents friction when the two membranes slide against each other during the breathing process.

Activity 8-2: Competency Verification

Lower Respiratory Tract

Review Figure 8–3, and check your labeling in Appendix C.

BREATHING PROCESS

As you read the following material, label Figure 8–4.

The entire process of gas exchange between the atmosphere and body cells is called *respiration.* Events of respiration include moving air into and out

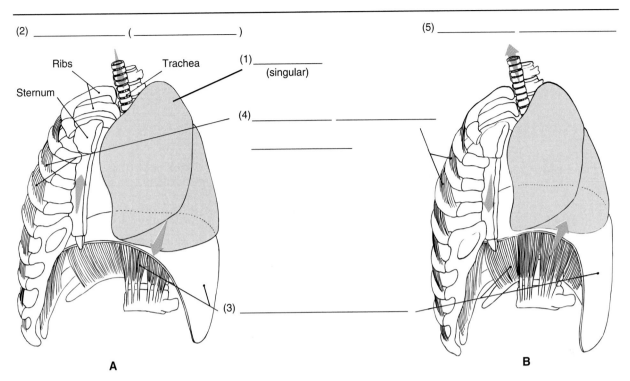

(2) _____ (_____)

Ribs   Trachea

Sternum

(1) _____
      (singular)

(4) _____ _____

_____

(3) _____

(5) _____ _____

A   **B**

Figure 8–4   *The actions of the respiratory muscles. (A) Inhalation: diaphragm contracts downward; intercostal muscles pull rib cage upward and outward; lungs are expanded. (B) Normal exhalation: diaphragm relaxes upward; rib cage falls down and in as external intercostal muscles relax; lungs are compressed. (Adapted from Scanlon, VC, and Sanders, TS: Essentials of Anatomy and Physiology, ed 3. FA Davis, Philadelphia, 1999, p 333, with permission.)*

of the (1) **lungs,** commonly called breathing or ventilation. The two types of respiration performed by the organs of the respiratory system are external respiration and internal respiration. External respiration refers to the exchange of oxygen and carbon dioxide within the lungs. This is the breathing process whereby a person breathes and exchanges air between the body and the outside environment. Internal respiration occurs in body tissues when oxygen (carried in blood from the lungs) is exchanged for carbon dioxide. This is the exchange of gases at tissue levels.

Breathing begins when the **phrenic nerve** stimulates the diaphragm to contract and flatten (descend). This causes an enlargement of the chest cavity, which creates a decrease in pressure within the thorax and draws air into the lungs. With each (2) **inhalation (inspiration)** of air, the (3) **diaphragm** contracts downward, and the (4) **external intercostal muscles** pull the rib cage upward and outward causing the lungs to expand. The diaphragm, a dome-shaped muscle, sep-

arates the thoracic cavity from the abdominal cavity. It is assisted by the intercostal muscles in changing the volume of the thoracic cavity by elevating and lowering the rib cage. The lungs are able to change capacity as the size of the thoracic cavity is altered. This ability is known as *compliance.* When the lung contains scar tissue or becomes diseased, compliance decreases and ventilation decreases. When the diaphragm relaxes, it moves upward into the thoracic cavity. This causes an increase in pressure within the thoracic cavity and forces air out of the lungs—the process of (5) **exhalation (expiration).**

Activity 8-3: Competency Verification
Breathing Process

Review the actions of the respiratory system in Figure 8–4, and check your labeling in Appendix C.

Activity 8–4: Competency Verification
Respiration

alveoli   nose
bronchi   olfactory
bronchioles   pharynx
larynx   pulmonary capillaries
lungs   trachea

Trace the respiration pathway by matching the terms listed above with the definitions given in the numbered list.

1. _____ the initial entryway for air into the respiratory system.

2. _____ referring to the receptors for the sense of smell.

3. _____ a passageway for both air and food.

4. _____ structure covered by the epiglottis during swallowing; another name for the *voice box*.

5. _____ structure that contains C-shaped cartilage rings; also called the *windpipe*.

6. _____ branching structures that lead to the lungs.

7. _____ structures that terminate in clusters of alveoli.

8. _____ the air sacs of the lungs.

9. _____ millions of structures that form the network encasing the alveoli.

10. _____ a pair of organs in the thorax, constituting the main component of the respiratory system.

Correct Answers _____ **× 10 =** _____ **% Score**

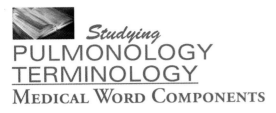

Studying
PULMONOLOGY
TERMINOLOGY
MEDICAL WORD COMPONENTS
Combining Forms

Combining Forms: Pulmonology

Combining Form	Meaning	EXAMPLE	
		Term/Pronunciation	Definition
UPPER RESPIRATORY TRACT			
nas/o	nose	**nas**/al NĀ-zl	pertaining to (-*al*) the nose
rhin/o		**rhin**/o/plasty RĪ-nō-plăs-tē	surgical repair (-*plasty*) of the nose to correct an anatomic defect or for cosmetic purposes
pharyng/o	pharynx (throat)	**pharyng**/o/scopy făr-ĭn-GŎS-kō-pe	visual examination (-*scopy*) of the throat
trache/o	trachea	**trache**/o/stomy trā-kē-ŎS-tō-mē	forming an opening (-*stomy*) by incising the skin over the trachea to permit an open airway *A tracheostomy is performed as an emergency procedure when the airway is blocked.*
LOWER RESPIRATORY TRACT			
alveol/o	alveolus (plural, alveoli)	**alveol**/ar ăl-VĒ-ō-lăr	pertaining to (-*ar*) the microscopic air sacs (alveoli) at the end of the bronchioles
bronch/o	bronchus (plural, bronchi)	**bronch**/o/spasm BRŎNG-kō-spăzm	involuntary contraction or twitching (-*spasm*) of the smooth muscle in the bronchi *This condition causes narrowing of the airway and occurs in asthma and bronchitis.*
bronchi/o		**bronchi**/ole BRŎNG-kē-ōl	smaller (-*ole*) tubular branches that are extensions of the bronchi

Combining Forms: Pulmonology (Continued)

Combining Form	Meaning	EXAMPLE	
		Term/Pronunciation	**Definition**
lob/o	lobe	**lob**/ectomy *lō-BĔK-tō-mē*	excision (-*ectomy*) of a lobe of any organ or gland *A lobectomy of the lung may be performed when cancer is localized in a particular lobe.*
pector/o	chest	**pector**/al *PĔK-tō-răl*	pertaining (-*al*) to the chest
steth/o		**steth**/o/scope *STĔTH-ō-skōp*	instrument (-*scope*) used to transmit to the examiner's ears sounds produced by the body *The stethoscope is used to hear breath and heart sounds as well as bowel sounds during the physical examination.*
thorac/o		**thorac**/o/centesis *thō-răk-ō-sĕn-TĒ-sĭs*	puncture (-*centesis*) of the chest to remove fluids *Excess fluid may need to be removed when it accumulates as a result of lung disease or as a common side effect of chemotherapy.*
pleur/o	pleura	**pleur**/itic *ploo-RĬT-Ĭk*	pertaining to (-*itic*) an inflammation of the pleura *The terms* pleurisy *and* pleuritis *are synonyms.*
pneum/o	air, lung	**pneum**/o/thorax *nū-mō-THŌ-răks*	collection of air or gas in the pleural cavity *Air enters as a result of a perforation through the chest wall or tear on the lung's surface. The suffix* -thorax *refers to the chest.*
pneumon/o	lung	**pneumon**/ia *nū-MŌ-nē-ă*	collection of air or gas in the pleural cavity
pulmon/o		**pulmon**/o/logist *pŭl-mō-NŎL-ō-jĭst*	specialist in the study of (-*logist*) pulmonary diseases
OTHER COMBINING FORMS			
anthrac/o	black, coal	**anthrac**/osis *ăn-thră-KŌ-sĭs*	condition of (-*osis*) coal dust in the lungs
atel/o	incomplete, imperfect	**atel**/ectasis *ăt-ĕ-LĔK-tă-sĭs*	incomplete expansion (-*ectasis*) of the lung; a collapsed lung

Combining Forms: Pulmonology (Continued)

Combining Form	Meaning	EXAMPLE	
		Term/Pronunciation	Definition
coni/o	dust	pneum/o/**coni**/osis *nū-mō-kō-nē-Ō-sĭs*	condition of (-*osis*) dust in the lung (*pneum/o*) *This is an occupational disorder that is caused by the inhalation of dust, especially during stone cutting or mining.*
hem/o	blood	**hem**/o/ptysis *hē-MŎP-tĭ-sĭs*	spitting (-*ptysis*) up blood
orth/o	straight	**orth**/o/pnea *ŏr-THŎP-nē-ă*	labored breathing (-*pnea*) that occurs when lying flat and is relieved by sitting up *Orthopnea is one of the classic symptoms of left ventricular heart failure.*
ox/o	oxygen	an/**ox**/ia *ăn-ŎK-sē-ă*	an abnormal condition (-*ia*) characterized by lack of oxygen *The prefix an- means "without," "not."*
phren/o	diaphragm, mind	**phren**/o/spasm *FRĔN-ō-spăzm*	involuntary contraction (-*spasm*) of the diaphragm.
spir/o	breathe	**spir**/o/metry *spī-RŎM-ĕ-trē*	measurement (-*metry*) or evaluation of air capacity of the lungs by means of a spirometer

Activity 8–5: Competency Verification
Medical Word Components

Check the box [✓] as you complete each numbered section.

[   ] **1.** Review the word components and their examples in the previous section. Then pronounce each word aloud.

[   ] **2.** For the following words, first write the suffix and its meaning. Then translate the meaning of the remaining components starting with the first part of the word.

> **Example:** nas/al
> **Answer:** *al*=pertaining to; nose

1. bronch/o/spasm   _____

2. pharyng/o/scopy   _____

3. rhin/o/plasty   _____

4. lob/ectomy   _____

5. pector/al   _____

6. pulmon/o/logist   _____

7. thorac/o/centesis   _____

8. trache/o/stomy   _____

9. alveol/ar   _____

10. bronchi/ole   _____

Correct Answers _____ **× 10 =** _____**% Score**

Prefixes and Suffixes

In this section, prefixes are listed alphabetically and
highlighted, whereas key suffixes are defined in the
right-hand column.

Prefixes

		EXAMPLE	
Prefix	**Meaning**	**Term/Pronunciation**	**Definition**
brady-	slow	**brady**/pnea _brăd-ĭp-NĒ-ă_	slow breathing (-_pnea_)
dys-	bad, painful, difficult	**dys**/phonia _dĭs-FŌ-nē-ă_	difficulty in speaking; hoarseness _The suffix_ -phonia _means "voice."_
eu-	good, normal	**eu**/pnea _ūp-NĒ-ă_	normal breathing (-_pnea_)
tachy-	rapid	**tachy**/pnea _tăk-ĭp-NĒ-ă_	rapid breathing (-_pnea_)
hyper-	excessive, above normal	hyper/**capnia** _hī-pĕr-KĂP-nē-ă_	excessive amount of carbon dioxide (-_capnia_) in the blood

Activity 8–6: Competency Verification

Prefixes and Suffixes

Check the box [✓] as you complete each numbered section.

[   ] **1.** Review the word components in the previous section. Then pronounce each word aloud.

[   ] **2.** For the following words, first write the suffix and its meaning. Then translate the meaning of the remaining components starting with the first part of the word.

> **Example:** hyper/capnia
> **Answer:** *capnia*=carbon dioxide (CO_2); excessive, above normal

1. phren/o/spasm _____

2. eu/pnea _____

3. anthrac/osis _____

4. tachy/pnea _____

5. an/ox/ia _____

6. brady/pnea _____

7. hem/o/ptysis _____

8. atel/ectasis _____

9. spir/o/metry _____

10. pneum/o/coni/osis _____

Correct Answers _____ **× 10 =** _____**% Score**

Pathological Conditions
Disorders Related to the Lungs, Bronchi, Pleural Cavity, and Pleural Membranes

PATHOLOGICAL CONDITION	DESCRIPTION
LUNG DISORDERS	
adult respiratory distress syndrome (ARDS) *ă-DŬLT RĔS-pĭ-ră-tō-rē dĭs-TRĔS SĬN-drōm*	A form of pulmonary edema in which dyspnea and tachypnea are followed by progressive hypoxemia. Also called *acute respiratory distress syndrome*, *wet lung*, and *shock lung*.
atelectasis *ăt-ĕ-LĔK-tă-sĭs* *atel=incomplete, imperfect* *ectasis=dilation, expansion*	A collapsed or airless condition of the lung or portion of the lung characterized by the collapse of the alveoli, preventing the respiratory exchange of carbon dioxide and oxygen. Some of the common causes include obstruction of the major airways and bronchioles, by compression on the lung from fluid or air in the pleural space, and a chest wound or tumor that causes air, fluid, or blood to accumulate in the pleural cavity. Immediate treatment includes reinflation of the lung to prevent necrosis, infection, and permanent lung damage.
consolidation *kŏn-sŏl-ĭ-DĀ-shŭn*	Process of becoming solid (solidification), as when the lungs become firm and inelastic from pneumonia.
chronic obstructive pulmonary disease (COPD) *KRŎ-nĭk ŏb-STRŬK-tĭv PŬL-mō-nĕ-rē dĭ-ZĒZ*	Any pathological process with chronic obstruction of the bronchial tubes and lungs. Diseases that may lead to COPD include emphysema, chronic bronchitis, chronic asthma, bronchiectasis, silicosis, and pulmonary tuberculosis. Smoking, prolonged exposure to polluted air, respiratory infections, and allergies are predisposing factors in the disease; synonymous with *chronic obstructive lung disease* (COLD).
emphysema *ĕm-fĭ-SĒ-mă* *emphys=to inflate* *ema=state, condition*	Chronic condition characterized by the destruction of the alveolar walls, which leads to permanently inflated alveolar air spaces. This condition results in poor ventilation, hypoxemia, and the use of accessory muscles to compensate for dyspnea, leading to a "barrel chest" appearance. Cigarette smoking is usually associated with this disease (Fig. 8–5A).
hyaline membrane disease, infant respiratory distress syndrome (IRDS) *HĪ-ă-lĭn MĔM-brān dĭ-ZĒZ, ĬN-fănt RĔS-pĭr-ă-tō-rē dĭs-TRĔS SĬN-drōm*	Atelectasis in the newborn, marked by cyanosis and dyspnea. This condition is caused by a lack of surfactant, a substance produced by the lungs to keep the alveoli inflated; usually related to premature births and infants born to diabetic mothers. This syndrome is the leading cause of death in prematurely born infants in the United States.

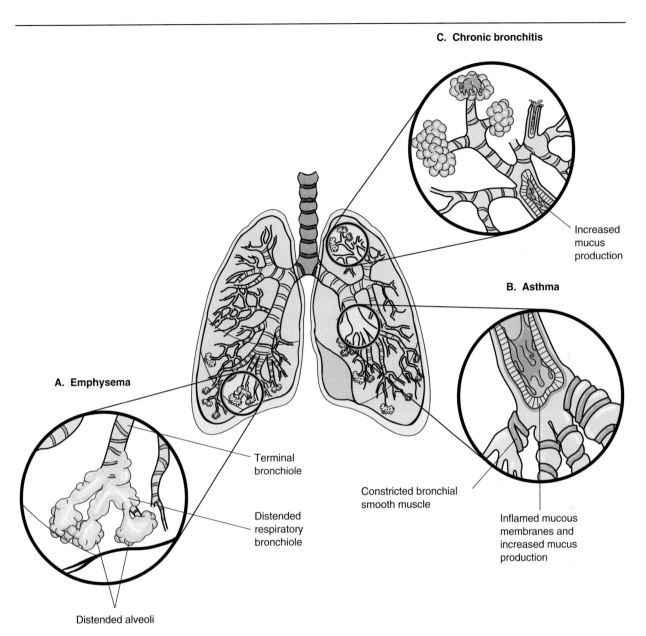

C. Chronic bronchitis

Increased
mucus
production

B. Asthma

A. Emphysema

Terminal
bronchiole

Distended
respiratory
bronchiole

Constricted bronchial
smooth muscle

Inflamed mucous
membranes and
increased mucus
production

Distended alveoli

Figure 8–5 *(A) Emphysema. Note distended bronchioles and alveoli. (B) Asthma. Note narrowed bronchial tubes and swollen mucous membranes. (C) Chronic bronchitis. Note inflamed airways and excessive mucus. (From Williams, LS, and Hopper, PD: Understanding Medical-Surgical Nursing. FA Davis, Philadelphia, 1999, p 529, with permission.)*

Disorders Related to the Lungs, Bronchi, Pleural Cavity, and Pleural Membranes (Continued)

PATHOLOGICAL CONDITION	DESCRIPTION
pneumoconiosis *nŭ-mō-kō-nē-Ō-sĭs* *pneumo=air, lung* *coni=dust* *osis=abnormal condition*	Lung disease resulting from prolonged inhalation of dust particles. The different types of pneumoconiosis are named according to the type of material that is inhaled; also known as *occupational lung disease*.
anthracosis *ăn-thră-KŌ-sĭs* *anthrac=black, coal* *osis=abnormal condition*	Accumulation of carbon deposits in the lung from inhalation of coal dust or smoke. Also known as *black lung disease* due to the black appearance of the lung.
asbestosis *ăs-bĕ-STŌ-sĭs* *asbest=asbestos* *osis=abnormal condition*	Lung disease resulting from inhalation of asbestos particles. This is linked to lung cancer, especially mesothelioma, and may take up to 20 years or more (latency period) to develop.
chalicosis *kăl-ĭ-KŌ-sĭs* *chalic=limestone* *osis=abnormal condition*	Lung disease resulting from the inhalation of dust produced by stone cutting.
silicosis *sĭl-ĭ-KŌ-sĭs* *silic=flint* *osis=abnormal condition*	Lung disease resulting from the inhalation of quartz dust.
pneumonia *nŭ-MŌ-nē-ă* *pneumon=lung, air* *ia=condition*	Infection of the lung caused by bacteria, virus, chemicals, or disease. Pneumonia can be classified by causative agent (etiologic agent) or by the anatomic location of the infection. Table 8–1 summarizes microorganisms that cause pneumonia. Table 8–2 lists four different types of pneumonia and the site at which the pneumonia occurs. Note that the type of pneumonia corresponds to the anatomic site in which it occurs.
pulmonary abscess *PŬL-mō-nĕ-rē ĂB-sĕs* *pulmon=lung* *ary=pertaining to, relating to*	Localized collection of pus in the lungs.
pulmonary cancer *PŬL-mō-nĕ-rē KĂN-sĕr*	A malignant tumor that frequently originates in the bronchi (bronchogenic). This type of cancer is the most common cause of cancer death in the United States for both men and women. Because it spreads (metastasizes) so rapidly, it is often diagnosed in the late stages and is difficult to control. Smoking is the most common cause of all types of pulmonary cancer.
pulmonary edema *PŬL-mō-nĕ-rē ĕ-DĒ-mă*	Accumulation of fluid in the alveoli and interstitial spaces; most common cause is left-sided congestive heart failure. Signs of mild pulmonary edema include orthopnea, cough, and rales. As congestion increases, hemoptysis occurs with worsening dyspnea and hypoxemia.
pulmonary embolus (PE) *PŬL-mō-nĕ-rē ĔM-bō-lŭs*	Blood clot or other material that travels through the bloodstream and lodges in the pulmonary vessels.

TABLE 8–1:   Causal Microorganisms of Pneumonia

VIRUS	BACTERIUM	PARASITE	FUNGUS
Adenovirus	*Escherichia coli*	*Pneumocystis carinii*	*Histoplasma capsulatum*
Cytomegalovirus	*Haemophilus influenzae*		*Candida*
Enterovirus	*Klebsiella pneumoniae*		*Coccidioides immitis*
Epstein-Barr virus	*Legionella pneumophila*		
Influenza viruses (A, B, C)	*Moraxella catarrhalis*		
Parainfluenza virus	*Mycoplasma pneumoniae*		
	Myobacterium tuberculosis		
	Neisseria meningitidis		
	Pseudomonas aeruginosa		
	Staphylococcus aureus		
	Streptococcus pneumoniae		
	Streptococcus pyogenes		

TABLE 8–2:   Infection Sites of Pneumonia

TYPE	SITE
Basal pneumonia	Consolidation at the base of the lung
Bronchopneumonia	Consolidation in the bronchus
Interstitial pneumonia	Inflammation involving tissue spaces within the lung
Lobar pneumonia	Partial or complete consolidation of one or more lobes of the lung

Disorders Related to the Lungs, Bronchi, Pleural Cavity, and Pleural Membranes (Continued)

PATHOLOGICAL CONDITION	DESCRIPTION
tuberculosis (TB) *tū-bĕr-kū-LŌ-sĭs* *tubercul=a little swelling* *osis=abnormal condition*	Infectious disease caused by the invasion of *Mycobacterium tuberculosis* into the lungs, which produces tubercles (granulomatous lesions) that usually remain dormant and asymptomatic until the immune system becomes impaired (immunocompromised) and then the active disease may occur. TB primarily affects the lungs but it can also infect any organ in the body. It is spread by inhaling droplets of respiratory secretions (aerosol transmission) or particles of dry sputum containing the TB organism. The incidence of this disease has decreased significantly until 1990, when multidrug-resistant strains began to appear. TB is seen most often in individuals with low incomes who are living in crowded conditions and in individuals with suppressed immune systems, such as those with HIV infection.

Disorders Related to the Lungs, Bronchi, Pleural Cavity, and Pleural Membranes (Continued)

PATHOLOGICAL CONDITION	DESCRIPTION
BRONCHIAL DISORDERS	
asthma ĂZ-mă	A respiratory disorder characterized by recurring episodes of paroxysmal dyspnea, wheezing on expiration/inspiration caused by constriction of the bronchi, coughing, and viscous mucoid bronchial secretions. The episodes may be precipitated by inhalation of allergens or pollutants, infection, cold air, vigorous exercise, or emotional stress. Treatment may include elimination of the causative agent, and various drugs, including inhaled agents that dilate the bronchi (Fig. 8–5*B*).
bronchiectasis brŏng-kē-ĔK-tă-sĭs *bronchi=bronchus* *ectasis=dilation, expansion*	Chronic dilation of a bronchus with a secondary infection that can result in destruction of the bronchial walls. Symptoms include expectoration of purulent sputum, coughing, and dyspnea.
bronchiolitis brŏng-kē-ō-LĪ-tĭs *bronchiol=bronchiole* *itis=inflammation*	Common infection in children under 18 months of age that is caused by the respiratory syncytial virus (RSV). Severity varies, and the virus causes inflammation and necrosis in the bronchioles with increased secretions, edema, and bronchospasm leading to small airway obstruction.
chronic bronchitis KRŎ-nĭk brŏng-KĪ-tĭs *bronch=bronchus* *itis=inflammation*	Inflammation of the bronchial tree characterized by hypersecretion of mucus, cough, and expectoration of sputum over a prolonged period of time. This condition is often caused by smoking, air pollution, or other environmental pollutants (Fig. 8–5*C*).
reactive airway disease (RAD) rē-ĂK-tĭv ĀR-wā dĭ-ZĒZ	Recurring episodes of paroxysmal (sudden) dyspnea and wheezing caused by constriction of the bronchi, coughing, and viscous mucoid bronchial secretions. The episodes may be triggered by inhalation of allergens or pollutants, infection, cold air, vigorous exercise, or emotional stress. It occurs most frequently in childhood or early adulthood, and is the leading cause of chronic illness in 5–10% of children. Treatment may include elimination of the causative agent, and drugs and aerosol treatments to dilate the bronchi and decrease bronchial inflammation. Also known as *asthma* (Fig. 8–5*B*).
PLEURAL CAVITY DISORDERS	
pneumothorax nū-mō-THŌ-răks *pneumo=air, lung* *thorax=chest*	Collection of air or gas in the pleural cavity. The presence of air at atmospheric pressure produces a separation of the membranes and prevents expansion of the lung, leading to atelectasis. Symptoms include dyspnea, tachycardia, and chest pain; other symptoms related to chest movements and mediastinal shift vary according to the type of pneumothorax.
open	A "sucking wound" caused by an injury such as a bullet or stab wound that creates an opening in the chest wall allowing air to enter the pleural cavity, resulting in immediate collapse of the lung (atelectasis) on the affected side (Fig. 8–6).

Disorders Related to the Lungs, Bronchi, Pleural Cavity, and Pleural Membranes (Continued)

PATHOLOGICAL CONDITION	DESCRIPTION

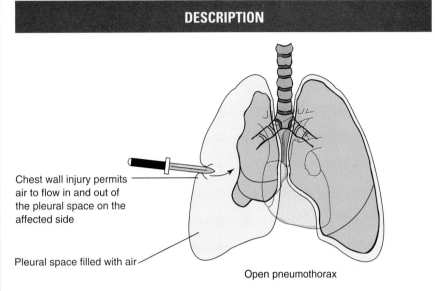

Chest wall injury permits air to flow in and out of the pleural space on the affected side

Pleural space filled with air

Open pneumothorax

Figure 8–6   *Open pneumothorax. (From Williams, LS, and Hopper, PD: Understanding Medical-Surgical Nursing. FA Davis, Philadelphia, 1999, p 541, with permission.)*

spontaneous, simple

Pneumothorax caused by an opening on the surface of the lung from the rupture of lesions as seen with lung abscess, carcinoma, emphysema, tuberculosis, or the spontaneous tear of the lung tissue (Fig. 8–7).

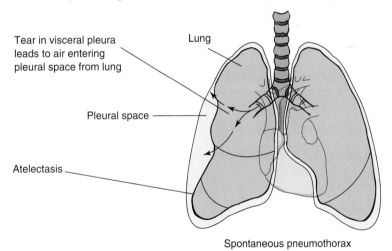

Tear in visceral pleura leads to air entering pleural space from lung

Lung

Pleural space

Atelectasis

Spontaneous pneumothorax

Figure 8–7   *Spontaneous pneumothorax. (From Williams, LS, and Hopper, PD: Understanding Medical-Surgical Nursing. FA Davis, Philadelphia, 1999, p 541, with permission.)*

tension

The most serious form of pneumothorax, which occurs when air enters the pleural cavity but is unable to escape.

This condition causes an increased intrapleural pressure, which leads to respiratory distress and hypoxia and becomes life-threatening if the increased pressure is not removed (Fig. 8–8). This type of pneumothorax is often related to high pressures caused by mechanical ventilation.

Disorders Related to the Lungs, Bronchi, Pleural Cavity, and Pleural Membranes (Continued)

PATHOLOGICAL CONDITION	DESCRIPTION
	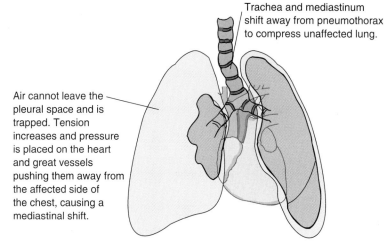

Figure 8–8 Tension pneumothorax with mediastinal shift. (From Williams, LS, and Hopper, PD: Understanding Medical-Surgical Nursing. FA Davis, Philadelphia, 1999, p 541, with permission.)

PATHOLOGICAL CONDITION	DESCRIPTION
pleural effusion PLOO-răl ě-FŪ-zhŭn	Passage of fluid into the pleural cavity. There are different types of effusions named according to the fluid.
empyema ěm-pī-Ē-mă	Pus in the pleural cavity.
hemothorax hē-mō-THŌ-răks *hemo=blood* *thorax=chest cavity, pleural cavity, thorax*	Blood in the pleural cavity.
hydrothorax hī-drō-THŌ-răks *hydro=water* *thorax=chest cavity, pleural cavity, thorax*	A noninflammatory collection of fluid in the pleural cavity that may cause dyspnea.

PLEURAL MEMBRANE DISORDERS

pleurisy, pleuritis PLOO-rĭs-ē, ploo-RĪ-tĭs *pleur=pleura* *isy=state, condition* *itis=inflammation*	Inflammation of the pleural membranes that causes them to rub together particularly during inspiration, producing severe, sharp pain (pleurodynia) and friction rub that can be heard or felt. Pleurisy may be caused by some other condition (secondary) or may be primary.

In the figure labels:

Trachea and mediastinum shift away from pneumothorax to compress unaffected lung.

Air cannot leave the pleural space and is trapped. Tension increases and pressure is placed on the heart and great vessels pushing them away from the affected side of the chest, causing a mediastinal shift.

Disorders Related to Respiration

PATHOLOGICAL CONDITION	DESCRIPTION
RESPIRATORY SOUND DISORDERS	
adventitious breath sounds *ăd-věn-TĬSH-ŭs brĕth sowndz*	Abnormal breath sounds heard on auscultation to the chest.
pleural friction rub *PLOO-răl FRĬK-shŭn rŭb*	Grating sound made by the motion of the pleural surfaces rubbing together; this can be heard by auscultation or felt through the fingertips when placed on the chest wall. This sound is associated with pleurisy, neoplasms, or other conditions and infections that result in a thickening of the pleura.
rales (crackles) *rāls*	Abnormal crackling sounds heard on auscultation of the chest during inspiration. The sounds are caused by passage of air through obstructed bronchi that contain secretions or exudates, or bronchi that are constricted by spasm. Although the term is commonly used, The American Thoracic Society now prefers the term *crackle* because it better describes the actual sound heard during examination.
stridor *strī-dor*	A high-pitched, harsh sound heard during respiration associated with obstruction of the larynx or bronchus; found in conditions such as croup.
rhonchus *RŎNG-kŭs*	A wheezing, snoring, or squeaking sound heard during auscultation of the chest of a person with partial airway obstruction.
wheeze *hwēz*	Continuous musical sound heard during expiration or inspiration produced by air passing through a partially obstructed airway. Wheeze occurs in asthma, croup, hay fever, and bronchitis.
RESPIRATORY PATTERN DISORDERS	
apnea *ăp-NĒ-ă* *a = without, not* *pnea = breathing*	Temporary cessation of breathing or respirations.
asphyxia *ăs-FĬK-sē-ă* *a = without* *sphyxia = pulse*	A condition caused by insufficient intake of oxygen. Some of the common causes of asphyxia are drowning, electrical shock, aspiration of vomitus, lodgment of a foreign body in the respiratory tract, inhalation of toxic gas or smoke, and poisoning. Artificial ventilation and oxygen are promptly administered to prevent brain damage. The underlying cause is then treated.
bradypnea *brăd-ĭp-NĒ-ă* *brady = slow* *pnea = breathing*	Abnormally slow breathing evidenced by a respiratory rate of less than 12 respirations per minute.
Cheyne-Stokes respiration *CHĀN STŌKS*	Abnormal breathing pattern marked by 10- to 60-second periods of apnea followed by deeper and more frequent respirations. This condition is often associated with impending death.

Disorders Related to Respiration (Continued)

PATHOLOGICAL CONDITION	DESCRIPTION
dyspnea dĭsp-NĒ-ă *dys=bad, painful, difficult*	Difficult or painful respiration; this can be due to exertion or a pathological condition or injury.
hyperpnea hī-pĕrp-NĒ-ă *hyper=excessive, above normal* *pnea=breathing*	An increase in the rate and depth of breathing.
hyperventilation hī-pĕr-vĕn-tĭ-LĀ-shŭn	Increased ventilation that results in high oxygen levels and decreased carbon dioxide levels (hypocapnia). Over a period of time this may cause chest pain, faintness, dizziness, and respiratory alkalosis.
hypopnea hī-pō-NĒ-ă *hypo=under, below* *pnea=breathing*	A decrease in the rate and depth of breathing.
Kussmaul breathing KOOS-mowl	Breathing pattern characterized by deep, gasping respirations; associated with severe diabetic acidosis. This type of respiration is associated with the body's attempt to counteract ketone build-up, which occurs with diabetic acidosis.
orthopnea or-thŏp-NĒ-ă *ortho=straight* *pnea=breathing*	Condition in which breathing is easier in an upright position, either sitting or standing.
paroxysmal nocturnal dyspnea (PND) păr-ŏk-SĬZ-măl nŏc-TŬR-năl dĭsp-NĒ-ă	Sudden, periodic attacks of shortness of breath (SOB) that occur at night and awaken the person.
tachypnea tăk-ĭp-NĒ-ă *tachy=rapid* *pnea=breathing*	Abnormally rapid breathing, evidenced by a respiratory rate of 40 or more respirations per minute; hyperventilation.
RESPIRATORY SECRETION DISORDERS	
hemoptysis hē-MŎP-tĭ-sĭs *hemo=blood* *ptysis=spitting*	Coughing or spitting up of blood.
mucus MŪ-kŭs	The viscous, slippery secretions of mucous membranes and glands containing mucin, white blood cells, water, inorganic salts, and exfoliated cells.

Disorders Related to Respiration (Continued)

PATHOLOGICAL CONDITION	DESCRIPTION
phlegm flĕm	Thick mucus secreted by the tissues lining the airways of the lungs.
sputum SPŪ-tŭm	Material coughed up from the lungs and expectorated through the mouth. Sputum contains mucus, cellular debris, or microorganisms, and it may also contain blood or pus.

Other Disorders

PATHOLOGICAL CONDITION	DESCRIPTION
anoxemia, **hypoxemia** ăn-ŏk-SĒ-mē-ă, hī-pŏks-Ē-mē-ă an = without, not hypo = under, below ox = oxygen emia = blood condition	Absence or deficiency of oxygen in the blood.
anoxia, hypoxia ăn-ŎK-sē-ă, hī-PŎKS-ē-ă an = without, not hypo = under, below ox = oxygen ia = condition	Absence or deficiency of oxygen in tissues.
anthrax ĂN-thrăks	A disease affecting primarily farm animals (cattle, goats, pigs, sheep, and horses), caused by the bacterium *Bacillus anthracis*. Anthrax in animals is usually fatal. Humans most often acquire it when a break in the skin has direct contact with infected animals and their hides, but they may also contract a pulmonary form by inhaling the spores of the bacterium. The cutaneous form begins with a reddish brown lesion that ulcerates and then forms a dark scab. The signs and symptoms that follow include internal hemorrhage, muscle pain, headache, fever, nausea, and vomiting. The pulmonary form is often fatal unless treated early. Treatment for both forms includes penicillin. A vaccine is available for veterinarians and for others for whom anthrax is an occupational hazard.
clubbing CLŬB-ĭng	Condition that affects the fingers and toes where soft tissue changes to firm, fibrotic enlargement at the end of the digits, and lateral and longitudinal curvature of the nails occurs (Fig. 8–9). This condition is found in many diseases of varying etiology, especially in lung diseases associated with chronic hypoxia.

Other Disorders (Continued)

PATHOLOGICAL CONDITION	DESCRIPTION
	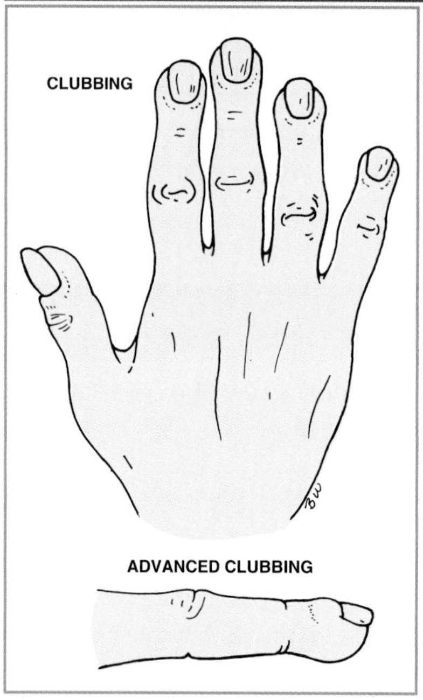 **Figure 8–9** *Clubbing. Note the lateral and longitudinal curvature of the nails. (From Venes, D: Taber's Cyclopedic Medical Dictionary, ed 19. FA Davis, Philadelphia, 1997, p 437, with permission.)*
cyanosis *sī-ă-NŌ-sĭs* *cyan=blue* *osis=abnormal condition*	Bluish discoloration of the skin and mucous membranes caused by the presence of reduced hemoglobin. This condition is caused by a deficiency of oxygen and an excess of carbon dioxide in the blood.
cystic fibrosis (CF) *SĬS-tĭk fĭ-BRŌ-sĭs*	Genetic disorder that produces a defect in the exocrine glands, causing abnormally thick, tenacious mucus. The glands most often affected are those of the respiratory system and the pancreas. The severity of this condition varies among individuals. In the lungs, the mucus obstructs air flow and stagnant mucus produces frequent bacterial infections. Improved treatment has increased the average life span to 30 years.
hypercapnia *hĭ-pĕr-KĂP-nē-ă* *hyper=excessive, above normal* *capnia=carbon dioxide (CO_2)*	Increased level of carbon dioxide in the blood.
mediastinal shift *mē-dē-ăs-TĬ-năl shĭft*	The effects of tension that increases in the pleural space, causing pressure on the heart and great vessels and pushing them away from the affected side of the chest (Fig. 8–8).
respiratory acidosis *RĔS-pĭ-ră-tō-rē ăs-ĭ-DŌ-sĭs*	This disorder occurs when there are above-normal levels of carbon dioxide (hypercapnia) in the body, which in turn causes a decrease in the pH of blood and body fluids.

Other Disorders (Continued)

PATHOLOGICAL CONDITION	DESCRIPTION
respiratory alkalosis *RĔS-pĭ-ră-tō-rē ăl-kă-LŌ-sĭs*	This disorder occurs when a person hyperventilates, which lowers the carbon dioxide level (hypocapnia) in the body and causes an increase in the pH of blood and body fluids.
sudden infant death syndrome (SIDS)	Unexpected and unexplained death of a healthy infant that typically occurs when the child is sleeping, usually between the ages of 2 weeks and 1 year.

Activity 8-7: Clinical Application
Pathological Conditions

adult respiratory distress syndrome (ARDS)
adventitious
anoxemia
anthracosis
asphyxia
atelectasis
bronchiectasis
bronchiolitis

consolidation
chronic obstructive pulmonary disease (COPD)
cystic fibrosis (CF)
dyspnea
emphysema
hemothorax
hydrothorax

hypercapnia
orthopnea
phlegm
pleurisy
pneumothorax
pulmonary embolus
tachypnea
tuberculosis (TB)

Match the terms listed above with the definitions given in the numbered list.

1. _____ difficult or painful respiration.

2. _____ material coughed up from the lungs and expectorated through the mouth.

3. _____ increased level of carbon dioxide (CO_2) in the blood.

4. _____ a group of lung diseases that is characterized by chronic persistent obstruction of the airway.

5. _____ abnormally rapid breathing; hyperventilation.

6. _____ chronic condition that develops slowly where there is destruction of alveolar walls and permanently inflated alveolar air spaces. Cigarette smoking is usually associated with this disease.

7. _____ solidification of the lungs caused by pneumonia.

8. _____ common infection in young children caused by the respiratory syncytial virus.

9. _____ condition caused by insufficient oxygen intake as in drowning, shock, inhalation of toxic smoke, or lodging of a foreign body in the respiratory tract.

10. _____ collapse of a lung or part of a lung.

11. _____ blood clot or other material that travels through the bloodstream and lodges in the pulmonary vessels.

12. _____ infectious disease that produces tubercles in the lung; contracted through aerosol transmission.

13. _____ inflammation of the pleural membranes.

14. _____ deficiency of oxygen in the blood.

15. _____ a form of pulmonary edema in which dyspnea and tachypnea are followed by progressive hypoxemia; also called *shock lung.*

16. _____ a noninflammatory accumulation of fluid in the pleural cavity.

17. _____ abnormal breath sounds heard on auscultation to the chest.

18. _____ genetic disorder that results in thick, tenacious mucus due to a defect in the exocrine glands.

19. _____ accumulation of carbon deposits in the lungs from inhalation of coal dust or smoke.

20. _____ collection of air or gas in the pleural cavity.

Correct Answers _____ × 5 = _____% Score

DIAGNOSTIC PROCEDURES AND TESTS

Imaging Procedures

PROCEDURE	DESCRIPTION
chest x-ray (CXR)	Radiograph of the chest taken from the anteroposterior (AP), posteroanterior (PA), or lateral projections.
	Used to diagnose atelectasis, masses, pleural fluid, air space disease (consolidation), pneumonia, interstitial changes, emphysema, and many other lung diseases.
chest computed tomography (CCT) *tō-MŎG-ră-fē*	Cross-sectional and three-dimensional imaging of the thorax; used to detect lesions in the lungs and thorax.
lung scan *lŭng skăn*	The use of radioactive substances or radiopharmaceuticals to image the lungs.
	This procedure is used effectively to diagnose blood clots in the lungs and pulmonary embolus (PE).

Imaging Procedures (Continued)

PROCEDURE	DESCRIPTION
magnetic resonance imaging (MRI) *măg-NĚT-ĭk RĔZ-ō-năns Ĭ-mă-jĭng*	This technique provides cross-sectional images of the thorax by exposure to magnetic and radio frequency energy sources. **Used to detect lesions in the thorax.**
pulmonary angiography *PŬL-mō-nĕ-rē ăn-jē-ŎG-ră-fē* *pulmon=lung* *ary=pertaining to* *angio=vessel* *graphy=process of recording*	Radiography of the blood vessels of the lungs after injection of a contrast medium.

Clinical Procedures

PROCEDURE	DESCRIPTION
tuberculin tests *tū-BĔR-kū-lĭn*	Diagnostic screening tests for tuberculosis..
Mantoux test *măn-TŪ*	Purified protein derivative (PPD) solution of *Myobacterium tuberculosis* is injected intradermally. A raised, red skin reaction after 48 to 72 hours confirms prior or present infection with tuberculosis.
tine test *tīn*	A four-pronged applicator that contains PPD solution is used to puncture the skin. A raised, red skin reaction is suggestive of tuberculosis. **A positive tine test result is followed up with the Mantoux test to confirm a positive tuberculosis diagnosis.**

Laboratory Tests

TEST	DESCRIPTION
arterial blood gas (ABG) *ăr-TĒ-rē-ăl blŭd găs*	A test that measures the oxygen and carbon dioxide in arterial blood by various methods to assess the adequacy of ventilation and oxygenation and the acid-base status.
culture and sensitivity (C&S)	Laboratory test that detects and identifies pathogenic bacteria and determines the appropriate antibiotic treatment. **Testing can be performed on sputum, blood, or any other body fluid specimen.**
sweat test	Analysis of a sweat sample to determine its chloride concentration; high levels are seen in children with cystic fibrosis.

Other Diagnostic Procedures

PROCEDURE	DESCRIPTION
auscultation *ăws-kŭl-TĀ-shŭn*	Use of a stethoscope to listen to sounds within the body, especially in the chest, neck, and abdomen; used to detect crackles or wheezes in the lungs, pleural rubs, and other physiological phenomena.
bronchoscopy *brŏng-KŎS-kō-pē* *broncho=bronchus* *scopy=visual examination*	Direct visualization of the bronchi using a flexible tube known as a bronchoscope, which is inserted through the mouth and trachea for the purpose of removing a foreign body, observing the air passages for disease, suctioning secretions, or obtaining a biopsy specimen or secretions for examination.
intubation *ĭn-tū-BĀ-shŭn*	Passage of a tube into a body aperture, specifically the insertion of a breathing tube through the mouth or nose into the trachea to maintain an airway or for the delivery of anesthetic gases and oxygen or both. Kinds of intubation include endotracheal intubation and nasotracheal intubation.
lung biopsy *lŭng BĪ-ŏp-sē*	Excision of a small piece of lung tissue for microscopic examination to confirm or establish a diagnosis; used to confirm a diagnosis of lung cancer.
mechanical ventilation	Use of a device referred to as a *mechanical ventilator*, which provides assisted breathing to the patient.
pulmonary function test (PFT)	Any of several different tests used to evaluate the condition of the respiratory system. Measures of expiratory flow and lung volume capacities are obtained. The forced vital capacity is one of the more important tests; it provides a measure of the amount of air that can be maximally exhaled after a maximum inspiration and the time required for that expiration. This test is commonly used to help diagnose and monitor chronic obstructive lung disease and other restrictive lung disorders.

SURGICAL AND THERAPEUTIC PROCEDURES

Surgical Procedures

PROCEDURE	DESCRIPTION
thoracentesis *thō-ră-sĕn-TĒ-sĭs*	Insertion of a needle between the ribs and into the pleural space. This procedure is often performed to aspirate fluid in patients with pleural effusion (excess fluid in the pleural space). The procedure may be diagnostic to obtain fluid samples from the pleural cavity for laboratory analysis, or therapeutic to remove fluid and reduce respiratory distress. If fluid accumulation is large or recurring, a chest tube might be placed to continuously drain the pleural space. It may also be performed to aspirate blood or air or to inject medication. Also called *thoracocentesis*.
thoracic surgery *thō-RĂS-ĭk SŬR-jĕr-ē*	Surgery involving the rib cage and structures contained within the chest.
thoracotomy *thō-răk-ŎT-ō-mē* *thorac=chest* *tomy=incision (of)*	A surgical incision that opens the chest for diagnostic or therapeutic purposes. Thoracic surgery may be performed for lung biopsy; for removal of tumors, lesions, or foreign objects; to repair trauma following penetrating or crushing injuries; or to repair or revise structural problems. Open-heart surgery also requires a thoracotomy and is discussed in Chapter 9.

Surgical Procedures (Continued)

PROCEDURE	DESCRIPTION
tracheostomy _trā-kē-ŎS-tō-mē_ _tracheo=trachea_ _stomy=forming an opening_ _(mouth)_	Surgical opening through the base of the neck into the trachea for the insertion of a tube to create an open airway (Fig. 8–10). The person breathes through this opening, bypassing the upper airways. Tracheostomy is performed on a variety of patients, including persons who have had a laryngectomy for cancer, persons with airway obstruction caused by trauma or tumor, persons who have difficulty clearing secretions from the airway, or persons who need prolonged mechanical ventilation. 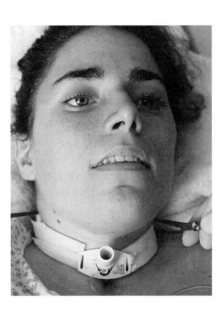 **Figure 8–10** _Patient with tracheostomy. (From Williams, LS, and Hopper, PD: Understanding Medical-Surgical Nursing. FA Davis, Philadelphia, 1999, p 494, with permission.)_

Therapeutic Procedures

PROCEDURE	DESCRIPTION
hyperbaric oxygenation _hī-pĕr-BĂR-ĭc ŏk-sĭ-jĕn-Ā-shŭn_	The administration of oxygen at greater-than-normal atmospheric pressure. The procedure is performed in specially designed chambers that permit the delivery of 100% oxygen at atmospheric pressure that is three times the normal level. This procedure is used to treat carbon monoxide poisoning, air embolism, smoke inhalation, acute cyanide poisoning, decompression sickness (formation of nitrogen bubbles in the tissues of divers and aviators who move too rapidly from environments of higher to those of lower atmospheric pressure), and other conditions. Also called _hyperbaric oxygen therapy._
nebulized mist treatments (NMTs) _NĔB-ū-līzd_	Use of a device for producing a fine spray (nebulizer) to deliver medication directly into the lungs. Topical use of this medication reduces systemic side effects. Bronchodilators, with or without oxygen, are most commonly administered. Other medications, including mucolytics and antibiotics, may also be given. Also called _aerosol therapy._
postural drainage _PŎS-tū-răl DRĀN-ĭj_	The use of body positioning to assist in the removal of secretions from specific lobes of the lung, bronchi, or lung cavities. The technique can be used in the treatment of pneumonias and other pulmonary infections, bronchiectasis, or chronic bronchitis, or for the removal of retained secretions.

Pharmacology

DRUG CLASSIFICATION	THERAPEUTIC ACTION
antibiotics ăn-tĭ-bī-ŎT-ĭks	Drugs that combat bacterial infection and have the ability to inhibit or kill foreign organisms within the body. Used in the treatment of bronchitis, pneumonia, and other respiratory tract infections.
anticoagulants ăn-tĭ-kō-ĂG-ū-lănts	Drugs used to inhibit blood clotting, and to treat a serious condition called *pulmonary embolism* (PE).
antifungals ăn-tĭ-FŬNG-găls	Drugs used to treat fungal infections. In the respiratory system, oral or intravenous drugs are used to treat lung infections.
antismoking agents ăn-tĭ-SMŌK-ĭng Ā-jents	Drugs that supply decreasing amounts of nicotine to help in the cessation of smoking. Different forms include nasal spray, chewing gum, and transdermal patches; also known as *nicotine replacement therapy*.
antituberculars ăn-tĭ-too-BĔR-kū-lărs	Drugs that inhibit the spread or progress of tuberculosis in the body.
antitussives ăn-tĭ-TŬS-ĭvs	Drugs that prevent or relieve coughing. They decrease coughing by anesthetizing the stretch receptors in the respiratory tract or by suppressing the brain's cough center.
bronchodilators brŏng-kō-DĪ-lā-tŏrs	Drugs used to expand the opening of the passages into the lungs, relaxing the smooth muscle of the bronchi, thereby increasing airflow. Used to treat asthma, emphysema, COPD, and exercise-induced bronchospasm.
corticosteroids kŏr-tĭ-kō-STĒR-oyds	Hormonal agents that reduce tissue edema and inflammation associated with chronic lung disease.
expectorants ĕk-SPĔK-tō-rănts	Agents that promote the clearance of mucus from the respiratory tract.
mucolytics mū-kō-LĬT-ĭks	A group of agents that liquefy sputum or reduce its viscosity so it can be coughed up more easily.

❖ ABBREVIATIONS

ABBREVIATION	MEANING	ABBREVIATION	MEANING
ABGs	arterial blood gases	mg	milligram (1/1000 grams)
AFB	acid fast bacillus (TB organism)	NMTs	nebulized mist treatments
ARDS	adult respiratory distress syndrome	PCP	*Pneumocystis carinii* pneumonia
		PE	physical examination, pulmonary embolism
BUN	blood urea nitrogen		
CBC	complete blood count	PEFR	peak expiratory flow rate
CF	cystic fibrosis	PFT	pulmonary function test
C&S	culture and sensitivity	pH	symbol for degree of acidity or alkalinity
CO_2	carbon dioxide		
COLD	chronic obstructive lung disease	pO_2	partial pressure oxygen
COPD	chronic obstructive pulmonary disease	PND	paroxysmal nocturnal dyspnea
		PPD	purified protein derivative
CPR	cardiopulmonary resuscitation	RAD	reactive airway disease
CXR	chest x-ray	RD	respiratory disease
FEF	forced expiratory flow	RDS	respiratory distress syndrome
FEV	forced expiratory volume	RSV	respiratory syncytial virus
FRC	functional residual capacity	RV	residual volume, right ventricle
FVC	forced vital capacity	SaO_2	arterial oxygen saturation
HCO_3^-	bicarbonate	SIDS	sudden infant death syndrome
HMD	hyaline membrane disease	SOB	shortness of breath
IPPB	intermittent positive-pressure breathing	TB	tuberculosis
		TPR	temperature, pulse, respiration
IRDS	infant respiratory distress syndrome	TV	tidal volume
		VC	vital capacity
L	liter, left, lumbar		

Activity 8–8: Clinical Application

Diagnostic Tests, Treatments, and Pharmacology

antitussives
arterial blood gas (ABG)
auscultation
chest computed tomography
expectorants
intubation

Mantoux test
nebulized mist treatment (NMT)
postural drainage
pulmonary angiography
thoracentesis
thoracotomy

Match the terms listed above with the definitions given in the numbered list:

1. _____ surgical incision to remove a tumor or obtain a lung biopsy from the lung.

2. _____ tuberculin test that is used to confirm a positive diagnosis of TB.

3. _____ insertion of an endotracheal tube through the nose or mouth into the trachea to maintain an airway.

4. _____ blood test to evaluate the levels of oxygen and carbon dioxide in the blood. It measures the adequacy of oxygenation.

5. _____ radiography of blood vessels of the lungs after injection of a contrast medium.

6. _____ use of a stethoscope to listen to sounds within the body, especially to detect crackles or wheezes in the lungs.

7. _____ treatment that uses gravity and patient positioning to remove secretions from the bronchi and lungs.

8. _____ agents that liquefy sputum or reduce its viscosity.

9. _____ insertion of a needle into the pleural space to drain air or fluid.

10. _____ a fine spray used to deliver medications directly to the lungs.

Correct Answers _____ **× 10 =** _____**% Score**

Activity 8–9: Build Medical Words
Diagnostic, Symptomatic, and Operative Terms

Use *rhin/o* (nose) to build medical words meaning:

1. discharge from the nose _____

2. inflammation of the (mucous membranes of the) nose _____

Use *bronch/o* (bronchus, bronchi) to build medical words meaning:

3. pertaining to the bronchi and alveoli _____

4. visual examination of the bronchi _____

5. calculus in a bronchus _____

Use *trache/o* (trachea) to build medical words meaning:

6. narrowing of the trachea _____

7. incision of the trachea _____

8. pertaining to the trachea and larynx _____

Use *thorac/o* (chest) to build medical words meaning:

9. surgical repair of the chest _____

10. forming an opening into the chest _____

Use *pneumon/o* (air, lung) to build medical words meaning:

11. disease of the lung _____

12. separation of the lung (from the pleura) _____

Use *pneum/o* (air, lung) to build medical words meaning:

13. suture of the lung _____

14. condition of dust in the lung _____

15. fixation of the lung _____

Use *pleur/o* (pleura) to build medical words meaning:

16. pain in the pleura _____

17. excision of the pleura _____

18. hernia of the pleura _____

Use *bronchiol/o* (bronchiole) to build medical words meaning:

19. inflammation of the bronchioles _____

20. dilation of the bronchioles _____

Correct Answers _____ **× 5 =** _____ **% Score**

MEDICAL RECORDS

Authentic medical records including a SOAP note, procedural report, discharge summary, and emergency report are presented in this section.

The following reading and dictionary exercise and medical record analysis will help you develop skills to abstract information and master the terminology in the reports. In turn, you will be able to understand the importance of accurately interpreting information from a medical record. Accurate interpretation is important because this information is used to initiate treatments, evaluate patient progress, and complete insurance claims for third-party reimbursements.

Reading and Dictionary Exercise

Place a check mark in the box [✓] after you complete the exercise.

[   ] **1.** Underline the following words in the reports as you read the SOAP note, procedural report, discharge summary, and the emergency report aloud. These medical records can be found at the end of the chapter.

[   ] **2.** Use a medical dictionary and Appendix F, Part 2 to define the terms below.

Note: You are not expected to fully understand all the parts of the medical records. The important aspect of this exercise is to use all available resources to complete it. Eventually you will master the terminology and format of these reports.

> > > MEDICAL RECORD 8-1: SOAP NOTE

Term	Pronunciation	Meaning
asthma	ĂZ-mă	_____
hypercholesterolemia	hī-pĕr-kō-lĕs-tĕr-ŏl-Ē-mē-ă	_____
dyspnea	dĭsp-NĒ-ă	_____
dysuria	dīs-Ū-rē-ă	_____
bilaterally	bī-LĂT-ĕr-ăl-lē	_____
rhonchi	RŎNG-kī	_____
wheezes	HWĒZ-ĕz	_____
nebulizer	NĔB-ū-lĭ-zĕr	_____
albuterol	ăl-BŪ-tĕr-ăl	_____
Solu-Medrol	SŎL-ū MĔD-rŏl	_____

> > > MEDICAL RECORD 8-2: PROCEDURAL REPORT

Term	Pronunciation	Meaning
bronchoscope	BRŎNG-kō-skōp	_____
transnasally	trănz-NĀ-zăl-lē	_____
carina	kă-RĪ-nă	_____
bronchopulmonary	brŏng-kō-PŬL-mō-nă-rē	_____
endobronchial	ĕn-dō-BRŎNG-kē-ăl	_____
friable	FRĪ-ă-bl	_____
mucosal	mū-KŌ-săl	_____
lesion	LĒ-zhŭn	_____
fluoroscopic	floo-or-ō-SKŌP-ĭk	_____
transbronchial	trănz-BRŎNG-kē-ăl	_____
needle aspiration	NĒ-dl ăs-pĭ-RĀ-shŭn	_____

brush biopsies	*brŭsh BĪ-ŏp-sēz*	_____
bronchial brush	*BRŎNG-kē-ăl brŭsh*	_____
cytology	*sī-TŎL-ō-jē*	_____
culture and sensitivity	*KŬL-tūr ănd sĕn-sĭ-TĬV-ĭ-tē*	_____
acid-fast bacilli	*Ă-sĭd-făst bă-SĬL-ī*	_____
Legionella	*lē-jĕ-NĔL-ă*	_____

> > > MEDICAL RECORD 8-3: DISCHARGE SUMMARY

Term	Pronunciation	Meaning
acute bronchitis	*a-KŪT brŏng-KĪ-tĭs*	_____
pneumonia	*nū-MŌ-nē-ă*	_____
acute renal failure	*a-KŪT RĒ-năl FĀL-yĕr*	_____
hyperkalemia	*hī-pĕr-kă-LĒ-mē-ă*	_____
desaturation	*dē-săt-ū-RĀ-shŭn*	_____
hypercapnia	*hī-pĕr-KĂP-nē-ă*	_____
Lasix	*LĀ-sĭks*	_____
nasal cannula	*NĀ-săl KĂN-ū-lă*	_____
afebrile	*ă-FĔB-rĭl*	_____
theophylline	*thē-ŌF-ĭ-lēn*	_____
tachycardia	*tăk-ĭ-KĂR-dē-ă*	_____
sinus arrhythmia	*SĪ-nŭs ă-RĬTH-mē-ă*	_____
prednisone	*PRĔD-nĭ-sōn*	_____
aerosol treatment	*ĔR-ō-sŏl*	_____
digoxin	*dĭ-JŎK-sĭn*	_____
electrolytes	*ē-LĔK-trō-līts*	_____
creatinine	*krē-ĂT-ĭn-ĭn*	_____

> > > MEDICAL RECORD 8-4: EMERGENCY REPORT

Term	Pronunciation	Meaning
periscapular	*pĕr-ĭ-SKĂP-ū-lăr*	_____

truncal	TRŬNG-kăl	_____
dyspnea	dĭsp-NĒ-ă	_____
palpation	păl-PĀ-shŭn	_____
excursions	ĕks-KŬR-zhŭns	_____
splinted	SPLĬNT-ĕd	_____
pleural	PLOO-răl	_____
oximetry	ŏk-SĬ-mĕ-trē	_____
cardiovascular	kăr-dē-ō-VĂS-kū-lăr	_____
benign	bē-NĬN	_____
ectopy	ĕk-TŌ-pē	_____
palpation	păl-PĀ-shŭn	_____
auscultation	aws-kūl-TĀ-shŭn	_____
pneumothorax	nū-mō-THŌ-răks	_____
anterolateral	ăn-tĕr-ō-LĂT-ĕr-ăl	_____
hemoglobin	hē-mō-GLŌ-bĭn	_____
Versed	VĔR-sĕd	_____
Demerol	DĔ-mĕr-ōl	_____
axillary	ĂK-sĭ-lār-ē	_____
nasal cannula	NĀ-săl KĂN-ū-lă	_____
intravenous	ĭn-tră-VĒ-nŭs	_____
thoracic	thō-RĂS-ĭk	_____
thoracostomy tube	thō-răk-ŎS-tō-mē tūb	_____

Critical Thinking: Analysis of Medical Records

This section provides experience in abstracting and analyzing information from medical records. At the same time, it reinforces the material presented in this chapter.

> > > MEDICAL RECORD 8–1: SOAP NOTE

1. What symptoms made the patient seek medical care?

_____

_____

2. What did the doctor find upon examination of the patient?

_____

> > > MEDICAL RECORD 8–2: PROCEDURAL REPORT

3. What does it mean that the bronchoscope was inserted transnasally?

_____

4. What was seen in the left lower bronchus?

_____

_____

5. What kinds of biopsy specimens were obtained during the procedure?

_____

_____

> > > MEDICAL RECORD 8–3: DISCHARGE SUMMARY

6. Why was the patient admitted to the hospital?

_____

_____

7. What caused the creatinine and BUN to be elevated?

_____

8. What contributed to the patient's episode of tachycardia and sinus arrhythmia, and what transpired to correct the problem?

_____

_____

_____

9. Is there any indication that the patient has an excessive amount of potassium in the blood?

_____

_____

> > > MEDICAL RECORD 8-4: EMERGENCY REPORT

10. What did the chest x-ray reveal?

_____

11. What procedure was performed to improve the patient's condition?

_____

_____

12. What complications would have occurred if this patient had not gone to the ER for treatment?

_____

_____

Audio Practice

Listen to the audio CD-ROM to practice the pronunciation of selected medical terms from this chapter.

Medical Record 8–1. SOAP Note

GENERAL HOSPITAL AND MEDICAL CENTER
2211 Fifth Avenue North • Healthy City, USA 12345 • (321) 123-4567

SOAP Note

Patient Name: Georgia Jones
Age: 68 yrs.

Patient Number: 55-78-43
Room Number: OP

DATE: March 5, 20xx

SUBJECTIVE:
She has had long history of asthma as well as carotid artery disease, hypercholesterolemia, depression, etc. She has had worsening asthma symptoms for 2 weeks, but for the last day it has been very, very bad. She has used her inhaler on a quite regular basis and has now started to develop some left-sided chest pain with severe dyspnea. She also has some dysuria.

OBJECTIVE:
She comes in with moderate respiratory distress. Respiratory rate is 30. She has very shallow, labored respirations with pursed-lip breathing and accessory muscle use. Air movement is very poor bilaterally with diffuse rhonchi and wheezes. She has not responded to two nebulizer treatments and, in fact, has worsened somewhat with those albuterol treatments. We have put her on 2 liters of oxygen, but the air movement is very, very poor, and respiratory muscle use has increased.

ASSESSMENT:
1. Severe asthma attack.

PLAN:
We will transfer her by rescue squad to Healthy City Hospital for further evaluation in the emergency department. We have given her 125 mg Solu-Medrol IV push. Additionally, we identified a urinary tract infection, which will be treated through the emergency room.

_____
Robert Scottsdale, M.D.

RS/dm
D: 03/05/xx
T: 03/06/xx

Medical Record 8–2. Procedural Report

GENERAL HOSPITAL AND MEDICAL CENTER
2211 Fifth Avenue North • Healthy City, USA 12345 • (321) 123-4567

Procedural Report

Patient Name: George Harrison   **Patient Number:** 55-78-33
Age: 53 yrs.   **Room Number:**   374

DATE: March 6, xx

PROCEDURE: BRONCHOSCOPY

The bronchoscope was passed transnasally. The vocal cords, larynx and trachea were all normal. The main carina was sharp. All bronchopulmonary segments were visualized. There was an endobronchial friable mucosal lesion seen in the left lower lobe bronchus, partially occluding the entire left lower lobe bronchus. No other endobronchial lesions or bleeding sites were noted.

Under fluoroscopic control, transbronchial biopsies of this left lower lung area were obtained, as well as transbronchial needle aspiration, bronchial brush biopsies and bronchial brush washings for cytology evaluation. Sterile brush cultures for culture and sensitivity, acid-fast bacilli, fungus and Legionella were also done.

The patient tolerated the procedure well.

_____
Ronald Horton, M.D.

RH/bab

D: 05/06/xx
T: 05/07/xx

Medical Record 8–3. Discharge Summary

GENERAL HOSPITAL AND MEDICAL CENTER
2211 Fifth Avenue North • Healthy City, USA 12345 • (321) 123-4567

Discharge Summary

Patient Name: Frank Forther
Date of Birth: 71 yrs.

Patient Number: 34-76-32
Room Number: 634

DISCHARGE SUMMARY
Date of Admission: 07/13/xx
Date of Discharge: 07/18/xx

PRINCIPAL DIAGNOSIS: Chronic obstructive pulmonary disease exacerbation.

SECONDARY DIAGNOSES:
    Acute bronchitis.
    Pneumonia.
    Acute renal failure.
    Severe hyperkalemia.
    Constipation.
    Depression.
    Coronary artery disease.

NARRATIVE SUMMARY: Mr. Forther was admitted because of severe shortness of breath and with a history of COPD and oxygen-dependency. He was found to be desaturating. His initial ABG on admission showed a pO_2 of 30, and he was on 2.5 L of oxygen, which was increased to 3.5 L of oxygen to improve his oxygenation. However, because he is a CO_2 retainer, his CO_2 also increased. The patient was transferred to the intensive care unit because of his desaturation, and hyperkalemia with hypercapnia. His initial laboratory evaluation also showed a potassium of 6.9, and he was given treatment to reduce his potassium. His kidney function also was not good, and his creatinine was up with BUN also very high. The patient was assessed to be dehydrated with acute renal failure. He was started on IV fluids. His potassium was held, also his Lasix was stopped. Over the next two or three days, the patient's condition improved. His pulmonary status improved gradually on antibiotics, steroids, and aerosol treatment. He was continued on 3.5 L of oxygen per nasal cannula, and the steroid was gradually decreased. His antibiotic was changed to oral antibiotic, and he remained afebrile.

The patient was started on theophylline, however on the third day of his being on theophylline, he did have an episode of tachycardia with heart rate of 130 to 140 with sinus arrhythmia. It was attributed to theophylline toxicity, and his theophylline was stopped. The level was above

Continued

Discharge Summary, page 2
Patient Name: Frank Forther   **Patient Number:** 34-76-32

therapeutic. Then his theophylline was restarted at a lower dose. The patient's heart rate improved, and his theophylline level came back to normal.

On July 18, 20xx, the patient was assessed to be in a stable condition. He was discharged home with home health care. He is to continue his antibiotic for five more days. Also he is to continue prednisone slowly, gradually decreasing the dose until he stops.

The patient's medication was detailed in the Community Referral form. He will continue on home oxygen and aerosol treatments. Follow up in about one week. Labs in one week: digoxin, theophylline, electrolytes, BUN, and creatinine.

On discharge, his potassium was coming down, and his BUN and creatinine were normal.

_____
Nicholas Louble, M.D.

NL/kje
D: 07/19/xx
T: 07/22/xx

Medical Record 8–4. Emergency Report

GENERAL HOSPITAL AND MEDICAL CENTER
2211 Fifth Avenue North • Healthy City, USA 12345 • (321) 123-4567

Emergency Report

Patient Name: Nancy Waters
Age: 23 yrs.

Patient Number: 45-22-12
Room Number: ER

DATE OF VISIT: 02/10/20xx

This 23-year-old female, who initially states that she is under the care of Dr. Jones, presents to the emergency department ambulatory, with complaint of severe right-sided chest pain with radiation to the right periscapular region. It is distinctly exacerbated with attempts at truncal movement and deep breathing. Onset was some two days ago with worsening this p.m. She further relates resting dyspnea with significant exertional component. She denies any left-sided discomfort. The patient has an essentially negative past medical history, with no current medications and no known history of allergy.

Physical examination finds markedly diminished breath sounds on the right. Trachea is thought to be midline to palpation, with excursions splinted due to pleural discomfort. Room air oximetry at 98% saturation. Her skin coloration is reasonably good, warm and dry to the touch. Cardio-vascular survey is otherwise benign. No clinical ectopy is present. Abdomen is benign to palpation and auscultation.

X-ray examination of the chest reveals the presence of an estimated 35 to 40% right pneumo-thorax. The patient was prepped on the right lateral and anterolateral chest wall. CBC obtained demonstrates white count of 10.9, with hemoglobin of 13.8. Following intravenous sedation with Versed and intramuscular Demerol, the patient had a chest tube inserted at the fifth intercostal space in the anterior axillary line. A #28 French tube was utilized and placed to underwater collection at negative 27 cm of water pressure. X-ray examination accomplished thereafter revealed good tube placement and lung re-inflation. The patient was maintained on oxygen by nasal cannula and intravenous hydration. She has tolerated the procedure extremely well and is both objectively and subjectively improved.

I discussed this case with a physician covering for Dr. Jones, who agrees with admission to the hospital in addition to consultation with Dr. Long, a thoracic surgeon on call. The case was discussed with Dr. Long, and he is in agreement to manage this patient on inpatient setting.

DIAGNOSIS: Acute right pneumothorax with thoracostomy tube placement.

Anthony Fitzwater, M.D.

AF/js
d&t: 02/10/20xx

sinoatrial node (SA node) sīn-ō-Ā-trē-ăl nōd	Area in the right atrium that generates electrical impulses that cause the muscle fibers of both atria to contract; also known as the *pacemaker of the heart.*
systemic circulation sĭs-TĔM-ĭk sĕr-kū-LĀ-shŭn	Circulation of blood from the body organs (except the lungs) to the heart and back again.
ventricle VĔN-trĭk-l	Lower chamber of the heart.

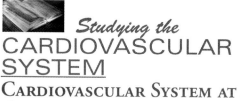

Studying the
CARDIOVASCULAR SYSTEM

Cardiovascular System at a Glance

The cardiovascular (CV) or circulatory system comprises the heart, which is essentially a muscular pump, as well as an extensive network of tubes, called *blood vessels.* The main purpose of the CV system is to deliver oxygen, nutrients, and other essential substances to the cells of the body and to remove the waste products of cellular **metabolism.** Delivery and removal of these products are achieved by a complex network of blood vessels: the arteries, capillaries, and veins that are connected to the heart. The heart pumps blood continuously through the body with the help of other body systems, especially the nervous and endocrine systems. Both the nervous and endocrine systems help to regulate the rate at which the heart beats and the blood pressure fluctuates. A healthy CV system maintains the continuous circulation of oxygen and food to the cells and rids the body of cellular waste materials. Without circulation, tissues are deprived of oxygen and nutrients, and waste removal stops. When this happens, an irreversible change in the cells takes place and may result in the person's death. Thus, the CV system is vital for survival.

The interrelationship of the CV system with other body systems is illustrated in Figure 9–1.

Structure and Function

Heart

The heart is a cone-shaped, muscular organ about the size of a fist. Its approximate weight is less than 1 pound. Located in the mediastinum, the area between the lungs in the thoracic cavity, it operates as two coordinated pumps, continuously sending blood around the body. The bulk of the heart lies beneath the sternum between the second and sixth ribs. The apex (tip) of the heart extends to the left of the sternum and lies

just above the diaphragm. The strongest beat of the heart can be heard or felt at the apex and is thus called the *apical pulse.* That is why we may think of the heart as being on the left side of the body.

Label Figure 9–2 as you read about the layers of the heart wall.

The heart wall comprises three layers: the endocardium, the myocardium, and the pericardium. All three layers are richly supplied with blood vessels. The innermost layer, the (1) **endocardium,** is a smooth layer of endothelial tissue. It lines the heart chambers and covers the connective tissue of the valves. The middle layer, the (2) **myocardium,** is composed mainly of cardiac muscle and forms the bulk of the heart. It is the layer that contracts, forcing the blood out of the heart chambers. The heart is enclosed in a membranous, fibrous, double-walled sac called the (3) **pericardium.** The pericardium comprises two serous layers: visceral and the parietal. The visceral layer, also called the (4) **epicardium,** is an integral part of the heart wall whereas the **parietal layer** lines the internal surface of the pericardium. Between the two layers (visceral and parietal) of pericardium is the (5) **pericardial cavity,** which contains serous pericardial fluid. The serous membranes, lubricated by the fluid, glide smoothly against one another during heart activity, allowing the mobile heart to work in a relatively friction-free environment.

 Activity 9–1: Competency Verification
Layers of the Heart Wall

Review Figure 9–2, and check your labeling in Appendix C.

Internal Structures of the Heart and Circulation of Blood

Label Figure 9–3 as you read the following material.

Internally, the heart comprises four chambers: two on the left side of the body and two on the right side of the body. The upper chambers are the (1)

Body System Connections
Cardiovascular System

THE DIGESTIVE SYSTEM
◆ The digestive system provides nutrients for absorption by the blood; the blood transports these nutrients to all body cells.

THE ENDOCRINE SYSTEM
◆ As hormones are transported in the blood, they influence the functions of the heart and blood vessels.

THE FEMALE REPRODUCTIVE SYSTEM
◆ The cardiovascular system transports vital substances to the organs of the reproductive system. ◆ The normal function of the sex organs, especially erectile tissue, is dependent on blood pressure.

THE INTEGUMENTARY SYSTEM
◆ To a great extent, body temperature is controlled by changes in the skin's blood flow.

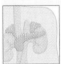

THE LYMPHATIC AND IMMUNE SYSTEMS
◆ Tissue fluids are returned to the bloodstream via the lymphatic system.

THE MUSCULOSKELETAL SYSTEM
◆ The cardiovascular system delivers needed oxygen and nutrients and carries away wastes. ◆ Bones protect cardiovascular organs by enclosure and help control blood calcium levels to maintain normal heart function.

THE NERVOUS SYSTEM
◆ The nervous system influences blood flow and blood pressure. ◆ To sustain life, the brain depends on a continuous blood flow.

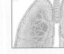

THE RESPIRATORY SYSTEM
◆ The heart pumps oxygen-deficient blood to the lungs, where the blood exchanges carbon dioxide for oxygen-rich blood.

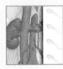

THE URINARY AND MALE REPRODUCTIVE SYSTEMS
◆ The kidneys eliminate waste products from the blood and control blood pressure and blood volume. ◆ The normal function of sex organs, especially erectile tissue, is dependent on blood pressure.

Figure 9–1   *The interrelationship of the cardiovascular system with other body systems.*

right atrium and the (2) **left atrium**. The lower two chambers are the (3) **right ventricle** and the (4) **left ventricle**. The internal partition that divides the heart is called either the **interatrial septum** (upper chambers) or the (5) **interventricular septum** (lower chambers), depending on which chambers it separates.

The *atria* (singular, **atrium**) are the receiving chambers for blood returning to the heart. Because the atria need contract only minimally to push blood into the ventricles, they provide little to the propulsive pumping activity of the heart.

Oxygen-poor blood enters the right atrium via two large veins, the vena cavae. The (6) **superior vena cava** returns blood from upper body. The (7) **inferior vena cava** returns blood from lower body. The *right atrium* contracts to force blood through the (8) **tricuspid valve** into the *right ventricle*. The tricuspid valve has three flexible cusps, or flaps, that prevents backflow of blood from the right ventricle into the right atrium and keeps the blood flowing in only one direction. The tricuspid valve stays shut as the right ventricle contracts to pump deoxygenated blood through the (9) **pulmonary valve**, into the **pulmonary artery.** The pulmonary artery branches into the (10) **right** and **left pulmonary arteries** after it leaves the right ventricle. Each branch carries deoxygenated blood to the lungs. It is the only artery in the body that carries deoxygenated blood. In the lungs, the pulmonary artery branches into millions of capillaries, each lying close to an air sac (alveolus). This is where the exchange of carbon dioxide (CO_2) and oxygen (O_2) takes place: carbon dioxide is expelled

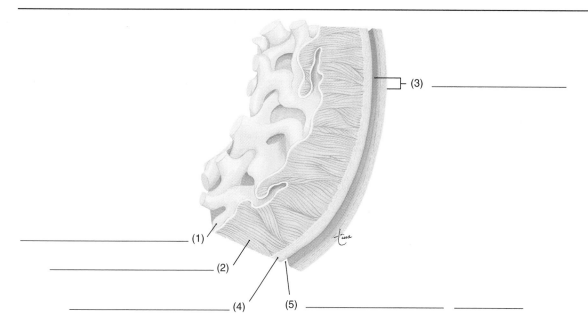

Figure 9–2 *The layers of the heart wall. (Adapted from Gylys, ME, and Masters, RM: Medical Terminology Simplified: A Programmed Learning Approach by Body Systems, ed 2. FA Davis, Philadelphia, 1998, p 380, with permission.)*

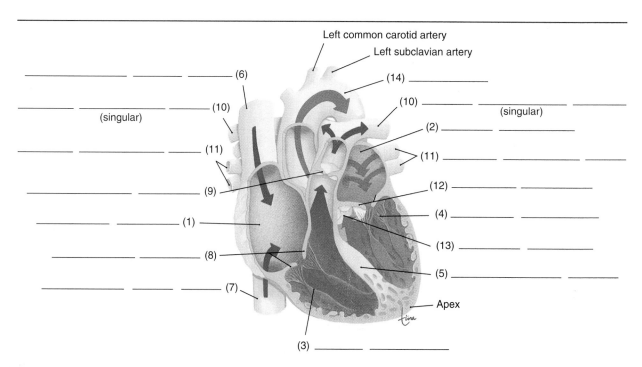

Figure 9–3 *The frontal section of the heart in anterior view, showing internal structures. (Adapted from Scanlon, VC, and Sanders, TS: Essentials of Anatomy and Physiology, ed 3. FA Davis, Philadelphia, 1999, p 260, with permission.)*

through exhalation and replaced with oxygen through inhalation. The blood is now oxygenated. The circulation of blood through the vessels from the heart to the lungs for oxygenation and then back to the heart again is known as **pulmonary circulation.**

The oxygen-rich blood returns to the heart via four pulmonary veins, (11) **two right** and **two left pulmonary veins** that deposit the blood into the left atrium. As the walls of the left atrium contract, blood is forced through the (12) **mitral valve** (bicuspid valve) into the left ventricle. The walls of the left ventricle are the thickest of all four chambers to enable it to contract more forcefully. This allows the blood to travel through the arteries to all parts of the body.

Oxygenated blood is pumped out of the left ventricle through the (13) **aortic valve** and into the (14) **aorta.** The aortic valve prevents a backflow of blood to the left ventricle once it has been pumped out. The aorta, the largest artery in the body, branches into numerous arteries that transport the freshly oxygenated blood to all parts of the body. Many of the arteries derive their names from the body parts near which they are located, such as the femoral arteries of the upper legs and the renal arteries of the kidneys, and the carotid arteries that supply blood to the head and neck. The circulation of blood from the body organs (except the lungs) to the heart and back again is known as **systemic circulation.**

Activity 9–2: Competency Verification
Internal Structures of the Heart

Check your labeling of Figure 9–3 in Appendix C.

Activity 9–3: Competency Verification
Blood Flow Through the Heart

Review the material on the internal structures of the heart and circulation of blood presented in the previous section, and label Flowchart 9–1 to trace the path of blood through the heart.

Coronary Arteries

Label Figure 9–4 as you read the following material.

The right and left coronary arteries are the first branches of the ascending aorta. The purpose of the coronary arteries is to supply blood to the myocardium because oxygen is essential for normal myocardial contractions to take place. The coronary arteries lie over the top of the heart much as a crown fits over a head—hence the name *coronary*, meaning "pertaining to a crown." The artery vascularizing the left side of the heart is the (1) **left coronary artery.** The (2) **right coronary artery** supplies oxygen to the right side of the heart, and divides into the (3) **left anterior descending artery** and the (4) **circumflex artery.** When a coronary artery becomes obstructed (usually by a clot or plaque), there is a disruption of the heart's activity. The blood supply in the affected area decreases (**ischemia**) or stops entirely. This leads to the death (**necrosis**) of part of the myocardium, leaving part of the heart muscle damaged and dysfunctional. The condition resulting in the death of myocardial tissue is called **infarction** (Fig. 9–5). This is a broad definition of a potentially devastating condition. In essence, the occluded coronary artery causes permanent damage to the heart muscle and the person suffers a myocardial infarction, or a heart attack. If prolonged ischemia takes place, the infarcted area can be quite large. The area that is affected by a myocardial infarction depends on which coronary artery is involved and the extent of the blockage. When there is a small blockage, necrosis may result in only a small portion of the heart that was directly fed by the blocked artery. The infarcted area is eventually replaced with scar tissue and the person is able to resume all normal activities.

Activity 9–4: Competency Verification
Coronary Arteries

Review Figure 9–4, and check your labeling in Appendix C.

Blood Vessels

The heart accomplishes its primary objective of feeding the body cells and removing waste materials through a network of vessels: the arteries, the veins, and the capillaries.

Blood vessels form a tubular network that permits blood to flow from the heart to all the living cells of the body and then back to the heart. Arteries carry blood away from the heart, whereas veins return blood to the heart. Arteries and veins are continuous with each other through smaller blood vessels called **arterioles** (minute arteries) and **venules** (tiny veins). The primary function of arteries, capillaries, and veins is to provide cells with vital nourishment and to remove waste substances. This process takes place at the capillary level.

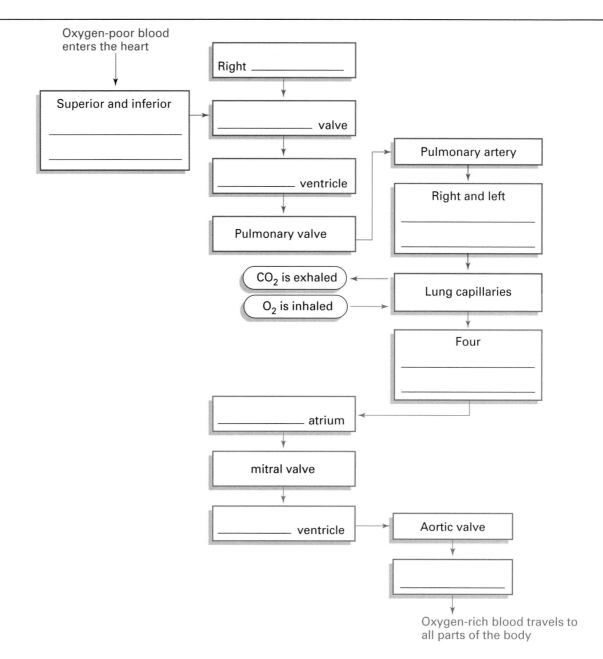

Flowchart 9–1 *Blood flow through the heart. The blue color indicates oxygen-poor blood, whereas the red color indicates oxygen-rich blood.*

Arteries

Because blood is propelled through arteries by the pumping action of the heart, its walls are thick and muscular in order to accommodate the surge of blood during the heart's contraction. This surge when blood is pumped from the heart is called **pulse.**

Label Figure 9–6 as you read the following material.

With the exception of the pulmonary artery, arterial blood contains oxygenated blood (blood with a high concentration of oxygen). Oxygenated blood

travels from (1) **arteries** to smaller vessels called (2) **arterioles,** and then to the microscopic (3) **capillaries.** Capillaries join the arterial system with the venous system as depicted in Figure 9–6.

Capillaries

Although capillaries are microscopic and have thin walls, they perform very important functions. For example, they form a network that enables cells to be provided with nourishment and waste products to be removed. Because of the thinness of their walls, differences in pressure enable substances, including

Combining Forms: Cardiology (Continued)

Combining Form	Meaning	EXAMPLE	
		Term/Pronunciation	**Definition**
cardi/o	heart	my/o/**cardi**/al mī-ō-KĂR-dē-ăl	pertaining to (-*al*) the heart muscle (*my/o*) *The middle layer of the heart is composed of muscle called the myocardium.*
hemangi/o	blood vessel	**hemangi**/ectasis hē-măn-jē-ĔK-tă-sĭs	dilation (-*ectasis*) of a blood vessel
phleb/o	vein	**phleb**/itis flĕ-BĪ-tĭs	inflammation (-*itis*) of a vein
ven/o		**ven**/ous VĒ-nŭs	pertaining to (-*ous*) a vein
scler/o	hardening, sclera	**scler**/osis sklĕ-RŌ-sĭs	abnormal condition of (-*osis*) hardening
sphygm/o	pulse	**sphygm**/o/meter sfĭg-MŎM-ĕt-ĕr	instrument for measuring (-*meter*) blood pressure
thromb/o	blood clot	**thromb**/us THRŎM-bŭs	condition (-*us*) of a stationary blood clot *A thrombus can obstruct a blood vessel or cavity of the heart and lead to a stroke or death.*
ventricul/o	ventricle (of heart or brain)	**ventricul**/ar vĕn-TRĬK-ū-lăr	pertaining to (-*ar*) a ventricle

Prefixes and Suffixes

In this section, prefixes are listed alphabetically and highlighted whereas suffixes are defined in the right-hand column on an as-needed basis.

Prefixes

Prefix	Meaning	EXAMPLE	
		Term/Pronunciation	**Definition**
brady-	slow	**brady**/cardi/ac brăd-ē-KĂR-dē-ăk	pertaining to (-*ac*) a slow heart (rate)
endo-	in, within	**endo**/cardi/um ĕn-dō-KĂR-dē-ŭm	structure (-*um*) within the heart (*cardi/o*) *The suffix -um means "structure," "thing."*

Prefixes (Continued)

Prefixes	Meaning	EXAMPLE	
		Term/Pronunciation	**Definition**
extra-	outside	**extra**/vascul/ar ĕks-tră-VĂS-kū-lăr	pertaining to (-*ar*) the area outside of a blood vessel (*vascul/o*)
peri-	around	**peri**/cardi/um pĕr-ĭ-KĂR-dē-ŭm	structure (-*um*) around the heart (*cardi/o*) The suffix -um *means "structure," "thing."*
tachy-	rapid	**tachy**/cardi/ac tăk-ē-KĂR-dē-ăk	pertaining to (-*ac*) a rapid heart (*cardi/o*) rate
trans-	through, across	**trans**/aort/ic trăns-ā-ŎR-tĭk	pertaining to (-*ic*) a surgical procedure performed through the aorta The combining form aort/o *refers to the aorta.*

In this section, suffixes are listed alphabetically and highlighted whereas key prefixes are defined in the right-hand column.

Suffixes

Suffix	Meaning	EXAMPLE	
		Term/Pronunciation	**Definition**
-gram	record, writing	electr/o/cardi/o/**gram** ē-lĕk-trō-KĂR-dē-ō-grăm	a record of the electrical (*electr/o*) activity of the heart (*cardi/o*)
-graph	instrument for recording	electr/o/cardi/o/**graph** ē-lĕk-trō-KĂR-dē-ō-grăf	instrument used to record the electrical (*electr/o*) activity of the heart (*cardi/o*) The combining form electr/o *means "electricity."*
-graphy	process of recording	electr/o/cardi/o/**graphy** ē-lĕk-trō-kăr-dē-ŎG-ră-fē	process of recording the electrical (*electr/o*) activity of the heart (*cardi/o*) This noninvasive test is used to diagnose abnormal cardiac rhythm and the presence of myocardial damage.
-stenosis	narrowing, stricture	arteri/o/**stenosis** ăr-tē-rē-ō-stĕ-NŌ-sĭs	narrowing of an artery (*arteri/o*) The narrowing of an artery can be caused by fatty plaque buildup (atheroma), scar tissue, or a blood clot (thrombus)

Activity 9-7: Competency Verification
Medical Word Components

Check the box [✓] as you complete each numbered section.

[   ] **1.** Review the word components for the cardiovascular system and their examples in the previous section. Then pronounce each word aloud.

[   ] **2.** For the words below, first write the suffix and its meaning. Then translate the meaning of the remaining components starting with the first part of the word.

> **Example:** cardi/al
> **Answer:** *al*=pertaining to, heart

1. phleb/itis   _____

2. scler/osis   _____

3. thromb/us   _____

4. aort/o/tomy   _____

5. sphygm/o/meter   _____

6. arteri/o/stenosis _____

7. tachy/cardi/ac   _____

8. my/o/cardi/um   _____

9. electr/o/cardi/o/gram_____

10. electr/o/cardi/o/graphy   _____

Correct Answers _____ **× 10 =** _____**% Score**

Pathological Conditions

PATHOLOGICAL CONDITION	DESCRIPTION

aneurysm
ĂN-ū-rĭzm

A localized dilation of the wall of a blood vessel, usually an artery, due to a congenital defect or weakness in the vessel wall.

Complications of an aneurysm include rupture, causing hemorrhage, thrombus, or embolus formation. Figure 9–9 illustrates different types of aortic aneurysms.

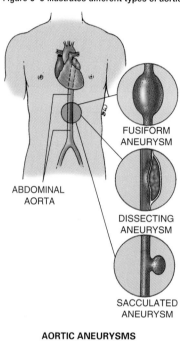

Figure 9–9 Aneurysms that may affect any part of the aorta. (From Venes, D: Taber's Cyclopedic Medical Dictionary, ed 19. FA Davis, Philadelphia, 2001, p 114, with permission.)

angina pectoris
ăn-JĪ-nă PĔK-tō-rĭs

Severe pain around the heart caused by a deficiency of oxygen supply to the heart muscle.

Pain or numbness typically radiates to the left shoulder and down the left arm and is frequently accompanied by a feeling of suffocation. Pain may be relieved by vasodilation of the coronary arteries by medication such as nitroglycerin (Fig. 9–10).

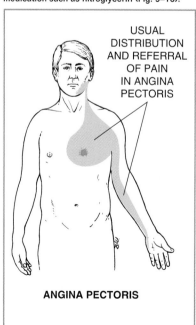

Figure 9–10 Angina pectoris. (From Venes, D: Taber's Cyclopedic Medical Dictionary, ed 19. FA Davis, Philadelphia, 2001, p 116, with permission.)

Pathological Conditions (Continued)

PATHOLOGICAL CONDITION	DESCRIPTION
arrhythmia ă-RĬTH-mē-ă	Any deviation from the normal pattern of the heartbeat. Also called *dysrhythmia*. Two common types of arrhythmias are flutter and fibrillation.
flutter FLŬT-ĕr	A rapid vibration or pulsation, especially of the heart, that may interfere with normal function.
fibrillation fĭ-brĭl-Ā-shŭn	Rapid, inefficient, random contractions of the heart that disrupt the normal sinus rhythm of the heart. Fibrillation is usually described by the part of the heart that is contracting abnormally, such as atrial fibrillation or ventricular fibrillation. To restore normal heart rhythm, a defibrillator (a device that delivers an electrical shock at a preset voltage to the myocardium through the chest wall) may be used (Fig. 9–11).

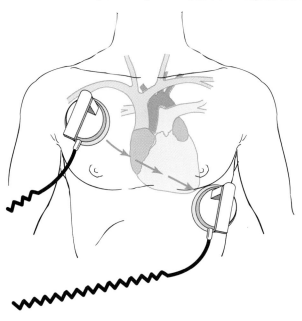

Figure 9–11   Placement of defibrillator paddles on chest. (From Williams, LS, and Hopper, PD: Understanding Medical-Surgical Nursing. FA Davis, Philadelphia, 1999, p 377, with permission.)

arteriosclerosis ăr-tē-rē-ō-sklĕ-RŌ-sĭs *arterio=artery* *scler=hardening, sclera* *osis=abnormal condition*	A common arterial disorder characterized by thickening, hardening, and loss of elasticity in the arterial walls.
atherosclerosis ăth-ĕr-ō-sklĕ-RŌ-sĭs *athero=fatty plaque* *scler=hardening, sclera* *osis=abnormal condition*	The most common form of arteriosclerosis, marked by cholesterol-lipid-calcium deposits in arterial linings. The condition begins as a fatty streak and gradually builds to a fibrous plaque or atheromatous (fatty) lesion. The plaque gradually creates a risk for thrombosis and is one of the major causes of coronary artery disease (CAD), angina pectoris, myocardial infarction (MI), and other cardiac disorders (Fig. 9–12).

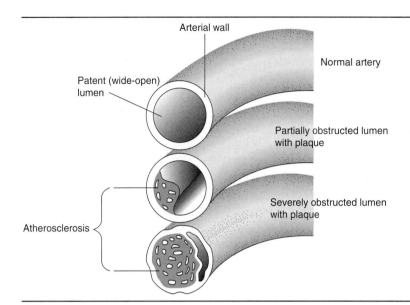

Figure 9–12 *Atherosclerosis obstructing blood flow in an artery. (From Gylys, BA, and Masters, RM: Medical Terminology Simplified: A Programmed Learning Approach by Body Systems, ed 2. FA Davis, Philadelphia, 1998, p 398, with permission.)*

PATHOLOGICAL CONDITIONS (CONTINUED)

PATHOLOGICAL CONDITION	DESCRIPTION
cardiomyopathy kăr-dē-ō-mī-ŎP-ă-thē *cardio=heart* *myo=muscle* *pathy=disease*	Any disease that affects the structure and function of the heart.
coarctation kō-ărk-TĀ-shŭn	A stricture (narrowing) or contraction of the walls of a vessel.
coarctation of the aorta	Congenital cardiac anomaly characterized by a localized narrowing of the aorta.
congestive heart failure (CHF)	Abnormal condition that reflects impaired cardiac pumping. This can eventually lead to left-sided heart failure, with the accumulation of fluid in the lungs (pulmonary edema), or right-sided heart failure, with accumulation of fluid (edema) in the abdominal organs and peripheral body areas. Causes may include MI, ischemic heart disease, and cardiomyopathy. Some of the prescribed treatments include drugs that strengthen the heart's contraction (such as digitalis) and diuretics to promote loss of fluid.
coronary artery disease (CAD) KŎR-ō-nă-rē ĂR-tĕ-rē dĭ-ZĒZ	Any one of the abnormal conditions that may affect the heart's arteries and produce various pathological effects, especially the reduced flow of blood and nutrients to the myocardium. The most common type of CAD is atherosclerosis, which is the leading cause of death in the Western world. Any other factor that limits blood flow through the coronary arteries may also be involved. Figure 9–13 illustrates a normal coronary artery compared with one that has progressed to a diseased state producing blockage and stenosis. Formerly called "coronary heart disease (CHD)."

Pathological Conditions (Continued)

PATHOLOGICAL CONDITION	DESCRIPTION
	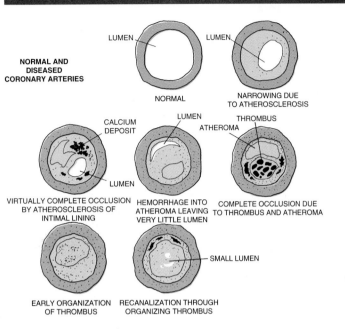

Figure 9–13 Normal and diseased coronary arteries. (From Thomas, CL: Taber's Cyclopedic Medical Dictionary, ed 18. FA Davis, Philadelphia, 1997, p 477, with permission.)

coronary artery spasm
KŎR-ō-nă-rē ĂR-tĕ-rē spăzm

Intermittent constriction of the large coronary arteries.

This may lead to angina pectoris in various conditions and is not necessarily associated with exertion.

deep vein thrombosis (DVT)
dēp vein thrŏm-BŌ-sĭs

A disorder involving a thrombus in one of the deep veins of the body, most commonly the lower leg.

Symptoms include tenderness, pain, warmth, and a red skin discoloration in the area where the clot is located. DVT is potentially life threatening if it dislodges and travels to the lungs or the brain. Treatment includes bed rest and use of anticoagulation and thrombolytic drugs to prevent movement of the thrombus toward the lungs.

embolus
ĔM-bō-lŭs
embol=plug
us=condition

A mass of undissolved matter, more commonly a blood clot, fatty plaque or air bubble, which travels through the bloodstream and becomes lodged in a blood vessel (Fig. 9–14).

Pathological Conditions (Continued)

PATHOLOGICAL CONDITION	DESCRIPTION

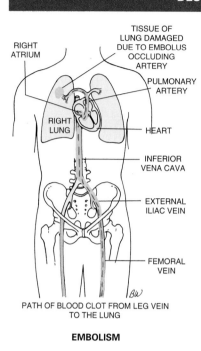

RIGHT ATRIUM

TISSUE OF LUNG DAMAGED DUE TO EMBOLUS OCCLUDING ARTERY

PULMONARY ARTERY

RIGHT LUNG

HEART

INFERIOR VENA CAVA

EXTERNAL ILIAC VEIN

FEMORAL VEIN

PATH OF BLOOD CLOT FROM LEG VEIN TO THE LUNG

EMBOLISM

Figure 9–14 *An obstruction of the pulmonary artery caused by a blood clot (thrombus) from the leg. The red dotted lines depict the path of the thrombus from the leg vein to the lung (pulmonary embolism). (From Venes, D: Taber's Cyclopedic Medical Dictionary, ed 19. FA Davis, Philadelphia, 2001, p 681, with permission.)*

---

endocarditis

ĕn-dō-kăr-DĪ-tĭs

endo =*in, within*

card =*heart*

itis =*inflammation*

Abnormal condition that affects the endocardium and heart valves and is characterized by lesions caused by a variety of diseases.

Kinds of endocarditis are bacterial endocarditis, nonbacterial thrombotic endocarditis, Libman-thrombotic endocarditis, and Libman-Sacks endocarditis.

---

heart block

A condition in which the conductive tissue of the heart fails to conduct impulses normally from the atrium to the ventricles, which results in an alteration of the rhythm of the heartbeat.

Heart block is further defined according to the location of the block and the type; for example, first-degree atrioventricular block occurs when all atrial impulses that should be conducted to the ventricles reach the ventricles but are delayed by a fraction of a second.

---

hemostasis

hē-MŎS-tă-sĭs

hemo =*blood*

stasis =*standing still*

The termination of bleeding by mechanical or chemical means, or by the coagulation process of the body.

---

hyperlipidemia

hī-pĕr-lĭp-ĕ-DĒ-mē-ă

hyper =*excessive, above normal*

lipid =*fat*

emia =*blood condition*

Excessive amounts of lipids in the blood.

PATHOLOGICAL CONDITIONS (CONTINUED)

PATHOLOGICAL CONDITION	DESCRIPTION
hypertension hī-pĕ-TĔN-shŭn *hyper=excessive, above normal* *tension=to stretch*	High blood pressure. In adults, a condition in which the blood pressure (BP) is higher than 140 mm Hg systolic or 90 mm Hg diastolic on three separate readings recorded several weeks apart. *Essential hypertension*, the most common kind, has no single identifiable cause but the risk is increased by obesity, high serum sodium level, hypercholesterolemia, and a family history of high blood pressure. Hypertension is one of the major risk factors for coronary artery disease, congestive heart failure, stroke, peripheral vascular disease, kidney failure, and retinopathy. Physical conditions, such as kidney disease, Cushing syndrome, or pregnancy complications may cause a type of hypertension called *secondary hypertension*.
ischemia ĭs-KĒ-mē-ă *isch= to hold back* *emia=blood condition*	Decreased supply of oxygenated blood to a body part or organ.
mitral valve prolapse (MVP) MĪ-trăl vălv prō-LĂPS	A common and occasionally serious condition in which a cusp or cusps of the mitral valve prolapse into the left atrium during systole. There may or may not be symptoms.
murmurs MŬR-mŭrz	Abnormal sounds heard on auscultation of the heart and adjacent large blood vessels. Murmurs range in sound from soft and blowing to loud and booming.
myocardial infarction (MI) mī-ō-KĂR-dē-ăl ĭn-FĂRK-shŭn *myo=muscle* *cardi=heart* *al=pertaining to*	Necrosis of a portion of cardiac muscle caused by partial or complete occlusion of one or more of the coronary arteries. Also called *heart attack*.
patent ductus arteriosus PĂT-ĕnt DŬK-tŭs ăr-tē-rē-Ō-sŭs	An abnormal opening between the pulmonary artery and the aorta caused by the failure of the ductus arteriosus to close after birth. It is seen primarily in premature infants.
palpitations păl-pĭ-TĀ-shŭns	A pounding or racing of the heart. It is associated with normal emotional responses or with heart disorders.
pericardial effusion pĕr-ĭ-KĂR-dē-ăl ĕ-FŪ-zhŭn *peri=around* *cardi=heart* *al=pertaining to*	A buildup of fluid in the pericardial space that is a common complication of *pericarditis*, and other various causes. Treatment includes pericardiocentesis.
peripheral arterial disease (PAD) pĕr-ĬF-ĕr-ăl ăr-TĒ-rē-ăl dĭ-ZĔZ	A systemic form of atherosclerosis in which blood flow is restricted by an intra-arterial accumulation of soft deposits of lipids and fibrin that harden over time. The incidence is highest among men with diabetes. Other risk factors include obesity and stress.

PATHOLOGICAL CONDITIONS (CONTINUED)

PATHOLOGICAL CONDITION	DESCRIPTION
Raynaud phenomenon *rā-NŌ*	Numbness in fingers or toes due to attacks of vasoconstriction of arterioles in the skin. The attacks, which can be triggered by exposure to cold or by emotional stimuli, may be an indicator of some other, more serious disorder.
rheumatic heart disease *roo-MĂT-ĭk*	Damage to heart muscle and heart valves caused by episodes of rheumatic fever.
septal defect *SĔP-tăl DĒ-fĕkt*	An abnormal, usually congenital defect in the wall separating the two chambers of the heart. Various amounts of oxygenated and deoxygenated blood mix, depending on the size and site of the defect, causing a decrease in the amount of oxygen carried in the blood to peripheral tissues. There are both atrial and ventricular septal defects.
tetralogy of Fallot *tĕ-TRĂ-lĕ-jē făl-Ō*	Congenital anomaly that consists of four defects: pulmonary artery stenosis, ventricular septal defect, malposition of the aorta so that it arises from the septal defect or right ventricle, and right ventricular hypertrophy. An infant with this condition is often described as a "blue baby," because of cyanosis and inefficient blood flow through the body. Surgical repair is required to correct the cardiac defects.
thrombus *THRŎM-bŭs* *thromb=blood clot* *us=condition*	An aggregation of platelets, fibrin, clotting factors, and the cellular elements of the blood attached to the interior wall of a vein or artery, sometimes occluding the lumen of the vessel. Also called *blood clot*.
thrombophlebitis *thrŏm-bō-flĕ-BĪ-tĭs* *thrombo=blood clot* *phleb=vein* *itis=inflammation*	Inflammation of a vein in conjunction with the formation of a thrombus. It usually occurs in an extremity, most frequently the lower leg.
varicose veins *VĂR-ĭ-kōs vānz*	A twisted, dilated vein with incompetent valves, most commonly found in the saphenous veins of the lower legs. Causes of varicose veins include congenitally defective valves, pregnancy, obesity and thrombophlebitis.

Activity 9–8: Clinical Application
Pathological Conditions

aneurysm	embolus	myocardial infarction (MI)
angina pectoris	fibrillation	palpitations
arrhythmia	hemostasis	septal defect
atherosclerosis	hyperlipidemia	thrombophlebitis
cardiomyopathy	hypertension	thrombus
coarctation	ischemia	varicose vein
congestive heart failure (CHF)	mitral valve prolapse (MVP)	

Match the terms listed above with the definitions given in the numbered list:

1. _____ excessive amount of lipids in the blood.

2. _____ synonymous with *heart attack.*

3. _____ a pounding or racing of the heart.

4. _____ a localized dilation, usually of an artery, due to a congenital defect or weakness in the vessel wall.

5. _____ a blood clot that obstructs a blood vessel by attaching itself to the interior wall of a vein or artery.

6. _____ any disease that affects the structure and function of the heart.

7. _____ inflammation of a vein in conjunction with the formation of a thrombus that occurs most frequently in the lower leg.

8. _____ any deviation from the normal pattern of the heartbeat; also known as a *dysrhythmia.*

9. _____ the most common form of arteriosclerosis, marked by cholesterol-lipid-calcium deposits in arterial linings.

10. _____ a stricture (narrowing) or contraction of the walls of a vessel.

11. _____ an abnormal, usually congenital, defect in the wall separating the two chambers of the heart.

12. _____ high blood pressure.

13. _____ a blood clot, fatty plaque, or air bubble that travels through the bloodstream.

14. _____ the termination of bleeding.

15. _____ a twisted, dilated vein with incompetent valves.

16. _____ decreased supply of oxygenated blood to a body part or organ.

17. _____ severe pain around the heart caused by a deficiency of oxygen supply to the heart muscle; pain or numbness typically radiates down the left arm.

18. _____ condition in which a cusp or cusps of the mitral valve prolapse into the left atrium during systole.

19. _____ a type of arrhythmia characterized by rapid, inefficient, random contractions of the heart that disrupt the normal sinus rhythm and that may need a defibrillator to restore the heart's normal rhythm.

20. _____ abnormal condition that reflects impaired cardiac pumping and can eventually lead to heart failure.

Correct Answers _____ × 5 = _____% **Score**

DIAGNOSTIC PROCEDURES AND TESTS
Imaging Procedures

PROCEDURE	DESCRIPTION
aortography ā-ŏr-TŎG-ră-fē *aorto =aorta* *graphy =process of recording*	Radiography of the aorta after the injection of an opaque contrast medium.
angiography ăn-jē-ŎG-ră-fē *angio =vessel* *graphy =process of recording*	Diagnostic or therapeutic radiography of the heart and blood vessels using a radiopaque contrast medium. Different types include magnetic resonance imaging, interventional radiography, and computed tomography.
digital subtraction angiography DĬ-jĭ-tăl sŭb-TRĂK-shŭn ăn-jē-ŎG-ră-fē	A computer technique used to investigate arterial blood circulation. A radiograph of blood vessels is produced and stored in a computer. Then a contrast medium is injected intravenously, and another radiograph is produced and stored in the computer. The two images are compared, and the computer "subtracts" the first image from the second; that is, it removes the structures not being studied, such as muscle or bone. The final image is an enhanced view of the contrast medium and the arteries.
Doppler ultrasonography DŎP-lĕr ŭl-tră-sŏn-ŎG-ră-fē	Technique for detecting the movement of blood flow. This technique allows the examiner to hear characteristic alterations in blood flow caused by vessel obstruction in various parts of an extremity.
duplex scanning DŪ-plĕks SKĂN-ĭng	Visualization of the venous system through an ultrasound machine (duplex scanner). The scanner can determine the direction of blood flow within the veins. It is especially useful in diagnosing thrombophlebitis.
echocardiography ĕ-kō-kăr-dē-ŎG-ră-fē *echo =a repeated sound* *cardio =heart* *graphy = process of recording*	Use of ultrasound to visualize internal cardiac structures and motion of the heart. Also called *ultrasonic cardiography*.
transesophageal echocardiography (TEE) trănz-ē-sŏf-ă-JĒ-ăl	Obtaining images through the chest wall by using a probe that is swallowed into the esophagus. TEE images are clearer than those using echocardiography and may be taken from several planes.

Laboratory Tests

TEST	DESCRIPTION
cardiac enzyme studies *KĂR-dē-ăk ĔN-zīm*	A battery of blood tests performed to determine the presence of cardiac damage.
coagulation tests *kō-ăg-ū-LĀ-shŭn*	A group of tests performed to determine the clotting ability of blood for purposes of diagnosis of clotting disorders and monitoring anticoagulant therapy.
lipid profile *LĬP-ĭd PRŌ-fĭl*	A battery of blood tests to measure fatty substances, including cholesterol, triglycerides, and lipoproteins. This test is used to evaluate the risk of developing coronary artery disease.
troponin I *TRŌ-pō-nĭn*	A blood test that measures protein that is released into the blood by damaged heart muscle (but not skeletal muscle) and therefore is a highly sensitive and specific indicator of recent MI.

Other Diagnostic Procedures

PROCEDURE	DESCRIPTION
cardiac catheterization *KĂR-dē-ăk* *kăth-ĕ-tĕr-ĭ-ZĀ-shŭn*	Insertion of a catheter (thin, flexible tube) through an incision into a large vein, usually of an arm (brachial approach) or leg (femoral approach); the catheter is threaded through the circulatory system into the heart. A contrast medium also may be injected and x-rays taken (angiography). This procedure can accurately identify and assess many conditions including congenital heart disease, valvular incompetence, blood supply, and myocardial infarction.
electrocardiography *ē-lĕk-trō-kăr-dē-ŎG-ră-fē* *electro=electricity* *cardio=heart* *graphy=process of recording*	The process of recording the electrical activity of the heart. This procedure is performed with an electrocardiograph and produces a graphic record, an electrocardiogram, which the cardiologist analyzes. It is of value in diagnosing cases of abnormal heart rhythm and myocardial damage.
Holter monitor test *HŌL-tĕr*	The use of a portable device small enough to be worn by a patient during normal activity. It consists of an electrocardiograph and a recording system capable of storing up to 48 hours of the individual's electrocardiogram record (Fig. 9–15). This test is particularly useful in obtaining a record of cardiac arrhythmia that would not be discovered by means of an ECG of only a few minutes' duration. The patient keeps a diary of activities and symptoms, which are then correlated with the ECG.

Other Diagnostic Procedures (Continued)

PROCEDURE	DESCRIPTION

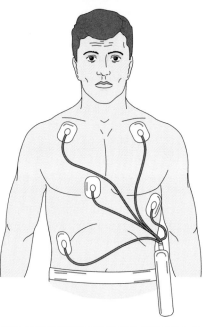

Figure 9–15 *Holter monitor. (From Williams, LS and Hopper, PD: Understanding Medical-Surgical Nursing, FA Davis, Philadelphia, 1999, p 279, with permission.)*

stress test strĕs tĕst	A method of evaluating cardiovascular fitness. While exercising, usually on a treadmill, the individual is subjected to steadily increasing levels of work. At the same time, the amount of oxygen consumed is measured while an electrocardiogram is administered.

SURGICAL AND THERAPEUTIC PROCEDURES

Surgical Procedures

PROCEDURE	DESCRIPTION
aneurysmectomy ĂN-ū-rĭzm-EK-tō-mē *aneurysm=a widening, a widened blood vessel* *ectomy=excision, removal*	Surgical removal of the sac of an aneurysm.
angioplasty ĂN-jē-ō-plăs-tē *angio=vessel* *plasty=surgical repair*	Any endovascular procedure that reopens narrowed blood vessels and restores forward blood flow. The blocked vessel is usually opened by balloon dilation.
laser coronary LĀ-zĕr KŌR-ō-nă-rē	The use of laser energy to vaporize an atherosclerotic plaque in a diseased coronary vessel.
percutaneous transluminal coronary (PTCA) pĕr-kū-TĀ-nē-ŭs trănz-LŪ-mĭ-năl KŌR-ō-nă-rē	A method of treating localized coronary artery narrowing. A special double-lumen catheter is designed so that a cylindrical balloon surrounds a portion of it. After the catheter is inserted transcutaneously in the artery, inflation of the balloon dilates the narrowed vessel. This procedure opens the passageway inside the blood vessel so that blood can flow freely (Fig. 9–16); also called *balloon angioplasty*. This technique may be used on narrowed arteries other than the coronaries.

Surgical Procedures (Continued)

PROCEDURE	DESCRIPTION
anastomosis ă-năs-tō-MŌ-sĭs	A surgical joining of two ducts, blood vessels, or bowel segments to allow flow from one segment to the other. A vascular anastomosis may be performed to bypass an aneurysm or a vascular or arterial occlusion.
atherectomy ăth-ĕr-ĔK-tō-mē *ather=fatty plaque* *ectomy=excision, removal*	Surgical removal of an atheroma in a major artery.
automatic implanted cardioverter defibrillator (AICD) KĂR-dē-ō-vĕr-tĕr dē-fĭb-rĭ-LĂ-tŏr	A surgically implanted device, about the size of a pacemaker, that automatically detects and corrects life-threatening dysrhythmias. When the defibrillator detects an abnormal complex or detects the heart rate outside of a preset rate, it automatically defibrillates to change the abnormal rhythm.
coronary artery bypass surgery (CABG) KŎR-ō-nărē ĂR-tĕr-ē	A procedure to create a detour or bypass around blockages. It increases the blood flow to the myocardial muscle and involves bypass grafts to the coronary arteries that reroute the blood flow around the occluded coronary artery. The operation involves the use of one or more of the patient's arteries or veins. Generally, the saphenous vein from the leg or the right or left internal mammary artery from the chest wall is used to bypass the blocked section (Fig. 9–17). Anastomosis (joining) of the vessel grafts to existing coronary arteries bypasses the blocked section and keeps the myocardium supplied with needed oxygenated blood. Resecting the mammary arteries for grafting is more difficult and time consuming than the saphenous vein, but the longevity of their patency is greater. More than one coronary artery bypass can be carried out at the same time depending on the number of blockages. For example, two blocked arteries may warrant a double bypass, whereas three blocked arteries may require a triple bypass, and so forth. This surgery is also called *coronary artery bypass graft* or *coronary bypass surgery*.
endarterectomy ĕnd-ăr-tĕr-ĔK-tō-mē *end=within* *arter=artery* *ectomy=excision, removal*	Surgical removal of the innermost lining of an artery. This procedure is performed to clear any major artery (carotid, femoral, or popliteal) that may be blocked by plaque accumulation.
intraluminal coronary artery stent placement ĭn-tră-LŪ-mĭ-năl	Surgical insertion of a stent (small, self-expanding meshlike tube) at the site of a blocked artery by a deflated balloon. Once the balloon is inflated, it expands and the stent opens up the blocked artery. The balloon is then deflated and removed. The expanded stent is left in place to keep the artery open. Its purpose is to prevent lumen closure (restenosis) following bypass surgery and to treat acute vessel closure after angioplasty.

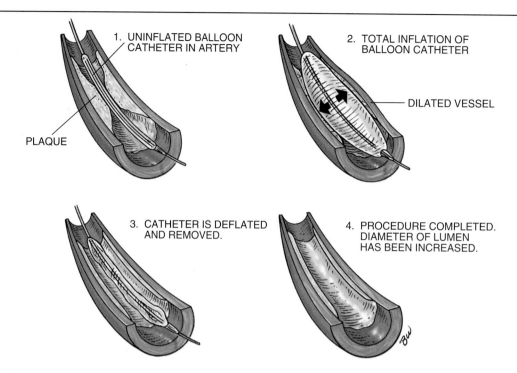

Figure 9–16 *Arterial balloon angioplasty. (From Venes, D: Taber's Cyclopedic Medical Dictionary, ed 19. FA Davis, Philadelphia, 2001, p 121, with permission.)*

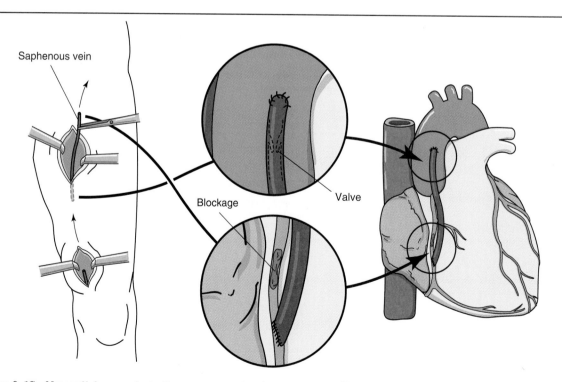

Figure 9–17 *Myocardial revascularization: coronary artery bypass surgery. (From Williams, LS, and Hopper, PD: Understanding Medical-Surgical Nursing. FA Davis, Philadelphia, 1999, p 408, with permission.)*

Surgical Procedures (Continued)

PROCEDURE	DESCRIPTION
pacemaker *PĂS-mā-kĕr*	Electrical device used to perform the function of the natural pacemaker of the heart. If the device uses electrodes inserted inside the body, it is called an *internal* or *implantable pacemaker*. Pacemakers are used to establish a normal heart rhythm and overcome heart block. They are set at a prescribed rate, usually 71 beats per minute, and are powered by batteries (which last up to 5 years) and a timer (Fig. 9–18). 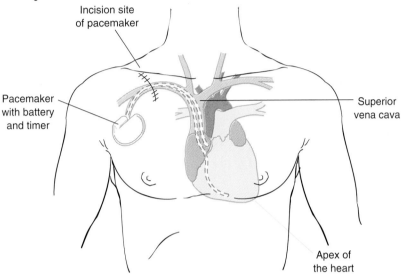 ***Figure 9–18*** *Permanent implantable pacemaker placed within the chest (Adapted from Williams, LS, and Hopper, PD: Understanding Medical-Surgical Nursing. FA Davis, Philadelphia, 1999, p 376, with permission.)*
pericardicentesis, pericardiocentesis *pĕr-ĭ-kăr-dĭ-sĕn-TĒ-sĭs,* *pĕr-ĭ-kăr-dē-ō-sĕn-TĒ-sĭs* *peri=around* *cardio=heart* *centesis= surgical puncture*	Surgical puncture of the pericardium to remove excess fluid in the pericardial sac.
valve replacement *vălv rē-PLĂS-mĕnt*	Replacement of a defective heart valve with a prosthesis.
valvuloplasty *VĂL-vū-lō-plăs-tē*	Plastic or restorative surgery on a valve, especially a cardiac valve.
balloon	Insertion of a balloon catheter to open a stenotic heart valve. Inflating the balloon decreases the constriction. This technique has been used to treat mitral or pulmonic stenosis.
vena cava filter *VĒ-nă KĀ-vă*	Surgical placement of a filter into the inferior vena cava. The filter prevents clots from traveling to the lungs without hindering blood flow.

Labels within figure:
Incision site of pacemaker
Pacemaker with battery and timer
Superior vena cava
Apex of the heart

Therapeutic Procedures

PROCEDURE	DESCRIPTION
cardiopulmonary resuscitation (CPR) *kăr-dē-ō-PŬL-mō-nĕ-rē rĭ-sŭs-ĭ-TĀ-shŭn*	The process of ventilating and circulating blood for a patient in cardiopulmonary arrest, usually by combining mouth-to-mouth ventilation with external chest compressions.
defibrillation, cardioversion *dē-fĭb-rĭ-LĀ-shŭn, KĂR-dē-ō-vĕr-zhŭn*	An electrical device called a *defibrillator* delivers shocks at a preset voltage to the heart to convert fibrillation and life-threatening dysrhythmias back to a normal rhythm (Fig. 9–11).
thrombolytic therapy (TT) *thrŏm-bō-LĬT-ĭk* *thrombo=blood clot* *lysis=separation, destruction, loosening*	The administration of drugs to dissolve an arterial clot(s).

Pharmacology

DRUG CLASSIFICATION	THERAPEUTIC ACTION
angiotensin-converting enzyme (ACE) inhibitors *ăn-jē-ō-TĔN-sĭn*	Drugs used to treat hypertension and congestive heart failure; decrease blood pressure, pulmonary resistance, and heart size.
antianginals *ăn-tē-ăn-JĬ-nălz*	Drugs that relieve angina pectoris by vasodilation. Drugs used to treat angina include nitrates, beta-adrenergic blockers, and calcium channel blockers.
antiarrhythmics *ăn-tē-ă-RĬTH-mĭks*	Drugs used to control irregular heartbeat. They exert a therapeutic effect by acting at different times during the electrical cycle of the heart; used in the treatment of atrial and ventricular arrhythmias.
anticoagulants *ăn-tĭ-kō-ĂG-ū-lănts*	Drugs that prevent clot formation. Used to decrease the risk of a stroke in patients who have had transient ischemic attacks; to prevent clots from forming postoperatively after heart, valve, or vascular surgery; and to prevent coagulation in stored blood that is later used for transfusions.
beta-adrenergic blockers *bā-tă-ăd-rĕn-ĔR-jĭk*	Drugs that decrease the rate and force of heart contractions, among other effects. Used to treat congestive heart failure, hypertension, angina, and arrhythmias; also called *beta blockers*.
calcium channel blockers	Drugs that control the rate and force of the heart's contractions by regulating the influx of calcium ions into the cells; they also cause dilation of blood vessels, making it easier for the heart to pump blood through the vessels.
cardiac glycosides, digitalis *KĂR-dē-ăk GLĬ-kō-sīdz, dĭj-ĭ-TĂL-ĭs*	Drugs that slow and strengthen heart muscle contractions. Used to treat congestive heart failure by allowing the heart to pump more slowly and more efficiently.

Pharmacology (Continued)

DRUG CLASSIFICATION	THERAPEUTIC ACTION
diuretics *dī-ū-RĔT-ĭks*	Drugs that eliminate fluid by increasing urine output by the kidneys. Used to treat congestive heart failure and sometimes hypertension.
thrombolytics *thrŏm-bō-LĬT-ĭks*	Drugs that dissolve clots. When thrombolytic enzymes were first introduced, they were the first drugs that could dissolve a clot. These drugs revolutionized the treatment of myocardial infarction and stroke; always given intravenously.

❖ ABBREVIATIONS

ABBREVIATION	MEANING	ABBREVIATION	MEANING
ACLS	advanced cardiac life support	LBBB	left bundle branch block
AICD	automatic implanted cardioverter defibrillator	LDL	low-density lipoprotein
		LDLC	low-density lipoprotein cholesterol
AS	aortic stenosis, left ear (auris sinistra)	LV	left ventricle
ASD	atrial septal defect	MI	myocardial infarction
ASHD	arteriosclerotic heart disease	mL	milliliter
AV	atrioventricular	MVP	mitral valve prolapse
BP	blood pressure	NIR	brand name of an arterial stent made by Medinol Ltd.
CABG	coronary artery bypass graft		
CAD	coronary artery disease	NSR	normal sinus rhythm
Cath	catheterization, catheter	NTG	nitroglycerin
CCU	coronary care unit	PAC	premature atrial contraction
CHD	coronary heart disease	PAD	peripheral arterial disease
CHF	congestive heart failure	PAT	paroxysmal atrial tachycardia
CK	creatine kinase	PTCA	percutaneous transluminal coronary angioplasty
CKMB	{not an abbreviation} [a creatinine kinase isoenzyme]		
		PVC	premature ventricular contraction
CPK	creatine phosphokinase		
CPR	cardiopulmonary resuscitation	RBBB	right bundle branch block
CV	cardiovascular	RV	residual volume, right ventricle
dL	deciliter	SA	sinoatrial
DOE	dyspnea on exertion	TEE	transesophageal echocardiography
DSA	digital subtraction angiography		
DVT	deep vein thrombosis	TOT CHOL	total cholesterol
ECG, EKG	electrocardiogram	TT	thrombolytic therapy
EMS	emergency medical service(s)	VSD	ventricular septal defect
HDL	high-density lipoprotein	VT	ventricular tachycardia
HPI	history of present illness		

Activity 9–9: Clinical Application
Diagnostic Tests, Treatments, and Pharmacology

anastomosis	balloon valvuloplasty	Holter monitor
angiography	cardiac catheterization	lipid profile
angioplasty	defibrillator	pacemaker
antianginals	diuretics	stent placement
anticoagulants	echocardiography	troponin I

Match the terms listed above with the definitions given in the numbered list:

1. _____ a battery of blood tests to measure levels of cholesterol, triglycerides, and lipoproteins; used to evaluate the risk of developing coronary artery disease.

2. _____ utilization of ultrasound to visualize internal cardiac structures and motion of the heart.

3. _____ insertion of a catheter through an incision into a large vein, usually of an arm or leg, that is threaded through the circulatory system into the heart.

4. _____ drugs that prevent clot formation and decrease the risk of a stroke.

5. _____ surgical procedure to reopen narrowed blood vessels and restore blood flow; usually with a balloon catheter.

6. _____ a portable device small enough to be worn by a patient during normal activity. It consists of a recording system capable of storing up to 48 hours of the individual's electrocardiogram.

7. _____ an electrical device that delivers shocks at a preset voltage to the heart to convert fibrillation and life-threatening dysrhythmias back to a normal rhythm.

8. _____ drugs that eliminate fluid by increasing urine output by the kidneys.

9. _____ diagnostic or therapeutic radiography of the heart and blood vessels using a radiopaque contrast medium.

10. _____ insertion of an inflatable balloon to open a stenotic heart valve.

11. _____ a permanent implantable device used to establish a normal heart rhythm and overcome heart block.

12. _____ blood test that measures protein that is released into the blood by damaged heart muscle (but not skeletal muscle); a highly sensitive and specific indicator of recent myocardial infarction.

13. _____ surgical joining of two blood vessels to bypass an aneurysm.

14. _____ drugs that relieve angina pectoris by vasodilation and include beta blockers and calcium channel blockers.

15. _____ surgical insertion of a small, self-expanding meshlike tube to treat acute vessel closure after angioplasty; opens up the blocked artery

Correct Answers _____ **× 6.67** _____ **% Score**

Activity 9–10: Build Medical Words
Diagnostic, Symptomatic, and Operative Terms

Use *cardi/o* (heart) to build medical words meaning:

1. pertaining to the heart _____

2. enlargement of the heart _____

3. any disease of the heart muscle _____

4. pain in the heart _____

Use *arteri/o* (artery) to build medical words meaning:

5. rupture of an artery _____

6. involuntary contraction or twitching of an artery _____

7. condition of hardening of the artery _____

Use *ven/o* (vein) to build medical words meaning:

8. pertaining to a vein _____

9. narrowing of a vein _____

10. suture of a vein _____

Use *phleb/o* (vein) to build medical words meaning:

11. incision of a vein _____

12. excision of a vein _____

Use *ather/o* (fatty plaque) to build medical words meaning:

13. removal of fatty plaque _____

14. a tumor of fatty plaque _____

Use *arteriol/o* (arteriole) to build medical words meaning:

15. inflammation of an arteriole (wall) _____

16. condition of hardening of the arterioles _____

Use *sphygm/o* (pulse) to build medical words meaning:

17. instrument to measure the pulse _____

18. resembling the pulse _____

Use *hemangi/o* (blood vessel) to build medical words meaning:

19. dilation of a blood vessel _____

20. tumor of blood vessels _____

Correct Answers _____ × 5 = _____ % Score

MEDICAL RECORDS

Authentic medical records for a patient who developed chest pain while playing tennis, and who was subsequently taken by ambulance to the emergency room and diagnosed with a heart attack, are presented in this section. They include an emergency room report, a laboratory report, a cardiac catheterization report, and a discharge summary.

The following dictionary exercise and medical record analysis will help you develop skills to abstract information and master the terminology in the reports. In turn, you will be able to understand the importance of accurately interpreting information from a medical record.

Reading and Dictionary Exercise

Place a check mark [✓] after you complete the exercise.

[ ] **1.** Underline the following words in the records as you read the emergency room note, the laboratory report, the cardiac catheterization report, and the discharge summary aloud. These medical records can be found at the end of the chapter.

[ ] **2.** Use a medical dictionary and Appendix F, Part 2 to define the terms below.

Note: You are not expected to fully understand all the parts of the medical records. The important aspect of this exercise is to use all available resources to complete it. Eventually you will master the terminology and format of these reports.

> > > MEDICAL RECORD 9–1: EMERGENCY ROOM REPORT

Term	Pronunciation	Meaning
diaphoresis	*dī-ă-fō-RĒ-sĭs*	_____
syncope	*SĬN-kō-pē*	_____
nitroglycerin	*nī-trō-GLĬS-ĕr-ĭn*	_____
Xanax	*ZĂN-ăks*	_____
inguinal	*ĬNG-gwĭ-năl*	_____
herniorrhaphy	*hĕr-nē-ŌR-ă-fē*	_____

anorexia	ăn-ō-RĔK-sē-ă	_____
pneumonia	nū-MŌ-nē-ă	_____
bronchitis	brŏng-KĪ-tĭs	_____
asthma	ĂZ-mă	_____
hemoptysis	hē-MŎP-tĭ-sĭs	_____
incontinence	ĭn-KŎN-tĭ-nĕns	_____
pruritus	proo-RĪ-tĭs	_____
hematologic	hē-mă-tō-LŎG-ĭk	_____
anemia	ă-NĒ-mē-ă	_____
neurologic	nū-rō-LŎG-ĭk	_____
vertigo	VĔR-tĭ-gō	_____
paresthesia	păr-ĕs-THĒ-zē-ă	_____
auscultation	ăws-kŭl-TĀ-shŭn	_____
carotid bruits	kă-RŎT-ĭd brwēs	_____
troponin	TRŌ-pō-nĭn	_____

> > > MEDICAL RECORD 9-2: LABORATORY REPORT

Term	Pronunciation	Meaning
ischemia	ĭs-KĒ-mē-ă	_____

> > > MEDICAL RECORD 9-3: CARDIAC CATHETERIZATION REPORT

Term	Pronunciation	Meaning
catheterization	kăth-ĕ-tĕr-ĭ-ZĀ-shŭn	_____
hypokinetic	hī-pō-kĭ-NĔT-ĭk	_____
ejection fraction	ē-JĔK-shŭn FRĂK-shŭn	_____
stented	STĔN-tĕd	_____
echocardiogram	ĕ-kō-KĂR-dē-ō-grăm	_____
Plavix	PLĂ-vĭks	_____
Lipitor	LĬP-ĭ-tŏr	_____

> > > MEDICAL RECORD 9-4: DISCHARGE SUMMARY

Term	Pronunciation	Meaning
angiographic	ăn-jē-ō-GRĂF-ĭk	_____
ventriculography	věn-trĭk-ū-LŎG-ră-fē	_____
anterolateral	ăn-těr-ō-LĂT-ěr-ăl	_____
valvular	VĂL-vū-lăr	_____
circumflex artery	SĚR-kŭm-flěks ĂR-těr-ē	_____
hematoma	hěm-ă-TŌ-mă	_____
femoral	FĚM-ŏr-ăl	_____

Critical Thinking: Analysis of Medical Records

This section provides experience in abstracting and analyzing information from medical records. At the same time, it reinforces the material presented in this chapter.

> > > MEDICAL RECORD 9-1: EMERGENCY ROOM REPORT

1. Why did the patient call the emergency medical service or ambulance?

_____

_____

2. What treatment did the EMS technicians administer once they arrived at the patient's home?

_____

3. What classification of drugs does nitroglycerin belong to? How does nitroglycerin relieve chest pain?

_____

_____

> > > MEDICAL RECORD 9-2: LABORATORY REPORT

4. Which laboratory test results under the lipid profile are abnormal and indicate an increased risk for coronary artery disease?

_____

5. What do the cardiac laboratory test results indicate?

_____

> > > MEDICAL RECORD 9-3: CARDIAC CATHETERIZATION REPORT

6. What are the significant findings of the cardiac catheterization?

_____

_____

_____

7. What drugs were prescribed to the patient?

_____

8. Does the patient have any limitations on activity levels? If yes, what are they?

_____

9. What lifestyle change is recommended for this patient to reduce his risk of future heart disease? Explain what this means.

_____

_____

> > > MEDICAL RECORD 9-4: DISCHARGE SUMMARY

10. What are the discharge diagnoses?

_____

_____

11. Which artery was found to be occluded? What procedure was then performed on it?

_____

Audio Practice

Listen to the audio CD-ROM to practice the pronunciation of selected medical terms from this chapter.

Medical Record 9-1. Emergency Room Report

GENERAL HOSPITAL AND MEDICAL CENTER
2211 Fifth Avenue North • Healthy City, USA 12345 • (321) 123-4567

Emergency Room Report

Patient Name: Edgar Robinson   **Patient Number:** 45-67-89
Birth Date: 04/01/xx   **Room Number:**   ER

DATE OF SERVICE: 10/28/xx

CHIEF COMPLAINT: Chest pain that started while playing tennis at approximately 1:30 p.m. today.

HISTORY OF PRESENT ILLNESS: Edgar Robinson is a 66-year-old Caucasian male who presents with onset of chest pain which occurred as he was playing tennis. The pain was initially low grade and quite subtle. He went home and as he was having lunch, his pain became more severe and associated with a tremendous feeling of weakness and with some nausea. He denies any vomiting, any dizziness, any diaphoresis or any syncope. His pain did not radiate to the shoulder, jaw or arm. EMS was called. They administered three nitroglycerin and four baby aspirin at the scene. The patient's pain dramatically improved. He was brought to General Hospital and Medical Center emergency department for evaluation and further treatment. Upon arrival at the emergency department, his pain was rated to be barely 1 on a scale of 1 to 10.

MEDICATION ALLERGIES: None.

CURRENT MEDICATIONS: Aspirin and Xanax.

PAST MEDICAL HISTORY: History of an anxiety disorder and right inguinal herniorrhaphy.

SOCIAL HISTORY: He does not smoke. Alcohol—social.

FAMILY HISTORY: Noncontributory.

REVIEW OF SYSTEMS: General: The patient denies malaise, fever, anorexia or weight loss. Respiratory: He denies shortness of breath, recent pneumonia, bronchitis, asthma, cough, hemoptysis, or sputum production. Cardiovascular: See HPI. GI: He denies vomiting. He admits to nausea. He denies abdominal pain, diarrhea, blood per rectum, change in color or caliber of the stool or tarry stools. GU: He denies itching or burning upon urination. He denies incontinence or urinary retention. Extremities: He denies redness, swelling or painful joints.

Continued

Medical Record 9–3. Cardiac Catheterization Report

GENERAL HOSPITAL AND MEDICAL CENTER
2211 Fifth Avenue North • Healthy City, USA 12345 • (321) 123-4567

Cardiac Catheterization Report

Patient Name: Edgar Robinson   **Patient Number:** 45-67-89
Date of Birth: 04/01/xx   **Room Number:** 750

October 29, 20xx

Thomas Booth, M.D.
2711 Goodard Road
Miami, FL 54321

Dear Thomas:

Your patient Edgar Robinson underwent emergency cardiac catheterization on 10/29/xx in response to an uncomplicated non-Q, high lateral MI that clinically was moderated by medical therapy, (CPK Max 1100). Single vessel CAD with mild LV dysfunction was found. The large, bifurcated, intermediate artery was totally occluded just beyond the origin and faintly collateralized. There was only mild irregularity of the other vessels. The intermediate artery territory was moderately hypokinetic, reducing the calculated ejection fraction to 53%. Immediately following that diagnostic procedure, the intermediate was successfully stented with a 2.5 mm NIR leaving an optimal result. An echocardiogram performed just prior to the procedure confirmed only mild to moderate hypokinesis of the affected segment; i.e., he may well experience full recovery. He will require one month of Plavix therapy in addition to aspirin. He was advised to refrain from vigorous athletic activity for 3-4 weeks to allow the ventricle to recover. His LDL was mildly elevated and HDL low (26) indicating the need for aggressive dietary measures. Lipitor 10 mg q.d. was initiated. He was referred to Dr. Dean Ornish's book "Reversing Heart Disease" for guidance in this regard. I look forward to following along with you.

Thomas, thanks again for allowing me to assist in Edgar's care. I enjoyed meeting him as well as working with you.

Sincerely,

Peter Carter, M.D.

PC/bab
D: 10/29/xx
T: 11/02/xx

Medical Record 9–4. Discharge Summary

GENERAL HOSPITAL AND MEDICAL CENTER
2211 Fifth Avenue North • Healthy City, USA 12345 • (321) 123-4567

Discharge Summary

Patient Name: Edgar Robinson   **Patient Number:** 45-67-89
Date of Birth: 04/01/xx   **Room Number:** ER

ADMISSION DATE: 10/28/xx

DISCHARGE DATE: 10/31/xx

ADMISSION DIAGNOSIS: Angina pectoris.

DISCHARGE DIAGNOSES:
1. High lateral non-Q wave myocardial infarction with associated angina pectoris.
2. Coronary artery disease.
3. Anxiety.

PROCEDURES: Cardiac catheterization 10/29/xx.

HISTORY: The patient is a 66-year-old Caucasian-European male who experienced lower mid sternal chest pain playing tennis, which increased in severity and radiated to the left and right chest after discontinuing his activity. He was treated with sublingual nitroglycerin, which completely relieved the pain. His history is significant for chest pain four years ago, which necessitated a cardiac catheterization at that time. This proved to be an essentially negative study. The patient also has a history of anxiety related to considerable occupational stress and hazards.

HOSPITAL COURSE: The patient was admitted to General Hospital and Medical Center where cardiac enzymes and serial EKGs were performed. Initial cardiac enzymes were normal; however, a repeat on 10/29/xx revealed elevated levels of CK at 1101, CKMB screen at 136.2, and troponin I at 238. EKG on 10/29/xx was suggestive of a non-Q wave high lateral myocardial infarction. This prompted Dr. Booth, the patient's attending physician, to consult with Dr. Dray. Dr. Dray found these indications required angiographic investigation and possible therapy and subsequently consulted with Dr. Carter. Dr. Carter performed a left heart catheterization on the morning of 10/29/xx. Diagnostic procedures included left ventriculography and coronary angiography. These diagnostic efforts revealed moderate anterolateral hypokinesis and a left ventricular ejection fraction estimated to be 53%. The valvular function was

Continued

Discharge Summary, page 2
Patient Name: Edgar Robinson   **Patient Number:** 45-67-89

determined to be normal as was the left main artery. Mild irregularity of the main circumflex artery as well as mild diffuse irregularity of the mid right coronary artery were noted. The intermediate artery was found to be occluded just beyond the origin with faint collaterals.

Dr. Carter successfully stented the origin and proximal portions of this vessel using a 2.5 mm 25 NIR. The patient tolerated the procedure well and experienced no complications during the immediate post procedure recovery phase. EKG the following day revealed persisting T wave inversion in Leads I and AV. Cardiac enzyme levels had decreased markedly. Physical examination of the patient one day post procedure revealed no hematoma in the femoral insertion site and no other significant physical findings. The patient progressed rapidly and without evidence of recurrent ischemia. Mr. Robinson was discharged home on 10/31/xx.

_____

Peter Carter, M.D.

PC/slm
D: 10/31/xx
T: 11/02/xx

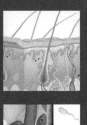
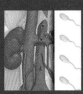
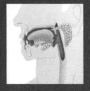
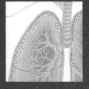

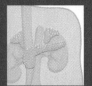
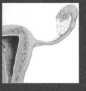
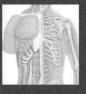
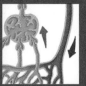
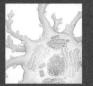
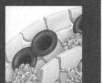

10 Endocrinology

Chapter Outline

Objectives

Upon completion of this chapter, you will be able to:

- Describe the type of medical treatment an endocrinologist provides.
- Name the organs of the endocrine system and discuss the functions of their hormonal secretions.
- Recognize, pronounce, build, and spell correctly medical terms related to the endocrine system.
- Describe pathological conditions, diagnostic tests, surgical procedures, and other treatments related to the endocrine system.
- Demonstrate your knowledge of this chapter by successfully completing the activities and analysis of medical records.

About Endocrinology

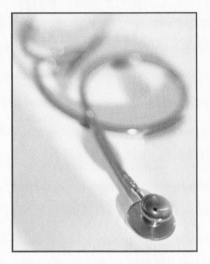

The medical practice of **endocrinology** encompasses the treatment of endocrine disorders and various hormonal disorders associated with body growth, sexual development, and function. **Endocrinologists** specialize in treating endocrine gland diseases and hormone production disorders. They evaluate the body's overall **metabolism,** calcium levels, the control of overall fluid concentrations, and disorders of blood sugar level and glucose metabolism. When surgery is required to treat an endocrine disorder, the endocrinologist works closely with the surgeon to provide the most advantageous patient care. Endocrinologists also play important roles related to their field of expertise in university-based academic research and in the pharmaceutical industry.

To grasp the scope of practice and the role of health-care practitioners in the medical specialty of endocrinology, it is essential to understand the structure and function of the endocrine system as well as the language of medicine that is related to this medical specialty.

Selected Key Terms

androgen
ĂN-drō-jĕn
andro=male
gen=forming, producing, origin

Generic term for an agent, usually a hormone (testosterone, androsterone) that stimulates activity of the accessory male sex organs or stimulates the development of male characteristics.

homeostasis
hō-mē-ō-STĀ-sĭs
homeo=same
stasis=standing still

A relative constancy or equilibrium in the internal environment of the body. This balance is maintained by the ever-changing processes of feedback and regulation in response to external or internal changes.

masculinization
măs-kū-lĭn-ĭ-ZĀ-shŭn

The normal development of secondary male sex characteristics that occurs during puberty; or the abnormal development of masculine characteristics that can occur in a woman.

metabolism
mĕ-TĂB-ō-lĭz-ĕm

The sum of all physical and chemical changes that take place within an organism; all energy and material transformations that occur within living cells.

prolactin
prō-LĂK-tĭn

A hormone produced by the pituitary gland. In humans, prolactin, in association with estrogen and progesterone, stimulates breast development and the formation of milk during pregnancy.

testis (plural, **testes**)
TĔS-tĭs
test=testis
is=noun ending

One of the paired male gonads or testicles.

virilism
VĬR-ĭl-ĭzm

The presence or development of male secondary sex characteristics in a woman.

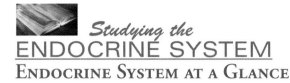

Studying the ENDOCRINE SYSTEM

ENDOCRINE SYSTEM AT A GLANCE

The internally secreting endocrine glands are ductless glands. They have a rich blood supply that enables the chemicals they produce to rapidly enter the bloodstream. These internal chemical messengers of the body are known as *hormones*. They are secreted directly into the bloodstream and transported by the circulatory system to all parts of the body. The production of hormones occurs at one site but their effects take place at various other sites in the body. For example, epinephrine is secreted by the adrenal glands (located above the kidneys) but has the capacity to influence the functions of other organs throughout the body. Epinephrine increases cardiac activity, dilates bronchial tubes, and increases the use of fats for energy. In contrast, exocrine glands, such as the sweat and oil glands, the liver (which secretes bile), and many others release their products through a duct onto body surfaces or into body cavities.

The endocrine and nervous systems are considered the dual regulatory systems of the body and coordinate each other's activities to maintain **homeostasis.** Both systems play an important role in coordinating hormone secretions. The nervous system fulfills this role by regulating body functions by means of nerve impulses. Certain parts of the nervous system either stimulate or inhibit the release of hormones. In turn, these hormone secretions are capable of stimulating or inhibiting the flow of nerve impulses. The complementary effects of both systems permit precise control of body functions in response to varied changes within and outside the body. The effects of the nervous system appear rapidly but may be short-lived. They are balanced by slower hormonal effects, which are longer lasting and usually occur at distant sites known as target sites or target organs. Some hormones, such as insulin (pancreatic secretion), have many target organs. Other hormones, such as calcitonin (thyroid secretion), have only one or a few target organs.

The release of hormones is controlled by different mechanisms that assist in maintaining a well-controlled blood level. Some hormones, such as thyroid hormone, are maintained at fairly constant levels, whereas others, such as epinephrine, are released intermittently as the demand occurs. Yet other hormones, such as estrogen in women, follow a cyclic pattern. In general, when hormone concentration rises and becomes too high, further production of that hormone must be inhibited. When hormone concentration decreases and becomes too low, the rate of production of that hormone must be increased. Therefore, a hormone deficiency can be corrected with a synthetic hormone medication to increase or replace the missing one. For example, if the pancreas does not produce insulin, medications are available to address this deficiency. The type of medication prescribed varies according to the patient's needs. Some patients with diabetes require periodic injections of insulin to maintain a normal blood sugar level, whereas others may be treated with oral antidiabetic drugs. These are discussed in greater detail in the Pathological Conditions and Pharmacology sections of this chapter.

The interrelationship of the endocrine system with other body systems is illustrated in Figure 10–1.

STRUCTURE AND FUNCTION

To learn the names and the respective locations of the endocrine glands, label Figure 10–2: the (1) **pituitary gland (hypophysis),** the (2) **thyroid gland,** the four (3) **parathyroid glands,** the paired (4) **adrenal glands (suprarenal),** the (5) **pancreas (islets of Langerhans),** the paired female (6) **ovaries,** the paired male (7) **testes,** the (8) **pineal gland,** and the (9) **thymus gland.** As you write the names of the glands, review their hormone secretions, which are summarized in Figure 10–2. These secretions are discussed in greater detail throughout the chapter. The hormone abbreviations can quickly be referenced in the Abbreviations section.

HORMONE SECRETION

The regulation of hormone secretion is achieved by *negative* and *positive feedback systems.* These mechanisms monitor and control the hormone levels in the body. The feedback mechanism that regulates most hormone secretions involves the hypothalamus, the pituitary gland, and the target organs (Fig. 10–3). The primary purpose of this mechanism is to regulate the balance of hormone secretions in the body in order to maintain homeostasis.

The main feedback mechanism in the endocrine system is the negative feedback mechanism. It can be compared to a thermostat in a central heating system. When a gland is working harder than the body needs it to work, the system switches the secretions off. Conversely, when the body needs to have the gland speed up, the system turns on the switch and the gland increases its secretions. Positive feedback, which occurs when the gland continues to trigger additional hormone secretions, is rarely seen in the endocrine system. In summary, positive feedback promotes the release of hormones, whereas negative feedback inhibits the release of hormones.

Body System Connections
Endocrine System

THE CARDIOVASCULAR SYSTEM
◆ As hormones are transported in the blood, they influence the functions of the heart and blood vessels.

THE DIGESTIVE SYSTEM
◆ Local hormones influence digestive activity; cholecystokinin stimulates contraction of the gall-bladder and secretion of pancreatic enzymes. ◆ The pancreas contains hormone-producing cells that play a role in the digestive process. ◆ The digestive system provides vital nutrients to endocrine organs.

THE FEMALE REPRODUCTIVE SYSTEM
◆ The development and function of the reproductive system are influenced by hormones. ◆ Sex hormones are the main influence on the development of the egg and the secondary sex characteristics.

THE INTEGUMENTARY SYSTEM
◆ Hormones activate either the decomposition or the synthesis of subcutaneous fat.

THE LYMPHATIC AND IMMUNE SYSTEMS
◆ Lymphocyte production is activated by hormones.

THE MUSCULOSKELETAL SYSTEM
◆ Due to hormone secretions, blood flow increases to muscles during exercise. ◆ Normal muscular and skeletal development requires adequate growth hormone. ◆ Blood calcium balance is governed by hormones.

THE NERVOUS SYSTEM
◆ The adrenal medulla and the posterior pituitary gland are controlled by nerve impulses. Likewise hormonal secretions influence nervous system functions.

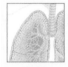

THE RESPIRATORY SYSTEM
◆ The release of certain hormones increases the rate of cellular respiration and dilates the bronchial tubes.

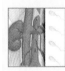

THE URINARY AND MALE REPRODUCTIVE SYSTEMS
◆ Water and electrolyte balance are controlled by the action of hormones on the kidneys. ◆ Specific hormones influence reproductive system development and function. ◆ Sex hormones are the main influence on the development of sperm.

Figure 10–1 *The interrelationship of the endocrine system with other body systems.*

Activity 10–1: Competency Verification
Endocrine Glands

Review the hormonal secretions that are summarized in Figure 10–2, and check your labeling of the endocrine glands in Appendix C.

PITUITARY GLAND

Located at the base of the brain, the pituitary gland is a small pea-shaped gland that is attached to the hypothalamus (see Fig. 10–2) by a short stalk. Often referred to as the "master gland" of the endocrine system, it is also known as the *hypophysis*. The pituitary

gland secretes hormones that govern hormonal secretions of other endocrine glands. Refer to Figure 10–3 for a graphic review of the pituitary gland's many target organs. The hormonal secretions of the pituitary, in a large part, are controlled by the hypothalamus.

The pituitary gland is functionally and structurally divided into an anterior lobe, or adenohypophysis, and a posterior lobe, or neurohypophysis. As their names imply, the adenohypophysis (*adeno*=gland) comprises glandular tissue, whereas the neurohypophysis (*neuro*=nerve) is composed, and is an extension, of the nerve tissue of the hypothalamus (Fig. 10–2), and the posterior pituitary gland. The hormone secretions of the adenohypophysis and neurohypophysis are discussed in the following sections.

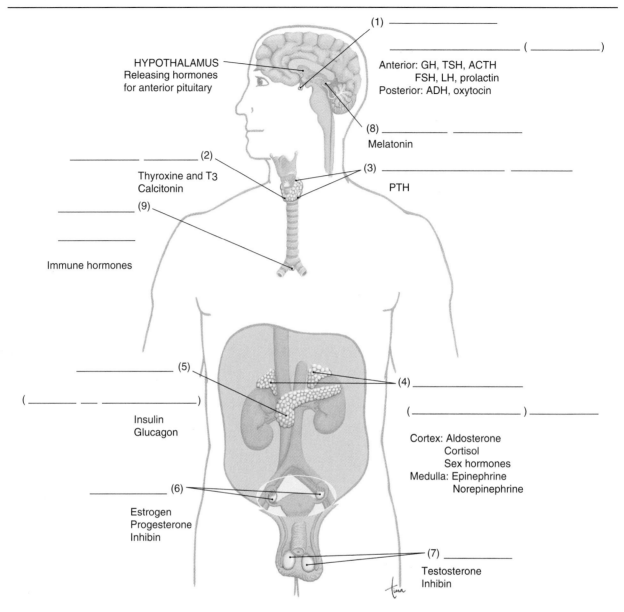

HYPOTHALAMUS
Releasing hormones
for anterior pituitary

(1) _____

_____ (_____)

Anterior: GH, TSH, ACTH
FSH, LH, prolactin
Posterior: ADH, oxytocin

(8) _____ _____
Melatonin

_____ _____ (2)
Thyroxine and T3
Calcitonin

(3) _____ _____
PTH

_____ (9)
_____
Immune hormones

(5) _____
(_____ __ _____)
Insulin
Glucagon

(4) _____
(_____) _____
Cortex: Aldosterone
Cortisol
Sex hormones
Medulla: Epinephrine
Norepinephrine

(6) _____
Estrogen
Progesterone
Inhibin

(7) _____
Testosterone
Inhibin

Figure 10–2 *The endocrine system. The names and locations of many endocrine glands. Both male and female gonads (testes and ovaries) are shown. (Adapted from Scanlon, VC, and Sanders, TS: Essentials of Anatomy and Physiology, ed 3. FA Davis, Philadelphia, 1999, p 211, with permission.)*

Adenohypophysis

1. **Adrenocorticotropic hormone (ACTH).**
   ACTH stimulates the adrenal cortex to release
   corticosteroid hormones, most importantly
   glucocorticoids, which help the body to resist
   any type of physiological stress situation such
   as injury, disease, exercise, or hypoglycemia
   (being hungry is stressful).

2. **Gonadotropic hormones.** The follicle-
   stimulating hormone (FSH) and *luteinizing*
   hormone (LH) are referred to collectively as
   gonadotropins. As their name implies, the

gonadotropins regulate the function of the
reproductive organs or gonads (ovaries and
testes). In both sexes, FSH stimulates **gamete**
(sperm or egg) production, whereas LH
promotes production of gonadal hormones. In
women, FSH initiates development of ova in the
ovarian follicles, induces estrogen production
by the follicle cells, stimulates ovulation, and
prepares the uterus for implantation and the
mammary glands for milk secretion.

3. **Growth hormone (GH).** Also known as
   somatotropin, GH stimulates the growth of
   bones and muscles, and of other organs.

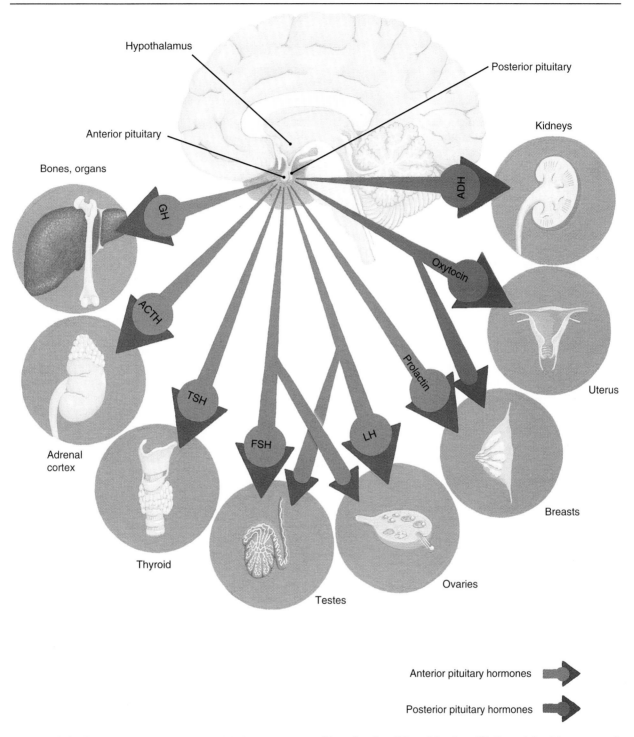

Figure 10–3 *Pituitary gland hormones and their target organs. (From Scanlon, VC, and Sanders, TS: Essentials of Anatomy and Physiology, ed 3. FA Davis, Philadelphia, 1999, p 183, with permission.)*

Hyposecretion of GH during childhood results in pituitary dwarfism. The possible cause is a congenital deficiency or destruction of the GH-producing cells. Conversely, hypersecretion of GH during childhood results in pituitary giantism. A possible cause may be a pituitary tumor present before puberty. When hypersecretion of

GH occurs during adulthood, the excess GH causes disproportionate increase in the size of bones. This includes the bones of the face, hands, and feet and results in acromegaly.

4. **Thyroid-stimulating hormone (TSH).** Also known as *thyrotropin*, TSH stimulates normal

development and secretory activity of the thyroid gland.

5. **Prolactin (PRL).** PRL enhances breast tissue growth and stimulates milk production by the mammary glands.

Neurohypophysis

1. **Antidiuretic hormone (ADH):** Also called vasopressin, ADH is produced by one of the specialized clusters of cells in the hypothalamus and is stored in the posterior pituitary until needed. This hormone prevents wide swings in water balance, helping to avoid dehydration or water overload.

2. **Oxytocin.** This hormone has no known function in men, but in women it triggers contractions of the pregnant uterus during labor and childbirth, and then later stimulates the release of breast milk.

A summary of hormones secreted by the pituitary gland is illustrated in Flowchart 10–1. Because this material may be difficult to grasp when you are first introduced to it, it is important to read the material on the pituitary gland again and refer to the figures and Flowchart 10–1 as you review the material.

THYROID GLAND

The thyroid gland is an H-shaped organ comprising two lobes that lie on either side of the trachea. The lobes are connected by a strip of tissue called *isthmus*. The thyroid gland is the largest gland of the endocrine system and is positioned just below the larynx.

The thyroid gland produces three hormones, **triiodothyronine** (T_3), **thyroxine** (T_4), and **calcitonin.**

1. **Triiodothyronine** and **thyroxine** are jointly known as *thyroid hormones*. T_3 contains three iodine atoms, whereas T_4 contains four iodine atoms. These hormones are produced in the thyroid gland and require iodine for their synthesis. The thyroid gland is extremely efficient in taking up iodine from the circulating blood and concentrating it within the cells.

The two hormones regulate cellular metabolic activity and serve as a general pacemaker by accelerating metabolic processes. They increase the rate of oxygen consumption and, in turn, the rate at which carbohydrates, proteins, and fats are metabolized. Thyroid hormones also influence cell replication and are important in brain development and normal growth. Because of their widespread effects on cellular metabolism, these hormones influence every major body organ.

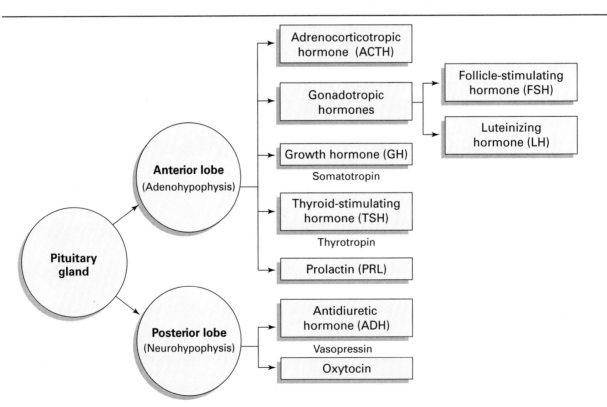

Flowchart 10–1 *The pituitary gland and its hormones: the anterior lobe (or adenohypophysis) and the posterior lobe (or neurohypophysis).*

Hyposecretion of thyroid hormones during childhood results in **cretinism;** hyposecretion of thyroid hormones during adulthood results in **myxedema.** Hypersecretion of thyroid hormones, most frequently due to **Graves disease,** is usually associated with an enlarged thyroid gland (goiter). **Goiter** (Fig. 10–4) also commonly occurs when there is a deficiency of iodine. These are discussed in the Pathological Conditions section of the chapter.

2. **Calcitonin** (or thyrocalcitonin) regulates the level of calcium in the blood and is known as a calcium-lowering hormone. When calcium levels in the blood are high, the thyroid gland responds by secreting calcitonin into the bloodstream. This causes bone cells known as *osteoclasts* to slow down their release of calcium into the bloodstream. Thus, blood calcium levels are lowered back to normal. Calcitonin exerts its most important effects during childhood years when bone growth is at its maximum rate.

The functions of thyroid gland hormones are illustrated in Flowchart 10–2. Because you may find this material difficult to understand when you are introduced to it, it is important to read the material on the thyroid gland again and refer to Flowchart 10–2 as you review the material.

PARATHYROID GLANDS

There are four parathyroid glands: a superior pair and an inferior pair, which are attached to each lateral thyroid lobe as illustrated in the posterior view of the thyroid glands in Figure 10–5. Only one hormone is produced by the parathyroid glands, the parathormone

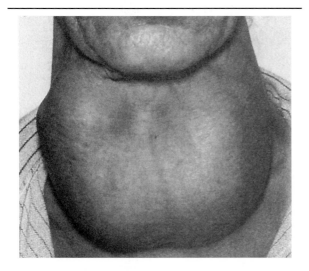

Figure 10–4 *Enlargement of the thyroid gland in goiter. (From Morton, PG: Health Assessment in Nursing. ed 2. FA Davis, Philadelphia, 1993, p 104, with permission.)*

hormone (PTH). PTH helps maintain homeostasis of *calcium* and *phosphate* levels by stimulating the bones, intestines, and kidneys. Increased secretion of PTH results in increased calcium absorption from the bones, small intestine, and kidneys. PTH's feedback mechanism adjusts calcium levels as it (1) stimulates the conservation of calcium by the kidneys; (2) stimulates the reabsorption of calcium and phosphate from bone to blood; and (3) stimulates the absorption of calcium by the intestine. The parathyroid hormones and their functions are illustrated in Figure 10–6. The following paragraph further illustrates the feedback mechanism of PTH.

Because of the actions of PTH, calcium and phosphate are released from bones, their concentration increasing in the blood. Thus, calcium that is necessary for the proper functioning of body tissues is available in the bloodstream. At the same time, PTH enhances absorption of calcium and phosphate from foods in the small intestine, which increases blood calcium and decreases blood phosphate. PTH causes the kidneys to conserve blood calcium and to accelerate excretion of phosphate in the urine. Excess PTH can result in markedly elevated levels of blood calcium, a potentially life-threatening situation. When blood calcium and blood phosphate become too high, calcium phosphate may accumulate in various organs of the body and cause tissue calcification. The overall effect of PTH is to regulate calcium and phosphate metabolism by raising blood calcium levels and lowering blood phosphate levels.

Because this new material may be difficult to grasp, it may be necessary to read this section again and review Figure 10–6, which illustrates the functions of parathyroid hormone.

ADRENAL GLANDS

Attached to the upper portion of each kidney are two adrenal glands. Because of their location above the kidneys, these glands are also known as the suprarenal glands (*supra* =above). As illustrated in Figure 10–2, they cover the superior surface of the kidneys. Each adrenal gland is structurally and functionally differentiated into an outer region, the *adrenal cortex,* and an inner region, the *adrenal medulla.* Each part generates different hormones that have distinctively different functions.

Adrenal Cortex

The adrenal cortex secretes three types of steroid hormones called *corticosteroids:* sex hormones, mineralocorticoids, and glucocorticoids.

1. **Sex hormones.** Estrogens and androgens are female and male hormones, which maintain

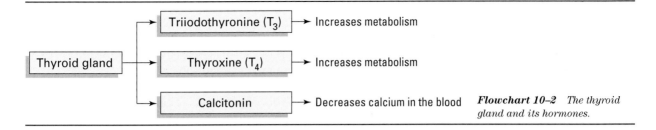

Triiodothyronine (T$_3$) → Increases metabolism

Thyroid gland → Thyroxine (T$_4$) → Increases metabolism

Calcitonin → Decreases calcium in the blood

Flowchart 10–2 The thyroid gland and its hormones.

secondary sex characteristics, such as breast development in the woman and facial hair in the man. Estrogens are produced primarily by the female ovaries and **androgens** are produced primarily by the male testes. Androgens are also secreted by the adrenal cortex in both women and men. In women, an oversecretion of adrenal androgen results in **virilism** or **masculinization.** In men, an oversecretion of adrenal estrogen and progestin results in **feminization.**

2. **Mineralocorticoids.** The essential function of mineralocorticoids is regulation of the electrolyte (mineral salt) concentrations in

extracellular fluids. They regulate sodium, water, and potassium balance by acting on the kidneys. *Sodium* (a positive electrolyte of salt) is one of the most important elements in the body and is essential to life. For the body to function normally, it is vital to have a normal balance of salts and water in the blood and tissues. *Aldosterone* is the most potent and essential mineralocorticoid. This hormone increases blood levels of sodium and water and decreases blood levels of an electrolyte called *potassium.*

3. **Glucocorticoids.** The glucocorticoids, mainly cortisol, help promote normal metabolism, resistance to stress, and counterinflammatory response. Pharmacological glucocorticoid preparations are frequently administered to reduce edema caused by the inflammatory response to tissue injury and also to suppress allergic manifestations. A synthetically prepared hormone known as *cortisone* resembles cortisol and is used in the treatment of inflammatory conditions such as arthritis. Hyposecretion of glucocorticoids results in Addison disease. Conversely, hypersecretion of glucocorticoids results in Cushing syndrome (Fig. 10–7). These are discussed in greater detail in the Pathological Condtions section of this chapter.

Adrenal Medulla

The adrenal medulla (Fig. 10–2) produces the hormones *epinephrine (adrenaline)* and *norepineph-rine (noradrenaline)*. Both hormones are sympathomimetic because they produce effects that mimic those brought about by the sympathetic nervous system. To a great extent, they are accountable for the fight-or-flight response and help the body resist stress. Epinephrine increases cardiac activity, dilates bronchioles, activates conversion of glycogen to glucose in the liver, increases use of fats for energy, increases the rate of cell respiration, decreases peristalsis, and causes vasoconstriction in the skin, viscera, and skeletal muscle. These hormones affect the body during stress. The most important function of norepinephrine is its ability to raise blood pressure by causing vasoconstriction in the skin, viscera,

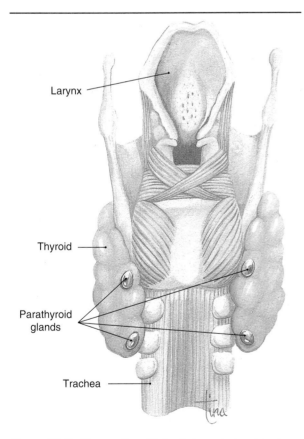

Larynx

Thyroid

Parathyroid glands

Trachea

Figure 10–5 The parathyroid glands in posterior view, on the lobes of the thyroid gland. (From Scanlon, VC, and Sanders, TS: Essentials of Anatomy and Physiology, ed 3. FA Davis, Philadelphia, 1999, p 219, with permission.)

Parathyroid hormone (PTH)

Stimulates the conservation of calcium by the kidneys
Stimulates the reabsorption of calcium and phosphate from
bone to blood
Stimulates the absorption of calcium by the intestine

The effect of PTH release is
to raise levels of calcium,
which in turn inhibits
further PTH release

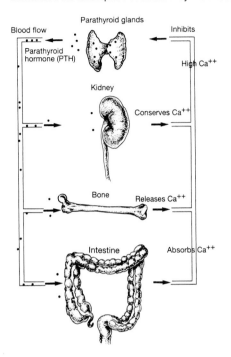

Figure 10–6 *The hormone released by the parathyroid glands. (From Glylys, BA, and Wedding, ME: Medical Terminology: A Systems Approach, ed 4. FA Davis, Philadelphia, 1999, p 297, with permission.)*

and skeletal muscles. The functions of the adrenal medulla and its hormones, epinephrine and norepinephrine, are illustrated in Flowchart 10–3.

A summary of the adrenal glands and their hormones is given in Flowchart 10–4. Because this material may be difficult to comprehend when you are first introduced to it, it is important to read the material on the adrenal glands again and refer to Flowchart 10–4.

PANCREAS

The pancreas is located posterior to the stomach, between the spleen and duodenum, as illustrated in Figure 10–2. It is a flattened organ with average length of 6 inches and its average weight is about 3 ounces. The pancreas functions both as an exocrine and an endocrine gland. A large pancreatic duct extends through the gland, carrying enzymes and other exocrine digestive secretions from the pancreas into the small intestine. The pancreas performs both exocrine (digestive) functions as well as endocrine functions, but only the endocrine functions are discussed here. For a discussion of exocrine functions, refer to Chapter 7.

Clusters of specialized cells within the pancreas called the **islets of Langerhans** produce two hormones: *glucagon* (produced by alpha cells) and *insulin* (produced by beta cells). These two important hormones help maintain the normal metabolism of sugars and starches in the body.

Glucagon

When the blood sugar level drops below normal, alpha cells release the hormone glucagon. Glucagon, in turn, stimulates the liver to break down glycogen and certain noncarbohydrates, like amino acids, into glucose. This breakdown increases the blood glucose that is released from the liver. Refer to Flowchart 10–5 to review the functions of insulin and glucagon that are related to the maintenance of the blood glucose level.

Two important pathological conditions related to blood glucose are **hypoglycemia** (low blood glucose) and **hyperglycemia** (high blood glucose), which are discussed in the Pathological Conditions section of this chapter.

Insulin

Insulin hormone has an opposite or **antagonistic** effect to that of glucagon. Insulin stimulates the liver to form *glycogen* (glycogenesis) from glucose and inhibits conversion of noncarbohydrates into glucose.

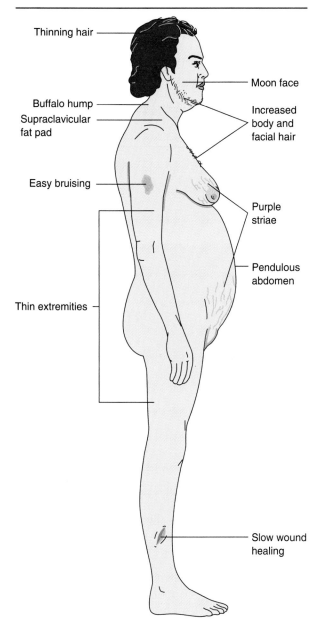

Thinning hair

Moon face

Buffalo hump

Supraclavicular fat pad

Increased body and facial hair

Easy bruising

Purple striae

Pendulous abdomen

Thin extremities

Slow wound healing

Figure 10–7 *Physical manifestations seen in Cushing syndrome.*

Insulin secretion is regulated by a negative feedback system sensitive to blood glucose concentration. After a meal, when blood glucose concentration rises to a relatively high level, *beta* cells release insulin. This action prevents high blood glucose concentration by stimulation of glycogen formation in the liver and the entrance of glucose into adipose and muscle cells. As insulin output is decreasing, glucagon secretion is increasing. So despite the great variation of carbohydrate ingestion, insulin and glucagon function together to maintain a relatively stable blood glucose concentration (Flowchart 10–5).

A facilitated-diffusion mechanism that is not stimulated by insulin provides all nerve cells, including those of the brain, with glucose. That is why nerve cells are particularly sensitive to changes in blood glucose concentration. Any condition that may cause such changes, such as oversecretion of insulin (hyperinsulinism), is likely to result in altered brain functions.

OVARIES

The ovaries (Fig. 10–2) are almond-shaped glands located in the pelvic cavity, one on each side of the uterus. The ovaries, also known as the *female gonads*, produce the female sex cell, the ovum (egg), as well as various important hormones.

Two hormones secreted by the ovaries, estrogen and progesterone, are responsible for the development of female sex characteristics and the regulation of the menstrual cycle. Both hormones play an important role in preparing the uterus for implantation of the fertilized egg, in maintaining pregnancy, and promoting growth of the placenta. The detailed structure and function of the ovaries are discussed in Chapter 11.

TESTES

The **testes** (Fig. 10–2) are two oval glands that lie in the scrotum. The testes, also known as the *male gonads*, produce *spermatozoa*, which are the male sex cells, as well as the male hormone *testosterone*. Male hormones secreted by the testes control sexual development and reproductive function. The detailed structure and function of the testes are discussed in Chapter 6.

Refer to Flowchart 10–7 for a summary of hormonal secretions of the ovaries and testes.

PINEAL GLAND

The pineal gland is a ductless gland attached to the posterior part of the third ventricle of the brain. It is

Insulin also produces the special effect of promoting facilitated diffusion of glucose across cell membranes with insulin receptors. These cells include those of cardiac muscle, adipose tissue, and resting skeletal muscle. The action of insulin decreases blood glucose concentration. Insulin secretion also increases protein synthesis, promotes transport of amino acids, and causes adipose cells to synthesize and store fat.

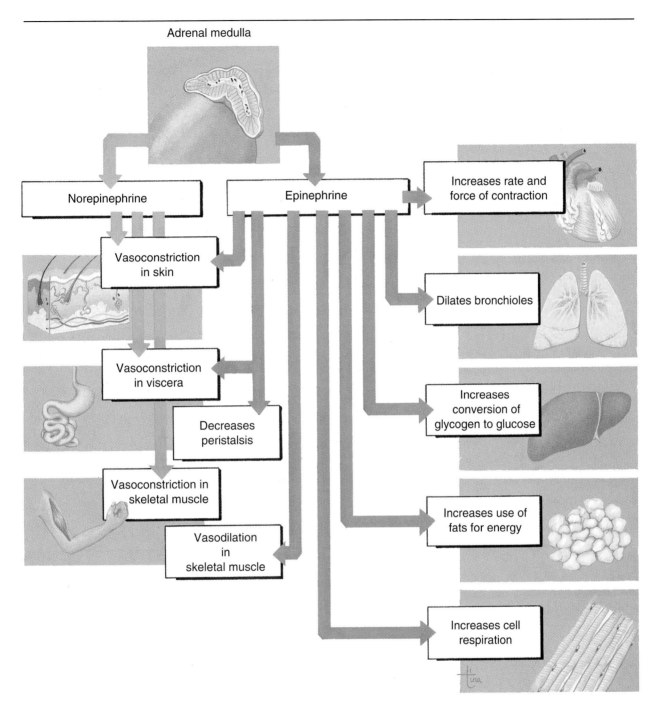

Flowchart 10–3 *The functions of norepinephrine and epinephrine, the adrenal medullary hormones. (From Scanlon, VC, and Sanders, TS: Essentials of Anatomy and Physiology, ed 3. FA Davis, Philadelphia, 1999, p 224, with permission.)*

encapsulated by the meninges covering the brain but lacks a direct connection to the rest of the brain. The pineal gland begins to regress in size at about age 7 years and in the adult appears as a thickened strand of fibrous tissue. Because of its anatomic structure as a ductless gland, it is included as an endocrine gland even though the exact functions of this gland have not been established. Many anatomic facts about the gland have been known for years, but its physiology or functions remain somewhat uncertain. There is some evidence that it secretes a hormone called *melatonin*. It is believed that this hormone influences reproductive activities by inhibiting gonadotropic hormones. As discussed previously, gonadotropins are hormones that stimulate the functions of the ovaries and testes.

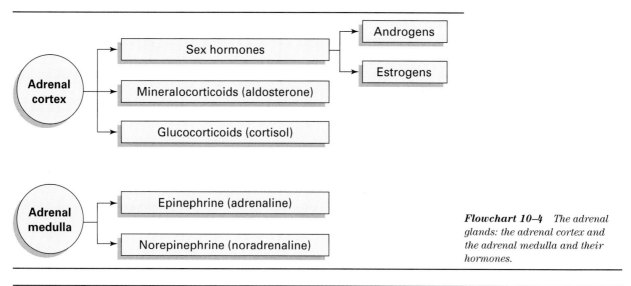

Flowchart 10–4 *The adrenal glands: the adrenal cortex and the adrenal medulla and their hormones.*

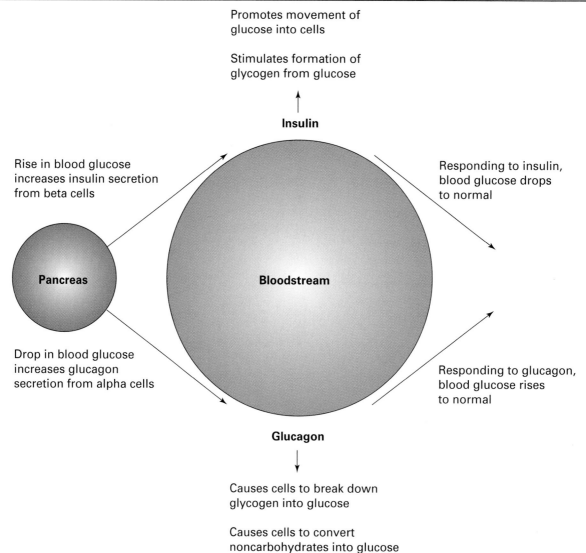

Flowchart 10–5 *Insulin and glucagon function together to help maintain a relatively stable blood glucose concentration. Negative feedback responding to blood glucose concentration controls the levels of both hormones.*

Combining Forms: Endocrinology (Continued)

Combining Form	Meaning	EXAMPLE	
		Term/Pronunciation	**Definition**
pancreat/o	pancreas	**pancreat/oma** *păn-krē-ăt-Ō-mă*	pancreatic tumor (*-oma*)
parathyroid/o	parathyroid glands	**parathyroid/ectomy** *păr-ă-thī-royd-ĔK-tō-mē*	surgical removal (*-ectomy*) of the parathyroid glands
thym/o	thymus gland	**thym/itis** *thī-MĪ-tĭs*	inflammation of the thymus gland
thyr/o	thyroid gland	**thyr/o/megaly** *thī-rō-MĔG-ă-lē*	enlargement (*-megaly*) of the thyroid gland
thyroid/o		**thyroid/ectomy** *thī-royd-ĔK-tō-mē*	surgical removal (*-ectomy*) of the thyroid gland
toxic/o	poison	**toxic/o/logist** *tŏks-ĭ-KŎL-ō-jĭst*	specialist in the study of (*-logist*) poisons or toxins

Prefixes and Suffixes

In this section, prefixes are listed alphabetically and highlighted, whereas key suffixes are defined in the right-hand column.

Prefixes

Prefix	Meaning	EXAMPLE	
		Term/Pronunciation	**Definition**
endo-	in, within	**endo/crine** *ĔN-dō-krīn*	to secrete (*-crine*) internally or within *Endocrine denotes a ductless gland that furnishes an internal secretion.*
exo-	outside, outward	**exo/crine** *ĔKS-ō-krīn*	to secrete (*-crine*) outwardly *Exocrine denotes a gland that secretes outwardly through excretory ducts.*
hyper-	excessive, above normal	**hyper/calc/emia** *hī-pĕr-kăl-SĒ-mē-ă*	excessive concentration of calcium (*calc/o*) in the blood (*-emia*)
hypo-	under, below	**hypo/kal/emia** *hī-pō-kăl-Ē-mē-ă*	lower-than-normal levels of potassium (*kal/o*) in the blood (*-emia*)
poly-	many, much	**poly/dipsia** *pŏl-ē-DĬP-sē-ă*	excessive thirst (*-dipsia*)

Activity 10–3: Competency Verification
Medical Word Components

Check the box [✓] as you complete each numbered section.

[   ] **1.** Review the word components in the previous section. Then pronounce each word aloud.

[   ] **2.** For the words below, first write the suffix and its meaning. Then translate the meaning of the remaining components starting with the first part of the word.

> **Example:** thyroid/itis
> **Answer:** *itis*=inflammation; thyroid gland

1. pancreat/oma   _____

2. parathyroid/ectomy _____

3. thyr/o/megaly   _____

4. thyroid/ectomy   _____

5. poly/dipsia   _____

6. adren/o/pathy   _____

7. kal/emia   _____

8. gonad/o/pathy   _____

9. endo/crine   _____

10. hyper/calc/emia   _____

Correct Answers _____ × 10 = _____% **Score**

PATHOLOGICAL CONDITIONS

PATHOLOGICAL CONDITION	DESCRIPTION
acidosis ăs-ĭ-DŌ-sĭs	Abnormal increase in hydrogen ion concentration of the blood due to an accumulation of acid, as in diabetic acidosis or renal disease.
acromegaly ăk-rō-MĔG-ă-lē *acro=extremity* *megaly=enlargement*	Chronic metabolic disease of middle-aged and older persons. It is characterized by enlarged features, particularly of the face, hands, and extremities. Overproduction of GH is seen in adenomas of the pituitary gland that occur during adulthood. Treatment involves lowering GH levels to normal and stabilizing or removing the underlying tumor while minimizing damage to the pituitary gland itself. Surgery may be attempted depending on the size and location of the tumor. Otherwise, radiation therapy or drug therapy may be used.

Pathological Conditions (Continued)

PATHOLOGICAL CONDITION	DESCRIPTION
Addison disease	A life-threatening condition caused by partial or complete failure of adreno-cortical function, often resulting from autoimmune processes, infection (especially tubercular or fungal), neoplasm, or hemorrhage in the gland. All three general functions of the adrenal cortex (glucocorticoid, mineralocorticoid, and androgenic) are lost.
aldosteronism ăl-dŏ-STĔR-ōn-ĭzm	A condition characterized by hypersecretion of aldosterone, occurring as a primary disease of the adrenal cortex, or more often, as a secondary disorder in response to various extra-adrenal pathological processes.
primary	Condition in which the blood contains high levels of aldosterone because of dysfunction of the adrenal gland. Also called *Conn syndrome*.
secondary	Condition in which the blood contains high levels of aldosterone because of dysfunction of organs other than the adrenal gland (e.g., the pituitary gland).
Cushing syndrome KOOSH-ĭng	A metabolic disorder caused by the chronic and excessive production of cortisol by the adrenal cortex or by the administration of glucocorticoids in large doses for several weeks or longer. When occurring spontaneously, the syndrome represents a failure in the body's ability to regulate the secretion of cortisol or ACTH. The most common cause of the syndrome is a pituitary tumor that increases secretion of ACTH. Characteristically the patient with Cushing syndrome has a decreased glucose tolerance; central obesity; round, "moon" face; edema; supraclavicular fat pads (buffalo hump); scant menstrual periods or decreased testosterone levels; muscular atrophy; skin infection; poor wound healing; hypokalemia; and emotional changes. Children with the disorder may stop growing. Hypertension, kidney stones, and psychosis may also occur (Fig. 10–7).
diabetes dī-ă-BĒ-tēz	A general term for diseases marked by excessive urination. Usually refers to *diabetes mellitus*.
diabetes mellitus (DM) dī-ă-BĒ-tēz MĔ-lĭ-tŭs	A chronic disorder of carbohydrate metabolism that is primarily a result of a deficiency or complete lack of insulin secretion by the beta cells of the pancreas or of defects of the insulin receptors in cells. This condition results in high levels of glucose in the blood (hyperglycemia).
insulin-dependent diabetes mellitus (IDDM), type 1	IDDM occurs mostly in children and adolescents (juvenile onset) and may be associated with a genetic predisposition to the disorder. It is characterized by destruction of beta cells of the islets of Langerhans with complete insulin deficiency in the body. Treatment includes daily injections of insulin (Fig. 10–8) in order to maintain a normal level of glucose in the blood. The maintenance of blood glucose levels is illustrated in Flowchart 10–5. You will also find additional information about the treatments of this disease in the Pharmacology section of this chapter.

Pathological Conditions (Continued)

PATHOLOGICAL CONDITION	DESCRIPTION

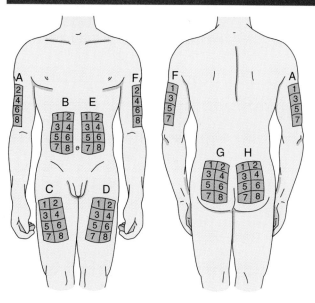

Rotation sites for injection of insulin.

Figure 10–8   Sample insulin rotation chart (From Williams, LS, and Hopper, PD: Understanding Medical-Surgical Nursing. FA Davis, Philadelphia, 1999, p 759, with permission.)

non–insulin-dependent diabetes mellitus (NIDDM), type 2

The onset of NIDDM is usually later in life (maturity onset). It is different from type 1, and its risk factors include a family history of diabetes and obesity. Although insulin is produced, insulin cannot exert its effects on cells because of the body's insensitivity to insulin.

Treatment includes medications that stimulate the release of pancreatic insulin and improve the body's sensitivity to insulin (oral hypoglycemic agents), weight reduction, and diet. Figure 10–8 shows rotation sites for insulin injections. You will also find additional information about treatment of this disease in the Pharmacology section of this chapter.

diuresis
dī-ū-RĒ-sĭs

di=double

ur=urine, urinary tract

esis=condition

Increased formation and secretion of urine.

Diuresis occurs in conditions such as diabetes mellitus, diabetes insipidus, and acute renal failure. Coffee, tea, certain foods, diuretic drugs, anxiety, fear, and some steroids cause diuresis.

dwarfism
DWŌRF-ĭzm

The condition of being abnormally small.

This condition may be hereditary or may be the result of various causes, such as endocrine dysfunction, deficiency diseases, renal insufficiency, or diseases of the skeleton. The opposite of gigantism (Fig. 10–9).

PATHOLOGICAL CONDITIONS (CONTINUED)

PATHOLOGICAL CONDITION	DESCRIPTION

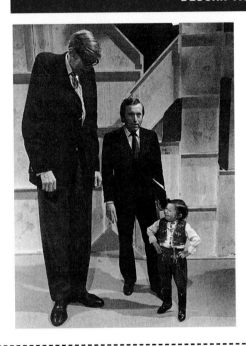

Figure 10–9 *Gigantism and dwarfism. (From Index Stock Imagery, Inc./Michael Serino, with permission.)*

exophthalmos
ĕks-ŏf-THĂL-mōs

Protrusion of the eyeballs; often a sign of hyperthyroidism (Fig. 10–10).

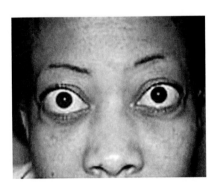

Figure 10–10 *Exophthalmos caused by Graves disease. (From Larry Sargent, MD, with permission.)*

gigantism
JĪ-găn-tĭzm

An abnormal condition characterized by excessive growth of the body.

This condition results from hypersecretion of the pancreatic GH. The opposite of dwarfism (Fig. 10–9).

glucosuria, glycosuria
gloo-kō-SŪ-rē-ă, glĭ-kō-SŪ-rē-ă
glucos = sugar, sweetness
uria = urine

Abnormal presence of glucose in the urine resulting from the ingestion of large amounts of carbohydrates or from a kidney disease such as nephrosis, or from a metabolic disease such as diabetes mellitus.

Pathological Conditions (Continued)

PATHOLOGICAL CONDITION	DESCRIPTION
goiter GOY-tĕr	Enlargement of the thyroid gland, possibly due to a lack of iodine in the diet, thyroiditis, inflammation from infection, tumors, or hyperfunction or hypofunction of the thyroid gland.
exophthalmic ĕks-ŏf-THĂL-mĭk *exo=outside, outward* *opthalm=eye* *ic=pertaining to*	Goiter accompanied by protrusion of the eyeballs, increased heart action, weight loss, and nervousness; synonymous with *thyrotoxicosis*. Also known as *Graves disease*.
Graves disease	Hyperthyroidism, also called *toxic goiter;* characterized by goiter and exophthalmos that may be due to an autoimmune reaction to thyroid tissue (Fig. 10–10).
hirsutism HŬR-sūt-ĭzm	Condition characterized by the excessive growth of hair or presence of hair in unusual places, especially in women. Hirsutism in women is usually caused by abnormalities of androgen production or metabolism.
hypercalcemia hī-pĕr-kăl-SĒ-mē-ă *hyper=excessive, above normal* *calc=calcium* *emia=blood condition*	Excess amount of calcium in the blood.
hyperglycemia hī-pĕr-glī-SĒ-mē-ă *hyper=excessive, above normal* *glyc=sugar, sweetness* *emia=blood condition*	Abnormally high levels of glucose in the blood, as in diabetes.
hypergonadism hī-pĕr-GŌ-năd-ĭzm *hyper=excessive, above normal* *gonad=gonads, sex glands* *ism=condition*	Excessive hormonal secretion of the sex glands.
hyperinsulinism hī-pĕr-ĬN-sŭ-lĭn-ĭzm	Excessive amount of insulin in the blood. It may be caused by administration of an higher insulin dose than required or the presence of an insulin-secreting tumor in the islets of Langerhans. Symptoms include hypoglycemia, hunger, shakiness, and diaphoresis.
hyperkalemia hī-pĕr-kă-LĒ-mē-ă *hyper=excessive, above normal* *kal=potassium (an electrolyte)* *emia=blood condition*	Excessive amount of potassium in the blood. This condition is seen frequently in acute renal failure, massive trauma, major burns, and Addison disease.

PATHOLOGICAL CONDITIONS (CONTINUED)

PATHOLOGICAL CONDITION	DESCRIPTION
hyperparathyroidism hī-pĕr-păr-ă-THĪ-roy-dĭzm *hyper=excessive, above normal* *parathyroid=parathyroid glands* *ism=condition*	High levels of parathyroid hormone in the blood resulting in elevated blood calcium levels and demineralization of bone.
hyperpituitarism hī-pĕr-pĭ-TŪ-ĭ-tăr-ĭzm *hyper=excessive, above normal* *pituitar=pituitary gland* *ism=condition*	Overactivity of the anterior lobe of the pituitary leading to such conditions as acromegaly, gigantism (Fig. 10–9), and Cushing syndrome (Fig. 10–7).
hyperthyroidism hī-pĕr-THĪ-royd-ĭzm *hyper=excessive, above normal* *thyroid=thyroid gland* *ism=condition*	A condition characterized by overactivity of the thyroid gland. The gland is usually enlarged, secreting higher-than-normal amounts of thyroid hormones, and the metabolic processes of the body are accelerated. Nervousness, exophthalmos, tremor, constant hunger, weight loss, fatigue, heat intolerance, palpitations, and other manifestations of thyroid storm may develop. This disorder is often caused by Graves disease, which is associated with exophthalmos.
hypervolemia hī-pĕr-vŏl-Ē-mē-ă *hyper=excessive, above normal* *vol=volume* *emia=blood*	An abnormal increase in the amount of intravascular fluid, particularly in the volume of circulating blood. This condition is often is caused when the kidneys retain large amounts of sodium and water. Manifestations include weight gain, edema, dyspnea, tachycardia, and pulmonary congestion.
hypoglycemia hī-pō-glī-SĒ-mē-ă *hypo=under, below* *glyc=sugar, sweetness* *emia=blood*	Deficiency of glucose in the blood, usually caused by administration of too much insulin, excessive secretion of insulin by islet cells in the pancreas, Addison disease, or dietary deficiency. This condition may cause weakness, headache, hunger, visual disturbances, ataxia, anxiety, personality changes, and if left untreated, delirium, coma, and death. The treatment is the administration of glucose in orange juice (or other fluids) by mouth if the person is conscious or in an intravenous glucose solution if the person is unconscious.
hypogonadism hī-pō-GŌ-năd-ĭzm *hypo=under, below* *gonad=gonads, sex glands* *ism=condition*	Underproduction of sex hormones by the ovaries or testes.
hyponatremia hī-pō-nă-TRĒ-mē-ă *hypo=under, below* *natr=sodium* *emia=blood*	A decreased concentration of sodium in the blood.

PATHOLOGICAL CONDITIONS (CONTINUED)

PATHOLOGICAL CONDITION	DESCRIPTION
hypoparathyroidism *hī-pō-păr-ă-THĪ-royd-ĭzm* *hypo = under, below* *parathyroid = parathyroid glands*	Insufficient secretion of PTH that leads to low calcium levels in the blood (hypocalcemia), which causes muscle twitching and spasms known as *tetany*.
hypothyroidism *hī-pō-THĪ-royd-ĭzm* *hypo = under, below* *thyroid = thyroid gland* *ism = condition*	Undersecretion of the thyroid gland, which results in a lowered metabolism with obesity, dry skin, slow pulse, sluggishness, and goiter. Treatment is replacement with synthetic thyroid hormone.
insulinoma *ĭn-sŭ-lĭn-Ō-mă*	Tumor of the islets of Langerhans in the pancreas, resulting in overproduction of insulin.
ketosis *kē-TŌ-sĭs* *ket = ketone bodies (acids and acetones)* *osis = abnormal condition*	The abnormal accumulation of ketones in the body as a result of excessive breakdown of fats caused by a deficiency or inadequate intake of carbohydrates. Fatty acids are metabolized instead, and the end products, ketones, begin to accumulate. This condition is seen in starvation. Untreated, ketosis may progress to ketoacidosis, coma, and death.
ketoacidosis *kē-tō-ă-sĭ-DŌ-sĭs*	Acidosis accompanied by an accumulation of ketones in the body, resulting from extensive breakdown of fats due to faulty carbohydrate metabolism. It occurs primarily as a complication of diabetes mellitus and is characterized by a fruity odor of acetone on the breath, mental confusion, dyspnea, nausea, vomiting, dehydration, weight loss, and if untreated, coma.
myxedema *mĭks-ĕ-DĒ-mă* *myx = mucus* *edema = swelling*	The most severe form of hypothyroidism. It is characterized by swelling of the hands, face, feet, and periorbital (around the eyes) tissues. At this stage the disease may lead to coma and death.
obesity *ō-BĒ-sĭ-tē*	An abnormal increase in the proportion of fat cells, mainly in the viscera and subcutaneous tissues of the body. Obesity may be exogenous or endogenous.
endogenous *ĕn-DŎJ-ĕ-nŭs* *endo = in, within* *gen = forming, producing, origin* *ous = pertaining to*	Obesity that originates within the body or is produced by an internal cause, such as the functional failure of an organ or system.
exogenous *ĕks-ŎJ-ĕ-nŭs* *exo = outside, outward* *gen = forming, producing origin* *ous = pertaining to*	Obesity that originates outside the body or is produced by external causes. This type of obesity is caused by a caloric intake significantly higher than the one needed to meet the metabolic requirements of the body.

PATHOLOGICAL CONDITIONS (CONTINUED)

PATHOLOGICAL CONDITION	DESCRIPTION
pancreatitis *păn-krē-ă-TĪ-tĭs* *pancreat=pancreas* *itis=inflammation*	An inflammatory condition of the pancreas that may be acute or chronic.
panhypopituitarism *păn-hī-pō-pĭ-TŪ-ĭ-tăr-ĭzm* *pan=all* *hypo=under, below* *pituitar=pituitary gland* *ism=condition*	Total pituitary impairment that brings about a progressive and general loss of hormonal activity.
pheochromocytoma *fē-ō-krō-mō-sī-TŌ-mă* *pheo=dusky, dark* *chromo=color* *cyt=cell* *oma=tumor*	A vascular tumor of chromaffin tissue, usually benign and usually located in the adrenal medulla. This condition is characterized by hypersecretion of epinephrine and norepinephrine.
polydipsia *pŏl-ē-DĬP-sē-ă* *poly=many, much* *dipsia=thirst*	Excessive thirst. It is characteristic of several different conditions, including diabetes mellitus, in which an excessive concentration of glucose in the blood osmotically increases the excretion of fluid via increased urination, which leads to hypovolemia and thirst.
polyuria *pŏl-ē-Ū-rē-ă* *poly=many, much* *uria=urine*	Excretion of an abnormally large quantity of urine. Some causes of polyuria are diabetes insipidus, diabetes mellitus, use of diuretics, excessive fluid intake, and hypercalcemia.
syndrome of inappropriate antidiuretic hormone (SIADH) secretion	An abnormal condition resulting in excess free water retention and release of ADH, which alters the body's fluid and electrolytic balances. SIADH develops in association with diseases that affect the osmoreceptors of the hypothalamus.
thyroid storm *THĪ-royd*	A severe, acute exacerbation of thyrotoxic symptoms. There is an abrupt onset of fever, sweating, tachycardia, pulmonary edema or congestive heart failure (CHF), and excessive restlessness. If left untreated, it may be fatal.
thyromegaly *thī-rō-MĔG-ă-lē* *thyro=thyroid gland* *megaly=enlargement*	Enlargement of the thyroid gland. Also referred to as *goiter*.
thyrotoxicosis *thī-rō-tŏks-ĭ-KŌ-sĭs* *thyro=thyroid gland* *toxic=poison* *osis=abnormal condition*	General term for any toxic reaction resulting from overactivity of the thyroid gland (hyperthyroidism).

Activity 10–4: Clinical Application
Pathological Conditions

acidosis	hyperglycemia	myxedema
acromegaly	hyperkalemia	pheochromocytoma
endogenous	hypervolemia	polydipsia
exophthalmos	hypogonadism	polyuria
hirsutism	hyponatremia	thyroid storm
hypercalcemia	IDDM	thyromegaly

Match the terms listed above with the definitions given in the numbered list:

1. _____ excessive growth of hair or presence of hair in unusual places, especially in women.

2. _____ protrusion of the eyeballs; often a sign of hyperthyroidism.

3. _____ occurs mostly in children and adolescents; characterized by destruction of beta cells of the islets of Langerhans with complete insulin deficiency in the body. Treatment includes daily injections of insulin.

4. _____ excessive amount of potassium in the blood.

5. _____ chronic disease of middle-aged persons characterized by enlarged features, particularly of the bone, face, hands, and extremities due to hypersecretion of GH.

6. _____ enlargement of the thyroid gland; also referred to as goiter.

7. _____ excretion of abnormally large amounts of urine.

8. _____ the most severe form of hypothyroidism. It is characterized by swelling of the hands, face, feet, and periorbital tissues.

9. _____ originating from within the body or produced from internal causes.

10. _____ excessive thirst characteristic of diabetes mellitus.

11. _____ thyrotoxic crisis. If left untreated, it may be fatal.

12. _____ abnormally high levels of glucose in the blood as in diabetes.

13. _____ abnormal increase in the amount of intravascular fluid, particularly in the volume of circulating blood.

14. _____ a decreased concentration of sodium in the blood.

15. _____ underproduction of sex hormones by the ovaries and testes.

Correct Answers _____ **× 6.67 =** _____ **% Score**	

DIAGNOSTIC PROCEDURES AND TESTS

Imaging Procedures

PROCEDURE	DESCRIPTION
computed tomography (CT) scan	Radiographic scan of endocrine organs to assist in the diagnosis of various pathologies; may also involve the use of radiographic contrast media.
magnetic resonance imaging (MRI) *măg-NĔT-ĭk RĔZ-ō-năns Ĭ-mă-jĭng*	Nonionizing images of magnetic resonance are used to identify abnormalities of pituitary, pancreatic, adrenal, and thyroid glands.
radioactive iodine uptake (RAIU) test *rā-dē-ō-ĂK-tĭv Ī-ō-dīn*	Procedure that measures levels of radioactivity in the thyroid following administration of radioactive iodine either orally (PO) or intravenously (IV). Used to monitor the ability of the thyroid to take up (uptake) iodine from the blood to determine thyroid function.
thyroid scan *THĪ-royd* *thyro=thyroid gland* *oid=resembling*	A radioactive substance is administered that is localized in the thyroid gland. The gland is then visualized with a scanning device to detect pathological formations such as tumors.

Laboratory Tests

PROCEDURE	DESCRIPTION
blood sugar (BS) test	Test to measure the level of glucose in the blood. Also called blood glucose; useful for diagnosis of diabetes mellitus and for adjusting medication dosages. Patients can monitor their blood glucose levels by purchasing monitoring equipment (Fig. 10–11). 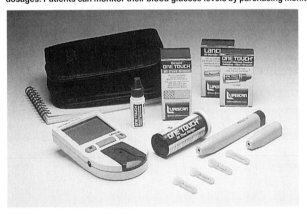 ***Figure 10–11*** *Home blood glucose monitoring. (From Williams, LS, and Hopper, PD: Understanding Medical-Surgical Nursing. FA Davis, Philadelphia, 1999, p 761, with permission.)*
electrolytes, measurement of *ē-LĔK-trō-līts*	Measurement of the level of ions, such as sodium, potassium, CO_2, and chloride in the blood. A normal electrolyte balance in the body is critical to body metabolism.

Laboratory Tests (Continued)

PROCEDURE	DESCRIPTION
fasting blood sugar (FBS)	Test to measure the level of glucose in the blood after a 12-hour fast.
glucose tolerance test (GTT) *GLOO-kōs*	A prescribed amount of glucose is administered either orally or intravenously, and blood samples are drawn and tested for glucose at specified intervals, usually for 3 to 6 hours. This test is most often used to assist in the diagnosis of diabetes mellitus or other disorders that affect carbohydrate metabolism.
ketone bodies *KĒ-tōn*	Test to determine the presence of ketone bodies in blood or urine; used as a screen for diabetic acidosis.
postprandial blood sugar (PPBS) *pōst-PRĂN-dē-ăl* *post=after, behind* *prandial=meal*	Test designed to measure blood glucose level immediately after a meal or after a designated number of hours after a meal.
radioimmunoassay (RIA) *rā-dē-ō-ĭm-ū-nō-ĂS-ā*	Method used to measure hormone levels in the blood by monitoring their ability to interfere with the binding of radioactive hormones to antibody molecules.
thyroid function tests	Tests used to determine the levels of T_3, T_4, and thyroid-stimulating hormone in the blood. Used to assist in diagnosing thyroid disorders and monitoring thyroid function.
total calcium	Measurement of the calcium concentration in the blood to detect bone and parathyroid disorders; hypercalcemia may indicate primary hyperparathyroidism or malignancy; hypocalcemia may indicate hypoparathyroidism.

SURGICAL AND THERAPEUTIC PROCEDURES

Surgical Procedures

PROCEDURE	DESCRIPTION
adenectomy *ăd-ĕn-ĔK-tō-mē* *aden=gland* *ectomy=excision, removal*	Excision of a gland.
adrenalectomy *ăd-rē-năl-ĔK-tō-mē* *adrenal=adrenal glands* *ectomy=excision, removal*	Excision of one or both adrenal glands.

Therapeutic Procedures

PROCEDURE	DESCRIPTION
hormone replacement therapy	Oral administration or injection of synthetic hormones to replace a hormone deficiency, such as of estrogen, testosterone, thyroid, and so forth.
hypophysectomy hī-pŏf-ĭ-SĔK-tō-mē	Excision of the pituitary gland (Fig. 10–12). This procedure may be performed to remove a pituitary tumor or to slow the growth and spread of a malignant tumor. 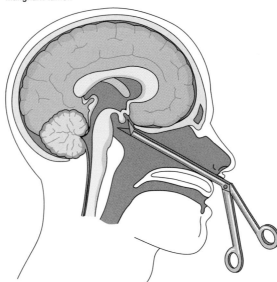 *Figure 10–12* *Transsphenoidal approach to pituitary for hypophysectomy. (From Williams, LS, and Hopper, PD: Understanding Medical-Surgical Nursing. FA Davis, Philadelphia, 1999, p 735, with permission.)*
lobectomy lō-BĔK-tō-mē *lob=lobe* *ectomy=excision, removal*	Excision of a lobe of an organ. In endocrine disorder treatments, *lobectomy* usually refers to the excision of one lobe of the thyroid gland.
radioiodine therapy rā-dē-ō-Ī-ō-dīn	Use of radioactive iodine to treat diseases, such as by destruction and removal of thyroid tumor cells.

Pharmacology

As discussed previously, the endocrine system comprises glands that secrete hormones directly into the bloodstream. When these glands malfunction because of disease processes, they release either a decreased or an increased level of hormone. Thus, drugs are prescribed either to normalize hormone levels or to counteract increased hormone levels.

DRUG CLASSIFICATION	THERAPEUTIC ACTION
anabolic steroids ăn-ă-BŎL-ĭk STĔR-oydz	Substances that change the natural balance in the body between tissue building (anabolism) and tissue breakdown (catabolism). These drugs increase tissue building and have been used for years by both female and male athletes to increase muscle mass, strength, and endurance. Even though these drugs are illegal in professional sports, many athletes continue to use them. In patients with AIDS, anabolic steroids have been legitimately prescribed to counteract the wasting syndrome. They are also used for male hormone replacement or to treat breast cancer in women.

Pharmacology (Continued)

DRUG CLASSIFICATION	THERAPEUTIC ACTION
antidiabetics *ăn-tĭ-dī-ă-BĔT-ĭks*	Oral antidiabetic drugs that stimulate the pancreas to produce and release insulin and to improve the action of insulin at its site of activity. Contrary to popular belief, these drugs are not a form of insulin and are not effective in the treatment of patients with type 1 diabetes mellitus. Another type of antidiabetic drugs inhibits an enzyme in the intestine that digests glucose. This causes delayed digestion of glucose, which, in turn, keeps the blood sugar lower after meals. This type does not stimulate the pancreas to produce more insulin.
antithyroids *ăn-tĭ-THĪ-roydz* *anti=against* *thyro=thyroid gland* *oids=resembling*	Agents that are used to treat hyperthyroidism by inhibiting the production of T_3 and T_4 in the thyroid gland.
corticosteroids *kŏr-tĭ-kō-STĒ-roydz*	Drugs from this class are widely used to treat inflammatory illnesses, including arthritis, asthma, and dermatitis. They are also used as replacement hormones in patients with adrenal insufficiency (Addison disease).
growth hormone replacements	Drugs used as a replacement therapy in patients with decreased levels or hyposecretion of growth hormone. Growth hormone deficiency retards skeletal growth in children.
insulins *ĭn-sū-linz*	A synthetic form of the insulin hormone, used by patients with type 1 diabetes mellitus. Patients with type 1 diabetes mellitus, also known as IDDM, are treated with daily subcutaneous injections of insulin. Traditionally, most insulin has been derived from beef or pork pancreas. Today, human insulin is also being produced using recombinant (altered) DNA techniques. The use of human insulin avoids the potential for allergic reactions. Regardless of the original source, all insulins are classified according to how quickly they act and how long their action lasts. There are three main categories: rapid-acting, also known as regular insulin; intermediate-acting, also known as NPH or lente; and long-acting, known as ultralente. There is also a fourth type that is a combination of regular and NPH. The time of action of any insulin varies considerably in different individuals. Duration of action depends on dose, injection site, blood supply, temperature, and physical activity.
thyroid supplements *THĪ-royd*	Supplements used in the treatment of hypothyroidism. These supplements are manufactured synthetically or they are obtained from natural sources such as desiccated (dried) ground beef or pork thyroid glands.
antidiuretics *ăn-tĭ-dī-ŭ-RĔT-ĭks*	Agents that inhibit the excretion of water by the kidneys. Antidiuretics such as vasopressin are used to control diabetes insipidus and subsequent polyuria resulting from antidiuretic hormone deficiency.

❖ ABBREVIATIONS

ABBREVIATION	MEANING	ABBREVIATION	MEANING
ACTH	adrenocorticotropic hormone	Na	sodium (an electrolyte)
ADH	antidiuretic hormone (vasopressin)	NIDDM	non–insulin-dependent diabetes mellitus
AKA	above-knee amputation	PBI	protein-bound iodine
BKA	below-knee amputation	PRL	prolactin
BMR	basal metabolic rate	PGH	pituitary growth hormone
Ca	calcium, cancer	PTH	parathyroid hormone (also called *parathormone*)
DI	diabetes insipidus; diagnostic imaging	RAI	radioactive iodine
DM	diabetes mellitus	RAIU	radioactive iodine uptake
FSH	follicle-stimulating hormone	T_3	triiodothyronine (thyroid hormone)
GH	growth hormone		
IDDM	insulin-dependent diabetes mellitus	T_4	thyroxine (thyroid hormone)
		TFT	thyroid function test
K	potassium (an electrolyte)	TSH	thyroid-stimulating hormone
LH	luteinizing hormone	VLDL	very-low-density lipoprotein
MSH	melanocyte-stimulating hormone		

Activity 10–5: Clinical Application

Diagnostic Procedures, Treatments, and Abbreviations

antidiuretics	glucose tolerance test (GTT)	radioimmunoassay (RIA)
anabolic steroids	hormone replacement therapy (HRT)	radioiodine therapy
antidiabetics	hypophysectomy	T_3, T_4
corticosteroids	insulin	thyroid scan
electrolytes	K	thyroidectomy
fasting blood sugar (FBS)	postprandial blood sugar (PPBS)	total calcium test

Match the terms listed above with the definitions given in the numbered list:

1. _____ measurement of the level of ions (sodium, potassium, carbon dioxide, and chlorine) in the blood.

2. _____ oral drugs that stimulate the pancreas to produce and release insulin.

3. _____ a natural hormone derived from beef or pork pancreas that is used to treat diabetic patients.

4. _____ test in which glucose is administered either orally or intravenously, and then blood and urine samples are measured at specific intervals to determine glucose levels.

5. _____ test to measure the level of glucose in the blood after a 12-hour fast.

6. _____ substance prescribed for AIDS patients to counteract wasting syndrome.

7. _____ excision of the thyroid gland.

8. _____ measurement of the glucose level after a meal.

9. _____ excision of the pituitary gland.

10. _____ drug classification for vasopressin.

11. _____ use of radioactive iodine to treat disease, such as destruction and removal of thyroid tumor cells.

12. _____ class of drugs used to treat inflammatory illnesses, including arthritis.

13. _____ hormones produced by the thyroid gland.

14. _____ drugs used to replace a hormone deficiency.

15. _____ imaging technique in which a radioactive substance is administered to visualize a gland with a scanning device; used to detect tumors.

Correct Answers _____ × **6.67 =** _____ **% Score**

Activity 10-6: Build Medical Words

Build Diagnostic, Symptomatic, and Surgical Terms

Use *adren/o* (adrenal glands) to build medical words meaning:

1. enlargement of the adrenal glands _____

2. disease of the adrenal glands _____

Use *pancreat/o* (pancreas) to build medical words meaning:

3. inflammation of the pancreas _____

4. any pancreatic disease _____

5. tumor of the pancreas _____

Use *thyr/o* (thyroid gland) to build medical words meaning:

6. enlargement of the thyroid gland _____

7. incision of the thyroid gland _____

Use *glyc/o* (sugar) to build medical words meaning:

8. condition of excessive sugar in the blood _____

9. condition of deficiency of sugar in the blood _____

10. formation of glycogen _____

Correct Answers _____ × 10 = _____ % Score		

MEDICAL RECORDS

Authentic medical records including a history and physical examination, a consultation, an operative report, and a discharge summary are presented in this section.

The following reading and dictionary exercise and medical record analysis will help you develop skills to abstract information and master the terminology in the reports. In turn, you will be able to understand the importance of interpreting information from a medical record accurately. Accurate interpretation is important because this information is used to initiate treatments, evaluate the patient's progress, and complete insurance claims for third-party reimbursements.

 Reading and Dictionary Exercise

Place a check mark [✓] after you complete the exercise.

[ ] **1.** Underline the following words in the records as you read the history and physical examination, consultation, operative report, and discharge summary aloud. These medical records can be found at the end of the chapter.

[ ] **2.** Use a medical dictionary to define the terms below.

Note: You are not expected to fully understand all the parts of the medical records. The important aspect of this exercise is to use all available resources to complete it. Eventually you will master the terminology and format of these reports.

> > > MEDICAL RECORD 10–1: HISTORY AND PHYSICAL EXAMINATION

Term	Pronunciation	Meaning
diabetes mellitus	dī-ă-BĒ-tēz MĔ-lĭ-tŭs	_____
sedentary	SĔD-ĕn-tā-rē	_____
anaerobic	ăn-ĕr-Ō-bĭk	_____
cellulitis	sĕl-ū-LĪ-tĭs	_____
conjunctivae	kŏn-jŭnk-TĪ-vā	_____
ausculation	aws-kŭl-TĀ-shŭn	_____
percussion	pĕr-KŬSH-ŭn	_____
scaphoid	SKĂF-oyd	_____

organomegaly	*ŏr-gă-nō-MĚG-ă-lē*	_____
trophic	*TRŎF-ĭk*	_____
bilaterally	*bī-LĂT-ĕr-ăl-ē*	_____
ulceration	*ŭl-sĕr-Ā-shŭn*	_____
erythema	*ĕr-ĭ-THĒ-mă*	_____
malleolus	*măl-Ē-ŏ-lŭs*	_____
calcaneal	*kăl-KĀ-nē-ăl*	_____
peripheral	*pĕr-ĬF-ĕr-ăl*	_____
neuropathy	*nū-RŎP-ă-thē*	_____
retinopathy	*rĕt-ĭn-ŎP-ă-thē*	_____
nephropathy	*nĕ-FRŎP-ă-thē*	_____

> > > MEDICAL RECORD 10–2: CONSULTATION

Term	Pronunciation	Meaning
gangrene	*GĂNG-grēn*	_____
carotids	*kă-RŎT-ĭdz*	_____
bruits	*brwēs*	_____
femoral	*FĔM-ŏr-ăl*	_____

> > > MEDICAL RECORD 10–3: OPERATIVE REPORT

Term	Pronunciation	Meaning
debridement	*dā-brēd-MŎN*	_____
supine	*sū-PĪN*	_____
nonambulatory	*nŏn-ĂM-bū-lă-tō-rē*	_____
atrophy	*ĂT-rō-fē*	_____
anterior	*ăn-TĒR-ē-ŏr*	_____
posterior	*pōs-TĒ-rē-ŏr*	_____
transected	*trăn-SĚK-tĕd*	_____
kanamycin	*kăn-ă-MĪ-sĭn*	_____
post	*pōst*	_____

> > > MEDICAL RECORD 1O-4: DISCHARGE SUMMARY

Term	Pronunciation	Meaning
hyperphosphatemia	*hī-pĕr-fōs-fă-TĒ-mē-ă*	_____
hyposmolarity	*hī-pŏz-mō-LĂR-ĭ-tē*	_____
vascular	*VĂS-kū-lăr*	_____
fetid	*FĒ-tĭd*	_____

Critical Thinking: Analysis of Medical Records

This section provides experience in abstracting and analyzing information from medical records. At the same time, it reinforces the material presented in this chapter.

> > > MEDICAL RECORD 1O-1: HISTORY AND PHYSICAL EXAMINATION

1. What brought Mr. Jones into the ER, and what was the history of his present illness?

_____

_____

2. Place a "+" in the space provided for positive findings and a "−" for negative findings. A positive finding indicates the patient had a history (Hx) of this condition; a negative finding indicates the patient did not have a history of this condition.

_____ thyromegaly   _____ diabetes

_____ organomegaly   _____ poor circulation

_____ ulceration and infection of left heel _____ neuropathy

> > > MEDICAL RECORD 1O-2: CONSULTATION

3. Explain what "left fifth toe metatarsal head amputation" means.

_____

_____

4. What two surgical procedures are recommended by Dr. Armani?

_____

5. Why did the surgeon recommend these two procedures?

_____

_____

> > > MEDICAL RECORD 10-3: OPERATIVE REPORT

6. What does it mean that the patient has not been ambulatory?

_____

7. Why did the surgeon perform an above-the-knee amputation (AKA) rather than a below-the-knee amputation (BKA)?

_____

_____

_____

8. Explain what a débridement is and whether or not the surgeon included débridement of the deep tissues.

_____

_____

_____

_____

> > > MEDICAL RECORD 10-4: DISCHARGE SUMMARY

9. What are the secondary diagnoses that indicate the patient has (a) an abnormally high concentration of phosphate in the circulating blood; (b) decreased osmolar concentration, especially of the blood or urine?

_____

_____

10. What complications did the patient experience because of his long-term, poorly controlled diabetes?

_____

_____

Audio Practice

Listen to the audio CD-ROM to practice the pronunciation of selected medical terms from this chapter.

Medical Record 10–1. History and Physical Examination

GENERAL HOSPITAL AND MEDICAL CENTER
2211 Fifth Avenue North • Healthy City, USA 12345 • (321) 123-4567

History and Physical Examination

Patient Name: Donald Jones
Birth Date: 04/03/xx

Patient Number: 43-23-77
Room Number: 232

HISTORY

REASON FOR ADMISSION: Infected foot.

HISTORY OF PRESENT ILLNESS: The patient is a 59-year-old individual with long-term type 1 diabetes mellitus never well controlled. The patient lives at home and is essentially sedentary. He developed a hot, swollen left heel and came in through the emergency room with what appeared to be an anaerobic infection with cellulitis. The patient's laboratory evaluation on admission revealed several significant issues. WBC was markedly elevated at 25,000, mild anemia with a hemoglobin of 10, hematocrit 29, platelets elevated at 730,000. The patient's neutrophil count was elevated at 22 with normal being 6. The patient's potassium was 6.0, glucose 337, bicarbonate 23, and glucose values were reasonable subsequent to this. BUN was elevated at 45. Creatinine was elevated at 2.6.

PHYSICAL EXAMINATION

HEENT: Pupils equal, round, regular, react to light and accommodation. Extraocular movements are intact. Lens and conjunctivae clear. Ears, nose, and throat are clear.

NECK: Supple. No thyroid enlargement. No carotid bruit.

HEART: Heart sounds are normal. There is an S4.

LUNGS: Clear to auscultation and percussion, although breath sounds were slightly distant.

ABDOMEN: Scaphoid. No organomegaly.

GENITALIA & RECTAL: Examination negative.

LOWER EXTREMITIES: Trophic changes in the feet bilaterally with amputation of the right great toe. There is a significant ulceration with early infection in the right heel.

Continued

History and Physical Examination, page 2
Patient Name: Donald Jones   **Patient Number:** 43-23-77

In the left heel, there is erythema to the level of the upper malleolus bilaterally and there is marked erythema at the entire calcaneal bed. There is an open foul ulceration of the heel that is reminiscent of an anaerobic/aerobic infection. There are no palpable pulses in either foot. No reflexes and no sensation to deep palpation.

ASSESSMENT:
1. Non-salvageable anaerobic/aerobic infection of the left heel in the context of peripheral diabetic neuropathy and poor circulation.

2. Diabetes mellitus with all complications: retinopathy proliferative, sensory motor neuropathy, and advancing diabetic nephropathy.

PLAN:
1. Vascular consultation for amputation.

2. Infectious disease consultation for appropriate antibiotic coverage.

_____

Vincent Armani, MD

VA/dw

D: 01/05/xx
T: 01/05/xx

Medical Record 10–2. Consultation

GENERAL HOSPITAL AND MEDICAL CENTER
2211 Fifth Avenue North • Healthy City, USA 12345 • (321) 123-4567

Consultation

Patient Name: Donald Jones   **Patient Number:** 43-23-77
Birth Date: 04/03/xx   **Room Number:** 232

DATE: 01/05/xx   **CONSULTING PHYSICIAN:** Vincent Armani, MD

This 59-year-old white male, an insulin-dependent diabetic and minimally ambulatory, with known renal insufficiency, was admitted with extensive gangrene and infection to the left heel and also in the area of gangrene and infection to the right heel. He is status post right first toe and left fifth toe and metatarsal head amputation years ago, having a significant diabetic neuropathy. He is being followed by Dr. Pratt from "Infectious Disease."

On exam, this well-developed, alert, right-handed white male has a brachial pressure of 110/70. The carotids have good pulses, and no bruits can be heard at any level. No apparent heart murmurs. Lungs are clear. There is no palpable aortic enlargement, masses, or organomegaly. He has good femoral and popliteal pulses as well as right dorsalis pedis and posterior tibial pulses, the dorsalis pedis and posterior tibial pulses being rather weak on the left. Both feet are warm. There is extensive gangrene and infection to the left heel, a well-healed left fifth toe metatarsal head amputation, and an area of breakdown at the amputation stump of the right great toe.

IMPRESSION:
1. Extensive gangrene and infection to the left heel.
2. Limited area of gangrene and infection to the right heel.
3. Insulin-dependent diabetes mellitus with neuropathy.
4. Renal insufficiency.

ADVISE:
1. Left below or above-the-knee amputation.
2. Debridement of the right heel.

The above procedures are to be scheduled when medically cleared for surgery.

Thank you for this consultation.

_____
Vincent Armani, MD

VA:lav
d&t: 01/04/xx

Medical Record 10–3. Operative Report

GENERAL HOSPITAL AND MEDICAL CENTER
2211 Fifth Avenue North • Healthy City, USA 12345 • (321) 123-4567

Operative Report

Patient Name: Donald Jones
Birth Date: 04/03/xx

Patient Number: 43-23-77
Room Number: 232

DATE OF OPERATION: 01/06/xx

PREOPERATIVE DIAGNOSIS:
1. Extensive gangrene and infection to the left heel.
2. Localized gangrene to the right heel.

POSTOPERATIVE DIAGNOSIS:
1. Extensive gangrene and infection to the left heel.
2. Localized gangrene to the right heel.

OPERATION:
1. Left above-knee amputation.
2. Debridement of the right heel.

SURGEON: Vincent Armani, MD

ANESTHESIA: Spinal.

SURGICAL INDICATIONS: This is a 59-year-old white male, insulin-dependent diabetic with renal insufficiency, admitted with extensive gangrene to the left heel and associated cellulitis and also a localized area of gangrene and infection to the right heel. He has not been ambulatory.

PROCEDURE: With the patient lying supine and under spinal anesthesia, the left leg up to the upper thigh was scrubbed with Betadine paint and Betadine solution, and sterile drapes were applied. A waterproof stockinet was used over the left lower leg. Because of the nonambulatory state and some degree of flexion contracture at the knee, as well as significant atrophy to the calf muscles, it was decided to perform an above-knee amputation. Anterior and posterior flaps were developed, and bleeders were electrocauterized. The muscle layers were transected and bleeders were electrocauterized; others ligated with #3-0 Vicryl and others suture ligated with #2-0 Vicryl. The femoral artery and vein were doubly clamped and severed and suture ligated with #0

Continued

Operative Report, page 2
Patient Name: Donald Jones   **Patient Number:** 43-23-77

Vicryl. The nerves were transected as high as could be reached. Using a periosteal elevator, the femur was exposed and transected using the Gigli saw. The edges were smoothed with a rasp. The stump was irrigated with kanamycin solution. Bleeders were electrocauterized. Closure was performed in layers. The deep fascia and muscles were approximated with interrupted sutures of #0 Vicryl, the superficial fascia and subcutaneous tissue with #2-0 Vicryl, and skin with staples.

The incision was painted with Betadine solution, covered with Xeroform gauze as well as Kerlix pads and wrapped with Kerlix wrap and then a 4-inch elastic bandage.

Following this, the right lower leg and foot were scrubbed with Betadine, painted with Betadine solution, and sterile drapes were applied. There was blistering to the heel with a localized area of gangrene. Debridement was done which did not include the deep tissues, and these may still be viable. A sterile dressing consisting of Xeroform gauze, Kerlix pads, and Kerlix wrap was then used. The patient tolerated the procedures well, and the blood loss was estimated at 150 mL. He was taken to the post anesthesia unit in satisfactory condition.

_____

Vincent Armani, MD

VA/dw

D: 01/06/xx
T: 01/06/xx

Medical Record 10–4. Discharge Summary

GENERAL HOSPITAL AND MEDICAL CENTER
2211 Fifth Avenue North • Healthy City, USA 12345 • (321) 123-4567

Discharge Summary

Patient Name: Donald Jones   **Patient Number:** 43-23-77
Birth Date: 04/03/xx   **Room Number:** 232

DATE OF ADMISSION: 01/03/xx

DATE OF DISCHARGE: 01/12/xx

REASON FOR ADMISSION: Infection in the foot.

PRINCIPAL DIAGNOSIS: Cellulitis of the foot.

SECONDARY DIAGNOSES:
    Extensive gangrene.
    Diabetes with neuropathy.
    Diabetes with retinopathy.
    Diabetes with nephropathy.
    Acute renal failure.
    Protein malnutrition.
    Hyperphosphatemia.
    Hyposmolarity.

PROCEDURES: Debridement with wound infection, Dr. Armani, 01/05/xx.
                  Above-the-knee amputation.

DISCHARGE SUMMARY: The patient is a 59-year-old individual, long-term poorly controlled type 1 diabetic with all the associated complications including peripheral vascular disease with neuropathy and peripheral diabetic neuropathy. The patient came in with a fetid foot, which was initially debrided and treated with antibiotics and conservative therapy. It became rapidly clear that this would not heal. The patient underwent an amputation. During the recovery phase, the patient did have difficulties in terms of his nutrition and his diabetes, which were adjusted, and the patient was transferred to a nursing home for further support and therapy.

_____

Samuel Edison, MD

SE/bab
d&t: 01/14/xx

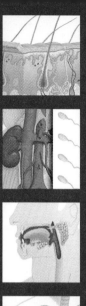
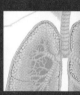

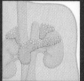

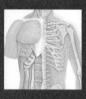

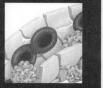

chapter

11 Obstetrics and Gynecology

Chapter Outline

Objectives

Upon completion of this chapter, you will be able to:

- Describe the types of medical treatment obstetricians and gynecologists provide.
- Name the organs of the female reproductive system and discuss their functions.
- Recognize, pronounce, build, and spell correctly terms related to the female reproductive system.
- Describe pathological conditions, diagnostic tests, surgical procedures, and other treatments related to the female reproductive system.
- Demonstrate your knowledge of this chapter by successfully completing the activities and analysis of medical records.

About Gynecology

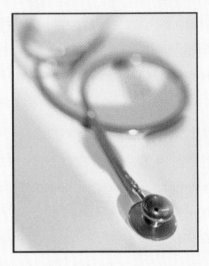

Obstetrics is the branch of medicine concerned with pregnancy and childbirth, including the study of the physiological and pathological functions of the female reproductive tract. It also involves the care of the mother and fetus throughout pregnancy, childbirth, and the immediate postpartum (after birth) period. An **obstetrician** is a physician who specializes in obstetrics.

Gynecology is the study of the health and diseases of the female reproductive organs, including the breasts. Unlike most medical specialties, gynecology encompasses surgical and nonsurgical expertise of the physician. A **gynecologist** is a physician who specializes in gynecology. Because obstetrics is studied in conjunction with gynecology, the physician's medical practice frequently encompasses both areas of expertise. This branch of medicine is called **obstetrics and gynecology (OB-GYN).** Both the obstetrician and gynecologist possess knowledge of endocrinology because hormones play an important role in the functions of the female reproductive system, especially the development of secondary sex characteristics, menstruation, pregnancy, and menopause. Therefore, infertility, birth control, and hormone imbalance are all part of the treatment provided by an OB-GYN physician.

To grasp the scope of practice and the role of health-care practitioners in the medical specialty of obstetrics and gynecology, it is important to understand the structure and function of the female reproductive system as well as the language of medicine that is related to this medical specialty.

Selected Key Terms

anteversion ăn-tĭ-VĔR-zhŭn *ante=before, in front* *version=turning*	A tipping forward of an organ as a whole, without bending. Also called *anteflexion.*
atrophy ĂT-rō-fē *a=without, not* *trophy=development, nourishment*	A wasting; a decrease in size of an organ or tissue due to disease or other influences.
CA 125	A glycoprotein found in the blood serum of patients with ovarian or other glandular cell carcinomas. Increasing levels of this antigen represent continuing tumor growth, which may indicate a poor prognosis.
carcinoma in situ kăr-sĭ-NŌ-mă ĭn SĬ-tū	A lesion characterized by cytological changes of the type associated with invasive carcinoma, but limited to a localized area without evidence of extension to adjacent structures.
fertilization fĕr-tĭl-ĭ-ZĀ-shŭn	The union of the male and female sex cells (gametes) to produce a fertilized egg (zygote) from which the embryo develops.
gestation jĕs-TĀ-shŭn	In mammals, the length of time from conception to birth. In humans, the average duration is 266 days from the onset of the last menstrual period. A gestation time of less than 37 weeks is regarded as premature.

graafian follicle GRĂF-ē-ăn FŎL-ĭ-kŭl	A mature follicle of the ovary that ruptures during ovulation to release an ovum (egg). Beginning with puberty and continuing until menopause, except during pregnancy, a graafian follicle develops at approximately monthly intervals.
gravida GRĂV-ĭ-dă	A pregnant woman. The term is used with numerals to indicate the number of times a woman has been pregnant—for example, gravida I or 1 indicates one pregnancy.
lactation lăk-TĀ-shŭn	The process of synthesis and secretion of milk from the breasts in nourishment of an infant or child.
orifice ŎR-ĭ-fĭs	The entrance or outlet of any anatomic structure, such as the mouth, vagina, or the anus.
ovulation ŏv-ū-LĀ-shŭn	The periodic ripening and rupture of the mature graafian follicle and the discharge of the ovum (egg) from the ovary as part of a monthly cycle that leads to fertilization or menstruation.
para PĂ-ră	A woman who has produced a viable infant (more than 20-weeks' gestation) regardless of whether the infant is alive at birth. The term is used with numerals to indicate the number of pregnancies carried to more than 20 weeks—for example, para 2 or II indicates a woman who has given birth twice.
parturition păr-tū-RĬSH-ŭn	The process of giving birth.
retroversion rĕt-rō-VĔR-shŭn retro=backward, behind version=turning	A turning, or a state of being turned back; especially the tipping of an entire organ. Also called *retroflexion*.
spermatozoa SPĔR-măt-ō-ZŌ-ă	Mature male germ cells that develop in the testes. Resembling a tadpole, each sperm cell has a head with a nucleus, a neck, and a tail that provides propulsion. Developed in vast numbers after puberty, sperm are the generative component of the semen, impregnating the ovum and resulting in fertilization.

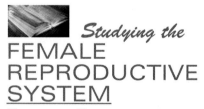

Studying the
FEMALE REPRODUCTIVE SYSTEM

FEMALE REPRODUCTIVE SYSTEM AT A GLANCE

Although the primary purpose of both the male and female reproductive systems is reproduction, the female reproductive system is much more complicated than that of the male. Not only must it produce the female sex cell, the ovum, which is capable of being fertilized; it must also prepare to nurture a developing fetus for approximately 9 months (40 weeks). The female and male gonads are the primary reproductive organs that are responsible for the production of gametes, also known as sex cells. The female gonads, the ovaries, produce ova. The male gonads, the testes, produce male sex cells (also called sperm or **spermatozoa**). Each month an *ovum* (plural, *ova*) is released and travels down one of the fallopian tubes where it may be fertilized by a sperm. If sperm does not fertilize the ovum (egg), hormone changes cause the uterine lining to shed and menstruation or bleeding occurs.

If fertilization takes place, the union of the female and male gametes produces a fertilized egg, known as a

Body System Connections
Female Reproductive System

 THE CARDIOVASCULAR SYSTEM
◆ The cardiovascular system transports vital substances to the organs of the reproductive system. ◆ The normal function of the sex organs, especially erectile tissue, is dependent on blood pressure.

 THE DIGESTIVE SYSTEM
◆ The reproductive system depends on the digestive system to provide adequate nutrients, including fats, to make conception and normal fetal development possible.

 THE ENDOCRINE SYSTEM
◆ The development and function of the reproductive system are influenced by hormones. ◆ Sex hormones are the main influence on the development of the egg and the secondary sex characteristics.

 THE INTEGUMENTARY SYSTEM
◆ The skin's sensory receptors influence the sucking reflex and erotic stimuli. ◆The skin's ability to stretch during pregnancy accommodates the growing fetus.

 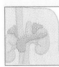 **THE LYMPHATIC AND IMMUNE SYSTEMS**
◆ Lymphatic vessels prevent edema by draining leaked tissue fluids. ◆ The female immune system has special mechanisms to inhibit its attack on sperm cells. ◆ Immune cells protect the reproductive organs from disease.

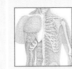 **THE MUSCULOSKELETAL SYSTEM**
◆ Muscular structures of the pelvic floor support the reproductive organs; abdominal muscles are active during childbirth. ◆ The pelvic bones enclose and protect some of the reproductive organs. ◆ A narrow pelvis may hinder the vaginal delivery of an infant.

 THE NERVOUS SYSTEM
◆ All the phases of the sexual response are regulated by the nervous system.

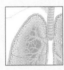 **THE RESPIRATORY SYSTEM**
◆ Respiration rate increases during sexual activity. ◆ Fetal respiration starts before birth.

 THE URINARY AND MALE REPRODUCTIVE SYSTEMS
◆ Kidneys remove wastes and maintain an acid-base balance of blood of mother and fetus. ◆ The male reproductive system produces sperm cells to fertilize the ovum.

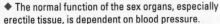

Figure 11–1 *The interrelationship of the female reproductive system with other body systems.*

zygote. Normally **fertilization** takes place in the fallopian tube when the ovum is about one-third of the way down the uterine tube. It usually occurs within 24 hours after ovulation when sperm cells (spermatozoa), discharged by the male during coitus (sexual intercourse, copulation), come in contact with and penetrate the ovum. Implantation and development of the new embryo take place in the uterus. The embryo contains an equal combination (half from each parent) of chromosomes, which contain DNA, the genetic material that controls the inheritance of traits from each parent.

Two hormones secreted primarily by the ovaries, estrogen and progesterone, not only prepare the uterus for implantation of the fertilized egg but also help maintain pregnancy and promote growth of the placenta. During the first 2 months, the developing human is called an embryo. After the 2nd month, the developing human is known as a fetus. The time from fertilization until birth is approximately 266 days from the onset of the last menstrual period and is known as the **gestation** period or pregnancy. A gestation time of less than 37 weeks is regarded as premature. Estrogen and progesterone also play an important role during adolescence in the development of secondary sex characteristics, such as general body shape, breast enlargement, and menstrual cycles.

The interrelationship of the female reproductive system with other body systems is illustrated in Figure 11–1.

STRUCTURE AND FUNCTION

The female reproductive system comprises the internal organs of reproduction and the external genitalia. The internal organs are the ovaries, fallopian tubes, uterus, and vagina. The external genitalia, also called the vulva, include the mons pubis, labia, clitoris, and Bartholin glands. The mammary glands (breasts) are also considered accessory organs of reproduction.

Internal Reproductive Organs
The Ovaries

Figure 11–2 illustrates the female reproductive system shown in lateral view, whereas Figure 11–3 illustrates the female reproductive system shown in anterior view. Various structures in the anterior view have been cross-sectioned in both figures to provide a better graphic understanding of the process of reproduction. Review the lateral and anterior figures simultaneously to gain a better visual understanding of the structural placement of the female reproductive organs.

Label Figures 11–2 and 11–3 as you read the following material.

The (1) **ovaries,** or female gonads, are almond-shaped glands located in the pelvic cavity, one on each side of the uterus. The (2) **ovarian ligaments** attach each ovary to the upper uterus. These ligaments help keep the ovaries in place. The ovaries contain thousands of tiny saclike structures called (3) **graafian follicles,** each of which encloses an ovum. The monthly series of events associated with the maturation of an ovum (a mature egg cell) is called the ovarian cycle. Once a month, during the ovarian cycle, the mature graafian follicle ruptures to the surface and the ovum leaves the ovary. The monthly release of the ovum is the process called **ovulation.** After ovulation, the empty follicle is transformed into a very different looking structure called the (4) **corpus luteum,** which ultimately degenerates at the end of a nonfertile cycle. The corpus luteum, a small yellowish mass, develops within a ruptured ovarian follicle after ovulation and secretes progesterone and estrogen.

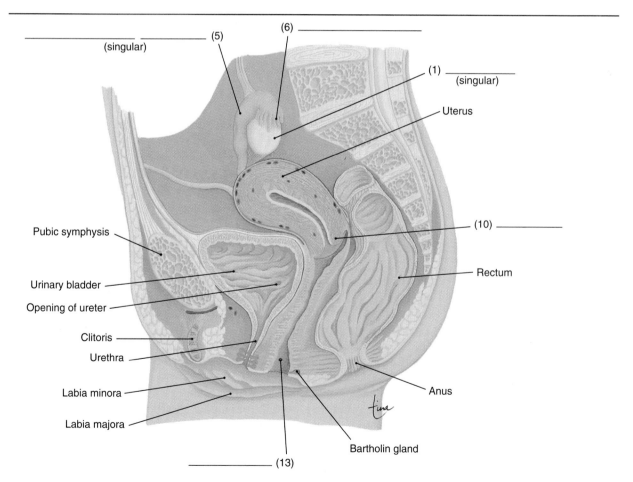

(singular) (5) (6) _____

(1) _____ (singular)

Uterus

Pubic symphysis

Urinary bladder

Opening of ureter

Clitoris

Urethra

Labia minora

Labia majora

(10) _____

Rectum

Anus

Bartholin gland

(13)

Figure 11–2 *The female reproductive system shown in lateral view. (Adapted from Scanlon, VC, and Sanders, TS: Essentials of Anatomy and Physiology, ed 3. FA Davis, Philadelphia, 1999, p 446, with permission.)*

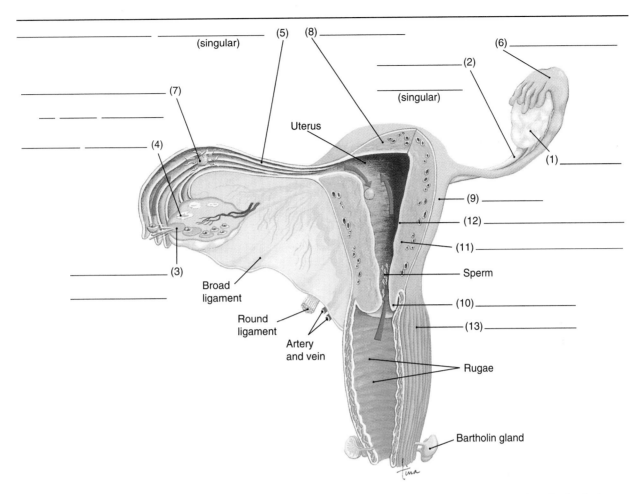

(5) (8) _____
(singular)

(7)

(4)

(3)

Uterus

Broad
ligament

Round
ligament

Artery
and vein

(6) _____

(2)
(singular)

(1) _____

(9) _____

(12) _____

(11) _____

Sperm

(10) _____

(13) _____

Rugae

Bartholin gland

Figure 11–3 *The female reproductive system shown in anterior view. The left ovary has been sectioned to show the developing follicles. The left fallopian tube has been sectioned to show fertilization. The uterus and vagina have been sectioned to show internal structures. Arrows indicate the movement of the ovum toward the uterus and the movement of sperm from the vagina toward the fallopian tube. (Adapted from Scanlon, VC, and Sanders, TS: Essentials of Anatomy and Physiology, ed 3. FA Davis, Philadelphia, 1999, p 447, with permission.)*

Fallopian Tubes

Two (5) **fallopian tubes** (oviducts, uterine tubes) open near the ovaries and extend laterally from superior angles of the uterus. Fingerlike projections, (6) **fimbriae,** encircle the open end of each fallopian tube. Their wavelike currents guide a released ovum into the fallopian tube. It is within the fallopian tube that (7) **fertilization of the ovum** takes place if spermatozoa are present. Many sperm cells may reach the egg cell, but only one actually fertilizes it. If fertilization or conception does not occur, the ovum disintegrates within 48 hours.

Uterus

The uterus (see Figs. 11–2 and 11–3) is a muscular, hollow, pear-shaped structure suspended in the pelvic cavity by bands of ligaments. When an ovum has been fertilized by sperm in the fallopian tube, it becomes implanted in the uterus and develops into an embryo.

In exceptional circumstances, two or more ova may be fertilized at a single time, a process resulting in multiple births (twins, triplets, quadruplets, etc.)

The uterus nourishes the embryo from the time the fertilized egg is implanted until the fetus is born. When an ovum is not fertilized, it passes directly through the uterus and lower reproductive organs and is eliminated from the body during menstruation.

Normally the uterus is flexed anteriorly where it joins the vagina, causing it to be in a position of **anteversion** (tilted forward). However, in older women, the organ is frequently in a position of **retroversion** (tilted back). The uterus comprises three parts: the (8) **fundus,** which is the upper and rounded part; the (9) **body,** which is the central part; and the inferior constricted portion that opens into the vagina, called the (10) **cervix** (cervix uteri). Its central opening allows the passage of sperm and menstrual blood. During childbirth, it dilates to allow passage of the newborn.

The uterine wall comprises three layers: the perimetrium, the outermost layer; the (11) **myometrium,** the bulky middle layer that contracts rhythmically during childbirth to expel the baby from the mother's body; and the (12) **endometrium,** the mucosal lining of the uterine cavity. Should fertilization occur, it is the endometrium that provides nourishment for the developing fetus. If fertilization does not occur, the endometrial lining is sloughed off and eliminated from the body during menstruation.

Vagina

The (13) **vagina** is a muscular tube that extends from the cervix to the exterior of the body. Its outer muscular wall widens during sexual intercourse and childbirth. During menstruation, it is the passageway for the elimination of endometrial tissue from the body.

Activity 11-1. Competency Verification
Female Reproductive System

Review Figures 11–2 and 11–3, and check your labeling in Appendix C.

External Genitalia

The combined structures of the external genitalia are known as the vulva. These include the mons pubis, the labia majora, labia minora, clitoris, and Bartholin glands. See Figure 11–2 for a lateral view of these structures.

Label Figure 11–4 as you read the following material about the external genitalia.

The (1) **mons pubis** is a fatty, rounded area overlying the pubic symphysis bone. This area develops pubic hair after puberty. Extending posteriorly from the mons are two elongated skin folds, the (2) **labia majora** and the (3) **labia minora.** The labia majora, the outer lips of the vagina, protect the labia minora and the clitoris. The labia minora lie underneath the labia majora and cover the (4) **urethral orifice** and (5) **vaginal orifice.** The (6) **clitoris,** an erectile structure, is generously supplied with sensory nerve fibers that are particularly sensitive to local stimulation. The culmination of such stimulation is orgasm. During sexual excitement, the vaginal orifice is lubricated by secretions from the (7) **Bartholin glands,** located within the wall immediately inside the vaginal orifice. A mucous membrane, the (8) **hymen,** partially closes

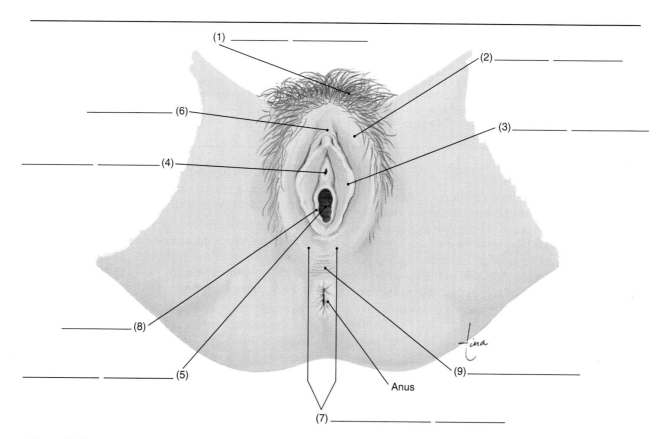

Anus

Figure 11–4 *The female external genitals (vulva) shown in inferior view of the perineum. (Adapted from Scanlon, VC, and Sanders, TS: Essentials of Anatomy and Physiology, ed 3. FA Davis, Philadelphia, 1999, p 450, with permission.)*

the vaginal orifice, and its durability varies among women. It may be ruptured during the first coitus (sexual intercourse), but it may also be disrupted earlier during a sports activity, tampon insertion, pelvic examination, or trauma.

The area between the anus and vaginal orifice is known as the (9) **perineum.** During childbirth, the perineum is stretched and may be torn, causing injury to the anus. To prevent excessive tearing of the perineum, or to hasten or facilitate birth of the baby, the obstetrician often incises the perineum by performing an episiotomy. After childbirth, the incision is closed or repaired.

Activity 11–2. Competency Verification
External Genitalia (Vulva)

Review Figure 11–4, and check your labeling of the vulva in Appendix C.

Mammary Glands

The mammary glands, or breasts, are accessory organs of the female reproductive system that are specialized to produce milk for nourishment of a newborn baby. They are located in the upper anterior aspect of the chest.

Label Figure 11–5 as you learn about the structures of the breast.

During puberty the woman's breasts develop as a result of periodic stimulation of ovarian hormones estrogen and progesterone. Estrogen is responsible for the development of (1) **adipose tissue** that increases the size of the breasts as they reach maturity at around 16 years of age. The size of the breast reflects the amount of fat around the glandular tissue, which is genetically determined. Breast size is not a factor in the ability to produce and secrete milk. The formation of milk is under hormonal control. During pregnancy, high levels of estrogen and progesterone prepare the glands for milk production.

Each breast has approximately 15 to 20 lobes of (2) **glandular tissue** that are responsible for milk production during **lactation.** Milk in these lobes is passed into the (3) **lactiferous duct** that opens on the tip of the raised (4) **nipple.** Circling the nipple is a border of slightly darker skin called the (5) **areola.** Under the areola, each lactiferous duct has a dilated region, called a (6) **lactiferous sinus** where milk accumulates during nursing. Because the main purpose of the breasts is to secrete milk for the nourishment of the newborn, pregnancy causes the breasts to enlarge for this function. Once the woman has nursed, her breasts return to their approximate size before pregnancy. At menopause, breast tissue begins to atrophy.

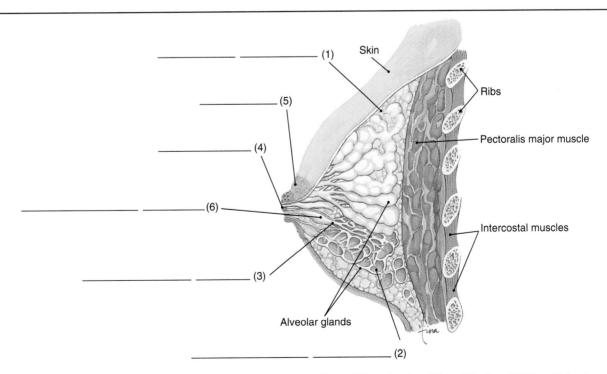

Figure 11–5 *The mammary gland shown in midsagittal section. (Adapted from Scanlon, VC, and Sanders, TS: Essentials of Anatomy and Physiology, ed 3. FA Davis, Philadelphia, 1999, p 451, with permission.)*

Activity 11-3. Competency Verification
Mammary Glands.

**Review Figure 11–5, and check your labeling
of the mammary gland in Appendix C.**

MENSTRUAL CYCLE

The initial menstrual period, **menarche,** occurs at puberty. The menstrual cycle is a series of cyclic changes that the uterine endometrium goes through each month as it responds to changing levels of ovarian hormones in the blood. The cycle duration is approximately 28 days. The uterine phases of the cycle are the menstrual phase, proliferative phase, and the secretory phase.

Menstrual Phase
Days 1–5

In this phase, the functional layer of the endometrium detaches from the uterine wall, a process that is accompanied by bleeding. The detached tissue and blood flow are discharged through the vagina as the menstrual flow. By day 5, several ovarian follicles begin to develop and produce more estrogen (Fig. 11–6).

Proliferative Phase
Days 6–14

In this phase, the endometrium rebuilds itself. As the estrogen level rises, several ova begin to mature in the graafian follicles with only one ovum reaching full maturity. On or about the 14th day, ovulation occurs when the graafian follicle ruptures. The egg then leaves the ovary and travels down the fallopian tube (see Fig. 11–6 and Flowchart 11–1).

Secretory Phase
Days 15–28

In this phase, the empty graafian follicle fills with a yellow material and now becomes the corpus luteum. Secretions of estrogen and progesterone by the corpus luteum stimulate the building of the endometrium

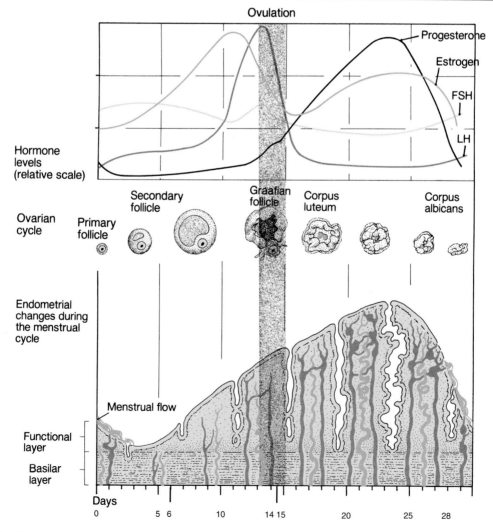

Figure 11–6 *The menstrual cycle. The levels of the important hormones are shown relative to one another throughout the cycle. Changes in the ovarian follicle are depicted. The relative thickness of the endometrium is also shown. (Adapted from Scanlon, VC, and Sanders, TS: Essentials of Anatomy and Physiology, ed 3. FA Davis, Philadelphia, 1999, p 453, with permission.)*

in preparation for the implantation of an embryo. If fertilization does not occur, the corpus luteum begins to degenerate at the end of the secretory phase as estrogen and progesterone levels decline. With the decrease of hormone levels, the uterine lining begins to shed and the menstrual cycle starts over again on this 1st day of the menstrual flow.

With a decrease in hormonal levels, some women experience symptoms called *premenstrual syndrome* (*PMS*). PMS usually occurs about 5 days after the fall in hormones with symptoms of nervous tension, irritability, headaches, breast tenderness, and a feeling of depression.

PREGNANCY

During pregnancy, the uterus changes its shape, size, and consistency. It grows large enough to accommodate the growing fetus, placenta, amniotic sac, and amniotic fluid. Usually it increases in weight to slightly over 2 pounds. From the moment of conception many changes occur, most of them controlled by the hormones estrogen and progesterone. The action of progesterone inhibits ovulation and ceases menstruation. A missed menstrual period is often the first sign of pregnancy. As pregnancy progresses, estrogen causes the softening and enlargement of the pubic joints, ligaments, and tissues in preparation for labor. This action brings its own discomforts, such as frequent urination, backache, and formation of stretch marks, as connective tissue loosens. Once the fertilized ovum becomes implanted in the uterine walls, two important

structures develop simultaneously with the developing embryo: the amnion and the placenta (Fig. 11–7).

The first structure, the *amnion*, is a thin membranous bag that eventually surrounds the embryo. It is the innermost of the two membranous layers of the amniotic sac surrounding the fetus. The outer layer of the sac is known as the *chorion*. As the embryo grows, the amnion entirely surrounds the embryo and becomes filled with amniotic fluid. Amniotic fluid serves as a cushion for the fetus against injury. The amnion with its fluid constitutes the "bag of waters," and usually ruptures just before birth as the labor process begins.

The second structure, the *placenta*, has the shape of a flat cake when fully developed and is formed by the chorion of the embryo and a portion of the endometrium of the mother. Thus, it originates from both embryonic and maternal tissues. The placenta provides an exchange of nutrients and wastes between fetus and mother and secretes several hormones necessary to maintain a normal pregnancy. The placental hormone, called *human chorionic gonadotropin* (HCG), normally prevents pregnancy loss. If the hormone is present in a urine sample, pregnancy is confirmed. The fetal side of the placenta contains the ar-

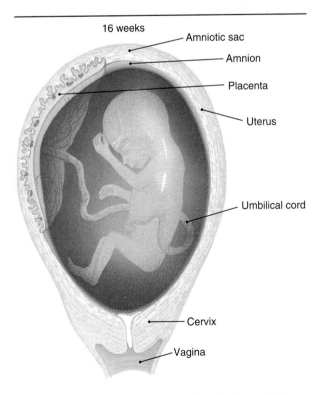

16 weeks
— Amniotic sac
— Amnion
— Placenta
— Uterus
— Umbilical cord
— Cervix
— Vagina

Figure 11–7   *Fetal development at 16 weeks. (Adapted from Scanlon, VC, and Sanders, TS: Essentials of Anatomy and Physiology, ed 3. FA Davis, Philadelphia, 1999, p 465, with permission.)*

Ovary

↓

Egg

↓

Fallopian tube

↓

Uterus

Egg is not fertilized

Egg is fertilized

↓

↓

Egg is expelled through menstruation

Egg is implanted in the uterus

Flowchart 11–1   *An egg during the ovarian cycle.*

teries and veins that form the umbilical cord. The umbilical cord holds the embryo in the amniotic cavity and includes three blood vessels that transport blood between the embryo and the placenta.

The average gestation lasts approximately 9 months or 266 days in duration or 280 days from the onset of the last menstrual period. The pregnancy is then concluded by childbirth (**parturition**). Up to the third month of pregnancy the product of conception is referred to as the embryo. After 8 weeks to the time of birth, the unborn offspring is referred to as the fetus. Toward the end of gestation, the myometrium begins to contract weakly at irregular intervals. At this time, the full-term fetus is usually positioned head down within the uterus.

LABOR AND CHILDBIRTH

Labor is the physiological process by which the fetus is expelled from the uterus. Labor occurs in three stages. The first is the stage of dilation, which begins with uterine contractions and terminates when there is complete dilation (10 cm) of the cervix. The second is the stage of expulsion. This is the time from complete cervical dilation to the birth of the baby. The last is the placental stage or afterbirth. It begins shortly after childbirth, when uterine contractions discharge the placenta from the uterus.

MENOPAUSE

After puberty, menstrual cycles usually continue at regular intervals into middle age, when they become increasingly irregular. Eventually the cycles cease altogether. This period in life is called **menopause** and signals the termination of ovulation and menstruation. Artificial menopause can occur when the ovaries are surgically removed, causing a reduction of estrogen and cessation of ovulation. Artificial menopause can also occur when the ovaries become dysfunctional because of the treatment of a disease with radiation or with some types of chemical agents.

With advancing age, estrogen levels fall and many women experience hot flashes, vaginal drying, and vaginal thinning (vaginal atrophy). Pharmacological replacement of estrogen, *estrogen replacement therapy* (ERT), is often prescribed to relieve the symptoms of menopause. ERT combined with low doses of progesterone is believed to play a role in the prevention of heart attacks, uterine cancer, and the development of porous bones (**osteoporosis**). Restraint in prescribing estrogens for long periods in all menopausal women arises from concern that there is an increased risk that long-term usage will induce **neoplastic** changes in estrogen-sensitive aging tissue. Thus, the use of ERT remains controversial.

Activity 11–4. Competency Verification
Gynecologic and Obstetrical Terms

estrogen	menarche	placental stage
fertilization	menopause	stage of dilation
gestation	myometrium	stage of expulsion
graafian follicles	para	vaginomycosis
lactation	parturition	

Match the terms listed above with their definitions in the numbered list:

1. _____ the union of female and male gametes to produce a fertilized egg (zygote).

2. _____ the process of giving birth.

3. _____ duration of pregnancy; in humans, approximately nine months.

4. _____ production and secretion of milk from the breasts for nourishment of an infant.

5. _____ the period that marks the cessation of a woman's reproductive ability.

6. _____ time from complete cervical dilation to birth of the baby.

7. _____ the beginning of the first menstrual period.

8. _____ begins with uterine contractions and terminates when the cervix uteri is completely dilated.

9. _____ hormone responsible for increased breast size as the breasts reach full maturity.

10. _____ the last stage of labor, also called afterbirth.

Correct Answers _____ × 10 = _____% Score

Studying
OBSTETRICS AND GYNECOLOGY TERMINOLOGY
MEDICAL WORD COMPONENTS

Combining Forms: Obstetrics and Gynecology

Combining Form	Meaning	EXAMPLE	
		Term/Pronunciation	**Definition**
amni/o	amnion (amniotic sac)	**amni**/o/centesis ăm-nē-ō-sĕn-TĒ-sĭs	transabdominal puncture (-*centesis*) of the amniotic sac using a needle and syringe to remove amniotic fluid for laboratory analysis
cervic/o	neck, cervix uteri (neck of uterus)	**cervic**/itis sĕr-vĭ-SĪ-tĭs	inflammation (-*itis*) of the cervix
colp/o	vagina	**colp**/o/scopy kŏl-PŎS-kō-pē	visual examination (-*scopy*) of the vagina
vagin/o		**vagin**/o/myc/osis văj-ĭn-ō-mī-KŌ-sĭs	abnormal (-*osis*) condition of a vaginal fungus (*myc/o*)
episi/o	vulva	**episi**/o/tomy ĕ-pĭs-ē-ŎT-ō-mē	incision (-*tomy*) of the perineum to avoid spontaneous laceration and facilitate delivery of a baby
vulv/o		**vulv**/o/pathy vŭl-VŎP-ă-thē	disease (-*pathy*) of the vulva
galact/o	milk	**galact**/o/rrhea gă-lăk-tō-RĒ-ă	discharge (-*rrhea*) from the nipple that is persistent and looks like milk
lact/o		**lact**/o/cele LĂK-tō-sēl	a cystic tumor of the breast caused by occlusion of a milk duct *The suffix* -cele *means* hernia, swelling. Lactocele *is synonymous with* galactocele.

Combining Forms: Obstetrics and Gynecology (Continued)

Combining Form	Meaning	EXAMPLE	
		Term/Pronunciation	**Definition**
gynec/o	woman, female	**gynec**/o/logy gī-nĕ-KŎL-ō-jē	study of (-*logy*) the diseases of the female reproductive organs and the breasts
hyster/o	uterus, womb	**hyster**/ectomy hĭs-tĕr-ĔK-tō-mē	removal (-*ectomy*) of the uterus *Unless otherwise specified, hysterectomy usually denotes complete removal of the uterus (corpus and cervix).*
metr/o		**metr**/o/rrhagia mē-trō-RĀ-jē-ă	excessive bleeding from the uterus occurring between periods *Uterine, ovarian tumors, and intrauterine devices or other foreign bodies can cause metrorrhagia. The suffix* -rrhagia *means* bursting forth (of) blood.
uter/o		**uter**/o/plasty ū-tĕr-ō-PLĂS-tē	surgical repair (-*plasty*) of the uterus
leiomy/o	smooth muscle (visceral)	**leiomy**/oma lī-ō-mī-Ō-mă	benign tumor (-*oma*) derived from smooth (nonstriated) muscle *Leiomyomas can occur in the uterus. A* leiomyoma uteri *is a benign neoplasm of the smooth muscle of the uterus.*
mamm/o	breast	**mamm**/o/gram MĂM-ō-grăm	x-ray record (-*gram*) of the breast
mast/o		**mast**/o/pexy MĂS-tō-pĕks-ē	fixation (-*pexy*) of the breast(s) *This type of plastic surgery is performed to lift sagging breasts to a more elevated normal position, often improving their shape.*
men/o	menses, menstruation	**men**/arche mĕn-ĂR-kē	first menstrual period *The suffix* -arche *means* beginning.
nat/o	birth	**nat**/al NĀ-tăl	pertaining to (-*al*) birth or the day of birth
oophor/o	ovary	**oophor**/oma ō-ŏf-ō-RŌ-mă	an ovarian tumor (-*oma*)
ovari/o		**ovari**/o/cyesis ō-vā-rē-ō-sī-Ē-sĭs	ovarian pregnancy (-*cyesis*)

Combining Forms: Obstetrics and Gynecology (Continued)

Combining Form	Meaning	EXAMPLE	
		Term/Pronunciation	**Definition**
perine/o	perineum	**perine**/o/rrhaphy pĕr-ĭ-nē-OR-ă-fē	suture of the perineum *This procedure is commonly done to repair a laceration that occurs or is made surgically during the delivery of the fetus.*
salping/o	tube (usually fallopian or eustachian [auditory] tubes)	**salping**/ectomy săl-pĭn-JĔK-tō-mē	removal (*-ectomy*) of the fallopian tube(s) *The fallopian tube is part of the female reproductive system; the eustachian (auditory) tube is related to the special sense of hearing. Keep the proper body system in mind when using this combining form.*

Activity 11–5. Competency Verification
Medical Word Components

Check off the box [✓] as you complete each numbered section.

[   ] **1.** Review the components and their examples in the previous section. Then pronounce each word aloud.

[   ] **2.** For the words below, first write the suffix and its meaning. Then translate the meaning of the remaining components starting with the first part of the word.

> **Example:** mamm/o/gram
> **Answer:** *gram*=record, writing; breast

1. cervic/itis   _____

2. galact/o/rrhea   _____

3. amni/o/centesis   _____

4. mast/o/pexy   _____

5. leiomy/oma   _____

6. vagin/itis   _____

7. vulv/o/pathy   _____

8. episi/o/tomy   _____

9. colp/o/scopy   _____

10. oophor/oma   _____

11. salping/ectomy _____

12. gynec/o/logy _____

13. hyster/ectomy _____

14. perine/o/rrhaphy _____

15. ovari/o/cyesis _____

Correct Answers _____ × 6.67 = _____% Score

Prefixes and Suffixes

In this section, prefixes are listed alphabetically and
highlighted whereas key suffixes are defined in the
right-hand column.

Prefixes: Obstetrics and Gynecology

		EXAMPLE	
Prefix	**Meaning**	**Term/Pronunciation**	**Definition**
ante-	before, in front	**ante**/version ăn-tĭ-VĔR-zhŭn	an abnormal position of an organ in which it is tilted forward on its axis, away from the midline *The suffix -version means "turning." When referring to the uterus, anteversion is the normal position of the uterus—tilted forward.*
dys-	bad, painful, difficult	**dys**/tocia dĭs-TŌ-sē-ă	difficult childbirth (*-tocia*)
endo-	in, within	**endo**/metr/itis ĕn-dō-mē-TRĪ-tĭs	inflammation (*-itis*) of the endometrium *The combining form metr/o means "uterus," "measure." The endometrium is the mucous membrane comprising the inner layer of the uterus.*
intra-		**intra**/uter/ine ĭn-tră-Ū-tĕr-ĭn	within the uterus *The suffix -ine means "pertaining to."*
multi-	many, much	**multi**/para mŭl-TĬP-ă-ră	a woman who has delivered more than one viable infant *The suffix -para means "to bear" (offspring).*
neo-	new	**neo**/nat/al nē-ō-NĀ-tăl	pertaining to (*-al*) birth (*nat/i*)

Prefixes: Obstetrics and Gynecology (Continued)

| Prefix | Meaning | EXAMPLE | |
		Term/Pronunciation	Definition
nulli-	none	**nulli**/gravida nŭl-ĭ-GRĂV-ĭ-dă	a woman who has never been pregnant *The suffix* -gravida *means* pregnant woman.
oxy-	quick, sharp	**oxy**/tocia ŏk-sē-TŌ-sē-ă	quick childbirth (-*tocia*)
pre-	before, in front of	**pre**/nat/al prē-NĀ-tl	pertaining to (-*al*) the period before birth (*nat/i*)
primi-	first	**primi**/para prī-MĬP-ă-ră	first birth *The suffix* -para *means* to bear (offspring).

Activity 11–6. Competency Verification

Prefixes and Suffixes

Check off the box [✓] as you complete each numbered section.

[   ] **1.** Review the prefix and suffix section and their examples. Then pronounce each word aloud.

[   ] **2.** For the words below, first write the suffix and its meaning. Then translate the meaning of the remaining components starting with the first part of the word.

> **Example:** neo/nat/al
> **Answer:** *al*=pertaining to, relating to; new; birth

1. pre/nat/al _____

2. dys/tocia _____

3. oxy/tocia _____

4. endo/metr/itis _____

5. intra/uter/ine _____

6. multi/para _____

7. primi/para _____

8. nulli/gravida _____

9. multi/gravida _____

10. ante/version _____

Correct Answers _____ × **10** = _____ **% Score**

Pathological Conditions
Female Reproductive Disorders

DISORDER	DESCRIPTION
MENSTRUAL DISORDERS	
amenorrhea ă-měn-ō-RĒ-ă *a=without, not* *meno=menses, menstruation* *rrhea=discharge, flow*	Absence of menstruation.
dysmenorrhea dĭs-měn-ō-RĒ-ă *dys=bad, painful, difficult* *meno= menses, menstruation* *rrhea= discharge, flow*	Painful menstruation.
menorrhagia měn-ō-RĀ-jē-ă *meno= menses, menstruation* *rrhagia= bursting forth (of blood)*	Increased amount and duration of menstrual flow.
metrorrhagia mě-trō-RĀ-jē-ă *metro=uterus, womb* *rrhagia= bursting forth (of blood)*	Bleeding between menstrual cycles.
oligomenorrhea ŏl-ĭ-gō-měn-ō-RĒ-ă *olig=scanty* *meno= menses, menstruation* *rrhea= discharge, flow*	An abnormally light menstrual flow or a reduction in menstruation.
polymenorrhea pŏl-ē-měn-ō-RĒ-ă *poly=many, much* *meno= menses, menstruation* *rrhea= discharge, flow*	An abnormally frequent recurrence of the menstrual cycle. **Also called** *polymenia.*
premenstrual syndrome (PMS) prē-MĚN-stroo-ăl SĬN-drōm	A syndrome of nervous tension, irritability, weight gain, edema, headache, mastalgia, dysphoria, and lack of coordination occurring during the last few days of the menstrual cycle before the onset of menses.

OTHER PATHOLOGICAL CONDITIONS (CONTINUED)

DISORDER	DESCRIPTION
PREGNANCY DISORDERS	
abruptio placentae ă-BRŬP-shē-ō plă-SĔN-tē	Premature detachment of a normally situated placenta after the 20th week of gestation. This can occur as a result of trauma, hypertension, cocaine use, pre-eclampsia, or without any known cause. Symptoms include severe hemorrhage, abdominal pain, and uterine contractions. This is an obstetrical emergency because it is a significant cause of maternal and fetal mortality.
breech presentation	Intrauterine position of the fetus in which the buttocks or feet present first (versus the head). Different types of breech presentations are illustrated in Figure 11–11. **TYPES OF BREECH PRESENTATIONS** A—FRANK; B—COMPLETE; C—INCOMPLETE; D—FOOTLING *Figure 11–11* Types of breech presentations. (From Venes, D: Taber's Cyclopedic Medical Dictionary, ed 18. FA Davis, Philadelphia, 1997, p 1556, with permission.)
eclampsia ĕ-KLĂMP-sē-ă	The gravest form of pregnancy-induced hypertension. It is characterized by convulsion, coma, hypertension, proteinuria, and edema. The cause is unknown, and it may be related to malnutrition, especially to lack of protein in the diet. It is usually fatal if left untreated. Treatment includes bed rest, close medical monitoring, and administration of medications to control hypertension and seizures.
ectopic pregnancy ĕk-TŎP-ĭk	Implantation of the fertilized ovum outside of the uterine cavity. This occurs in approximately 1% of pregnancies, mostly in the oviducts (tubal pregnancy), as seen in Figure 11–12A. Complications of this condition include rupture within the fallopian tube leading to hematosalpinx and peritonitis. Surgery is indicated to remove the implant and preserve the fallopian tube before rupture occurs. Other sites of ectopic pregnancies are illustrated in Figure 11–12B.
hydramnios hī-DRĂM-nē-ŏs *hydr=water* *amnios=a caul (the intact amniotic sac surrounding the fetus at birth)*	An excess of amniotic fluid that leads to an overdistension of the uterus and the possibility of malpresentation of the fetus. The pressure of the enlarged uterus gives rise to maternal breathlessness, edema, cyanosis, and varicose veins. Amniocentesis is necessary to reduce the amount of amniotic fluid.

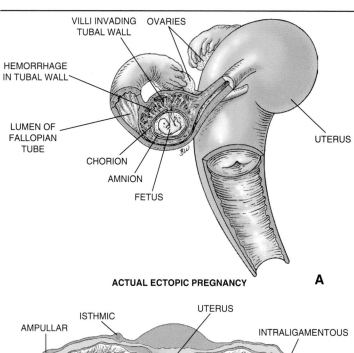

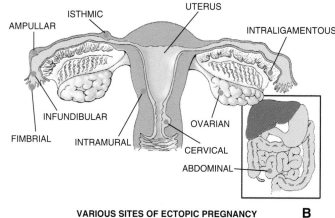

Figure 11–12 *(A) Actual ectopic pregnancy. (B) Various sites of ectopic pregnancy. (From Venes, D: Taber's Cyclopedic Medical Dictionary, ed 19. FA Davis, Philadelphia, 2001, p 1736, with permission.)*

Other Pathological Conditions (Continued)

DISORDER	DESCRIPTION
placenta previa plă-SĔN-tă PRĒ-vē-ă	A placenta that is abnormally implanted in the uterus so that it impinges on or covers the internal os (opening) of the uterine cervix. This may result in a decreased oxygen supply to the fetus and an increased risk of hemorrhage and infection to the mother. The cause is unknown. Maternal symptoms include painless bleeding usually occurring during the last trimester, hemorrhage, and premature labor. Cesarean delivery is often performed.
pre-eclampsia prē-ē-KLĂMP-sē-ă *pre=before, in front* *ec=out, out from* *lampsia=to shine*	A complication of pregnancy characterized by hypertension, proteinuria, and edema. The condition may progress rapidly from mild to severe and if untreated, it can lead to eclampsia or toxemia. Bed rest can manage mild pre-eclampsia. Severe pre-eclampsia needs additional treatment that often includes medications to prevent premature labor and seizures.

OTHER PATHOLOGICAL CONDITIONS (CONTINUED)

DISORDER	DESCRIPTION
NEONATAL DISORDERS	
Down syndrome, trisomy 21 *TRĪ-sō-mē*	Chromosomal abnormality that results in mild to severe mental retardation and other abnormalities. It is marked by a sloping forehead, small ear canals, gray or light yellow spots at the periphery of the iris, short broad hands and feet, a flat nose or absent bridge, low-set ears, and generally dwarfed physique. The incidence is approximately 1 in 80 for offspring of women above 40 years of age.
hyaline membrane disease (HMB) *HĪ-ă-lĭn*	Respiratory condition that primarily occurs in the premature neonate. A lack of protein in the lining of the lungs causes them to collapse. Also known as *respiratory distress syndrome (RDS)*.
hydrocephalus *hī-drō-SĔF-ă-lŭs* *hydro=water* *cephal=head* *us=condition*	An abnormal accumulation of cerebrospinal fluid (CSF) in the ventricles of the brain. In infants the head enlarges because the bones of the skull are not fused together at birth. Surgical intervention is necessary to insert a shunt to drain the excess fluid to the peritoneal cavity, correct the ventricular obstruction, or reduce the production of CSF.
kernicterus *kĕr-NĬK-tĕr-ŭs* *kern= kernel (nucleus)* *icterus= jaundice*	An abnormal toxic accumulation of bilirubin in the central nervous system tissues caused by high levels of bilirubin in the bloodstream (*hyperbilirubinemia*) of a neonate; jaundice appears; the more serious effects include brain damage and mental retardation.
pyloric stenosis *pī-LOR-ĭk stĕ-NŌ-sĭs* *pylor=pylorus* *ic=pertaining to* *stenosis=narrowing, stricture*	A congenital defect in which narrowing of the pyloric sphincter at the outlet of the stomach causes an obstruction that blocks the flow of food into the small intestine. Diagnosis is made in infants by the presence of forceful projectile vomiting and palpitation of a hard prominent pylorus. Pyloromyotomy and pyloroplasty are the surgical procedures to correct the condition.

Activity 11–7. Clinical Application
Pathological Conditions

breech presentation
carcinoma of the breast
eclampsia
endometrial cancer
endometriosis
fibrocystic breast disease
hyaline membrane disease
hydatidiform mole

hydramnios
pelvic inflammatory disease (PID)
placenta previa
polymenorrhea
premenstrual syndrome (PMS)
sexually transmitted diseases (STDs)
toxic shock syndrome

Match the diagnoses listed above with an explanation of their pathological condition in the numbered list:

1. _____ an excess of amniotic fluid with an overdistension of the uterus.

2. _____ infection of the uterus, ovaries, fallopian tubes, and adjacent pelvic structures.

3. _____ an intrauterine polycystic mass in which the chorionic villi have undergone cystic degeneration causing rapid growth of the uterus with hemorrhage.

4. _____ a group of diseases spread by sexual intercourse or genital contact; diseases include chlamydia, genital herpes, gonorrhea, human papillomavirus (HPV), syphilis, and trichomoniasis.

5. _____ a placenta that is abnormally implanted in the uterus so that it impinges on or covers the internal os of the uterine cervix. This may result in decreased oxygen supply to the fetus and an increased risk of hemorrhage and infection to the mother.

6. _____ the most prevalent gynecologic malignancy, most often occurring in the fifth or sixth decade of life; the major symptom is postmenopausal bleeding.

7. _____ disease caused by toxin-producing strains of *Staphylococcus aureus;* leads to hypovolemia, hypotension, and shock.

8. _____ the presence of single or multiple cysts that give a nodular consistency to the breast.

9. _____ the gravest form of pregnancy-induced hypertension characterized by grand mal seizure, coma, proteinuria, and edema.

10. _____ nervous tension, irritability, weight gain, edema, headache, mastalgia, and dysphoria during the last few days of the menstrual cycle before the onset of menses.

11. _____ intrauterine position in which the fetal buttocks or feet present first.

12. _____ abnormal growth of endometrial tissue outside the uterine cavity that may cause dysmenorrhea, infertility, and painful intercourse.

13. _____ a malignant breast tumor. Surgical treatments include lumpectomy, simple or total mastectomy, and modified radical mastectomy.

14. _____ an abnormally frequent recurrence of the menstrual cycle.

15. _____ respiratory condition that primarily occurs in premature neonates; the lack of protein in the lining of the lung causes lung collapse; also known as RDS.

Correct Answers _____ **× 6.67 =** _____ **% Score**

DIAGNOSTIC PROCEDURES AND TESTS
Imaging Procedures

PROCEDURE	DESCRIPTION
GYNECOLOGICAL AND BREAST-RELATED PROCEDURES	
hysterosalpingography *hĭs-tĕr-ō-săl-pĭn-GŎG-ră-fē* *hystero= uterus, womb* *salpingo= tube (usually fallopian or eustachian [auditory] tubes)* *graphy=process of recording*	Radiography of the uterus and oviducts after injection of a contrast medium.
mammography *măm-ŎG-ră-fē* *mammo=breast* *graphy=process of recording*	Radiography of the breast that is used to diagnose benign and malignant tumors. A routine mammogram consists of two views of each breast (see Figs. 11–8 and 18–6). The American Cancer Society (ACS) recommends a baseline mammogram for women between the ages of 35 and 40 years, and a mammogram every 2 years after the age of 40. After the age of 50, the ACS recommends a mammogram be taken for all women every year. However, women identified to be in a risk group, such as those with a history of breast cancer or those with a family member positive for breast cancer, should have a mammogram every year.
pelvic ultrasonography *PĔL-vĭk ŭl-tră-sŏn-ŎG-ră-fē* *pelv=pelvis* *ic=pertaining to* *ultra=beyond, excess* *sono=sound* *graphy=process of recording*	An image of sound waves as they reflect off the organs in the pelvic area. The use of sound waves (versus x-rays) is called *ultrasonography* or *ultrasound*. The recorded image is called a *sonogram*. Figure 11–13 shows a sonogram of a fetus showing the fetal abdominal aorta. 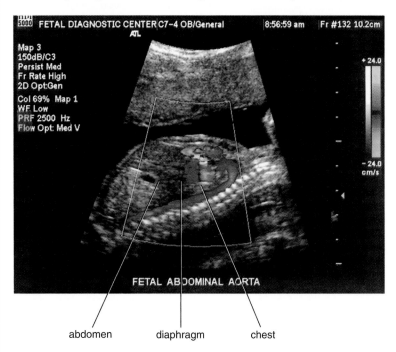

Figure 11–13 Sonogram showing the fetal abdominal aorta. (Courtesy of Medical College of Ohio, Radiology Department.)

Imaging Procedures (Continued)

PROCEDURE	DESCRIPTION
transvaginal ultrasonography *trăns-VĂJ-ĭn-ăl ŭl-tră-sŏn-ŎG-ră-fē* *trans=through, across* *vagin=vagina* *al=pertaining to* *ultra=beyond, excess* *sono=sound* *graphy=process of recording*	Insertion of a sound probe into the vagina to produce a closer, more accurate ultrasound image of the structures within the pelvis.

PREGNANCY AND CHILDBIRTH

fetal monitoring	The use of electrocardiography and ultrasonography to record the fetal heart rate (FHR) during labor.

Other Diagnostic Procedures

PROCEDURE	DESCRIPTION
amniocentesis *ăm-nē-ō-sĕn-TĒ-sĭs* *amnio=amnion (amniotic sac)* *centesis=surgical puncture*	Removal of a small amount of amniotic fluid for laboratory analysis. The fluid is studied chemically and cytologically to detect genetic abnormalities, fetal maturity, and gender of the fetus.
breast biopsy	Obtaining a tissue sample for microscopic analysis to detect the presence of carcinoma. The sample may be obtained surgically or through a needle and syringe (*aspiration biopsy*).
chorionic villus sampling (CVS)	A procedure for withdrawing bits of the chorionic villi (placental tissue) from the placenta for examination. A small tube is inserted through the vagina and cervical canal and guided by ultrasound to an area where a piece of placental tissue can be removed. CVS allows earlier testing (at 8 weeks, but it is usually recommended after the 10th week) than amniocentesis, and is much faster. It is used to obtain prenatal evaluation data early in a pregnancy and to diagnose potential genetic defects.
colposcopy *kŏl-PŎS-kō-pē* *colp=vagina* *scopy=visual examination*	Examination of the vagina and cervix with an optical magnifying instrument (*colposcope*). It is commonly performed after a Pap smear to evaluate cervical dysplasia and obtain biopsy specimens of the cervix.
culdocentesis *kŭl-dō-sĕn-TĒ-sĭs* *culdo=cul-de-sac* *centesis=surgical puncture*	Needle aspiration through the vagina to remove intraperitoneal fluid for examination or diagnosis. Aspiration of blood may indicate a ruptured ectopic pregnancy.
Papanicolaou test, Pap smear *pă-pă-NĬ-kō-lā-oo tĕst, păp smēr*	Microscopic analysis of cells taken from the cervix and vagina to detect the presence of carcinoma. The cells are obtained after the insertion of a vaginal speculum (Fig. 11–14) and the use of a cotton swab, wooden spatula, or special brush (*cytobrush*) to scrape a small tissue sample from the cervix and vagina.

Other Diagnostic Procedures (Continued)

PROCEDURE	DESCRIPTION
	 Figure 11–14 *A vaginal speculum. After insertion of the vaginal speculum, the two opposing portions can be pushed apart for examining the vagina and cervix. The speculum should be warmed before use. (From Williams, LS, and Hopper, PD: Understanding Medical Surgical Nursing. FA Davis, Philadelphia 1999, p 783, with permission.)*
pelvimetry pĕl-VĬM-ĕ-trē *pelvi=pelvis* *metry=act of measuring*	Measurement of the pelvic dimensions and proportions to determine whether or not it will be possible to deliver a fetus through the birth canal.
pregnancy test	Test performed on blood or urine that detects the presence of human chorionic gonadotropin (HCG) produced by the placenta. The presence of HCG confirms that conception has occurred.

SURGICAL AND THERAPEUTIC PROCEDURES

Surgical Procedures

PROCEDURE	DESCRIPTION
GYNECOLOGICAL AND BREAST-RELATED PROCEDURES	
breast reconstruction	Plastic surgical procedure performed following mastectomy. The type of material used to reconstruct the breast includes silicone implants or transplanted tissue (*graft*) from one part of the body (such as the hips or thighs) to the breast.
TRAM flap	A plastic surgical procedure called a transrectus abdominis musculocutaneous (TRAM) flap, in which a muscle from the lower abdomen is tunneled under the abdominal and thoracic wall to the mastectomy scar. After the muscle is tucked under the chest skin, a silicone implant may be inserted before the skin flap is sewn in place. Nipple reconstruction is usually performed at a later time (Fig. 11–15).

Surgical Procedures (Continued)

PROCEDURE	DESCRIPTION
	TRAM (transrectus abdominis musculocutaneous) flap Muscle tucked under chest skin Skin flap sewn in place Rectus flap pulled through tunnel under skin **Additional procedures** Silicone implant behind muscle and skin flap Nipple reconstructed with skin from thigh, labia or other site *Figure 11–15 Mastectomy reconstruction. (Adapted from Williams, LS, and Hopper, PD: Understanding Medical Surgical Nursing, FA Davis, Philadelphia 1999, p 798, with permission.)*
conization kŏn-ĭ-ZĀ-shŭn	Excision of a cone of tissue, such as the mucous membrane of the cervix, for biopsy.
cryosurgery krī-ō-SĔR-jĕr-ē *cryo=cold*	The use of subfreezing temperature to destroy tissue. A probe containing liquid nitrogen produces the freezing temperature. Cryosurgery is frequently used to treat abnormal tissue of the cervix. Also known as *cryocauterization*.
dilation and curettage (D&C)	Dilation of the uterine cervix canal of the uterus and scraping (curettage) of the endometrium of the uterus. Used to diagnose uterine disease, correct heavy or prolonged uterine bleeding, or to empty uterine contents of the products of conception; also called *dilatation and curettage*.
hysterectomy hĭs-tĕr-ĔK-tō-mē *hyster=uterus, womb* *ectomy=excision, removal*	Removal of the uterus through the abdominal wall or vagina. The presence of benign or malignant tumors is the most frequent reason for hysterectomy.
lumpectomy lŭm-PĔK-tō-mē	Surgical excision of a tumor, such as a breast tumor, without removing large amounts of surrounding tissue.
mastectomy măs-TĔK-tō-mē *mast=breast* *ectomy=excision, removal*	Surgical removal of one or both breasts, most commonly performed to remove a malignant tumor.

Surgical Procedures (Continued)

PROCEDURE	DESCRIPTION
modified radical	Mastectomy with the preservation of the large chest muscles that move the arm.
radical	Mastectomy with removal of the large chest muscles together with removal of all of the axillary lymph nodes.
simple	Mastectomy in which only breast tissue is removed.
salpingo-oophorectomy săl-pĭng-gō-ō-ŏf-ō-RĔK-tō-mē *salpingo=tube (usually* *fallopian or eustachian* *[auditory] tubes)* *oophor=ovary* *ectomy=excision, removal*	Surgical removal of a fallopian tube and an ovary.
tubal ligation TŪ-băl lī-GĀ-shŭn	Sterilization procedure that involves blocking both fallopian tubes by cutting or burning them and tying them off.
PREGNANCY AND CHILDBIRTH	
abortion ă-BOR-shŭn *abort=to miscarry* *ion=the act of*	The termination of pregnancy before the fetus reaches the stage of viability; may be spontaneous (*miscarriage*) or induced.
cesarean section (C-section) sĕ-SĂR-ē-ăn	Removal of the fetus by abdominal incision into the uterus. This procedure is performed when abnormal maternal or fetal conditions are judged likely to make vaginal delivery hazardous.
episiorrhaphy ĕ-pĭz-ĭ-OR-ră-fē *episio=vulva* *rrhaphy=suture*	Suturing of a lacerated perineum.
episiotomy ĕ-pĭs-ē-ŎT-ō-mē *episio=vulva* *tomy=incision (of)*	Surgical procedure in which an incision is made in a woman's perineum to enlarge her vaginal opening for delivery. This procedure is performed most often to prevent tearing of the perineum and to hasten or facilitate childbirth.

Therapeutic Procedures

PROCEDURE	DESCRIPTION
GYNECOLOGICAL PROCEDURES	
cauterization *kaw-tĕr-ĭ-ZĀ-shŭn*	The use of chemicals (such as silver nitrate) or an electrically heated instrument to burn and destroy abnormal tissue. This procedure is used to treat cervical erosion and cervical dysplasia. Loop electrocautery excision procedure (LEEP) is a type of cauterization used to biopsy cervical tissue.
cerclage *sār-KLŌZH*	An obstetric procedure in which a nonabsorbable suture is used for holding the cervix closed to prevent spontaneous abortion in a woman who has an incompetent cervix. The band is usually released when the pregnancy is at full term to allow labor to begin.
epidural anesthesia *ĕp-ĭ-DŪ-răl ăn-ĕs-THĒ-zē-ă* *epi =above, upon* *dur= dura matter, hard* *al =pertaining to* *an =without, not* *esthes = feeling* *ia = condition*	Pain management by injection of an anesthetic into the epidural space, usually in the lumbar area, during labor.
intrauterine device (IUD) *ĭn-tră-Ū-tĕr-ĭn* *intra =in, within* *uter =uterus, womb* *ine =pertaining to*	Contraceptive device that consists of a bent strip of radiopaque plastic with a fine monofilament tail that is inserted into the uterus by a gynecologist. The exact action of the IUD is not understood, but it is thought that the presence of a foreign object in the uterus prevents implantation of the ovum.

Pharmacology

DRUG CLASSIFICATION	THERAPEUTIC ACTION
antibiotics *ăn-tĭ-bī-ŎT-ĭks* *anti =against* *bio =life* *tic =pertaining to*	Drugs that inhibit the growth of microorganisms; various classes include those effective against gram-negative and gram-positive bacteria. Used in the treatment of various infections affecting the female reproductive system and sexually transmitted diseases.
antiestrogens *ăn-tĭ-ĔS-trō-jĕnz*	Agents used to prevent the recurrence of breast cancer and to treat metastatic breast cancer.
antifungals *ăn-tĭ-FŬNG-gǎls*	Agents used to treat fungal infections. In the female reproductive system they are used to treat vaginal yeast infections caused by *Candida albicans*.

Pharmacology (Continued)

DRUG CLASSIFICATION	THERAPEUTIC ACTION
estrogen hormones *ĔS-trō-jĕn HOR-mōns*	Agents used in estrogen replacement therapy (ERT) during menopause to correct estrogen deficiency and as chemotherapy for some types of cancer. The long-term use of ERT effectively reduces the symptoms of menopause, reduces the risk of osteoporosis, and keeps cholesterol levels low. Estrogen may be given orally, transdermally, by injection, or as a topical cream (to treat vaginal symptoms only).
oral contraceptives *OR-ăl kŏn-tră-SĔP-tĭvs*	Birth control pills that exert a hormonal influence to prevent pregnancy. Most contain a combination of estrogen and progestin (a group name for progesterone and progesterone derivatives) that is taken for 21 days every month. Other oral contraceptives contain only progestin.
oxytocins *ŏk-sē-TŌ-sĭns*	Agents that stimulate the uterus to contract, thus inducing labor. Also used to rid the uterus of unexpelled placenta or a dead fetus, and act on the mammary gland to stimulate the release of milk.
progestins *prō-JĔS-tĭns*	A large group of synthetic drugs that have a progesterone-like effect on the uterus; used to treat abnormal uterine bleeding due to hormonal imbalance. When prescribed in combination with estrogen, progestins are used in hormone replacement therapy and oral contraceptives.
selective estrogen receptor modulators (SERMs) *sĕ-LĔK-tĭv ĔS-trō-jĕn rē-SĔP-tor MŎD-ū-lā-tors*	Drugs that function like estrogen in some tissues but block the effect of estrogen in others; have estrogen-like effects on bone, increasing bone mineral density and decreasing cholesterol levels.

❖ ABBREVIATIONS

GYNECOLOGIC ABBREVIATION	MEANING	ABBREVIATION	MEANING
AB, ab	abortion, antibodies	**Hb, Hbg, Hgb**	hemoglobin
ACS	American Cancer Society	**HSG**	hysterosalpingography
AI	artificial insemination	**HSV**	herpes simplex virus
BSE	breast self-examination	**HPV**	human papillomavirus
CA 125	cancer cell surface antigen 125	**IUD**	intrauterine device (a contraceptive device)
CIS	carcinoma *in situ*		
D&C	dilation, dilatation and curettage	**LEEP**	loop electrocautery excision procedure
DC	discharge		
DUB	dysfunctional uterine bleeding	**LH**	luteinizing hormone
ERT	estrogen replacement therapy	**LMP**	last menstrual period
FSH	follicle-stimulating hormone	**L, l**	liter, left, lumbar
G	gravida (pregnant)	**lt**	left
GC	gonorrhea	**MH**	marital history
GYN	gynecology	**LSO**	left salpingo-oophorectomy

ABBREVIATION	MEANING	ABBREVIATION	MEANING
OCPs	oral contraceptive pills	**FHT**	fetal heart tone
Pap	Papanicolaou smear (test for cervical or vaginal cancer)	**FTND**	full-term normal delivery
		HCG	human chorionic gonadotropin
Path	pathology	**HDN**	hemolytic disease of newborn
PID	pelvic inflammatory disease	**HMD**	hyaline membrane disease
PMP	previous menstrual period	**IUGR**	intrauterine growth rate, intrauterine growth retardation
PMS	premenstrual syndrome		
R	respiration, right	**IVF**	in vitro fertilization
R/O	rule out	**IVF-ET**	in vitro fertilization and embryo transfer
RSO	right salpingo-oophorectomy		
rt	right	**LBW**	low birth weight
SERMs	selective estrogen receptor modulators	**NB**	newborn
		OB	obstetrics
STD	sexually transmitted disease	**RDS**	respiratory distress syndrome
TAH	total abdominal hysterectomy	**UC**	uterine contraction
TOH	total abdominal hysterectomy	**XX**	female sex chromosomes
TRAM	trans-rectus abdominis musculocutaneous	**XY**	male sex chromosomes
TSS	toxic shock syndrome		
TVH	total vaginal hysterectomy		
VD	venereal disease		

OBSTETRIC AND FETUS-RELATED

ABBREVIATION	MEANING
CPD	cephalopelvic disproportion
CS, C-section	cesarean section
CSF	cerebrospinal fluid
CVS	chorionic villus sampling
CWP	childbirth without pain
DOB	date of birth
EDC	estimated date of confinement
FECG; FEKG	fetal electrocardiogram
FHR	fetal heart rate

OTHER

ABBREVIATION	MEANING
CA	cancer, chronological age, cardiac arrest
cc	cubic centimeter
cm	centimeter
F	Fahrenheit
Hgb	hemoglobin
mg	milligram (1/1000 gram)
para 1, 2, 3	unipara, bipara, tripara (number of viable births)
prn	as needed, as required
SC, subcu, sub q	subcutaneous (injection)
tid	three times a day

Activity 11–8. Clinical Application
Diagnostic Tests, Treatments, and Abbreviations

abortion	hysterosalpinography
amniocentesis	oral contraceptives
cerclage	oxytocins
chorionic villus sampling (CVS)	Pap smear
dilation and curettage (D&C)	pregnancy test
hysterectomy	tubal ligation

Match the diagnostic procedures and treatments listed above with the definitions given in the numbered list:

1. _____ detects the presence of human chorionic gonadotropin (HCG) in a urine or blood sample.

2. _____ drugs that exert a hormonal influence to prevent pregnancy.

3. _____ radiography of the uterus and oviducts after injection of contrast medium.

4. _____ procedure in which a nonabsorbable suture is used for holding the cervix closed to prevent spontaneous abortion.

5. _____ microscopic analysis of cells taken from the cervix and vagina to detect the presence of carcinoma.

6. _____ the termination of pregnancy before the fetus reaches the stage of viability; it can be spontaneous or induced.

7. _____ removal of amniotic fluid for laboratory analysis to detect genetic abnormalities, fetal maturity, and sex of the fetus.

8. _____ drugs that stimulate contraction of the uterus.

9. _____ dilation of the uterine cervix canal and the scraping of the endometrium; used to detect pathological conditions of the uterus.

10. _____ placental tissues are obtained for prenatal diagnosis of potential genetic defects.

Correct Answers _____ × 10 = _____ **% Score**

Activity 11–9. Build Medical Words
Diagnostic, Symptomatic, and Surgical Terms

Use *hyster/o* (uterus, womb) to build medical words meaning:

1. disease of the uterus _____

2. radiography of the uterus and oviducts _____

3. myoma of the uterus _____

Use *uter/o* (uterus, womb) to build medical words meaning:

4. relating to the uterus and cervix _____

5. herniation of the uterus _____

6. pertaining to the uterus and rectum _____

Use *oophor/o* (ovary) to build medical words meaning:

7. pain in an ovary _____

8. inflammation of an ovary and oviduct _____

9. excision of the ovaries _____

Use *salping/o* tube (usually fallopian or eustachian [auditory] tubes) to build medical words meaning:

10. inflammation of the fallopian tubes _____

11. fixation of a fallopian tube _____

12. incision of a fallopian tube _____

Use *colp/o* (vagina) to build medical words meaning:

13. instrument used to examine the vagina _____

14. narrowing of the vagina _____

Use *vagin/o* (vagina) to build medical words meaning:

15. inflammation of the vagina _____

16. abnormal condition due to a vaginal fungus _____

17. relating to the vagina and labia _____

Use *gynec/o* (woman, female) to build medical words meaning:

18. study (of diseases) of the female _____

19. physician who specializes in diseases of the female _____

20. disease of females_____

Correct Answers _____ **× 5 =** _____ **% Score**

MEDICAL RECORDS

Authentic records of a delivery note, emergency room report, operative report, and a discharge summary are included in this section.

The following dictionary exercise and medical record analysis will help you develop skills to abstract information and master the terminology in the reports. Accurate interpretation is important because information of this type is used in numerous areas of the medical practice, such as initiation of treatments, evaluation of patients' progress, and completion of insurance claims.

 Reading and Dictionary Exercise

Place a check mark [✓] after you complete the exercise.

[ ] **1.** Underline the following words in the reports as you read the delivery note, the emergency room report, the operative report, and the discharge summary aloud. These medical records can be found at the end of the chapter.

[ ] **2.** Use a medical dictionary and Appendix F, Part 2 to define the following terms.

Note: You are not expected to fully understand all the parts of the medical records. The important aspect of this exercise is to use all resources that are available to complete it. Eventually you will master the terminology and format of these reports.

> > > MEDICAL RECORD 11−1: DELIVERY NOTE

Term	Pronunciation	Meaning
effaced	ĕ-FĀSD	_____
Pitocin	pĭ-TŌ-sĭn	_____
vertex	VĔR-tĕks	_____
occiput	ŎK-sĭ-pŭt	_____
periurethral	pĕr-ē-ū-RĒ-thrăl	_____
perineal	pĕr-ĭ-NĒ-ăl	_____
Apgars	ĂP-gărs	_____
nuchal cord	NŪ-kăl kord	_____
Vicryl	VĪ-krĭl	_____
placenta	plă-SĔN-tă	_____
eccentric	ĕk-SĔN-trĭk	_____
epidural anesthesia	ĕp-ĭ-DŪ-răl ăn-ĕs-THĒ-zē-ă	_____

> > > MEDICAL RECORD 11-2: EMERGENCY ROOM REPORT

Term	Pronunciation	Meaning
vaginal	*VĂJ-ĭn-ăl*	_____
gonorrhea	*gŏn-ō-RĒ-ă*	_____
Monistat	*MŎN-ĭ-stăt*	_____
cyanosis	*sī-ă-NŌ-sĭs*	_____
suprapubic	*soo-pră-PŪ-bĭk*	_____
erythematous	*ĕr-ĭ-THĒ-mă-tŭs*	_____
purulent	*PŪR-ū-lĕnt*	_____
ulceration	*ŭl-sĕr-Ā-shŭn*	_____
trichomonads	*trĭk-ō-MŌ-nădz*	_____
adnexal	*ăd-NĔK-săl*	_____
pelvic inflammatory disease	*PĔL-vĭk ĭn-FLĂM-ă-tor-ē dĭ-ZĒZ*	_____
trichomoniasis	*trĭk-ō-mō-NĪ-ă-sĭs*	_____
Suprax	*SŪ-prăks*	_____
Zithromax	*ZĬTH-rō-măks*	_____
Flagyl	*FLAG-ĕl*	_____
doxycycline	*dŏk-sē-SĪ-klēn*	_____

> > > MEDICAL RECORD 11-3: OPERATIVE REPORT

Term	Pronunciation	Meaning
uterine fibroids	*Ū-tĕr-ĭn FĪ-broydz*	_____
menorrhagia	*mĕn-ō-RĀ-jē-ă*	_____
vaginal hysterectomy	*VĂJ-ĭn-ăl hĭs-tĕr-ĔK-tō-mē*	_____
bilateral salpingo-oophorectomy	*bī-LĂT-ĕr-ăl săl-pĭng-gō-ō-ŏf-ō-RĔK-tō-mē*	_____
gravida	*GRĂV-ĭ-dă*	_____
para	*PĂ-ră*	_____

dorsal lithotomy	*DOR-săl lĭth-ŎT-ō-mē*	_____
speculum	*SPĔK-ū-lŭm*	_____
tenaculum	*tĕn-ĂK-ū-lŭm*	_____
lidocaine	*LĪ-dō-kān*	_____
epinephrine	*ĕp-ĭ-NĔF-rĭn*	_____
circumferentially	*sĕr-kŭm-fĕr-ĔN-shăl-ē*	_____
uterosacral	*ū-tĕr-ō-SĀ-krăl*	_____
morcellation	*mor-sĕl-Ā-shŭn*	_____
pedicles	*PĔD-ĭ-kls*	_____
infundibulopelvic	*ĭn-fŭn-dĭb-ū-lō-PĔL-vĭk*	_____
ligament	*LĬG-ă-mĕnt*	_____
hemostasis	*hē-MŎS-tă-sĭs*	_____
Foley catheter	*FŌ-lē KĂTH-ĕ-tĕr*	_____

> > > MEDICAL RECORD 11–4: DISCHARGE SUMMARY

Term	Pronunciation	Meaning
abdominal	*ăb-DŎM-ĭ-năl*	_____
hysterectomy	*hĭs-tĕr-ĔK-tō-mē*	_____
pelvic washings	*PĔL-vĭk WĂSH-ĭngs*	_____
pelvic	*PĔL-vĭk*	_____
periaortic	*pĕr-ē-ā-OR-tĭk*	_____
lymphadenopathy	*lĭm-făd-ĕ-NŎP-ă-thē*	_____
omentectomy	*ō-mĕn-TĔK-tō-mē*	_____
appendectomy	*ăp-ĕn-DĔK-tō-mē*	_____
intraperitoneally	*ĭn-tră-pĕr-ĭ-tō-NĒ-ăl-ē*	_____
jugular	*JŬG-ū-lăr*	_____
erythema	*ĕr-ĭ-THĒ-mă*	_____
magnesium sulfate	*măg-NĒ-sē-ŭm SŬL-fāt*	_____
voiding	*VOYD-ĭng*	_____

flatus	*FLĀ-tŭs*	_____
afebrile	*ă-FĔB-rĭl*	_____
serosanguineous	*sē-rō-săn-GWĬN-ē-ŭs*	_____
Dulcolax	*DŬL-kō-lăks*	_____
epithelial	*ĕp-ĭ-THĒ-lē-ăl*	_____
Percocet	*PĔR-kō-sĕt*	_____
Senokot	*SĔN-ŏ-kŏt*	_____
Climara	*klī-MĂ-ră*	_____

Critical Thinking: Analysis of Medical Records

This section provides experience in abstracting information from medical records. At the same time, it reinforces the material presented in this chapter.

> > > MEDICAL RECORD 11–1: DELIVERY NOTE

1. What type of delivery did the mother have?

_____

2. a. What types of tears were repaired?

_____

   b. How were they repaired?

_____

_____

3. What specific drug was used to induce labor? What classification does this drug belong to?

_____

> > > MEDICAL RECORD 11–2: EMERGENCY ROOM REPORT

4. Place a "+" in the space provided for positive findings and a "−" for negative findings. A positive finding indicates the patient had these symptoms; a negative finding indicates the patient did not have the symptoms.

____ hematuria   ____ skin rash

____ vaginal irritation   ____ vaginal drainage

____ fever   ____ foul-smelling drainage

5. What were the diagnoses of this patient?

_____

_____

6. What are the possible complications if the patient does not treat her STDs?

_____

_____

_____

> > > MEDICAL RECORD 11–3: OPERATIVE REPORT

7. What type of surgery was performed?

_____

8. What position was the patient in during the surgery?

_____

9. How much blood did the patient lose during surgery?

_____

> > > MEDICAL RECORD 11–4: DISCHARGE SUMMARY

10. Why was surgery performed on the patient?

_____

11. What did the pathology report confirm?

_____

12. What were the patient's discharge instructions?

_____

_____

_____

_____

Audio Practice

Listen to the audio CD-ROM to practice the pronunciation of selected medical terms from this chapter.

Medical Record 11–1. Delivery Note

GENERAL HOSPITAL AND MEDICAL CENTER
2211 Fifth Avenue North • Healthy City, USA • (321) 123-4567

Delivery Note

Patient Name: Bonnie Jones	**Patient Number:** 34-34-15
Birth Date: 05/10/xx	**Room Number:** 432

Date of Delivery: September 10, 20xx

The patient, a 30-year-old gravida 2 para 1, 40+ weeks gestation, was brought for elective induction/augmentation of labor. She had been contracting intermittently and had a great change of pelvic pressure over the last four days. Her cervix had changed from 2 to 3 cm; it was 50% effaced, very soft posterior, and the head was at –2 station. I had stripped the membranes twice, but still she did not go into labor. I then brought her for induction of labor. Pitocin infusion was begun at 8 p.m. on September 9. She progressed to complete by 5 a.m. on September 10. She delivered around 6:00 in the morning on September 10. She had a spontaneous vaginal delivery from vertex occiput anterior over a first-degree periurethral tear and a first-degree perineal tear. The baby was a live-born girl, 8 pounds 5 ounces, with Apgars 8 at one minute and 9 at five minutes. There was a nuchal cord x1. This could not be slipped over the head and I delivered the baby through the loop of cord. The cord had three vessels. The tears were repaired with interrupted sutures of 4-0 Vicryl, one for the periurethral tear and four for the perineal tear. The placenta delivered with gentle traction on the cord. The cervix was inspected; there were no tears. The placenta was intact. It did have an eccentric insertion of the cord. Mother and baby were left in the delivery room in good condition. Mother had adequate epidural anesthesia for the repair.

_____

Michael J. Allen, M.D.

MJA/ps

D: 09/10/xx
T: 09/11/xx

Medical Record 11–2. Emergency Room Report

GENERAL HOSPITAL AND MEDICAL CENTER
2211 Fifth Avenue North • Healthy City, USA 12345 • (321) 123-4567

Emergency Room Report

Patient Name: Mona Roman   **Patient Number:** 02-22-41
Birth Date: 04/15/xx   **Room Number:** ER

DATE OF VISIT: 04/01/20xx

CHIEF COMPLAINT: Vaginal irritation and drainage.

HISTORY OF PRESENT ILLNESS: This is a 20-year-old female who says that for the past weeks she has had lower abdominal pressure, a lot of vaginal discharge, and burning with urination. Her last menstrual period was May 13. She says it was normal in duration and intensity. No real other specific complaints, except that she states that her boyfriend said that he thinks he has gonorrhea, and she wants to be checked.

REVIEW OF SYSTEMS: No fever or chills, vomiting, diarrhea, or rashes.

MEDICATIONS: She says that she has been using over-the-counter Monistat without improvement.

PHYSICAL EXAMINATION: A well-developed 20-year-old female who is in no apparent distress. Her vitals are stable. She is afebrile. Her skin is without cyanosis or rashes. Chest is clear. Heart regular rate and rhythm. Her abdomen is soft with active bowel sounds. She has tenderness in the suprapubic area. Pelvic examination reveals normal external genitalia, although the vaginal mucosa is markedly erythematous, and she has a lot of foul-smelling, purulent drainage. There is no gross ulceration. Cervical cultures were obtained. Wet mount was obtained and showed some trichomonads. Bimanual examination shows uterine motion tenderness. There is no adnexal mass or tenderness.

DIAGNOSIS: Probable pelvic inflammatory disease. Trichomoniasis. Possible gonorrhea exposure.

PLAN: She was given 400 mg Suprax here, 1 g Zithromax, and a prescription for Flagyl 250 mg t.i.d. for 10 days, as well as doxycycline 100 mg b.i.d. for 10 days. She should follow up with the clinic in 2-3 days and return if any problems occur.

_____

M. Wolf, M.D.

MW/js
D&T: 04/02/xx

Medical Record 11–3. Operative Report

GENERAL HOSPITAL AND MEDICAL CENTER
2211 Fifth Avenue North • Healthy City, USA 12345 • (321) 123-4567

Operative Report

Patient Name: Maureen Staples   **Patient Number:** 33-23-15
Birth Date: 03/17/xx   **Room Number:** 327

DATE OF OPERATION: 03/25/xx

PREOPERATIVE DIAGNOSIS: Uterine fibroids, menorrhagia.

POSTOPERATIVE DIAGNOSIS: Uterine fibroids, menorrhagia.

OPERATION: Vaginal hysterectomy, bilateral salpingo-oophorectomy.

ANESTHESIA: General.

SURGEON: Ann Thrush, M.D.   **ASSISTANT:** Thomas Juniper, M.D.

CLINICAL INDICATIONS: The patient, a 45-year-old gravida 2 para 2, who presented with uterine fibroids which were causing urinary retention and menorrhagia.

PROCEDURE: The patient was brought to the operating room where general anesthesia was administered. She was prepped and draped in the usual sterile fashion. The patient was placed in the dorsal lithotomy position. A posterior weighted speculum was placed, and the anterior lip of the cervix was grasped with a single-toothed tenaculum. Lidocaine 1% with epinephrine was injected circumferentially around the cervix. A scalpel was used to make a circumferential incision around the cervix to push the bladder and rectum away from the uterus. The posterior cul-de-sac was entered sharply and posterior cul-de-sac was placed.

At this time, the uterosacral ligaments were clamped, cut and tied with suture of 0 Vicryl. The bladder was sharply and bluntly taken away from the uterus, and the anterior cul-de-sac was entered. Clamps were then placed across the uterine vessels bilaterally, and these were secured with 0 Vicryl suture. At this time, it was noted the uterus was very large, at least 12 weeks' size, and there were multiple large fibroids extending down to the cervix. Morcellation was carried out, and the fibroids were removed in pieces. Finally all the pedicles were clamped and secured with suture of 0 Vicryl, and the uterus was removed. Infundibulopelvic ligaments were then clamped bilaterally, and the ovaries and fallopian tubes were removed. Again the pedicles were secured with 0 Vicryl suture. Adequate hemostasis was assured. Estimated blood loss was 450 cc. The peritoneum was closed in pursestring fashion using 2-0 Vicryl suture. The uterosacral

Continued

Operative Report, page 2
Patient Name: Maureen Staples   **Patient Number:**   33-23-15

ligaments were suspended to the vaginal cuff bilaterally. The vaginal cuff was closed with interrupted figure-of-eight sutures of 0 Vicryl. The Foley catheter was placed and noted to be draining clear, yellow urine. The patient went to the recovery room in stable condition.

_____

Ann Thrush, M.D.

AT/fje

D: 03/25/xx
T: 03/26/xx

Medical Record 11–4. Discharge Summary

GENERAL HOSPITAL AND MEDICAL CENTER
2211 Fifth Avenue North • Healthy City, USA 12345 • (321) 123-4567

Discharge Summary

Patient Name: Jolene Fritter   **Patient Number:** 03-44-19
Birth Date: 08/03/xx   **Room Number:** 909

Date of Admission: 10/30/xx

Date of Discharge: 11/04/xx

PRINCIPAL DIAGNOSIS: Pelvic mass with possible ovarian cancer.

PROCEDURE: Total abdominal hysterectomy, bilateral salpingo-oophorectomy, pelvic washings, pelvic and periaortic lymphadenectomy, partial omentectomy, appendectomy.

SUMMARY: The patient is a 47-year-old white female with large pelvic abdominal mass measuring approximately 16 cm with minimally elevated CA-125 of 66 who was referred by Dr. Martha Smith. She is gravida 0, para 0, with no current past medical history. On 10/30/xx she underwent hysterectomy and staging procedure for possible ovarian cancer without complication. Estimated blood loss was 1500 cc. Two Jackson-Pratt drains were draining, one intraperitoneally and one with a right subcu as well as a right internal jugular central line.

On 10/31/xx, postoperative day 1, the patient complained of some pain but no nausea or vomiting. The Jackson-Pratt drain had a small amount of output. Electrolytes normal. HGB 9.3; the night before it was 10.2. Urine output was adequate. Her Foley catheter was discontinued, and she was instructed to ambulate.

On 11/01/xx, postoperative day 2, the patient complained of some minor back pain. Ambulated without difficulty. Still no flatus. Urine output was 1700 cc. Incision was clean, dry and intact without erythema. Later that day her temperature came down to 37.9, HGB 8.8. She was transfused 2 units of packed red blood cells. Magnesium sulfate was also replaced which was found to be low at 1.5. Bowel stimulation per rectum was performed with small amount of results. Pathology was still pending.

On postoperative day 3, the patient was ambulating and voiding without difficulty. Still no flatus. Bowel sounds were hypoactive. She was afebrile, vital signs stable. Right Jackson-Pratt drain was pulling large amount of serosanguineous fluid, approximately 1 liter. Later that day, the patient received Dulcolax suppositories x2 without significant results.

Continued

Discharge Summary, page 2
Patient Name: Jolene Fritter   **Patient Number:** 03-44-19

On postoperative day 4, 11/03/xx, the patient was doing well. Continued to complain of being bloated, still no flatus except for after using a Dulcolax suppository. She was afebrile, vital signs stable. Right Jackson-Pratt drain continued to put out 950 cc. Her pathology came back revealing a mixed epithelial borderline tumor with negative lymph nodes. We continued bowel stimulation with milk of magnesia and also with suppositories. Her left Jackson-Pratt drain was taken out.

On 11/04/xx, postoperative day 5, the patient was doing much better. Two bowel movements overnight. Afebrile. Vital signs stable. Incision clean, dry and intact. She was discharged home later that morning on a soft diet. Encouraged fluid intake. Discharge medications include Percocet p.r.n., Senokot-S once a day, Climara patch to be changed q. week. She has an appointment with my office later this week for staple removal. She is to call for any severe abdominal pain, vaginal bleeding, or temperature greater than 100.4.

_____
Franklin Doe, M.D.

FD/jk

D: 11/05/xx
T: 11/07/xx

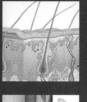
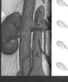
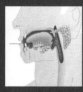
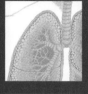

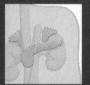
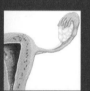
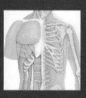

chapter

12 Orthopedics

Chapter Outline

Objectives

Upon completion of this chapter, you will be able to:

- Describe the type of medical treatment orthopedists provide.
- Name and locate the major bones of the skeletal system.
- Identify the differences among the three types of muscles and provide an example of how each type functions.
- Recognize, pronounce, build, and spell correctly medical terms related to the musculoskeletal system.
- Describe pathological conditions, diagnostic tests, surgical procedures, and other treatments related to the musculoskeletal system.
- Demonstrate your knowledge of this chapter by successfully completing the activities and the analysis of medical records.

About Orthopedics

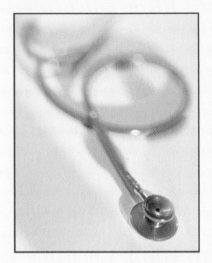

Orthopedics, also spelled **orthopaedics,** is the branch of medicine concerned with the prevention, diagnosis, care, and treatment of musculoskeletal disorders. These include injury to, or disease of, the body's bones, joints, ligaments, muscles, and tendons. Orthopedists are medical doctors who specialize in orthopedics. They employ medical, physical, and surgical methods to restore function that has been lost as a result of injury or disease to the musculoskeletal system. Orthopedists coordinate their treatment methods with other health-care practitioners such as physical therapists, occupational therapists, and sports medicine physicians. Besides the orthopedist, the **rheumatologist** (also an MD) specializes in the treatment of joint diseases—specifically, various forms of arthritis.

Another health-care practitioner, the **osteopathic physician (DO),** provides medical treatment of musculoskeletal disorders. The osteopathic philosophy maintains that good health requires proper alignment of bones, muscles, ligaments, and nerves. Like the MD, osteopathic physicians provide state-of-the-art methods of medical treatment, including prescribing drugs and performing surgeries.

Still another health-care practitioner, the **chiropractor,** is certified and licensed to provide chiropractic care in treating musculoskeletal disorders. Unlike medical doctors and osteopaths, the chiropractor is not a physician. They do not employ drugs or surgery, the primary basis of treatment used by medical doctors. **Chiropractic medicine** is a system of therapy based on the theory that disease is caused by pressure on nerves. In most cases, treatment provided by chiropractors involves the physical manipulation of the spinal column. Some practitioners employ radiology for diagnosis and diet in addition to spinal manipulation.

To grasp the scope of practice and the role of health-care practitioners in the medical specialty of orthopedics, it is important to understand the structure and function of the musculoskeletal system as well as the language of medicine that is related to this medical specialty.

Selected Key Terms

articulation ăr-tĭk-ū-LĀ-shŭn	The place of union between two or more bones; a joint.
articular cartilage ăr-TĬK-ū-lăr KĂR-tĭ-lĭj	A type of hyaline connective tissue that covers the articulating surfaces of bones within synovial joints.
bursa BŬR-să	A padlike sac or cavity found in connective tissue, usually near joints. It is lined with a synovial membrane and secretes synovial fluid that acts to reduce friction between tendon and bone, tendon and ligament, or between other structures where friction is likely to occur.
collagen KŎL-ă-jĕn	A strong, fibrous, insoluble protein found in the connective tissue of tendons, ligaments, bone, cartilage, and deep fascia.
collagenous fiber kŏl-LĂJ-ĕ-nŭs FĪ-bĕr	Any one of the tough, white, protein fibers that constitute much of the intercellular substance and the connective tissue of the body, including bones. Collagenous fibers contain collagen; they are often arranged in bundles that strengthen the tissues in which they are embedded.

fontanel fŏn-tă-NĔL	An unossified membrane or soft spot lying between the cranial bones of the skull of a fetus or infant. Also spelled *fontanelle.*
hematopoiesis hē-mă-tō-poy-Ē-sĭs *hemato=blood* *poiesis=formation, production*	The production and development of blood cells, normally in the bone marrow.
ligament LĬG-ă-mĕnt	A strong, flexible band of fibrous tissue that connects bones, cartilage, and other structures to provide support or to attach fascia or muscles.
manubrium mă-NŪ-brē-ŭm	The upper segment of the sternum articulating with the clavicle and first pair of costal cartilages.
suture SŪ-chŭr	The line of union in an immovable articulation, such as those between the skull bones.
synovial joint sĭn-Ō-vē-ăl joynt	A freely movable joint in which the bony surfaces are covered by articular cartilage and connected by a fibrous, connective-tissue capsule that is lined with a synovial membrane; also called *diarthrosis.*
tendon	Band of dense, fibrous connective tissue that attaches muscle to bone.

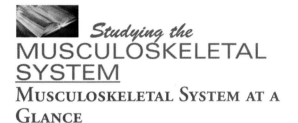

Studying the MUSCULOSKELETAL SYSTEM

MUSCULOSKELETAL SYSTEM AT A GLANCE

The musculoskeletal system consists of bones, joints, and muscles. Together with soft tissue, many vital organs are enclosed and protected from injury by bones. For example, the bones of the skull protect the brain; the rib cage protects the heart and lungs. In addition to support and protection, the skeletal system has several other important functions. Movement is possible because bones provide points of attachment for muscles, tendons, and ligaments. The marrow of larger bones continuously produces blood cells, a function called **hematopoiesis.** Bones also serve as a storage site for minerals, particularly phosphorus and calcium. When the body experiences a need for a certain mineral, such as calcium during pregnancy, the mineral is withdrawn from the bones and put into the bloodstream for the body to use. Calcium in the blood is necessary for blood clotting and for the proper functioning of nerves and muscles.

Muscles perform several important functions for the body, such as producing movement, maintaining posture, and stabilizing joints. All muscles, through contraction, provide the body with motion or body posture. Less apparent muscle movement is involved in the passage and elimination of food through the digestive system, the propulsion of blood through the arteries, and the contraction of the bladder to eliminate urine.

Muscle size and shape vary greatly, from the massive triangles of the upper back to the slender cables of the small, dexterous hand. The size and shape of a muscle determine the strength with which it contracts, and thus influence its specific function. The most powerful muscles are those that run along the spine; they maintain posture and provide the strength for lifting and pushing. The smallest muscle, the stapedius, is located inside the ear. It acts reflexively in response to loud sounds to reduce excessive vibrations that could injure the internal ear.

The interrelationship of the musculoskeletal system with other body systems is shown in Figure 12–1.

STRUCTURE AND FUNCTION

Bones

Bone Tissue

Bone, also known as **osseous tissue,** is a specialized form of dense connective tissue composed of bone cells (osteocytes) within a strong, nonliving matrix made of calcium salts and the protein **collagen.** Unlike other connective tissues, the intercellular substance of bone contains abundant mineral salts, primarily calcium phosphate, and **collagenous fibers.** As these salts are deposited in the framework formed by the collagenous fibers of the intercellular

Body System Connections
Musculoskeletal System

THE CARDIOVASCULAR SYSTEM
◆ The cardiovascular system delivers needed oxygen and nutrients and carries away wastes.
◆ Bones protect cardiovascular organs by enclosure and help control blood calcium levels to maintain normal heart function.

THE DIGESTIVE SYSTEM
◆ Muscles play an important role in the digestive system. They facilitate mastication, swallowing, and the movement of digestive ingredients throughout the entire gastrointestinal tract. ◆ Dietary calcium is absorbed by the digestive system to help normal bone development.

THE ENDOCRINE SYSTEM
◆ Due to hormonal secretions, blood flow increases to muscles during exercise. ◆ Normal muscular and skeletal development requires adequate growth hormone. ◆ Blood calcium balance is governed by hormones.

THE FEMALE REPRODUCTIVE SYSTEM
◆ Muscular structures of the pelvic floor support the reproductive organs; abdominal muscles are active during childbirth. ◆ The pelvic bones enclose and protect some of the reproductive organs. ◆ A narrow pelvis may hinder the vaginal delivery of an infant.

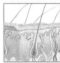
THE INTEGUMENTARY SYSTEM
◆ The skin protects muscles and bones. ◆ Body temperature is regulated by involuntary muscle contractions (shivering). ◆ The skin's ability to absorb vitamin D helps to provide calcium for bones.

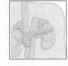
THE LYMPHATIC AND IMMUNE SYSTEMS
◆ The immune system protects the musculoskeletal system from disease. ◆ Bone marrow produces cells of the immune system.

THE NERVOUS SYSTEM
◆ The brain and spinal cord are protected by bones.
◆ Nervous impulses control movement and provide information about the position of body parts.

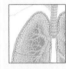
THE RESPIRATORY SYSTEM
◆ Muscles related to breathing help the respiratory system expel carbon dioxide and inhale oxygen-rich air.
◆ The rib cage protects the lungs from injury and provides attachments for muscles involved in breathing.

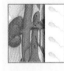
THE URINARY AND MALE REPRODUCTIVE SYSTEMS
◆ Muscle tissue controls voluntary urine elimination from the bladder. ◆ The rib cage provides some protection to the kidneys. ◆ Both the kidneys and bone tissue work together to control blood calcium levels.

Figure 12–1 *The interrelationship of the musculoskeletal system with other body systems.*

substance, the tissue hardens or becomes ossified. The hardness of bone is largely due to the inorganic calcium phosphate deposited within the intercellular matrix. Numerous collagenous fibers, also embedded within the matrix, give some flexibility to bone. During the growing process, and after an injury, bone tissue continually breaks down and rebuilds, renewing its shape and proportion.

Structure and Types

Bones come in many shapes and sizes. Generally they can be classified into four principal types: long, short, flat, and irregular. Varying shapes of bones reflect their different roles in the body.

Long bones include the bones of the arms, legs, hands, and feet, but do not include the bones of the wrists and ankles. Most long bones are slightly curved, which helps to increase the ability of the bones to absorb shocks and distribute stresses. All long bones have the same general structure and are discussed here.

Label Figure 12–2 as you learn about the parts of a long bone.

The (1) **diaphysis** is the shaft or long, main portion of a bone. The (2) **distal epiphysis** and (3) **proximal epiphysis** are the two ends of a bone. Both have a somewhat bulbous shape to provide space for muscle and ligament attachments near the joints. The structural unit of (4) **compact bone,** also called the **osteon** or (5) **haversian system,** forms a cylinder that is very hard and dense. Even though it appears very dense, a

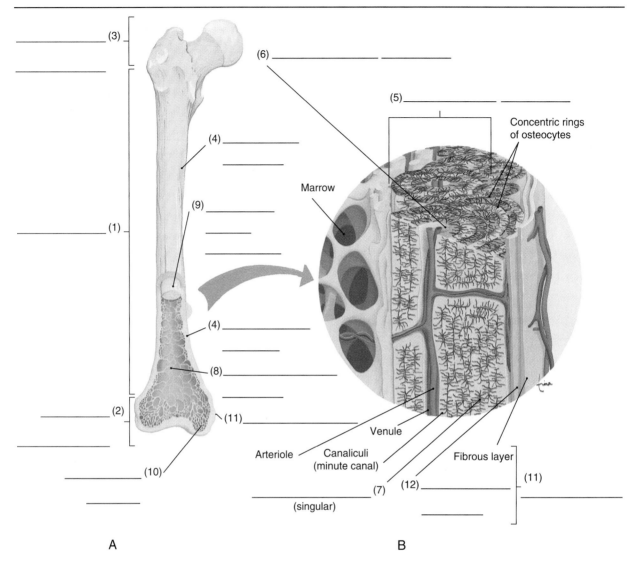

Figure 12–2 *The bone tissue. (A) Femur with distal end cut in longitudinal section. (B) Compact bone showing haversian systems. (Adapted from Scanlon, VC, and Sanders, TS: Essentials of Anatomy and Physiology, ed 3. FA Davis, Philadelphia, 1999, p 99, with permission.)*

microscope reveals that it is riddled with canals that serve as passageways for nerves and blood vessels. These numerous canals, one of which is the (6) **haversian canal,** enable nutrients and oxygen to reach the (7) **osteocytes.** The (8) **medullary cavity** is continuous with the spaces of the spongy bone. It lies within the central shaft of the long bones and contains (9) **yellow bone marrow** composed primarily of fat cells. The epiphyses are made up largely of (10) **spongy bone** surrounded by a layer of compact bone. Red bone marrow is found within the porous chamber of spongy bone. This marrow is richly supplied with blood and consists of immature and mature blood cells in various stages of development. In an adult, the production of red blood cells (*erythropoiesis*) occurs in red bone marrow. Red bone marrow is also responsible for the

formation of white blood cells (*leukopoiesis*) and platelets (the production of all blood cells taken together is called *hematopoiesis*). The (11) **periosteum,** a dense, white, fibrous membrane, covers the remaining surface of the bone. It contains numerous blood and lymph vessels and nerves. In growing bones, the inner layer, called the (12) **osteogenic layer,** contains the bone-forming cells, osteoblasts. Because blood vessels and *osteoblasts* are located here, the periosteum provides a means for bone repair and general bone nutrition. It also serves as a point of attachment for muscles, ligaments, and tendons.

Short bones are somewhat cubical. They consist of a core of spongy bone, also known as *cancellous bone*, that is enclosed in a thin layer of compact tissue. Bones of the wrists, ankles, and toes are short bones. **Flat bones** are exactly what their name suggests. They provide broad surfaces for muscular attachment or protection for internal organs. Bones of the skull, shoulder blades, and sternum are flat bones. **Irregular bones** include the bones that cannot be grouped under the previous headings because of their complex shapes. They include the bones of the vertebrae, the ilium, the middle ear, and some bones of the face.

Activity 12–1: Competency Verification
Bone Tissue

Review Figure 12–2, and check your labeling in Appendix C.

Bone Surfaces

External surfaces of bones are rarely smooth and are formed with projections, depressions, and openings. These surfaces serve as sites of muscle, ligament, and tendon attachment, as points of articulation, or to provide cavities and pathways for blood vessels and nerves. Various types of projections are evident in bones. They may be rounded, sharp, narrow, or have a large ridge, called a *crest*. Depressions are cavities and openings in a bone. Surfaces of bones are named in different ways, and each has a certain distinguishing feature and function. The anatomic terms for the most common types of projections, depressions, and openings are summarized in Table 12–1.

Joints

To allow for body movements, bones must have surfaces that join together **(articulate).** These articulating surfaces form joints that have various degrees of mobility. Some are freely movable **(diarthrosis);** others are only slightly movable **(amphiarthrosis);** and the remaining are totally immovable **(synarthrosis).** All three types are necessary for smooth, coordinated body movements.

In structural terms, diarthroses (singular, diarthrosis) are **synovial joints,** joints in which articulating bones are separated by a fluid-containing joint capsule filled with lubricating synovial fluid. In most synovial joints, the capsule is strengthened by **ligaments** (fibrous bands, or sheets, of connective tissues) that lash the bones together, providing additional strength to the joint capsule.

A **bursa** (plural, **bursae**) is a padlike sac or cavity found in connective tissue, usually in the vicinity of joints. It is lined with a synovial membrane that secretes synovial fluid. The bursa acts as a small cushion that allows the tendon to move over the bone as it contracts and relaxes. Some common locations of bursae are at the shoulder joint (*subacromial bursa*), elbow joint (*olecranon bursa*), and knee joint (*patellar bursa*).

Skeleton

The human skeleton is divided into two parts: the axial skeleton and the appendicular skeleton. The skeleton consists of approximately 206 bones of varying shapes and sizes (Fig. 12–3).

Axial Skeleton

The **axial skeleton,** as illustrated in off white (Fig. 12–3), consists of the bones of the skull, vertebral column, and the bony thorax (ribs and sternum). This part of the skeleton supports the head, neck, and trunk. It also protects the brain, the spinal cord, and the internal organs of the thorax from injuries. All these bones are flat and contain red bone marrow.

The combining forms of bones are derived from the names of the bones. Learn the combining forms and write them next to the labeled bones of the axial skeleton in Figure 12–3.

1. **crani/o** refers to the cranium or skull.

2. **stern/o** refers to the sternum (breastbone). The sword-shaped inferior portion of the sternum is known as the *xiphoid process* (*xiph/o=sword*).

3. **cost/o** refers to the ribs, which are attached to the sternum.

4. **vertebr/o** refers to the vertebrae (backbone). The vertebral column is also called the *spinal column* and is composed of 26 bones called *vertebrae* (singular, vertebra).

Appendicular Skeleton

The **appendicular skeleton** consists of the bones of the arms and legs along with those of the scapula, the clavicle, and the pelvis. These bones attach to the axial skeleton as appendages. Learn the combining forms as you label the bones of the appendicular skeleton in Figure 12–3.

5. **humer/o** refers to the humerus (upper arm bone). It articulates with the *scapula* at the shoulder and with the *radius* and *ulna* at the elbow.

6. **carp/o** refers to the carpus (wrist bone), the eight wrist bones.

7. **metacarp/o** refers to the metacarpus (hand bone), which radiates from the wristlike spokes and forms the palm of the hand.

8. **phalang/o** refers to the phalanges (bones of the fingers and toes).

TABLE 12–1: Projections, Depressions, and Openings

PROJECTION	DESCRIPTION	EXAMPLE
Condyle	Rounded, knucklelike process at the joint; usually covered by articular cartilage	Condyle of the humerus
Head	A prominent, rounded, articulating end of a bone	Head of the femur
Process	Any bony prominence	Mastoid process of the temporal bone
Spine	Sharp, slender, often pointed projection	Spine of the scapula
Trochanter	Massive, irregularly shaped process found only on the femur	Greater trochanter of the femur
Tubercle	Small rounded projection or process	Tubercle of the femur
Tuberosity	A large roughened process or projection	Tuberosity of the humerus
DEPRESSIONS AND OPENINGS		
Foramen	Rounded opening through a bone to accommodate blood vessels and nerves	Foramen of the skull through which cranial nerves pass
Fossa	Shallow, basinlike depression in a bone	Axillary (armpit)
Groove	Slight depression, or fissure	Deep furrows in the brain
Meatus, Canal	A tubelike passageway into a bone	External auditory meatus of the temporal bone
SINUS	A cavity or hollow space in a bone	Frontal sinus

9. **pelv/i** and **pelv/o** refer to the pelvis. The pelvis provides attachment for the legs and also supports the soft organs of the abdominal cavity.

10. **femor/o** refers to the femur (thigh bone). The femur is the longest and strongest bone in the body. It articulates with the hip bone and the bones of the lower leg.

11. **patell/o** refers to the patella (kneecap). It articulates with the femur but essentially is a "floating bone." The main function of this bone is to protect the knee joint but its exposed position makes it vulnerable to dislocation and fracture.

12. **tibi/o** refers to the tibia (larger inner bone of the lower leg). The tibia is the weight-bearing bone of the lower leg.

13. **fibul/o** refers to the fibula (smaller, outer bone of lower leg). The fibula is not a weight-bearing bone but is important because muscles are attached and anchored to it.

14. **calcane/o** refers to the calcaneum (heel bone).

Activity 12–2: Competency Verification
Bones of the Skeleton

Review Figure 12–3, and check your labeling in Appendix C.

Skull

Two separate sets of bones form the complex bony structure of the skull: the **cranial bones** and the **facial bones.** With the exception of one facial bone, all other bones of the skull are joined together by **sutures.** Sutures, also known as **suture joints,** are the lines of junction between two bones, especially of the skull, and are usually immovable. At birth, membrane-filled spaces called **fontanels,** or **fontanelles,** are found between cranial bones. The fontanels, also called "soft spots," are areas where the bone-making process is not yet complete. In very young children, the sutures are flexible to allow for growth, but with age they ossify and become virtually fixed. The only facial bone that moves is the **mandible** (bone of the lower jaw). This movement is necessary for speaking and to complete the chewing process, known as *mastication.*

Cranial Bones

The eight cranial bones, collectively known as the **cranium,** enclose and protect the brain and the organs of hearing and equilibrium. The cranium also provides a site of attachment for head muscles. The major bones of the cranium are shown in Figures 12–4*A* and *B.* Label the bones as you read the following material.

The (1) **frontal bone** forms the anterior portion of the skull above the eyes. One (2) **parietal bone** is sit-

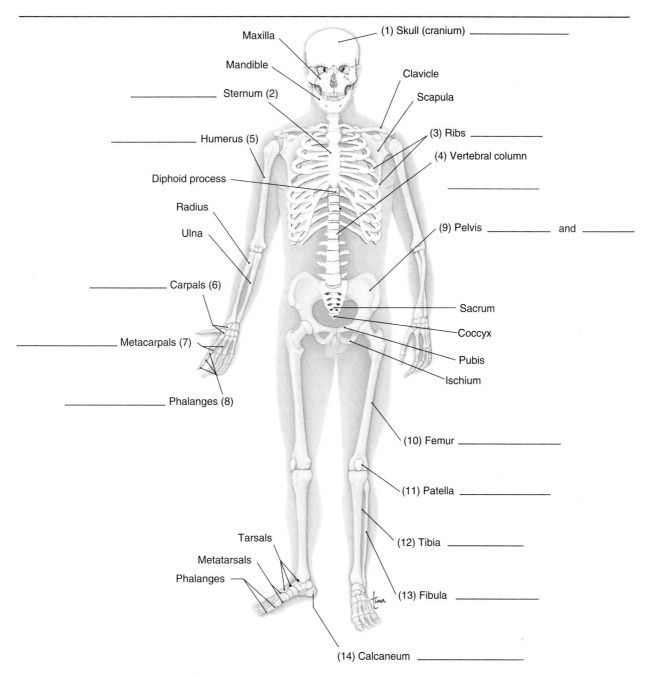

Maxilla

Mandible

Sternum (2) _____

Humerus (5) _____

Diphoid process

Radius

Ulna

Carpals (6) _____

Metacarpals (7) _____

Phalanges (8) _____

Tarsals

Metatarsals

Phalanges

(1) Skull (cranium) _____

Clavicle

Scapula

(3) Ribs _____

(4) Vertebral column

_____

(9) Pelvis _____ and _____

Sacrum

Coccyx

Pubis

Ischium

(10) Femur _____

(11) Patella _____

(12) Tibia _____

(13) Fibula _____

(14) Calcaneum _____

Figure 12–3 *The anterior view of the skeleton. The axial skeleton is indicated in off-white. (Adapted from Scanlon, VC, and Sanders, TS: Essentials of Anatomy and Physiology, ed 3. FA Davis, Philadelphia, 1999, p 106, with permission.)*

uated on each side of the skull just behind the frontal bone. Together, the parietal bones form the upper sides and roof of the cranium. Each parietal bone meets the frontal bone along the (3) **coronal suture,** routing down the midline to the upper part of the (4) **lambdoid suture.** The (5) **occipital bone** forms the back of the skull and the base of the cranium. It joins the parietal bones along the lambdoidal suture. A large occipital opening on its lower surface, called the *foramen magnum*, provides a passage for nerve fibers from the brain, which enter the vertebral canal to be-

come part of the spinal cord. The rounded processes, known as *occipital condyles*, located on each side of the foramen magnum, articulate with the first vertebra (atlas) of the vertebral column. Two (6) **temporal bones,** one on each side of the skull, form part of the lower cranium. Each temporal bone has a complicated shape that contains various cavities and recesses associated with the internal ear, the essential part of the organ of hearing. A rounded projection of the temporal bone, the (7) **mastoid process,** is located posterior to the (8) **external auditory meatus**

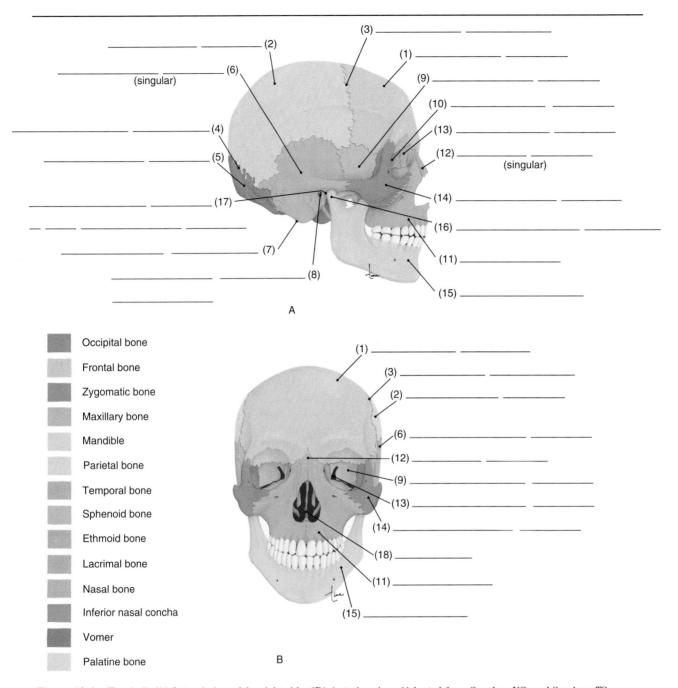

Figure 12–4 *The skull. (A) Lateral view of the right side. (B) Anterior view. (Adapted from Scanlon, VC, and Sanders, TS: Essentials of Anatomy and Physiology, ed 3. FA Davis, Philadelphia, 1999, p 107, with permission.)*

(ear canal). This process provides a point of attachment for several neck muscles. The (9) **sphenoid bone,** located at the middle part of the base of the skull, resembles a bat with its wings extended. The sphenoid is considered the keystone of the cranium because it forms a central wedge that joins with all other cranial bones, holding those skull bones together. A very light and spongy bone, the (10) **ethmoid bone,** forms most of the bony area between the nasal cavity and parts of the orbits of the eye.

Facial Bones

The facial skeleton consists of 13 immovable bones and 1 movable lower jaw. Facial bones are responsible for several important functions: they form the basic shape of the face; secure the teeth; provide muscle attachments that move the jaw and control facial expressions; contain openings for passage of food and air; and provide cavities for the sense organs of smell, sight, and taste.

Continue to label Figures 12–4*A* and 12*B* as you read about the descriptions of facial bones.

The (11) **maxilla,** a paired bone, forms the upper jaw and the central portion of the facial skeleton. Portions of these bones comprise the anterior roof of the mouth (*hard palate*), the floors of the orbits, the sides and floor of the nasal cavity, and the sockets of the upper teeth. Inside the maxillae, lateral to the nasal cavity, are the *maxillary sinuses*, the largest paranasal sinuses. All facial bones except the mandible (lower jaw) articulate with the maxillae. Two thin and nearly rectangular bones, the (12) **nasal bones,** lie side by side and are fused medially, forming the bridge of the nose. Two small (13) **lacrimal bones** are located at the corner of each eye. These thin, small bones unite to form the groove for the lacrimal sac and canals through which the tear ducts pass into the nasal cavity. The paired (14) **zygomatic bone,** the bone on either side of the face below the eye, forms the high portion of the cheeks below and to the sides of the eyes. It is commonly referred to as the *cheekbone.* The largest, strongest facial bone, the (15) **mandible,** is the only movable skull bone. The posterior (16) **mandibular condyle** joins the (17) **mandibular fossa of the temporal bone,** forming the *temporomandibular joint* (*TMJ*) on the same side. The thin, flat bone called the (18) **vomer** forms a part of the nasal septum. If the vomer is deviated (pushed to one side), the nasal chambers are of unequal size, which may cause breathing difficulties.

Activity 12–3: Competency Verification
Cranial and Facial Bones

Review Figure 12–4, and check your labeling in Appendix C.

Thorax

Two important internal organs of the **thorax** (chest) are the heart and lungs. Together with other soft tissue, the internal organs are enclosed and protected from injury by the thorax, or chest. As you read the following paragraph, label Figure 12–5.

The ribs, the (1) **sternum** (chest plate), and the thoracic vertebrae (see Fig. 12–5) form the skeletal framework of the rib cage. There are 12 pairs of ribs; each pair is attached posteriorly to a thoracic vertebra. The first seven pairs of ribs are called the (2) **true ribs.** They articulate with the (3) **manubrium** and body of the sternum by means of (4) **costal cartilage.** The costal cartilage of the next five pairs of ribs, known as the (5) **false ribs,** is not fastened directly to the sternum. The last two pairs of false ribs are not attached in any way to the sternum but are attached posteriorly to the thoracic vertebrae and called the (6) **floating ribs.**

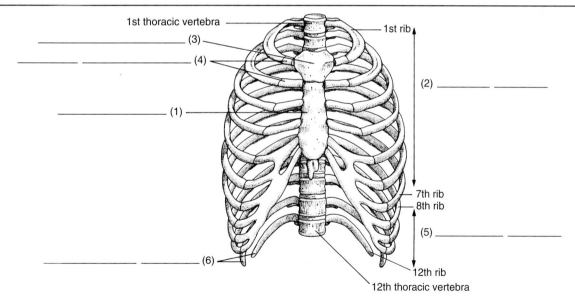

Figure 12–5   *The thorax. (Adapted from Gylys, BA, and Wedding, ME: Medical Terminology: A Systems Approach, ed 3. FA Davis, Philadelphia, 1999, p 209, with permission.)*

Activity 12–4: Competency Verification
Thorax

Review Figure 12–5, and check your labeling in Appendix C.

Vertebral Column

The **vertebral column,** also known as the **spinal column** or **backbone,** of the adult is composed of 26 bones called vertebrae (singular, vertebra). Five regions of bones—the cervical vertebrae, the thoracic vertebrae, the lumbar vertebrae, the sacrum, and the coccyx—comprise the vertebral column. Each region derives its name from its location along the length of the spinal column and is discussed below.

Label Figure 12–6 as you read the following information about the vertebral column.

The seven (1) **cervical vertebrae** form the skeletal framework of the neck. The first cervical vertebra, the (2) **atlas,** supports the skull. The second cervical vertebra, the (3) **axis,** makes possible the rotating movements of the head. Under the seventh cervical vertebra are twelve (4) **thoracic vertebrae** that support the chest and serve as a point of **articulation** for the ribs. The next five vertebrae, the (5) **lumbar vertebrae,** are situated in the lower back area and carry most of the weight of the torso. Below this area, the five sacral vertebrae are fused into a single bone in the adult, which is referred to as the (6) **sacrum.** The tail of the vertebral column consists of four or five fragmented vertebrae that are also fused together and referred to as the (7) **coccyx.**

Vertebrae are separated by flat, round structures, the (8) **intervertebral disks,** which are composed of a fibrocartilaginous substance with a gelatinous mass in the center *(nucleus pulposus).* When disk material protrudes into the neural canal, pressure on the adjacent nerve root causes pain. This condition is referred to as herniation of an intervertebral disk, **herniated nucleus pulposus (HNP),** ruptured disk, or slipped disk.

Activity 12–5: Competency Verification
Vertebral Column

Review Figure 12–6, and check your labeling in Appendix C.

Pelvic Bones

The **pelvic (hip) girdle,** a basin-shaped structure along with its associated ligaments, supports the weight of the body from the vertebral column (Fig. 12–7). It also supports the sigmoid colon, the rectum, the urinary bladder, and other soft organs of the abdominopelvic cavity. The pelvic bones provide points of attachment for the legs, as shown in Figure 12–3.

The male and female pelves (singular, pelvis) differ considerably in size and shape. Some of the differences are attributable to the function of the female pelvis during the stages of childbearing. The female pelvis is shallower than the male pelvis but wider in every direction. The female pelvis not only supports the enlarging uterus as the fetus matures, but also provides a large opening to allow the infant to pass through during birth.

Label Figures 12–7A and B as you read the following material.

Both the female and male pelves are divided into the (1) **ilium,** (2) **ischium,** and (3) **pubis.** These are fused together in the adult to form a single bone called the *innominate bone.* The bladder is located behind the (4) **symphysis pubis;** the rectum is in the curve of the (5) **sacrum** and (6) **coccyx.** In the female, the uterus, fallopian tubes, ovaries, and vagina are located between the bladder and the rectum.

Activity 12–6: Competency Verification
Pelvic Girdle

Review Figure 12–7, and check your labeling in Appendix C.

Muscles

Muscles make up the bulk of the body and account for about half its weight. All muscles have the ability to contract from excitation by a stimulus and to relax and return to their original size and shape. All muscles, through contraction, provide the body with motion or body posture. Muscle motion that is less apparent includes the motion of muscles that control the passage of food through the digestive system and the propulsion of blood through the arteries, and the contraction of the bladder to eliminate urine. Muscles are of three types: skeletal, smooth, and cardiac.

Skeletal muscles (voluntary or **striated muscles)** are muscles the action of which is controlled by will. Some examples of voluntary muscles are the muscles that move the eyeballs, tongue, and bones. Except for cardiac muscle, all striated muscles are voluntary.

Smooth muscles (involuntary or **visceral muscles)** are muscles the action of which is not controlled by will. They are found principally in the visceral organs, in the walls of arteries, in the walls of respiratory passages, and in the urinary and repro-

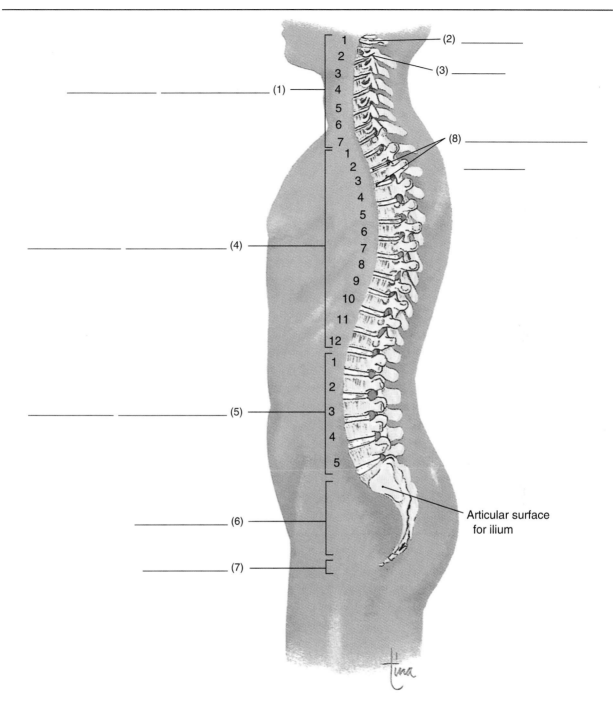

Figure 12–6 *The vertebral column. Lateral view of left side. (Adapted from Scanlon, VC, and Sanders, TS: Essentials of Anatomy and Physiology, ed 3. FA Davis, Philadelphia, 1999, p 112, with permission.)*

ductive ducts. These muscles are constantly at work performing tasks such as propelling food throughout the alimentary canal, keeping the eyes in focus, and controlling the diameter of the arteries. The contraction of smooth muscle is under *autonomic* (involuntary) *nervous control.*

The **cardiac muscle** is found only in the heart and is unique for its branched interconnections. Like skeletal muscle, cardiac muscle is striated; but unlike skeletal muscle, it experiences rhythmical involuntary contractions.

If a muscle loses its nerve supply, it will shrink to about two-thirds of its bulk within a few months. Many diseases affecting muscles, such as poliomyelitis and **myasthenia gravis,** are really diseases of the nervous system rather than the muscles.

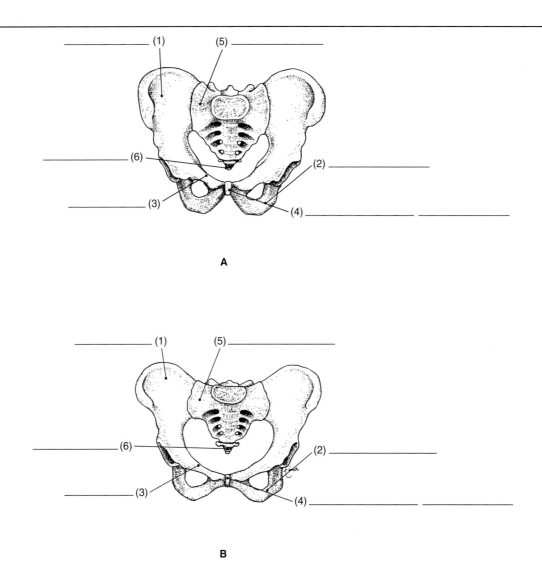

A

B

Figure 12–7 *The pelvic (hip) girdle. (A) Male pelvis, anterior view. (B) Female pelvis, anterior view. (Adapted from Scanlon, VC, and Sanders, TS: Essentials of Anatomy and Physiology, ed 3. FA Davis, Philadelphia, 1999, p 118, with permission.)*

Muscles are more often injured than diseased and are capable of self-repair. If a muscle is partly destroyed, the remaining part will grow larger and stronger in an effort to compensate.

Figure 12–8 along with Table 12–2 illustrates the actions performed by muscles. Most are in pairs and provide opposing functions (**antagonists**).

Attachments

Muscles attach to bones by either fleshy or fibrous attachments. In **fleshy attachments,** muscle fibers arise directly from bone. These fibers distribute force over wide areas. In **fibrous attachments,** the connective tissue converges at the end of the muscle to become continuous and indistinguishable from the periosteum. In some instances, this connective tissue penetrates the bone itself. Connective tissue fibers that form a cord or strap are referred to as **tendons.** This construction localizes a great deal of force in a small area of bone. In this way, a fibrous attachment is much stronger than a fleshy attachment. Ligaments are composed of connective tissue and attach one bone to another. When the fibrous attachment spans a large area of a particular bone, the attachment is called an **aponeurosis.** Such attachments are found in the lumbar region of the back. To become familiar with the names of major muscles, review Figure 12–9.

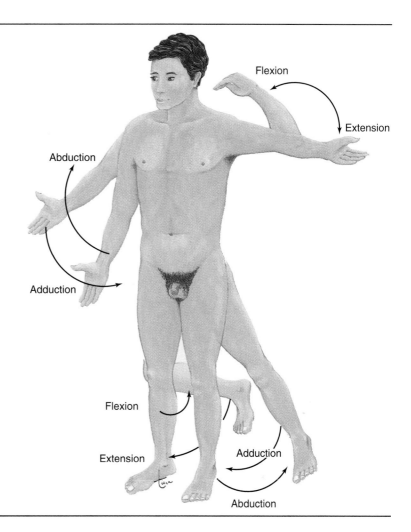

Figure 12–8 *The actions of muscles. (From Scanlon, VC, and Sanders, TS: Essentials of Anatomy and Physiology, ed 3. FA Davis, Philadelphia, 1999, p 139, with permission.)*

TABLE 12–2:	Muscle Actions
ACTION	**DEFINITION**
Flexion	Decreases the angle of a joint
Extension	Increases the angle of a joint
Adduction	Moves closer to the midline
Abduction	Moves away from the midline
Pronation	Turns the palm down
Supination	Turns the palm up
Dorsiflexion	Elevates the foot
Plantar flexion	Lowers the foot (points the toes)
Rotation	Moves a bone around its longitudinal axis

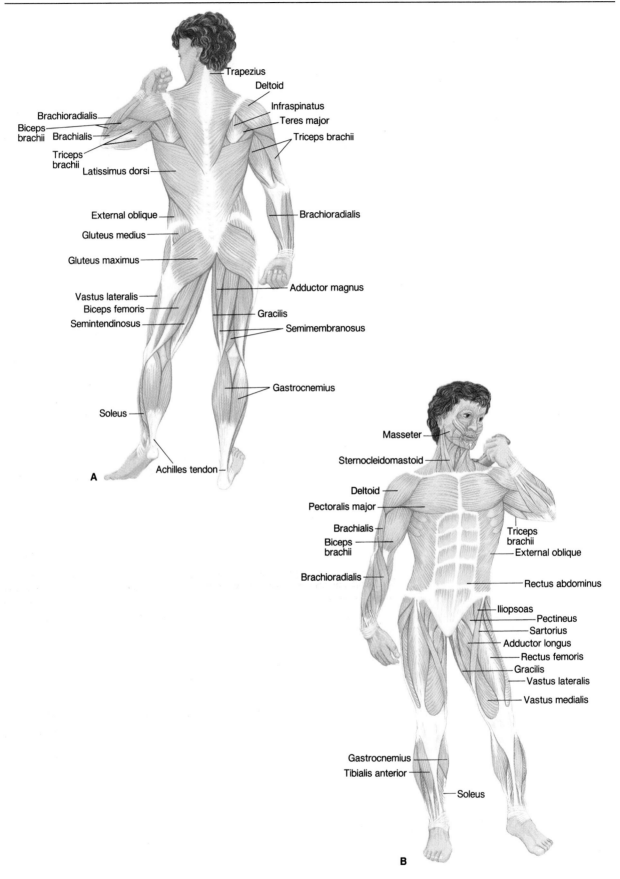

Figure 12–9 *The major muscles of the body. (A) Posterior view. (B) Anterior view. (From Scanlon, VC, and Sanders, TS: Essentials of Anatomy and Physiology, ed 3. FA Davis, Philadelphia, 1999, pp 140–141, with permission.)*

Activity 12–7: Competency Verification

Actions of Muscles

Refer to Figure 12–8 and Table 12–2 to choose the action of muscles that best describe each numbered statement below. The terms may be used more than once in the answer column.

abduction	plantar flexion
adduction	pronation
dorsiflexion	rotation
extension	supination
flexion	

1. _____ movement toward the midline of the body.

2. _____ to turn the palm upward.

3. _____ to increase the angle of a joint.

4. _____ to decrease the angle of a joint.

5. _____ to elevate the foot.

6. _____ movement away from the midline of the body.

7. _____ to lower the foot (point the toes).

8. _____ to turn the palm downward.

9. _____ movement of the arm in a circular motion.

10. _____ the opposite of extension.

Correct Answers _____ × 10 = _____% Score

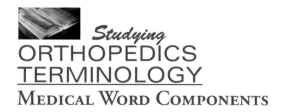

Studying ORTHOPEDICS TERMINOLOGY
MEDICAL WORD COMPONENTS

The combining forms related to specific bones of the axial and appendicular skeleton are illustrated in Fig-

ure 12–3. Use it as a reference when you study the medical word components in this section.

Combining Forms
Axial Skeleton

The axial skeleton consists of the bones of the skull, ribs, vertebral column, and thorax. These bones provide a framework to support the body and to protect the internal organs housed within them. They are summarized here.

Combining Forms: Axial Skeleton

Combining Form	Meaning	EXAMPLE	
		Term/Pronunciation	**Definition**
cephal/o	head	**cephal**/ad SĔF-ă-lăd	toward (-*ad*) the head
cervic/o	neck	**cervic**/al SĔR-vĭ-kăl	pertaining to (-*al*) the neck of the body or the neck of the uterus
cost/o	ribs	sub/**cost**/al sŭb-KŎS-tăl	pertaining to (-*al*) the area under (*sub*-) the ribs
crani/o	cranium	**crani**/o/tomy krā-nē-ŎT-ō-mē	incision (-*tomy*) of the skull *This procedure can be performed to remove tumors or to control cranial bleeding.*
lamin/o	lamina (part of the vertebral arch)	**lamin**/ectomy lăm-ĭ-NĔK-tō-mē	excision (-*ectomy*) of the lamina *This operation is performed to relieve compression of the spinal cord, as caused by a degenerated or displaced disk or by a bone displaced in an injury.*
myel/o	bone marrow, spinal cord	**myel**/o/pathy mī-ĕ-LŎP-ă-thē	any pathological condition (-*pathy*) of the spinal cord
orth/o	straight	**orth**/o/ped/ist or-thō-PĒ-dĭst	one who specializes (-*ist*) in the treatment and diagnosis of musculo-skeletal conditions *The combining forms ped/o and ped/i mean "foot" or "child"; orth/o means "straight." Originally, an orthopedist corrected bone deformities in children.*
oste/o	bone	**oste**/o/porosis ŏs-tē-ō-pō-RŌ-sĭs	porous (-*porosis*) bone
rachi/o	spine	**rachi**/o/meter rā-kē-ŎM-ĕ-tĕr	instrument used to measure (-*meter*) spinal curvature

Combining Forms: Axial Skeleton (Continued)

Combining Form	Meaning	EXAMPLE	
		Term/Pronunciation	**Definition**
spondyl/o	vertebrae (backbone)	**spondyl**/o/ptosis *spŏn-dĭ-lō-TŌ-sĭs*	prolapse (*-ptosis*) of a vertebra. Spondyloptosis *is also known as a "slipped disk" and is synonymous with* spondylolisthesis.
vertebr/o		inter/**vertebr**/al *ĭn-tĕr-VĔRT-ĕ-brĕl*	relating to (*-al*) the area between (*inter-*) two adjacent vertebrae
stern/o	sternum (breastbone)	**stern**/o/cost/al *stĕr-nō-KŎS-tăl*	pertaining to (*-al*) the sternum and ribs (*cost/o-*)
thorac/o	chest	**thorac**/ic *thō-RĂS-ĭk*	pertaining to (*-ic*) the chest

Appendicular Skeleton

The appendicular skeleton contains the bones that support the appendages or limbs found in the upper and lower extremities. The bones of the upper and lower extremities, plus the bones called girdles, the *shoulder girdle* (*pectoral girdle*) and the *pelvic girdle*, form the appendicular skeleton (see Fig. 12–3).

Combining Forms: Appendicular Skeleton

Combining Form	Meaning	EXAMPLE	
		Term/Pronunciation	**Definition**
UPPER EXTREMITIES			
brachi/o	arm	**brachi**/al *BRĀ-kē-ăl*	pertaining to (*-al*) the arm
carp/o	carpus (wrist bones)	**carp**/al *KĂR-păl*	pertaining to (*-al*) the wrist bones *There are eight bones that make up the wrist.*
clavicul/o	clavicle (collar bone)	supra/**clavicul**/ar *soo-pră-klă-VĬK-ū-lăr*	pertaining to (*-ar*) the area above (*supra-*) the collar bone
dactyl/o	fingers, toes	**dactyl**/o/spasm *DĂK-tĭ-lō-spăzm*	a cramp of the finger or toe *The combining form -spasm means "involuntary contraction, twitching."*
humer/o	humerus (upper arm bone)	**humer**/al *HŪ-mĕr-ăl*	pertaining to (*-al*) the humerus *The humerus is the upper bone of the arm from the elbow to the shoulder joint.*
acromi/o	acromion (projection of the scapula)	**acromi**/o/clavicul/ar *ă-krō-mē-ŏ-klă-VĬK-ū-lăr*	pertaining to (*-ar*) the acromion and the clavicle (*clavicul/o*)

Combining Forms: Appendicular Skeleton (Continued)

Combining Form	Meaning	EXAMPLE	
		Term/Pronunciation	Definition
metacarp/o	metacarpus (hand bones)	**metacarp**/al *mĕt-ă-KAR-păl*	pertaining to (*-al*) the metacarpus *There are five bones that make up the hand.*
phalang/o	phalanges (bones of fingers and toes)	**phalang**/ectomy *făl-ăn-JĔK-tō-mē*	excision (*-ectomy*) of one or more phalanges
radi/o	radiation, x-ray, radius (lower arm bone on thumb side)	**radi**/al *RĀ-dē-ăl*	pertaining to (*-al*) the radius bone
uln/o	ulna (lower arm bone on thumb side)	**uln**/ar *ŬL-năr*	pertaining to (*-ar*) the ulna *The ulna is the inner and larger bone of the forearm on the opposite side of the thumb.*
LOWER EXTREMITIES			
calcane/o	calcaneum (heel bone)	**calcane**/o/dynia *kăl-kā-nē-ō-DĬN-ē-ă*	pain (*-dynia*) in the calcaneum
femor/o	femur (thigh bone)	**femor**/al *FĔM-or-ăl*	pertaining to (*-al*) the femur *The femur is the longest and strongest bone in the skeleton.*
fibul/o	fibula (smaller, outer bone of the lower leg)	**fibul**/ar *FĬB-ū-lăr*	pertaining to (*-ar*) the fibula
ili/o	ilium (lateral, flaring portion of the hip bone)	**ili**/ac *ĬL-ē-ăk*	pertaining to (*-ac*) the ilium
ischi/o	ischium (lower portion of the hip bone)	**ischi**/al *ĬS-kē-ăl*	pertaining to (*-al*) the ischium
lumb/o	loins (lower back)	**lumb**/ar *LŬM-băr*	pertaining to (*-ar*) the loin area or lower back
patell/o	patella (kneecap)	**patell**/ectomy *păt-ĕ-LĔK-tō-mē*	excision (*-ectomy*) of the patella
ped/i	foot, child	**ped**/i/algia *pĕd-ē-ĂL-jē-ă*	pain (*-algia*) in the foot
pelv/i **pelv**/o	pelvis	**pelv**/ic *PĔL-vĭk*	pertaining to (*-ic*) the pelvis

Combining Forms: Appendicular Skeleton *(Continued)*

Combining Form	Meaning	EXAMPLE	
		Term/Pronunciation	**Definition**
pod/o	foot	**pod**/iatry pō-DĪ-ă-trē	branch of medicine specializing in disorders of the feet *The suffix* -iatry *means "physician, medicine, treatment."*
pub/o	pelvis bone (anterior part of the pelvic bone)	pub/is PŪ-bĭs	the pelvic bone *The suffix* -is *is a noun ending.*
tibi/o	tibia (larger inner bone of the lower leg)	**tibi**/al TĬB-ē-ăl	pertaining to (-*al*) the tibia *The tibia is also known as the* shin bone.

Activity 12–8: Competency Verification
Medical Word Components: Axial and Appendicular Skeleton

Check off the box [✓] as you complete each numbered section.

[ ] **1.** Review the medical components and their examples in the previous section. Then pronounce each word aloud.

[ ] **2.** For the words below, first write the suffix and its meaning, then translate the meaning of the remaining components starting with the first part of the word.

> **Example:** tibi/al
> **Answer:** *al* = pertaining; tibia (larger inner bone of the lower leg)

1. cervic/al _____

2. myel/o/pathy _____

3. thorac/ic _____

4. lamin/ectomy _____

5. spondyl/o/ptosis _____

6. sub/cost/al _____

7. phalang/ectomy _____

8. pedi/algia _____

9. pelv/ic _____

10. acromi/o/clavicul/ar _____

| Correct Answers _____ × 10 = _____% Score |

Joints, Muscles, and Related Structures

Combining Forms: Joints, Muscles, and Related Structures

Combining Form	Meaning	EXAMPLE	
		Term/Pronunciation	Definition
JOINTS			
ankyl/o	stiffness, bent, crooked	ankyl/osis ăng-kĭ-LŌ-sĭs	condition (-osis) of a stiff joint, usually resulting from a disease *Immobility and stiffness of a joint most often occur in rheumatoid arthritis.*
arthr/o	joint	**arthr**/o/desis ăr-thrō-DĒ-sĭs	surgical immobilization of a joint to relieve pain or provide support *The suffix -desis means "binding" or "fixation."*
chondr/o	cartilage	**chondr**/o/malacia kŏn-drō-măl-Ā-shē-ă	softening (-malacia) of the articular cartilage, usually the patella, which occurs in young adults after knee injury
condyl/o	condyle (rounded protuberance at end of a bone that forms an articulation)	**condyl**/oid KŎN-dĭ-loyd	resembling (-oid) a condyle
synov/o	synovial membrane, synovial fluid	**synov**/itis sĭn-ō-VĪ-tĭs	inflammation (-itis) of the synovial membrane
MUSCLES			
lei/o	smooth	**lei**/o/my/oma lī-ō-mī-Ō-mă	tumor (-oma) consisting primarily of smooth muscle (my/o)
my/o	muscle	**my**/o/pathy mī-ŎP-ă-thē	diseased (-pathy) muscle or muscle tissue
rhabd/o	rod-shaped (striated)	**rhabd**/o/my/oma răb-dō-mī-Ō-mă	tumor (-oma) consisting of primarily striated muscular (my/o) tissue

Combining Forms: Joints, Muscles, and Related Structures (Continued)

Combining Form	Meaning	EXAMPLE	
		Term/Pronunciation	Definition
RELATED STRUCTURES			
fasci/o	band, fascia (fibrous membrane supporting and separating muscles)	**fasci**/ectomy *făsh-ē-ĔK-tō-mē*	excision (*-ectomy*) of strips of fascia *This surgical procedure is often performed when excessive growth of fibrous tissue occurs around the joints, causing immobility (fibrous ankylosis).*
fibr/o	fiber, fibrous tissue	**fibr**/o/my/algia *fĭ-brō-mī-ĂL-jē-ă*	pain (*-algia*) in fibrous and muscle (*my/o*) tissue *This is a chronic condition that occurs most frequently in the tissues of the neck, shoulders, back, knees, and hips.* *This condition was previously labeled as fibrositis or rheumatism.*
ten/o	tendon	**ten**/o/rrhaphy *tĕn-OR-ă-fē*	suturing of a tendon
tend/o		**tend**/o/lysis *tĕn-DŎL-ĭ-sĭs*	process of freeing a tendon from adhesions *The suffix -lysis means "separation," "destruction," "loosening."*
tendin/o		**tendin**/itis *tĕn-dĭn-Ī-tĭs*	inflammation (*-itis*) of a tendon

Prefixes and Suffixes

In this section, prefixes are listed alphabetically and highlighted, whereas key suffixes are defined in the right-hand column.

Prefixes

Prefix	Meaning	EXAMPLE	
		Term/Pronunciation	Definition
dia-	through, across	**dia**/physis *dī-ĂF-ĭ-sĭs*	the shaft or middle region of a long bone *The suffix -physis means "to grow."*
epi-	above, upon	**epi**/physis *ĕ-PĬF-ĭ-sĭs*	the end of a long bone *The suffix -physis means "to grow."*
endo-	in, within	**endo**/lumb/ar *ĕn-dō-LŬM-băr*	in the lower back or lumbar (*lumb/o*) portion of the spinal cord *The suffix -ar means "pertaining to."*

Prefixes (Continued)

Prefix	Meaning	EXAMPLE	
		Term/Pronunciation	**Definition**
peri-	around	**peri**/oste/al pĕr-ē-ŎS-tē-ăl	pertaining to (-*al*) the periosteum. *The periosteum is a strong, fibrous membrane that covers the surface of a long bone.*

Activity 12–9: Competency Verification
Medical Word Components: Joints, Muscles, and Related Structures

Check off the box [✓] as you complete each numbered section.

[   ] **1.** Review the components and their examples in the previous section. Then pronounce each word aloud.

[   ] **2.** For the words below, first write the suffix and its meaning. Then translate the meaning of the remaining components starting with the first part of the word.

> **Example:** ten/o/rrhaphy
> **Answer:** *rrhaphy*=suture; tendon

1. tendin/itis   _____

2. endo/lumb/ar   _____

3. arthr/o/desis   _____

4. rhabd/o/my/oma   _____

5. chondr/o/malacia   _____

6. peri/oste/al   _____

7. synov/itis   _____

8. ankyl/osis   _____

9. fasci/ectomy   _____

10. fibr/o/my/algia   _____

Correct Answers _____ × 10 = _____% Score

PATHOLOGICAL CONDITIONS

Bone and Joint Disorders

DISORDER	DESCRIPTION
ankylosis ăng-kĭ-LŌ-sĭs *ankyl=stiffness, bent, crooked* *osis=abnormal condition*	The stiffening and immobility of a joint as the result of disease, trauma, surgery, or abnormal bone fusion.
arthritis ăr-THRĪ-tĭs *arthr=joint* *itis=inflammation*	Inflammation of a joint usually accompanied by pain, swelling, and frequently, changes in structure.
ankylosing spondylitis ĂNG-kĭ-lōs-ĭng spŏn-dĭl-Ī-tĭs *spondyl=vertebrae* *(backbone)* *itis=inflammation*	A chronic, progressive arthritis that first affects the spine and adjacent structures. As the disease progresses, the spine becomes increasingly stiff, with fusion of the spine into a position of *kyphosis* (humpback). Also called *rheumatoid spondylitis*.
gouty GOWT-ē	Arthritis caused by excessive uric acid in the body. A defect in uric acid metabolism causes accumulation of uric acid in the blood (*hyperuricemia*), joints, and surrounding tissue, with damage to the synovial membrane and articular cartilage. Any joint may be affected, but gout usually begins in the big toe. Treatment consists of a diet low in uric acid and the administration of drugs to lower uric acid production, relieve pain, and decrease inflammation.
osteoarthritis ŏs-tē-ō-ăr-THRĪ-tĭs *osteo=bone* *arthr=joint* *itis=inflammation*	A progressive, degenerative joint disease characterized by bone spurs (*osteophytes*) and destruction of articular cartilage.
rheumatoid ROO-mă-toyd	A chronic, systemic disease marked by inflammatory changes in joints and related structures that result in crippling deformities. Onset may vary, but it usually occurs in middle age. The pathological changes in the joints are generally thought to be caused by an autoimmune disease. Treatment consists of the administration of drugs—large doses of aspirin, corticosteroids, and gold compounds—as well as heat application, exercise, and physical therapy to maintain full range of motion (ROM) of affected joints. Figure 12–10 shows joint abnormalities in the hands of a patient with rheumatoid arthritis. 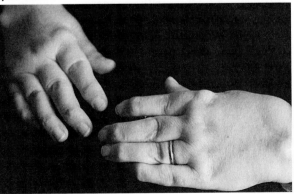 ***Figure 12–10*** *Joint abnormalities in hands of a patient with rheumatoid arthritis. (From Williams, LS, and Hopper, PD: Understanding Medical Surgical Nursing. FA Davis, Philadelphia, 1999, p 890, with permission.)*

Bone and Joint Disorders (Continued)

DISORDER	DESCRIPTION
bursitis *bŭr-SĪ-tĭs*	Inflammation of a bursa, particularly those located between bony prominences and muscle or tendons, such as the shoulder, elbow (also known as *tennis elbow*), and knee. Analgesics, heat, and diathermy often relieve symptoms, but in more severe cases, the injection of local anesthetics or cortisone may be required. In chronic cases, surgical removal of calcifications may be necessary.
bunion *BŬN-yŭn*	An abnormal enlargement of the joint at the base of the great toe. This disorder is caused by the inflammation of the bursa, usually the result of chronic irritation and pressure from tight-fitting shoes, by degenerative bone disease, or by heredity. Treatment includes padding around the toes to relieve pressure, medications for pain and swelling, or *bunionectomy*.
carpal tunnel syndrome (CTS) *KĂR-păl TŬN-ĕl SĬN-drōm*	A common, painful disorder produced by compression on the median nerve as it passes between the ligament and the bones and tendons of the wrist (carpal tunnel). It is often seen in cumulative overuse of the wrist. Symptomatic treatment includes the use of drugs to reduce pain and inflammation. Surgical treatment that releases the carpal ligament is performed when the pain cannot be relieved with medication.
dislocation *dĭs-lō-KĀ-shŭn*	Displacement of a bone from its normal location within a joint, causing loss of function in the joint.
subluxation *sŭb-lŭks-Ā-shŭn*	A partial dislocation; this can occur in any synovial joint, but it is more common in the fingers, shoulders, knees, and hips.
Ewing sarcoma *Ū-ĭng săr-KŌ-mă*	A malignant tumor that develops from bone marrow, usually in long bones or the pelvis. It occurs most frequently in adolescent boys and is characterized by pain, swelling, fever, and leukocytosis. Treatment includes surgery, chemotherapy, and radiotherapy.
fracture *FRĂK-chŭr*	A break in the bone. Some examples of fractures are described next, and illustrated in Figure 12–11.
complicated	A fracture in which the broken bone injures an internal organ, such as a broken rib piercing the lung.
compound (open)	A fracture with an external wound in the skin.
comminuted	A fracture in which the bone is broken or splintered into pieces.
impacted	A fracture in which the bone is broken and one end is wedged into the interior of the other.
incomplete	A break in the bone in which the line of fracture does not include the whole bone.
greenstick	A fracture in which the bone is partially bent and partially broken (as when a green stick breaks); occurs in children.

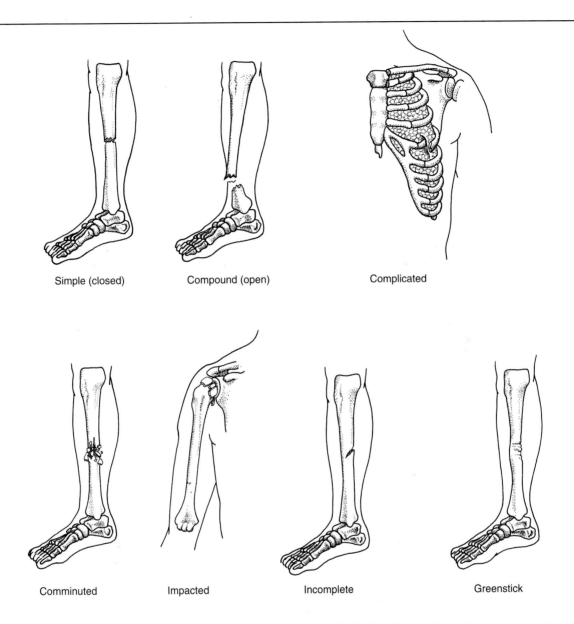

Simple (closed) Compound (open) Complicated

Comminuted Impacted Incomplete Greenstick

Figure 12–11 *Types of fractures. (Adapted from Gylys, BA, and Wedding, ME. Medical Terminology: A Systems Approach, ed 4. FA Davis, Philadelphia, 1999, p 203, with permission.)*

Bone and Joint Disorders (Continued)

DISORDER	DESCRIPTION
pathological	A fracture of a diseased or weakened bone produced by a force that would not have fractured a healthy bone. The underlying disease may be metastasis from a cancer that originated elsewhere, primary cancer of the bone, or osteoporosis.
simple (closed)	A fracture without an external wound.
ganglion GĂNG-lē-ŏn	A cyst that develops from the joint capsule or a tendon, usually in the wrist. Treatment is only necessary when the ganglion becomes painful or bothersome to wrist function. Treatment includes a ganglionectomy or a needle aspiration to remove the fluid from the cyst.

Bone and Joint Disorders (Continued)

DISORDER	DESCRIPTION
Lyme disease *līm dĭ-ZĒZ*	An acute, recurrent inflammatory infection transmitted through the bite of an infected deer tick. It is initially characterized by a circular rash and flulike symptoms and progresses within a period of a few days or weeks to other sites of the body to produce malaise, myalgia, arthritis, and neurologic and cardiac symptoms. When treated early, the results are good. Antibiotic therapy is the main mode of treatment.
osteochondroma *ŏs-tē-ō-kŏn-DRŌ-mă* *osteo=bone* *chondr=cartilage* *oma=tumor*	Benign tumor composed of bone and cartilage. The tibia and femur are most frequently involved, with onset usually in childhood, but it may not be diagnosed until adulthood.
osteomalacia *ŏs-tē-ō-măl-Ā-shē-ă* *osteo=bone* *malacia=softening*	A vitamin D deficiency in adults marked by increasing softness of the bones, to the point of their becoming flexible and brittle, and thus causing deformities. When the disease occurs in children, it is called rickets, which is rarely seen in the United States.
osteomyelitis *ŏs-tē-ō-mī-ĕl-Ī-tĭs* *osteo=bone* *myel=bone marrow, spinal cord* *itis=inflammation*	Local or generalized infection of the bone and bone marrow. This disorder is usually caused by bacteria introduced through trauma or surgery, by direct extension from a nearby infection, or via the bloodstream. *Staphylococci* are the most common causative agents.
osteoporosis *ŏs-tē-ō-por-Ō-sĭs* *osteo=bone* *porosis=porous*	A disorder characterized by abnormal loss of bone density. It occurs most frequently in postmenopausal women, sedentary or immobilized individuals, and patients on long-term steroid therapy. Pain, especially in the lower back, pathological fractures, loss of stature, and various deformities are typically associated with osteoporosis. Increased calcium intake and estrogen replacement therapies are often used for the prevention and management of postmenopausal osteoporosis.
osteosarcoma *ŏs-tē-ō-săr-KŌ-mă* *osteo=bone* *sarc=flesh (connective tissue)* *oma=tumor*	The most common malignant tumor of the bone. Also known *as osteogenic sarcoma.*
Paget disease *PĂJ-ĕt di-ZEZ*	A skeletal disease of unknown cause usually affecting the middle-aged and elderly that is characterized by excessive bone destruction and unorganized bone repair. Also known as *osteitis deformans* because the unorganized bone repair can result in a *bowing* and deformity of the bone.
talipes *TĂL-ĭ-pēz*	Any of several deformities of the foot that are usually congenital, where the foot is in a relatively fixed, twisted, abnormal position. Also known as *clubfoot.*

Spinal Disorders

DISORDER	DESCRIPTION
herniated disk HĔR-nē-ā-tĕd dĭsk	A rupture of the fibrocartilage surrounding an intervertebral disk, releasing the nucleus pulposus into the vertebral canal. This often results in pressure on a spinal nerve, which causes lower back pain that may radiate down the leg (sciatica). This most frequently occurs in the lumbar region. Bed rest, pain medication, and physical therapy are initial treatments. Surgery such as *laminectomy* and *spinal fusion* may be performed on patients with recurrent or chronic disc herniation. Also known as *herniated nucleus pulposus, ruptured disk, slipped disk.* Figure 12–12 illustrates the difference between a normal, healthy spinal disk and a herniated spinal disk.
kyphosis kī-FŌ-sĭs *kyph=hill, mountain* *osis=abnormal condition*	An abnormal curvature of a portion of the spine, commonly known as *hump-back* or *hunchback.* Treatment consists of spine-stretching exercises, sleeping with a board under the mattress, and wearing a brace to straighten the kyphotic curve; surgery is rarely required.
lordosis lor-DŌ-sĭs *lord=curve, swayback* *osis=abnormal condition*	An abnormal, inward curvature of a portion of the spine, commonly called *swayback.* This may be caused by increased weight of the abdominal contents, resulting from obesity or excessive weight gain during pregnancy.
scoliosis skō-lĭ-Ō-sĭs *scoli=crooked, bent* *osis=abnormal condition*	An abnormal sideward curvature of the spine, either to the left or to the right. Some rotation of a portion of the vertebral column also may occur. Scoliosis often occurs in combination with *kyphosis* and *lordosis*. Treatment depends on the severity of the curvature and may vary from exercises, physical therapy, and back braces to surgical intervention.

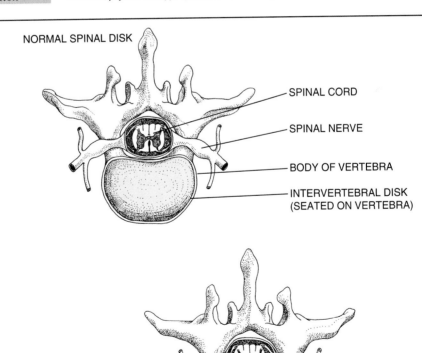

NORMAL SPINAL DISK

SPINAL CORD

SPINAL NERVE

BODY OF VERTEBRA

INTERVERTEBRAL DISK
(SEATED ON VERTEBRA)

GELATINOUS INTERIOR OF THE RUPTURED DISK PROTRUDES INTO THE VERTEBRAL CANAL AND PUSHES AGAINST THE SPINAL NERVE.

HERNIATED SPINAL DISK

Figure 12–12 *Normal and herniated spinal disks. (From Venes, D: Taber's Cyclopedic Medical Dictionary, ed 19. FA Davis, Philadelphia, 2001, p 979, with permission.)*

Muscular Disorders

DISORDER	DESCRIPTION
muscular dystrophy *MŬS-kū-lăr DĬS-trō-fē* *muscul=muscle* *ar=pertaining to* *dys=bad, painful, difficult* *trophy=development,* *nourishment*	A group of genetic diseases characterized by progressive weakness and atrophy of muscles without the involvement of the nervous system. Treatment consists primarily of supportive measures, such as physical therapy, and orthopedic procedures to reduce deformity.
Duchenne *dū-SHĔN*	The most common form of muscular dystrophy that usually appears between 3 and 5 years of age and spreads from the leg and pelvic muscles to the involuntary muscles. Muscles rapidly deteriorate as fat replaces functional muscle cells. Usually, by the age of 12 the person is confined to a wheelchair. There is no cure for this disease and most die from Duchenne muscular dystrophy within 10 to 15 years of symptom onset.
polymyositis *pŏl-ē-mī-ō-SĪ-tĭs* *poly=many, much* *myos=muscle* *itis=inflammation*	The chronic inflammation of a number of muscles simultaneously, usually accompanied by deformity, pain, edema, sweating, tension, and insomnia. The cause is unknown, but evidence suggests that it is an *autoimmune disorder*. Treatment consists of supportive therapy and corticosteroids.
rhabdomyosarcoma *răb-dō-mī-ō-săr-KŌ-mă* *rhabdo=rod-shaped (striated)* *myo=muscle* *sarc=flesh (connective tissue)* *oma=tumor*	A highly malignant tumor derived from primitive striated muscle cells that occurs most frequently in the head and neck. Also called *rhabdomyoblastoma, rhabdosarcoma.*
sprain *sprān*	Traumatic injury to the tendons, muscles, or ligaments around a joint, characterized by pain, swelling, and discoloration of the skin over the joint. The duration and severity of the symptoms vary with the extent of damage to the supporting tissues. Treatment consists of cold compresses, application of a bandage for support, elevation of the joint, and rest. The ankle joint is the most common site for a sprain.
strain *strān*	Trauma to the muscles and/or tendons from excessive use.

Activity 12–10: Clinical Application
Pathological Conditions

bunion	kyphosis	polymyositis
comminuted	lordosis	rhabdomyosarcoma
compound	Lyme disease	scoliosis
dislocation	muscular dystrophy	sprain
ganglion	osteoarthritis	strain
gouty	osteoporosis	subluxation
greenstick	Paget disease	talipes

Match the diagnoses listed above with an explanation of their pathological condition in the numbered list:

1. _____ arthritis caused by excessive uric acid in the body.

2. _____ an abnormal sideward curvature of the spine, either to the left or right.

3. _____ any of several deformities of the foot.

4. _____ an abnormal, inward curvature of a portion of the spine, commonly called swayback.

5. _____ an abnormal enlargement of the joint at the base of the great toe.

6. _____ a partial dislocation.

7. _____ trauma to the muscles and/or tendons from excessive use.

8. _____ a disorder characterized by abnormal loss of bone density.

9. _____ a progressive, degenerative joint disease characterized by bone spurs and destruction of articular cartilage.

10. _____ traumatic injury to the tendons, muscles, or ligaments around a joint characterized by pain, swelling, and discoloration of the skin over the joint.

11. _____ a skeletal disease of unknown cause, usually affecting the middle-aged and elderly, that is characterized by excessive bone destruction and unorganized bone repair.

12. _____ chronic inflammation of a number of muscles simultaneously, usually accompanied by deformity, pain, edema, sweating, tension, and insomnia.

13. _____ an acute, recurrent inflammatory infection transmitted through the bite of an infected deer tick.

14. _____ a group of genetic diseases characterized by progressive weakness and atrophy of muscles without the involvement of the nervous system.

15. _____ a cyst that develops from the joint capsule or a tendon, usually in the wrist.

16. _____ an exaggeration of angulation in the normal posterior curve of the thoracic spine; also known as humpback or hunchback.

17. _____ a highly malignant tumor derived from primitive, striated muscle cells.

18. _____ a fracture in which the bone is partially bent and partially broken; occurs in children.

19. _____ a fracture with an external wound in the skin.

20. _____ a fracture in which the bone is broken or splintered into pieces.

Correct Answers _____ × 5 = _____ **% Score**

Diagnostic Procedures and Tests

Imaging Procedures

PROCEDURE	DESCRIPTION
arthrography *ăr-THRŎG-ră-fē* *arthro=joint* *graphy=process of recording*	Radiography of joint after injection of a contrast medium.
bone scan	The injection of radiopharmaceuticals to enable visualization of a bone using the image produced by the emission of radioactive particles (see Fig. 18–7). Used in nuclear medicine department.
dual energy x-ray absorptiometry (DEXA) *ăb-sorp-shē-ŎM-ĕ-trē*	An imaging technique to measure bone density for purposes of diagnosis and management of osteoporosis.
electromyography (EMG) *ē-lĕk-trō-mī-ŎG-ră-fē* *electro=electricity* *myo=muscle* *graphy=process of recording*	The process of recording the strength of the contraction of a muscle when it is stimulated by electric current.
myelography *mī-ĕ-LŎG-ră-fē* *myelo=bone marrow, spinal cord* *graphy=process of recording*	Radiography of the spinal cord after injection of a contrast medium into the spinal canal. It is used to identify spinal disorders caused by disease or trauma such as tumors, cysts, and herniated intervertebral disks.

Laboratory Tests

TEST	DESCRIPTION
erythrocyte sedimentation rate (ESR or sed rate) *ĕ-RĬTH-rō-sīt* *sĕd-ĭ-mĕn-TĀ-shŭn rāt* *erythro=red* *cyte=cell*	Test to measure the rate at which RBCs settle to the bottom of a narrow tube. Elevated ESRs are not specific for any disorder but indicate the presence of inflammation, as seen in rheumatoid arthritis.
rheumatoid factor (RF) *ROO-mă-toyd FĂK-tor*	Blood test to detect the presence of the rheumatoid factor. Rheumatoid factors are antibodies often found in the serum of patients with a clinical diagnosis of rheumatoid arthritis.
calcium (Ca) level	Measures the amount of calcium in the blood.
creatine phosphokinase (CPK) *KRĒ-ă-tĭn fŏs-fō-KĪ-nās*	Blood test that measures the level of the enzyme creatine phosphokinase. This test is used as a reliable measure of skeletal and inflammatory muscle diseases and can be helpful in diagnosing muscular dystrophy. It is also a test used to diagnose myocardial infarction.

Laboratory Tests (Continued)

TEST	DESCRIPTION
phosphorus level *FŎS-fō-rŭs*	Test to measure the amount of phosphorus in the blood; useful in the diagnosis of bone disorders.
uric acid test *Ū-rĭk*	Test to measure the amount of uric acid in the blood. **High levels are associated with gouty arthritis.**

SURGICAL AND THERAPEUTIC PROCEDURES

Surgical Procedures

PROCEDURE	DESCRIPTION
arthrocentesis *ăr-thrō-sĕn-TĒ-sĭs* *arthro=joint* *centesis=surgical puncture*	Surgical puncture of a joint space with a needle to remove accumulated fluid.
arthrodesis *ăr-thrō-DĒ-sĭs* *arthro=joint* *desis=binding, fixation (of a bone or joint)*	Surgical immobilization of a joint; artificial ankylosis.
arthrolysis *ăr-THRŎL-ĭ-sĭs* *arthro=joint* *lysis=separation, destruction, loosening*	Surgical procedure to restore mobilization to an ankylosed joint.
arthroplasty *ĂR-thrō-plăs-tē* *arthro=joint* *plasty=surgical repair*	The surgical reconstruction or replacement of a painful, degenerated joint to restore mobility in rheumatoid or osteoarthritis, or to correct a congenital deformity.
total hip	Replacement of the femoral head and acetabulum with prostheses, such as a metallic femoral head and a plastic-coated metal acetabulum. **This is performed because of severe joint deterioration. Figure 12–13A is a radiograph of an arthritic right hip. Figure 12–13B is a radiograph of the same hip after arthroplasty with the prostheses in place.**
arthroscopy *ăr-THRŎS-kō-pē* *arthro=joint* *scopy=visual examination*	Visual examination of the interior of a joint performed by inserting an endoscope through a small incision. **This procedure is performed to repair and remove joint tissue especially of knee, ankle, and shoulder.**

Surgical Procedures (Continued)

PROCEDURE	DESCRIPTION

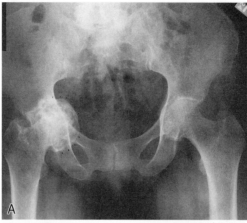

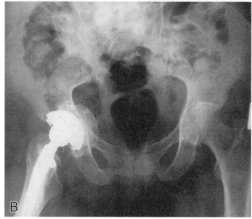

Figure 12–13 (A) Arthritis of right hip. (B) Total hip arthroplasty of arthritic hip. (From Williams, LS, and Hopper, PD: Understanding Medical Surgical Nursing, FA Davis, Philadelphia, 1999, p 898, with permission.)

laminectomy lăm-ĭ-NĔK-tō-mē *lamin=lamina (vertebral arch)* *ectomy=excision, removal*	Surgical removal of the bony arches of one or more vertebrae. This procedure is performed to relieve compression of the spinal cord as caused by a ruptured intervertebral disk.
open reduction of fractures	The treatment of bone fractures by a surgical procedure to place the bone(s) in proper alignment. Devices such as pins, screws, wires, or nails may be used internally to maintain the bone alignment while healing takes place. These devices are called *internal fixation devices*.
sequestrectomy sē-kwĕs-TRĔK-tō-mē *sequestr=a separation* *ectomy=excision, removal*	Excision of a necrosed piece of bone (*sequestrum*); synonymous with *sequestrotomy*.

Therapeutic Procedures

PROCEDURE	DESCRIPTION
closed reduction of fractures	The treatment of bone fractures by manipulating the bones into proper position (*reduction*) without making an incision into the skin. After reduction, the bone is then immobilized with an external device to maintain proper alignment while healing occurs. Examples of external devices used are *casting, splinting,* and *traction.*
casting	The application of a solid, stiff dressing formed with plaster of Paris or other material to a limb or body part to immobilize it during healing.
splinting	The use of an orthopedic device to an injured body part for immobilization, stabilization, and protection during the healing process.
traction	The process of putting a bone, limb, or group of muscles under tension by means of weights and pulleys to align or immobilize the part, or to relieve pressure on it.

Pharmacology

DRUG CLASSIFICATION	THERAPEUTIC ACTION
corticosteroids *kor-tĭ-kō-STĒR-oyds*	Drugs that reduce the inflammation associated with arthritis, bursitis, and tendinitis. Some corticosteroids can be injected directly into the joint (*intra-articular* administration), or they can be given orally.
gold salts	Drugs that contain actual gold (from 29% to 50% of the total drug) in capsules or in solution for injection; used to treat active rheumatoid arthritis. Rheumatoid arthritis is an autoimmune disease in which the patient's own macrophages attack and damage cartilage. Gold salts inhibit the activity of macrophages but cannot reverse past damage.
minerals	Over-the-counter calcium supplements are used to supplement the diet and increase calcium to prevent osteoporosis.
nonsteroidal anti-inflammatory drugs (NSAIDs) *nŏn-stē-ROYD-ăl ăn-tĭ-ĭn-FLĂM-ă-tŏr-ē*	Agents that exert antipyretic and analgesic effects in addition to their anti-inflammatory effects. These drugs are very effective for the relief of mild-to-moderate pain of varied origin as well as for the inhibition of platelet aggregation in the prevention of a cerebrovascular accident (CVA). Aspirin, *acetylsalicylic acid (ASA)*, included in this category, is the oldest drug used to treat arthritis. This is the first line of treatment for rheumatoid arthritis, but if NSAIDs fail, gold salts may be added to the treatment regimen.
skeletal muscle relaxants	Agents that relieve muscle spasm and stiffness and are prescribed to treat acute musculoskeletal conditions such as strains, sprains, and "pulled muscles."

❖ ABBREVIATIONS

ABBREVIATION	MEANING	ABBREVIATION	MEANING
ACL	anterior cruciate ligament	mcg	microgram
ASA	acetylsalicylic acid	MG	myasthenia gravis
C1, C2, etc.	first cervical vertebra, second cervical vertebra, etc.	MS	musculoskeletal, multiple sclerosis, mental status
Ca	calcium, cancer	NSAIDs	nonsteroidal anti-inflammatory drugs
CDH	congenital dislocation of the hip		
CTS	carpal tunnel syndrome	ORTH, ortho	orthopedics
DEXA	dual energy x-ray absorptiometry	P	phosphorus
DJD	degenerative joint disease	RA	rheumatoid arthritis
EMG	electromyography	RF	rheumatoid factor
ESR	erythrocyte sedimentation rate	ROM	range of motion
Fx	fracture	SD	shoulder disarticulation
HD	hemodialysis, hip disarticulation, hearing distance	T_1, T_2, etc.	first thoracic vertebra, second thoracic vertebra, etc.
HNP	herniated nucleus pulposus (herniated disk)	THA	total hip arthroplasty
		THR	total hip replacement
HP	hemipelvectomy	TKA	total knee arthroplasty
IS	intracostal space	TKR	total knee replacement
KD	knee disarticulation	TMJ	temporomandibular joint
L1, L2, etc.	first lumbar vertebra, second lumbar vertebra, etc.		

Activity 12–11: Clinical Application

Diagnostic Tests, Treatments, and Abbreviations

calcium
casting
corticosteroids
DEXA
EMG
internal fixation devices

laminectomy
phosphorus level
sequestrectomy
skeletal muscle relaxants
traction
uric acid test

Match the terms listed above with the definitions given in the numbered list:

1. _____ the process of recording the strength of the contraction of a muscle when it is stimulated by electric current.

2. _____ an imaging technique to measure bone density that is used to diagnose osteoporosis.

3. _____ an abnormally high reading on this laboratory test is associated with gouty arthritis.

4. _____ excision of a necrosed piece of bone.

5. _____ surgical procedure performed to relieve compression of the spinal cord as in the case of a ruptured disk.

6. _____ devices such as pins, screws, wires, and nails that are used to align the bone in the open reduction of fractures.

7. _____ the use of devices, such as weights and pulleys, to align or immobilize a body part, or to relieve pressure on it.

8. _____ the application of a solid, stiff dressing—formed with plaster of Paris or other material—to a limb or body part for the purpose of immobilization during healing.

9. _____ reduce inflammation associated with arthritis, bursitis, and tendinitis.

10. _____ used as a supplement to prevent osteoporosis.

Correct Answers _____ × 10 = _____% Score

Activity 12–12: Build Medical Words
Diagnostic, Symptomatic, and Surgical Terms

Use *oste/o* (bone) to build medical words meaning:

1. beginning or formation of bones_____

2. bone cells _____

3. pain in the bones _____

4. disease of the bones and joints _____

5. tumor of bone and cartilage _____

Use *cervic/o* (neck) to build medical words meaning:

6. pertaining to the neck and arm _____

7. pertaining to the neck and face _____

Use *stern/o* (breastbone) to build medical words meaning:

8. resembling the breastbone _____

9. pertaining to the sternum and ribs _____

Use *myel/o* (bone marrow, spinal cord) to build medical words meaning:

10. herniation of the spinal cord _____

11. softening of the spinal cord _____

Use *arthr/o* (joint) to build medical words meaning:

12. inflammation of the joint _____

13. visual examination of a joint _____

14. surgical puncture of a joint _____

Use *pelv/i* (pelvis) to build medical words meaning:

15. instrument for measuring the pelvis _____

16. measurement of the pelvis _____

Use *my/o* (muscle) to build medical words meaning:

17. any disease of muscles _____

18. suture of a muscle _____

19. pain in the muscle _____

20. instrument to cut muscle _____

Correct Answers _____ × 5 = _____% **Score**

MEDICAL RECORDS

Authentic reports from the medical records of four different patients are included in this section.

The following dictionary exercise and medical record analysis will help you develop skills to abstract information and master the terminology in the reports. Accurate interpretation is important because information of this type is used in numerous areas of the medical practice, such as initiation of treatments, evaluation of patients' progress, and completion of insurance claims.

Reading and Dictionary Exercise

Place a check mark in the box [✓] after you complete the exercise.

[   ] **1.** Underline the following words in the reports as you read the consultation, the operative report, the pathology report, and the discharge summary aloud. These medical records can be found at the end of the chapter, just before the Glossary of Medical Word Components.

[   ] **2.** Use a medical dictionary and Appendix F, Part 2, to define the terms below.

Note: You are not expected to fully understand all parts of the medical records. The important aspect of this exercise is to use all available resources to complete it. Eventually you will master the terminology and format of these reports.

> > > MEDICAL RECORD 12–1: OPERATIVE REPORT

Term	Pronunciation	Meaning
rotator cuff	*rō-TĀ-tor kŭf*	_____

acromionectomy	*ă-krō-mē-ŏ-NĔK-tō-mē*	_____
postoperative	*pōst-ŎP-ĕr-ă-tĭv*	_____
scalene block	*skā-LĒN blŏk*	_____
arthrogram	*ĂR-thrō-grăm*	_____
biceps	*BĪ-sĕps*	_____
supraspinatus	*soo-pră-SPĬN-ă-tŭs*	_____
infraspinatus	*ĭn-fră-SPĬN-ă-tŭs*	_____
debrided	*dā-BRĒD-ĕd*	_____
supine	*sū-PĪN*	_____
deltoid	*DĔL-toyd*	_____
subacromial	*sŭb-ă-KRŌ-mē-ăl*	_____
bursa	*BŬR-să*	_____
spur	*spŭr*	_____
humeral	*HŪ-mĕr-ăl*	_____
coracoacromial	*kor-ă-kō-ă-KRŌ-mē-ăl*	_____
subcutaneous	*sŭb-kū-TĀ-nē-ŭs*	_____
subcuticular	*sŭb-kū-TĬK-ū-lăr*	_____
intrascalene block	*ĭn-tră-skā-LĒN blŏk*	_____

> > > MEDICAL RECORD 12-2: CONSULTATION

Term	Pronunciation	Meaning
laminectomy	*lăm-ĭ-NĔK-tō-mē*	_____
posterolateral	*pŏs-tĕr-ō-LĂT-ĕr-ăl*	_____
Propulsid	*prō-PŬL-sĭd*	_____
Prilosec	*PRĪ-lō-sĕk*	_____
Norvasc	*NOR-văsk*	_____
Xanax	*ZĂN-ăks*	_____
Darvocet	*DĂR-vō-sĕt*	_____
dorsiflexion	*DOR-sĭ-flĕk-shŭn*	_____

lumbosacral	*lŭm-bō-SĀ-krăl*	_____
epidural	*ĕp-ĭ-DŪR-ăl*	_____
fluoroscopy	*floor-ŎS-kō-pē*	_____

> > > MEDICAL RECORD 12–3: OPERATIVE REPORT

Term	Pronunciation	Meaning
osteoarthritis	*ŏs-tē-ō-ăr-THRĪ-tĭs*	_____
total hip arthroplasty	*ĂR-thrō-plăs-tē*	_____
decubitus position	*dē-KŪ-bĭ-tŭs*	_____
orthopedic	*or-thō-PĒ-dĭk*	_____
lateral	*LĂT-ĕr-ăl*	_____
anterior	*ăn-TĒ-rē-or*	_____
superior	*sū-PĒ-rē-or*	_____
iliac spine	*ĬL-ē-ăk spīn*	_____
distally	*DĬS-tăl-ē*	_____
greater trochanter	*GRĀ-tĕr trō-KĂN-tĕr*	_____
femur	*FĒ-mŭr*	_____
tensor fascia	*TĔN-sŏr FĂSH-ē-ă*	_____
retractor	*rĭ-TRĂK-tor*	_____
abductor	*ăb-DŬK-tor*	_____
capsulectomy	*kăp-sū-LĔK-tō-mē*	_____
femoral head	*FĔM-or-ăl*	_____
adduct	*ă-DŬKT*	_____
reamer	*RĒ-mĕr*	_____
acetabular	*ăs-ĕ-TĂB-ū-lăr*	_____
cartilage	*KĂR-tĭ-lĭj*	_____
cystic lesions	*SĬS-tĭk LĒ-zhŭns*	_____
prosthesis	*PRŎS-thē-sĭs*	_____
reduction	*rĭ-DŬK-shŭn*	_____

subcuticular   *sŭb-kū-TĬK-ū-lăr*   _____

> > > MEDICAL RECORD 12–4: EMERGENCY ROOM REPORT

Term	Pronunciation	Meaning
normocephalic	*nor-mō-sĕ-FĂL-ĭk*	_____
atraumatic	*ā-traw-MĂT-ĭk*	_____
supple	*SŬ-pl*	_____
auscultation	*aws-kŭl-TĀ-shŭn*	_____
angulation	*ăng-ū-LĀ-shŭn*	_____
capillary refill	*KĂP-ĭ-lăr-ē RĒ-fĭl*	_____
anatomical snuffbox	*ăn-ă-TŎM-ĭ-kăl* *SNŬF-bŏks*	_____
distal	*DĬS-tăl*	_____
radius	*RĀ-dē-ŭs*	_____
ulna	*ŬL-nă*	_____
abduct	*ăb-DŬKT*	_____
neurovascularly	*nū-rō-VĂS-kū-lăr-lē*	_____
comminuted	*KŎM-ĭ-nū-tĕd*	_____
intra-articular	*ĭn-tră-ăr-TĬK-ū-lăr*	_____
Colles fracture	*kŏ-LĒZ FRĂK-chŭr*	_____
apex volar	*Ā-pĕks VŌ-lăr*	_____
ulnarly	*ŬL-năr-lē*	_____
splint	*splĭnt*	_____
fentanyl	*FĔN-tă-nĭl*	_____

Critical Thinking: Analysis of Medical Records

This section provides experience in abstracting information from medical records. At the same time, it reinforces the material presented in this chapter.

> > > MEDICAL RECORD 12-1: OPERATIVE REPORT

1. What type of diagnostic test verified the presence of a right rotator cuff tear?

_____

2. What type of surgical procedure was performed to correct the rotator cuff tear?

_____

3. Why wasn't the rotator tear repaired?

_____

_____

_____

4. What was done to improve the range of motion of the rotator cuff?

_____

_____

> > > MEDICAL RECORD 12-2: CONSULTATION

5. What type of previous medical treatment did the patient receive for back pain?

_____

6. What medication is the patient taking for his back pain?

_____

> > > MEDICAL RECORD 12-3: OPERATIVE REPORT

7. Why was a total hip arthroplasty performed?

_____

8. What position was the patient in during the surgical procedure?

_____

9. What prostheses were inserted to replace the left hip?

_____

> > > MEDICAL RECORD 12-4: EMERGENCY ROOM REPORT

10. What brought the patient into the emergency room?

_____

11. What type of fracture does the patient have?

_____

12. What treatment did she receive for her injury?

_____

Audio Practice

Listen to the audio CD-ROM to practice the pronunciation of selected medical terms from this chapter.

Medical Record 12–1. Operative Report

GENERAL HOSPITAL AND MEDICAL CENTER
2211 Fifth Avenue North • Healthy City, USA 12345 • (321) 123-4567

Operative Report

Patient Name: Matthew Joiner   **Patient Number:** 32-17-48
Birth Date: 05/10/xx   **Room Number:** 317

DATE OF OPERATION: 11/10/20xx

PREOPERATIVE DIAGNOSIS: Right rotator cuff tear.

POSTOPERATIVE DIAGNOSIS: Massive chronic right rotator cuff tear.

OPERATION: Right shoulder open partial acromionectomy.

SURGEON: Richard Geldinger, M.D.

ANESTHESIA: General with postoperative scalene block.

SURGICAL INDICATIONS: The patient is a 60-year-old gentleman with a long history of right shoulder pain after a fall. An arthrogram had confirmed the presence of a rotator cuff tear. The patient was treated conservatively for an extended period of time, but due to persistent pain and weakness, presents now for attempted rotator cuff repair.

OPERATIVE FINDINGS: Before the surgery the patient had an excellent full range of motion. However, during the surgery a large tear was discovered. The biceps tendon could not adequately be identified. The supraspinatus was entirely torn back to the infraspinatus, and this was not repairable. The joint was debrided, and a partial acromionectomy was performed.

PROCEDURE: The patient was brought to the operating room, placed on the operating table in the supine position. After the induction of general anesthesia, he was then placed in the semi-sitting position. The right shoulder and upper extremity were then prepped and draped. After this was performed, an anterior incision was made extending down through the deltoid and split in line with its muscle fibers off the anterior acromion distally about 1-1/2 inches. This was taken down to the subacromial bursa. The bursa was entered and joint fluid was identified. A massive rotator cuff tear was identified. A limited debridement was done. It was determined that this tear was not repairable. Even a partial repair would have left him with fairly significant limitations in external rotation. It was decided then to debride the joint. Spurs of the anterior surface of the acromion and over the humeral head were debrided. The wound was

Continued

Operative Report, page 2

Patient Name: Matthew Joiner   **Patient Number:** 2-17-48

irrigated. A limited subacromial decompression in attempting to save the coracoacromial ligament was performed. The patient had the joint again irrigated. A portion of the subacromial bursa was reapproximated. The deltoid was reapproximated with 3-0 and #1 Ethibond suture.

The subcutaneous tissue was closed with 3-0 Vicryl suture. The skin was closed with 2-0 subcuticular Prolene suture. Steri-Strips were applied. A sterile dressing was applied. An intrascalene block was then administered and then the patient was awakened from general anesthesia and taken to the recovery room in stable condition, having tolerated this procedure well. Sponge and needle counts were correct.

_____

Richard Geldinger, M.D.

RG/alm
D: 11/10/xx
T: 11/11/xx

Medical Record 12–2. Consultation

GENERAL HOSPITAL AND MEDICAL CENTER
2211 Fifth Avenue North • Healthy City, USA 12345 • (321) 123-4567

Consultation

Patient Name: Patrick Bridges
Birth Date: 06/23/xx

Patient Number: 77-34-77
Room Number: 215

CONSULTATION

This is a 56-year-old male who is referred for evaluation and treatment of chronic low back pain and had been seen several times in our clinic who is status post laminectomy with pain across his lower back and towards his left posterolateral portion of his leg. He has had no change in weakness or numbness and continued to have good relief for several months following his previous block and is here for continued treatment.

ALLERGIES: None

MEDICATIONS: Propulsid, Prilosec, Norvasc, Xanax, Darvocet.

PHYSICAL EXAMINATION: He is afebrile. His vital signs are stable. He again shows fairly stable exam with decreased dorsiflexion and weakness in the left side of his foot and slight decrease in pinprick sensation in this region, but otherwise is without change.

IMPRESSION: Lumbosacral disk disease and chronic pain status post laminectomy.

PLAN: Epidural via fluoroscopy and Arrow Theracath.

The risks and options of the procedure were discussed, and he wished to proceed.

ADDENDUM: He tolerated the procedure well with good pain relief and was discharged with a prescription for Darvocet as well as follow up and return instructions.

_____

Henry Blackford, M.D.

HB/emb
d&t: 02/02/xx

Medical Record 12–3. Operative Report

GENERAL HOSPITAL AND MEDICAL CENTER
2211 Fifth Avenue North • Healthy City, USA 12345 • (321) 123-4567

Operative Report

Patient Name: John Royers
Birth Date: 08/14/xx

Patient Number: 23-65-34
Room Number: 534

DATE: 03/02/xx

PREOPERATIVE DIAGNOSIS: Osteoarthritis, left hip.

POSTOPERATIVE DIAGNOSIS: Osteoarthritis, left hip.

OPERATION: Left total hip arthroplasty.

SURGEON: Mary Snyder, D.O.

ASSISTANT: John Rogers, P.A.

ANESTHESIA: General.

PROCEDURE: The patient was brought into the operating room and transported to the operating table without incident. Under satisfactory general anesthesia, he was positioned in a right lateral decubitus position, prepped with Betadine, scrubbed and draped in the usual orthopedic fashion. Direct lateral incision was made, extending from a point level with the anterior superior iliac spine and carried distally to the midpoint of the greater trochanter, and subsequently distally along the lateral aspect of the femur. Careful dissection was then carried out to the level of the underlying tensor fascia which was split the full length of the incision. We subsequently then placed the Charnley retractor and dissected free the abductor musculature, leaving a cuff of tissue for reattachment. We then performed a partial capsulectomy and because of the severe deformity of the femoral head and neck, we were forced to utilize an oscillating saw for cutting the femoral head from the neck, remove the head, and then we were able to adduct and externally rotate the femoral head and neck. Thereafter we gained entry to the femoral canal utilizing the starter reamer. This was followed by reamers of increasing size, up to a Press-Fit 10. We then utilized broaches of increasing size up to a Press-Fit 10 as well. We then turned our attention to the acetabular side, utilizing acetabular reamers up to a 58 outside diameter, then placed the appropriate cup and found that indeed we had a good fit. Being satisfied that we had, in fact, removed all cartilage and also cystic lesions within the acetabulum

Continued

Operative Report, page 2
Patient Name: John Royers   **Patient Number:** 23-65-34

proper, we then placed the final metal cup and secured it with two additional screws. We then turned our attention once again to the femur, removed the trial prosthesis and subsequently inserted a Press-Fit 10 final prosthesis, then carried out trial reductions, accepting a +5 neck. This was indeed set into place. The plastic liner was inserted into the acetabular cup, and the head then positioned and reduction and stability through a full range of motion. We then copiously irrigated once again, placed the leg on a May stand in an abducted position, and then commenced closure in layers utilizing 0 Vicryl over a Hemovac drain. The subcuticular tissue was closed with 2-0 Vicryl, and the skin was then closed with staples. Dry dressing was applied, and the patient was subsequently awakened and was transported to the recovery room in good condition, having tolerated the procedure well.

_____

Mary Snyder, D.O.

MS/bab
D: 03/02/xx
T: 03/03/xx

Medical Record 12–4. Emergency Room Report

GENERAL HOSPITAL AND MEDICAL CENTER
2211 Fifth Avenue North • Healthy City, USA 12345 • (321) 123-4567

Emergency Room Report

Patient Name: Irma Kennedy
Birth Date: 03/01/xx

Patient Number: 02-02-34
Room Number: ER

DATE OF VISIT: 05/10/20xx

CHIEF COMPLAINT: Left wrist injury.

HISTORY OF PRESENT ILLNESS: An 82-year-old white female presents with a left wrist injury. The patient states that her shrubs have not been trimmed, and she was trying to get in between them on a ladder, and fell. She fell against her left hand. She complains of pain over the left wrist. There is no numbness or tingling in the hand. The patient does have limited range of motion secondary to pain.

PHYSICAL EXAMINATION: Temperature 36.3, pulse 85, respirations 18, blood pressure 158/88. General: Alert, well-developed, well-nourished, elderly white female in no acute distress. HEENT: Normocephalic, atraumatic. Neck is supple, nontender. Lungs are clear to auscultation. Heart regular rate and rhythm. Abdomen soft, nontender. Extremities are warm and dry. The patient does have gross obvious deformity to her left wrist with swelling and posterior angulation. The pulses were palpable. She had brisk capillary refill and sensation in all her fingers. There is no tenderness over the anatomical snuffbox. Her pain was over the distal radius and ulna. Range of motion was limited secondary to pain. The patient could not fully flex, extend, or abduct her fingers secondary to pain. Otherwise, she was neurovascularly intact.

TREATMENT: X-rays of the left wrist, 3 views, showed a comminuted, intra-articular Colles fracture. There is 10 degrees of angulation, apex volar, wrist is shortened by 2-3 cm, displaced approximately 1 cm ulnarly.

Dr. Michael, the orthopedic surgeon, was called, and he reduced the fracture and put her in a splint. The patient was initially given fentanyl 25 mcg IM for pain. During the reduction, she was given an additional 25 mcg of fentanyl. Please refer to Dr. Michael's dictation for details of the procedure.

Continued

Emergency Room Report, page 2
Patient Name: Irma Kennedy   **Patient Number:** 02-02-34

DIAGNOSIS: LEFT COMMINUTED, INTRA-ARTICULAR COLLES FRACTURE.

_____

Thomas Short, M.D.

TS/jc

D&T: 05/10/xx

Structure and Function

Lymphatic System

The lymphatic system consists of lymph, lymph vessels, a number of lymphoid tissue masses known as lymph nodes, and three organs—the tonsils, thymus, and spleen. All these organs, structures, and tissues, including bone marrow, play an important role in the immune response.

As stated earlier, the major function of the lymphatic system is to drain fluid from tissue spaces and return it to the blood (Fig. 13–2). Other important functions of the lymphatic system are to transport fats from the digestive tract to the blood, to produce lymphocytes, and to develop antibodies that are important to immunity. The structures related to the lymphatic system are discussed first.

Lymph Vessels

Lymph capillaries, just like blood capillaries, are thin-walled tubes that form complex networks that carry lymph from tissue spaces to larger **lymphatic vessels.** The thin walls allow the interstitial fluid to enter the lymphatic capillaries. Basically, lymph is tissue fluid that has entered a lymphatic capillary. Once lymph enters a lymphatic capillary, it passes through larger lymphatic vessels with walls that are similar to those of veins but are slightly thinner. Just like veins, lymphatic vessels have valves that eliminate lymph backflow and guarantee the flow of lymph in one direction, toward the thoracic cavity.

Label Figure 13–3 as you read the following material about the system of lymph vessels. At the same time, observe the location of the major groups of lymph nodes.

The larger lymphatic vessels lead to specialized organs called **lymph nodes** (masses of lymph tissue) surrounded by a fibrous, connective tissue capsule. After leaving the nodes, the vessels merge to form even larger vessels called (1) **lymphatic trunks,** which drain lymph and are named for the region they serve. Lymphatic trunks join one of two collecting ducts, the (2) **right lymphatic duct** or the (3) **thoracic duct.** The thoracic duct is the larger and longer of the two. After leaving the collecting ducts, lymph enters the venous system through the (4) **left subclavian vein.**

Lymph Nodes

Small oval bodies of lymphatic tissue—lymph nodes—occur in clusters along the lymphatic vessels of the body. Lymph nodes vary in both shape and size, but each node is surrounded by a dense, fibrous connective tissue capsule. The two basic functions of lymph nodes are concerned with body protection.

1. Lymph nodes act as lymph "filters." The nodes contain special **phagocytes** that help in the purification of the lymph fluid. Phagocytes, also known as *macrophages,* remove bacteria, foreign substances, and cell debris from the lymph. This process effectively prevents them from being delivered to the blood and spreading further into the body (Fig. 13–4). The process of engulfing and destroying the bacteria is called **phagocytosis** (Fig. 13–5). Besides lymph nodes, macrophages are also located in the tonsils, spleen, liver, lungs, bones, brain, and spinal cord. About 50 percent of all macrophages are found in the liver as **Kupffer cells.** Along with **neutrophils,** macrophages are the major phagocytic cells of the immune system.

2. Lymph nodes play an important role in activating the immune system. Lymphocytes, the main warriors of the immune system, are located in the lymph nodes. As stated earlier, they monitor the lymphatic stream for the presence of *antigens* and mount an attack against them.

Continue to label the lymph nodes in Figure 13–3, and note their specific location in various regions of the body. Some of the principal groups of lymph nodes are the (5) **popliteal nodes,** the (6) **inguinal nodes,** and the (7) **iliac nodes** of the lower extremity; the (8) **lumbar nodes** of the pelvic region; the (9) **cubital** and (10) **axillary nodes** of the upper extremity; the (11) **thoracic nodes** of the chest; the (12) **cervical** and (13) **submaxillary nodes** around the neck.

Lymph nodes of the pharynx are called **tonsils.** They provide protection against bacteria and other harmful substances that enter the body through the nose or mouth. Some children experience persistent infections in the **pharyngeal** region causing the tonsils to become chronically infected. At that stage the tonsils may become the source of infection, and treatment may require a **tonsillectomy.** If tonsillectomy is performed, there are many other lymph nodes in the pharynx to take over the functions of the surgically removed tonsils.

 Activity 13-1: Competency Verification
Major Groups of Lymph Vessels and Lymph Nodes

Review the major groups of lymph nodes in Figure 13–3, and check your labeling of these structures in Appendix C.

Spleen

The soft, blood-rich spleen is the largest lymphatic organ in the body. It is situated between the upper

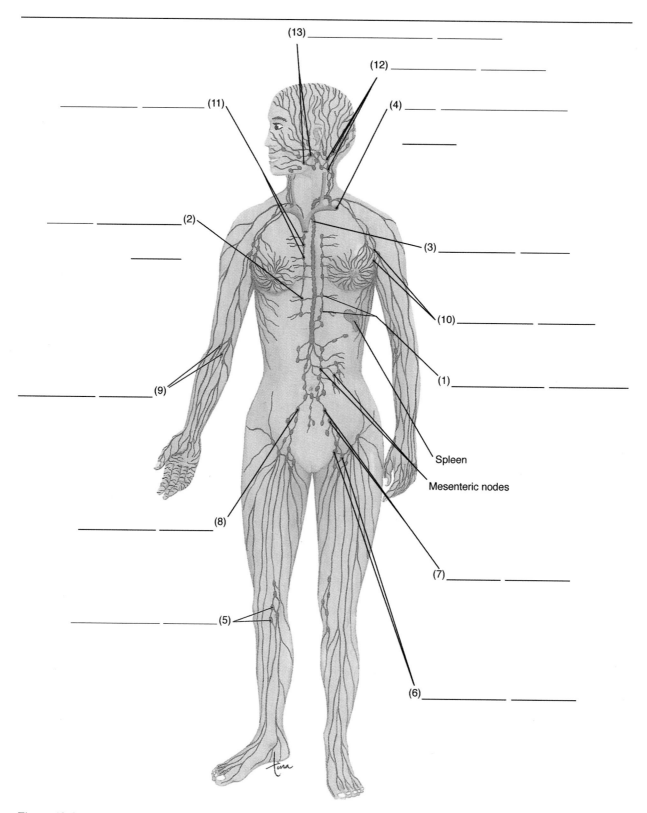

Figure 13–3 *The system of lymph vessels and the major groups of lymph nodes. Lymph is returned to the blood in the right and left subclavian veins. (Adapted from Scanlon, VC, and Sanders, TS: Essentials of Anatomy and Physiology, ed 3. FA Davis, Philadelphia, 1999, p 307, with permission.)*

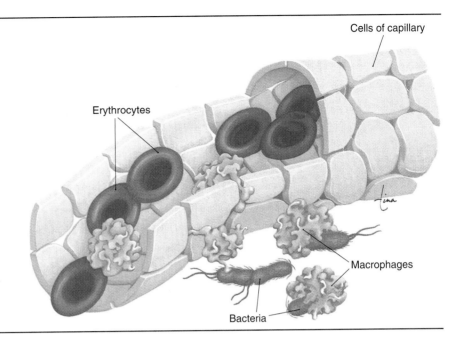

Cells of capillary

Erythrocytes

Macrophages

Bacteria

Figure 13–4 *A white blood cell (leukocyte) leaving a capillary to destroy pathogens in surrounding tissue. (From Scanlon, VC, and Sanders, TS: Essentials of Anatomy and Physiology, ed 2. FA Davis, Philadelphia, 1995, p 252, with permission.)*

left quadrant of the abdomen, just below the diaphragm and behind the stomach. The lower rib cage protects the spleen from physical trauma.

Besides providing a site for lymphocyte proliferation and immune surveillance, the spleen plays an important role in the immune response by filtering the blood and destroying old erythrocytes by macrophages (see Fig. 13–4). The spleen also removes **pathogens** of various kinds from the blood that flow through its sinuses. Despite its large size and many important functions, an excision of the spleen, known as **splenectomy,** seems to create few problems because the liver and bone marrow take over most of its functions. Nonetheless, postsplenectomy patients are more susceptible to some bacterial infections, such as pneumonia and meningitis. In a child younger than 12, the spleen will regenerate if a small part of it is left in the body.

Thymus

The thymus is located in the anterior thorax just beneath the sternum. In infants the thymus is large and extends under the sternum (Fig. 13–6). With progression of puberty, the size of the thymus tends to regress so that there is very little thymus tissue found in adults.

Although the endocrine functions of the thymus are rather obscure, it does secrete a hormone called **thymosin,** which is important in the development of immune responses in children. This hormone stimulates the red bone marrow to produce **T lymphocytes** or **T cells.** The thymus also stores lymphocytes and converts some of them into T cells. T cells play an important role in the immune system as discussed in the following section.

Immune System
Antigens and Antibodies

Antigens are **markers** on the surface of cells that identify cells as being the body's own cells or as being foreign cells. Cells of an individual person have their own unique antigens, which are identified as **self.** Antigens of foreign substances are identified as intruders, invaders, or **nonself.** Each and every pathogen, or foreign substance, has its own unique antigens. Appearance of nonself substances induces an immune response for their eventual destruction or neutralization. A single bacterium, or a single molecule of a toxin, may have several antigens or markers. In this case the body will be induced to release several kinds of **antibodies.** Viruses, bacteria, protozoa, fungi, allergens, malignant cells, transplanted tissue, and organs can trigger immune responses.

Antibodies, also known as **immunoglobulins (Igs),** constitute the **gamma globulin** part of blood proteins. The gamma globulins are divided into five classes of antibodies: immunoglobulin M (IgM), immunoglobulin A (IgA), immunoglobulin D (IgD), immunoglobulin G (IgG), and immunoglobulin E (IgE). (To remember the five Ig types, think of the word *MADGE.*) Each class of antibodies has a different structure (Fig. 13–7). They also have different locations and functions in the body (Table 13–1).

The antibodies are secreted by plasma cells in response to an antigen. They do not themselves destroy foreign antigens but become attached to such antigens to "label" them for destruction. Each antibody is specific for only one antigen, and the plasma cells of

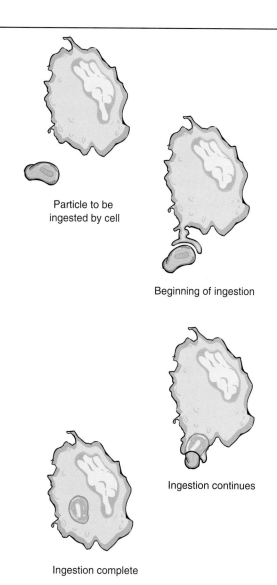

Particle to be ingested by cell

Beginning of ingestion

Ingestion continues

Ingestion complete

Figure 13–5 *Phagocytosis. (From Williams, LS, and Hopper, PD: Understanding Medical-Surgical Nursing. FA Davis, Philadelphia, 1999, p 103, with permission.)*

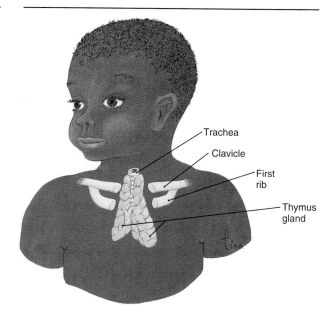

Figure 13–6 *The location of the thymus in a young child. (From Scanlon, VC, and Sanders, TS: Essentials of Anatomy and Physiology, ed 3. FA Davis, Philadelphia, 1999, p 305, with permission.)*

an individual are capable of producing millions of different antibodies, or **antigen-specific** antibodies. Figure 13–8 illustrates how antibodies bind with the antigen like two pieces of a jigsaw puzzle.

Immune Response

The body's immune system is a specific defense system that tracks down and destroys almost any type of pathogen that invades the body. As a *functional system*, it identifies specific foreign substances and acts to immobilize, neutralize, or eliminate them. A healthy immune system protects us from a variety of infectious agents as well as abnormal body cells. It recognizes a foreign antigen and activates an immune response. A disabled, or malfunctioning, immune system may result in some of the most devastating diseases, such as rheumatoid arthritis, cancer, and AIDS. The activity of the immune system is known as the *immune response.*

The lymphocytes known as T cells and B cells are the major disease fighters involved in specific immune responses. This means that each cell is genetically programmed to respond to one specific kind of foreign antigen. It is estimated that the human immune system can respond to hundreds of millions of different foreign antigens. Less than 1 percent of lymphocytes reside in the circulating blood; the rest lie in the lymph nodes, spleen, and other lymphoid organs, where they can maximize contact with foreign antigens. Each type performs different functions.

In the fetus, both T cells and B cells develop in the bone marrow. T cells originate from bone marrow **stem cells** and migrate to the thymus, where the thymic hormones bring about their maturation. The T cells then migrate to the lymph nodes and nodules throughout the body and to the spleen. B cells originate from bone marrow stem cells and migrate directly to lymphatic tissue. During an immune response some B cells become plasma cells and have the capacity to produce antibodies, which eventually bind to a specific foreign antigen.

The involvement of T cells in cell-mediated immunity and B cells in humoral immunity is discussed next.

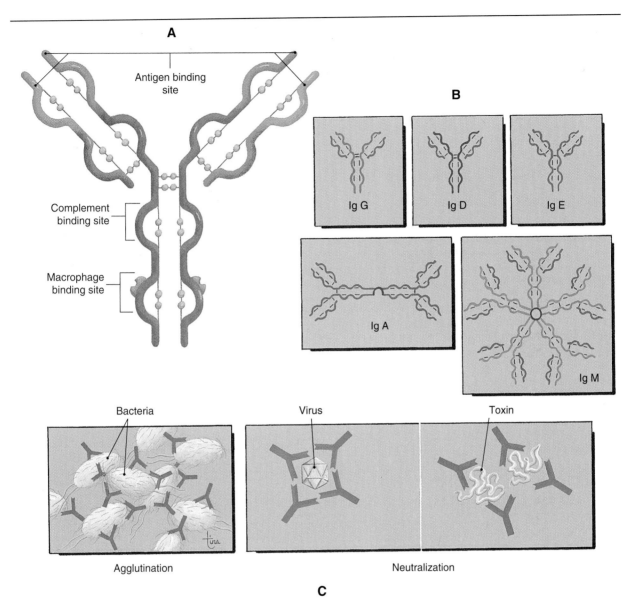

Figure 13–7 *Antibodies. (A) Structure of an antibody. (B) Structure of the five classes of antibodies. (C) Antibody activity: agglutination of bacteria and neutralization of viruses or toxins. (From Scanlon, VC, and Sanders, TS: Essentials of Anatomy and Physiology, ed 3. FA Davis, Philadelphia, 1999, p 310, with permission.)*

Cell-Mediated Immunity

When lymphocytes defend the body, the immunity is known as **cell-mediated immunity** because the protective factor is living cells. Cell-mediated immunity does not involve the production of antibodies and is essentially directed against intracellular pathogens, such as parasites, bacteria, viruses, malignant cells, fungi, and grafts of foreign tissue. The sensitized circulating lymphocytes, upon their return to the nearest node, stimulate the residing lymphocytes to become various types of sensitized T cells. These lymphocytes are referred to as "T" because they have spent some time in the thymus gland of the developing fetus

where they were programmed to become T cells. The newly created army of T cells becomes specialized to perform several activities. **Killer T cells,** also known as **cytotoxic cells,** are programmed to lyse (disintegrate) cells such as cancer cells or those infected by viruses or other intracellular parasites. They also release chemicals that activate phagocytes, such as macrophages and neutrophils (see Fig. 13–5). **Helper T cells** function to chemically or directly stimulate the proliferation of other T cells and B cells. **Memory T cells** have the ability to remember specific antigens and quickly activate the immune response if they reappear on a future occasion. **Suppressor T cells**

TABLE 13–1: Classes of Antibodies

NAME	LOCATION	FUNCTION
Immunoglobulin M (IgM)	Blood	Produced first by the maturing immune system of infants Produced first during an infection (IgG production follows)
Immunoglobulin A (IgA)	External secretions (e.g., tears, saliva)	Present in breast milk; provides passive immunity for breast-fed infants Found in secretions of all mucous membranes
Immunoglobulin D (IgD)	B lymphocytes (B cells)	Antigen-specific receptors on B lymphocytes (B cells)
Immunoglobulin G (IgG)	Blood, extracellular fluid	Crosses the placenta to provide passive immunity for newborns Provides long-term immunity following recovery or a vaccination
Immunoglobulin E (IgE)	Mast cells or basophils	Important in allergic reactions; mast cells release histamine

Note: Immunoglobulins, also called gamma globulins, are antibodies that play an important role in immunity. To remember the five Ig types, think of the word MADGE.

are responsible for determining the quantity of T cells and B cells to be produced, so that the immune response is only as strong as the need dictates.

Humoral Immunity

Humoral immunity is provided by antibodies present in the body's "humors," or fluids, such as the blood or lymph. Antibodies produced by lymphocytes circulate freely in the blood and lymph, where they bind primarily to bacteria and their toxins and to free viruses, inactivating them temporarily and marking them for destruction. Humoral immunity is characterized by production of antibodies in response to a specific antigen. When a B cell is confronted with a specific type of antigen, it transforms into a plasma cell. These cells produce antibodies known as im-

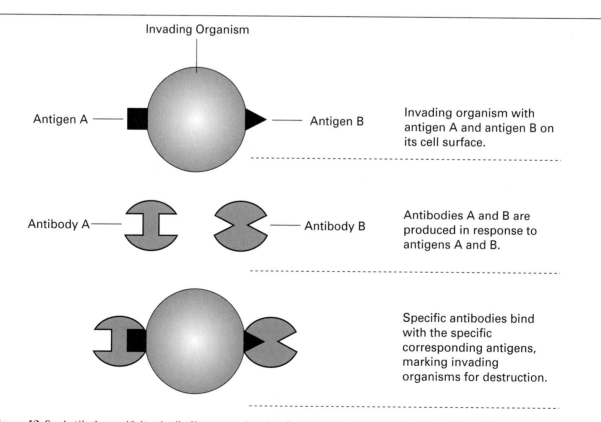

Invading Organism

Antigen A — Antigen B

Invading organism with antigen A and antigen B on its cell surface.

Antibody A — Antibody B

Antibodies A and B are produced in response to antigens A and B.

Specific antibodies bind with the specific corresponding antigens, marking invading organisms for destruction.

Figure 13–8 *Antibody specificity. Antibodies are produced by B-cell lymphocytes to bind with specific antigens.*

ABBREVIATION	MEANING	ABBREVIATION	MEANING
FISH	fluorescence in situ hybridization (newer cytogenetic technique that can detect cryptic abnormalities not evident by standard cytogenetic banding studies)	**MAI**	*Myobacterium avium intracellulare*
		RS	Reed-Sternberg (cells)
		Toxo	toxoplasmosis (parasitic infection associated with AIDS)
Histo	histoplasmosis (fungal infection seen in AIDS virus in serum)	**WBC, wbc**	white blood cell, white blood count
LDL	low-density lipoprotein		

Activity 13–5: Clinical Application
Diagnostic Procedures and Treatments and Pharmacology

AIDS cocktail
antiglobulin test
antivirals
bone marrow aspiration biopsy
chemotherapy
ELISA

immunosuppressants
immunotherapy
PCP
tissue typing
vaccination
Western blot

Match the terms listed above with the definitions given in the numbered list:

1. _____ a laboratory test used to detect the presence of HIV; more precise than ELISA.

2. _____ injection of attenuated microorganisms; administered to induce immunity or to reduce the effects associated with infectious diseases.

3. _____ a test for the presence of antibodies that coat and damage RBCs as a result of any of several diseases or conditions; also called *Coomb test.*

4. _____ agents that significantly suppress the body's natural immune response to an antigen; administered in treatment of transplant patients.

5. _____ a combination of drugs used to retard HIV replication and mutation.

6. _____ removal of living tissue from the bone marrow by suction through a fine needle attached to a syringe; used for microscopic evaluation.

7. _____ technique used to determine the histocompatibility of tissues to be used in grafts and transplants with the recipient's tissues and cells.

8. _____ the application of immunologic knowledge and techniques to prevent and treat disease.

9. _____ treatment of disease by means of chemical agents.

10. _____ drugs used to treat various viral conditions such as herpes virus infection, chickenpox, and influenza A.

Correct Answers _____ × 10 = _____% Score

Activity 13–6: Build Medical Words
Diagnostic, Symptomatic, and Surgical Terms

Use *aden/o* (gland) to build medical words meaning:

1. inflammation of a gland _____

2. disease of a gland _____

3. excision of a gland _____

Use *angi/o* (vessel) to build medical words meaning:

4. disease of a vessel _____

5. forming, producing, or origin of a (blood) vessel _____

6. suture of any vessel _____

Use *agglutin/o* (clumping, gluing) to build medical words meaning:

7. process of clumping or gluing _____

8. forming, producing, or origin of clumping or gluing _____

Use *immun/o* (immune, immunity) to build medical words meaning:

9. study of immunity _____

10. specialist in the study of immunity _____

11. producing immunity _____

Use *phag/o* (swallowing, eating) to build medical words meaning:

12. a cell that ingests _____

13. pertaining to a cell that ingests _____

Use *splen/o* (spleen) to build medical words meaning:

14. enlargement of the spleen _____

15. enlargement of the spleen and liver _____

Use *thym/o* (thymus gland) to build medical words meaning:

16. tumor of the thymus gland _____

Use -*asthenia* (weakness, debility) to build a medical word meaning:

17. weakness or debility of muscles _____

Use lymph/o (lymph) to build medical words meaning:

18. tumor of lymph tissue _____

19. disease of the lymph glands _____

Use -*phylaxis* (protection) to build a medical word meaning:

20. against protection _____

Correct Answers _____ × 5 = _____ % Score

MEDICAL RECORDS

Authentic medical records of a patient diagnosed with HIV and a patient who had a bone marrow transplant are presented in this chapter. The records include a discharge summary, chart notes, and clinical team notes.

The following dictionary exercise and medical record analysis will help you develop skills to abstract information and master the terminology in the reports. Accurate interpretation is important because this type of information is utilized in numerous areas of the medical practice, such as initiation of treatments, evaluation of patient's progress, and completion of insurance claims.

Reading and Dictionary Exercise

Check the box [✓] after you complete the exercise.

[   ] **1.** Underline the following words in the reports as you read the discharge summary, chart notes, and clinical team notes aloud. These medical records can be found at the end of the chapter.

[   ] **2.** Use a medical dictionary; and Appendix F, Part 2 to define the terms below.

Note: You are not expected to fully understand all the parts of the medical records. The important aspect of this exercise is to use all available resources to complete it. Eventually you will master the terminology and format of these reports.

> > > MEDICAL RECORD 13–1: DISCHARGE SUMMARY

Term	Pronunciation	Meaning
Pneumocystis carinii	*nū-mō-SĬS-tĭs kă-RĬ-nē-ī*	_____
ganciclovir	*găn-SĪ-klō-vēr*	_____
Neupogen	*NŪ-pō-jĕn*	_____
bronchoscopy	*brŏng-KŎS-kō-pē*	_____

Term	Pronunciation	Meaning
cystomegalovirus	*sī-tō-MĔG-ă-lō-vī-rŭs*	_____
antiretroviral therapy	*ăn-tĭ-rĕ-trō-VĪ-răl THĔR-ă-pē*	_____
AZT		_____
3TC		_____
Viracept	*VĪ-ră-sept*	_____
Kaposi sarcoma	*KAP-ō-sē săr-KŌ-mă*	_____
asymptomatic	*ā-sĭmp-tō-MĂT-ĭk*	_____
diarrhea	*dī-ă-RĒ-ă*	_____
thrush	*thrŭsh*	_____
vaginal candidiasis	*VĂJ-ĭn-ăl kăn-dĭ-DĪ-ă-sĭs*	_____
tachypneic	*tăk-ĭp-NĒ-ĭk*	_____
Bactrim	*BĂK-trĭm*	_____
auscultation	*aws-kŭl-TĀ-shŭn*	_____
antimicrobials	*ăn-tĭ-mī-KRŌ-bē-ăls*	_____

> > > MEDICAL RECORD 13-2: CHART NOTES

Term	Pronunciation	Meaning
zidovudine	*zĭ-DŌ-vū-dēn*	_____
lamivudine	*lă-MĒ-vū-dĭn*	_____
maculopapular	*măk-ū-lō-PĂP-ū-lăr*	_____
differential	*dĭf-ĕr-ĕn-shăl*	_____
neutropenia	*nū-trō-PĒ-nē-ă*	_____
phenotype	*FĒ-nō-tīp*	_____
supraclavicular	*soo-pră-klă-VĬK-ū-lăr*	_____
palpated	*PĂL-pā-tĕd*	_____
hepatosplenomegaly	*hĕp-ă-tō-splē-nō-MĔG-ă-lē*	_____
floaters	*FLŌ-tĕrs*	_____
quadrant	*KWŎD-rănt*	_____

wasting	_WĀST-ĭng_	_____
immunosuppression	_ĭm-ū-nō-sŭ-PRĔSH-ŭn_	_____
immunocompetent	_ĭm-ū-nō-KŎM-pĕ-tĕnt_	_____
Epogen	_ĔP-ō-jĕn_	_____
Sustiva	_sŭs-TĬ-vă_	_____

> > > MEDICAL REPORT 13-3: CLINICAL TEAM NOTES

Term	Pronunciation	Meaning
allogenic	_ăl-ō-JĔN-ĭk_	_____
stem cell	_stĕm sĕl_	_____
Actigall	_ĂK-tĭ-gawl_	_____
cyclosporine	_sī-klō-SPOR-ĭn_	_____
Septra	_SĔP-tră_	_____
supple	_SŬ-pĕl_	_____
adenopathy	_ăd-ĕ-NŎP-ă-thē_	_____
gallop	_GĂL-ŏp_	_____
ovoid	_Ō-voyd_	_____
hepatosplenomegaly	_hĕp-ă-tō-splē-nō-MĔG-ă-lē_	_____
maculopapular	_măk-ū-lō-PĂP-ū-lăr_	_____
erythematous	_ĕr-ĭ-THĔM-ă-tŭs_	_____

Critical Thinking: Analysis of Medical Records

This section provides experience in abstracting and analyzing information from medical records. At the same time, it reinforces the material presented in this chapter.

> > > MEDICAL RECORD 13-1: DISCHARGE SUMMARY

1. What type of infection does this patient have? What was the most likely mode of transmission?

_____

_____

2. Place a "+" in the space provided for positive findings and a "−" for negative findings. A positive finding indicates the patient had a history (Hx) of this condition; a negative finding indicates the patient did not have a history of this condition.

____ vaginal candidiasis   ____ Kaposi sarcoma

____ tachypnea and tachycardia   ____ AIDS-wasting syndrome

____ *Pneumocystis carinii* pneumonia   ____ bronchitis

3 How was her child affected by her disease? Is the child being monitored by a physician?

_____

_____

> > > MEDICAL RECORD 13-2: CHART NOTES

4. What are the results of her CBC? What do the results mean?

_____

_____

_____

_____

5. Explain what it means when the patient complains of "floaters" in her visual field.

_____

_____

6. What was the "Plan of Care" for pneumococcal vaccination, PICC line, and Pap?

_____

_____

_____

_____

> > > MEDICAL RECORD 13-3: CLINICAL TEAM NOTES

7. What is CML? What segment of the population is most at risk for contracting this disease?

_____

_____

_____

8. What subjective symptoms is the patient experiencing?

_____

_____

_____

9. What abnormalities were found during the physical examination with the integumentary system?

_____

_____

_____

10. What is the probable cause of the patient's integumentary problem?

_____

_____

11. What treatment is prescribed to reduce the chances of infection while the patient is taking immunosuppressants?

_____

12. Why is the doctor performing a biopsy on Mr. Salem?

_____

_____

Audio Practice

Listen to the audio CD-ROM to practice the pronunciation of selected medical terms from this chapter.

Medical Record 13–1. Discharge Summary

GENERAL HOSPITAL AND MEDICAL CENTER
2211 Fifth Avenue North • Healthy City, USA 12345 • (321) 123-4567

Discharge Summary

Patient Name: Shanna Davis

Patient Number: 34-22-09

Birth Date: 09/14/xx

Admission Date: 3/28/xx

Discharge Date: 3/31/xx

ADMISSION DIAGNOSES:
Human immunodeficiency virus (HIV) infection
Presumptive Pneumocystis carinii pneumonia (PCP) with acute respiratory distress.
Wasting.

FINAL DIAGNOSES:
Pneumocystis carinii pneumonia.
Human immunodeficiency virus infection.
Wasting.

COMPLICATIONS: None.

OPERATIONS AND SPECIAL PROCEDURES:
Bronchoscopy on 3/29/xx
PICC line for ganciclovir therapy, 3/30/xx

CONDITION ON DISCHARGE: Improved.

DISPOSITION: Home with visiting nurse service for Neupogen and cytomegalovirus therapy

HISTORY OF PRESENT ILLNESS: The patient is a 26-year-old female who had been diagnosed as having an HIV infection 13 months ago. At that time she was started on triple drug antiretroviral therapy: AZT, 3TC, and Viracept. Her adherence to the regimen has been intermittent, and antiretroviral resistance is a concern. She presented to the ER with fever and chest pain, symptoms she had experienced for the last two weeks. She had been seen in a local emergency room for these symptoms on 3/3/xx and 3/12xx.   A chest x-ray performed on last visit was read as normal.

SOCIAL HISTORY: Her husband is deceased from AIDS one year ago with progressive multifocal leukoencephalopathy (PML) and Kaposi sarcoma. She has one child, age 3, who was diagnosed at the time when the patient was diagnosed. The child is being managed by a pediatric infectious disease specialist. The child is asymptomatic at this time except for failure to thrive.

Continued

Discharge Summary, page 2
Patient Name: Shanna Davis   **Patient Number:** 34-22-09

She denies any history of injecting drug use, transfusion, and identifies three lifetime sexual partners.

Her past medical history is significant for HIV and several episodes of diarrhea, sinusitis, thrush and vaginal candidiasis. Her fever was 102. She exhibited shortness of breath on exertion. Her oxygen saturation was 97 at rest but dropped to 95 on ambulation. She was tachypneic and mildly tachycardic. She gave a history of a 20-pound weight loss. The chest x-ray showed diffuse lower lobe infiltrates, and she was diagnosed with presumptive Pneumocystis carinii pneumonia and placed on Bactrim. She was admitted for a bronchoscopy with alveolar lavage to confirm the diagnosis. The antiretroviral treatment was re-initiated and she was counseled as to the need to strictly adhere to her therapeutic regimen.

A CBC with differential, T-cell subset, HIV viral load, and HIV phenotype were drawn. The bronchoscopy was performed on the morning after admission with no complications. On discharge she is able to ambulate without shortness of breath. Her lungs are clear to auscultation, and the most recent x-ray revealed resolving infiltrates.

HOSPITAL COURSE: The patient was admitted and bronchoscopy performed the following morning. No complications. Antimicrobials for PCP and her antiretrovirals were started. She was discharged 2 days post admission and has been given an appointment to follow up with the infectious disease physician in 1 week.

DISCHARGE MEDICATIONS: AZT, 3TC, Viracept, Bactrim.

DIET AND ACTIVITY: Activity as tolerated. Regular diet with increased protein and calories. Dietary consult at next clinic visit.

_____
Melvin Jamison, D.O.

MJ/slr

D: 03/31/xx
T: 04/02/xx

Medical Record 13–2. Chart Notes

GENERAL HOSPITAL AND MEDICAL CENTER
2211 Fifth Avenue North • Healthy City, USA 12345 • (321) 123-4567

Chart Notes

Patient Name: Shanna Davis   **Patient Number:** 34-22-09
Birth Date: 09/14/xx   **Room Number:** Clinic

DATE OF VISIT: 04/15/xx

Weight: 98 pounds
BP: 110/92
RR: 24
HR: 112

<u>Meds</u>: Bactrim b.i.d.
        zidovudine (AZT)
        lamivudine (3TC)
        Viracept (nelfinavir)

SUBJECTIVE:
Complains of shortness of breath on occasion, tires easily, rash and diarrhea.

OBJECTIVE:
The patient "No Showed" for her infectious disease appointment but does return to the clinic for her rescheduled appointment today, two weeks post discharge. At this time she reports severe diarrhea, fatigue, and continued weight loss. She has developed a fine maculopapular rash indicative of a hypersensitivity reaction, presumptively to Bactrim. The T cell subset values from her admission were 120 (9%). Her CBC with differential reveals profound neutropenia, and her viral load is 257,000. The bronchoscopy specimen was positive for Pneumocystis on silver stain. The phenotype indicates resistance to AZT and Viracept.

On physical exam, she demonstrates shotty lymphadenopathy in the anterior cervical region, but no axillary or supraclavicular nodes are palpated. Abdominal exam reveals hepatosplenomegaly at 4 fingerbreadths. Her respiratory status has improved though she has some shortness of breath on exertion. She is complaining of "floaters" in her visual field. Her retinal exam reveals some cotton wool spots in the right lower quadrant visual field. She has lost another 10 pounds since discharge, and her temporal lobe wasting is more prominent.

Continued

Chart Notes, page 2
Patient Name: Shanna Davis   **Patient Number:** 34-22-09

ASSESSMENT:
Profound immunosuppression. Resolving PCP. Continued wasting. Presumptive
cytomegalovirus retinitis. Allergic reaction to Bactrim. Neutropenia. May not be
immunocompetent to respond to vaccinations.

PLAN:
1. Ophthalmology consult.
2. Pneumococcal vaccination. Follow up Pneumococcal immunoglobulin testing in 6 weeks
   to measure for adequate antibody production.
3. Skin anergy test battery for immunocompetence.
4. Discontinue Bactrim, initiate aerosolized pentamidine treatments q month, starting with a
   treatment today.
5. Start ganciclovir intravenous therapy and continue for the next ten days.
6. PICC line to be placed for ganciclovir therapy and ongoing monitoring of neutropenia.
7. Arrange for Epogen injection 3 times per week through visiting nurse services.
8. Discontinue Viracept and AZT and start d4T and Sustiva at a b.i.d. dosing regimen.
9. Repeat viral load at this visit to establish baseline for new regimen.
10. Pap on next clinic visit; not done today due to stage of menstrual cycle.
11. Patient counseled as to the need for contraception on Sustiva due to the teratogenic
    effects of this drug.
12. Labs today to include hepatitis battery; (partner was HIV positive) liver profile, chem-20
    and amylase.

_____

Melvin Jamison, D.O.

MJ/art
D: 04/15/xx
T: 04/16/xx

Medical Record 13–3. Clinical Team Notes

GENERAL HOSPITAL AND MEDICAL CENTER
2211 Fifth Avenue North • Healthy City, USA 12345 • (321) 123-4567

Clinical Team Notes

Patient Name: Eugene Salem   **Patient Number:** 34-22-12
Birth Date: 08/23/xx   **Room Number:** 893

DIAGNOSIS: CML status post allogenic peripheral blood stem cell transplant on 1/18/xx from his brother.

CURRENT MEDICATIONS: Magnesium Oxide two tablets p.o. q.i.d., Actigall 300 mg p.o. t.i.d., cyclosporine 75 mg p.o. q.a.m., 50 mg p.o. q.p.m., Septra DS one p.o. Saturday, Sunday, and Monday.

SUBJECTIVE: Mr. Salem states that he has one loose stool per week. He has had a decreased appetite since starting Actigall 7/25 and he has also had a corresponding weight loss 1.8 kg over the past month. He continues to have a coating on his tongue and the inside of his mouth feels rough. He denies pain, nausea, vomiting, fever, sweats, chills, cough, sore throat, bleeding or urinary symptoms, headaches, visual changes, and shortness of breath.

OBJECTIVE: Vital signs: Temperature 36.3, blood pressure 116/81, heart rate 70, respiratory rate 20, weight 104.7 kg. Well developed, well nourished white male in no apparent distress. Pupils equally round and reactive to light. Mildly injected sclera. EOMI. Oral mucosa with white reticular coating, bilateral buccal mucosa with thick coating on tongue. Neck supple without adenopathy and chest clear to auscultation. Cardiovascular: Regular rate and rhythm without murmur, rub, or gallop. Abdomen soft, ovoid, nontender, nondistended. Normal bowel sounds times four without hepatosplenomegaly. Extremities without edema. Skin: Maculopapular erythematous rash on entire back, upper chest, upper arms with an erythematous flush to the patient's face. Maculopapular rash involves approximately 20 to 25% of the body surface area.

LABORATORY DATA: WBC 4.5, hemoglobin 14.3, hematocrit 41.2, platelets 78, 39%, neutrophils, 23% lymphocytes, 10% monos, 27% eosinophils, 1% bands, sodium 136, potassium 4.0, chloride 103, CO_2 29, BUN 10, creatinine 1.2, glucose 101, calcium 8.4, magnesium 2.0, total protein 6.4, albumin 3.2, total bilirubin 1.0, alkaline phosphatase 112, LDH 665, AST 155, ALT 158.

Continued

clude **acetylcholine, epinephrine,** and **dopamine.** Each neuron has contact with up to 20 synapses. This makes the total number of possible synaptic contacts among the 50 billion neurons in the body about one trillion. This should give you some idea of how complex this system is, as well as how neural information is transmitted seemingly instantaneously.

Many axons in both the PNS and CNS are covered with a white, fatty (lipoid) sheath made of **myelin,** which acts as an electrical insulator to keep the impulse traveling down the axon. This sheath accelerates the impulse to the terminals and keeps the impulse from stimulating adjacent nerves and short-circuiting. This covering is called the (6) **myelin sheath.** The sheath gives the white appearance to the axons of the brain and spinal cord is known as **white matter.** Unmyelinated fibers, dendrites, and nerve cell bodies make up what is known as the **gray matter.** When axons that should be myelinated lose their sheaths, significant problems can arise, such as multiple sclerosis (see the Pathology section of this chapter).

Peripheral nerves have an additional cellular membrane that covers the myelin sheath. This additional covering is called the (7) **neurolemma,** or neurolemmal sheath, and is made up of layers of (8) **Schwann cells.** This covering permits a damaged axon to regenerate. Because neurolemma is not found in the CNS, damaged or severed nerves in the spinal cord and brain cannot regenerate, and nerve function is permanently lost.

Activity 14–1: Competency Verification
Structures of the Neuron

Review Figure 14–2, and check your labeling of the various neuron structures in Appendix C.

The Classification of Neurons

There are three types of neurons that may be classified according to their structure or function: **sensory** neurons, **motor** neurons, and **mixed** neurons (also called **interneurons**). The various types of neurons are bundled together to form nerves and are referred to as sensory nerves, motor nerves, and mixed nerves.

The **sensory neurons,** also known as **afferent nerves,** carry impulses from receptors in the skin, skeletal muscles, joints, and internal organs *toward* the spinal cord and brain (*af=toward; ferent=to carry*). This pathway conducts *sensory* information, that is, information regarding what the peripheral receptors are "sensing." This would include sensations of heat, cold, pain, pressure, brightness, etc. The mes-

sages that originate in these peripheral receptors are sent *toward* the brain. When the brain receives these messages via the sensory pathway, it interprets the information as a sensation. Then it responds to the sensation by sending impulses back toward the peripheral muscles and glands telling them to respond in a particular way. These outgoing impulses are sent by way of the **motor neurons,** also known as **efferent nerves** (*ef=away from; ferent=to carry*). Motor nerves conduct the messages *away from* the central nervous system.

An example of this process of incoming and outgoing information is described in the following example. Imagine that you have been so intent on reading this chapter that you have not realized that your neck was beginning to hurt. The receptors in your neck begin to ache because those muscles have been contracted for so long. The message of pain is sent from the muscles to the brain by way of the *sensory nerves.* Once the brain receives the message, it responds in order to restore equilibrium by getting rid of the pain. Thus, it sends a message back to those neck muscles to move and change position. It sends this message by way of the *motor nerves.*

There are also **interneurons,** or **mixed nerves,** that are composed of *both* sensory and motor fibers. For example, the facial nerve has both types of fibers. When the tongue receptors transmit a taste, the facial nerve is operating as a sensory nerve. When this muscle contracts to move food around in the mouth, the facial nerve is functioning as a motor nerve.

Neuroglia

Neuroglia provide many supportive and protective functions for the neurons. They are generally smaller than neurons and outnumber them 5 to 13 times. It was once thought that neuroglia served only a support role for neurons. Although many do function this way by twining around neurons forming support networks, it is now known that there are other types of neuroglia that serve functions other than support. There are four types of neuroglia: **astrocytes, oligodendrites, microglia,** and **ependymocytes,** as illustrated in Figure 14–3.

- **Astrocytes** (*astro=star, cyte=cell*) are star-shaped cells that twine around neurons to form a supporting network in the brain and spinal cord and attach neurons to their blood vessels. They also form a selective barrier, known as the *blood-brain barrier,* that slows the passage of some drugs and keeps harmful substances from leaving the blood and crossing the capillary walls into the brain tissues. It serves as a protective mechanism that helps maintain a stable environment for the brain.

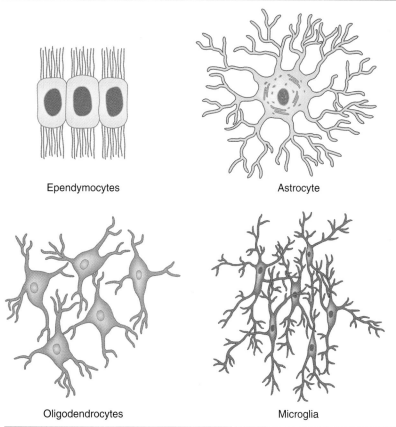

Ependymocytes

Astrocyte

Oligodendrocytes

Microglia

Figure 14-3   *The four types of neuroglia.*

- **Oligodendrites** (*oligo=scanty, dendr=tree*) resemble astrocytes, but their projections are fewer and shorter. They help to develop the myelin sheath around axons of CNS neurons.

- **Microglia** (*micro=small, glia=glue, neuroglia tissue*) are the smallest neuroglia. They are capable of movement, as well as of phagocytosis of damaged tissue and pathogens during infection.

- **Ependymocytes** (*ependyma=upper garment, wrap, cytes=cells*) are epithelial cells, many of which are ciliated. They are arranged in a single layer lining the ventricles of the brain and are involved in the circulation of the cerebrospinal fluid. Also called *ependymal cells.*

Neuroglia are a common source of gliomas (tumors). It is estimated that gliomas account for 40 to 45 percent of brain tumors (see pathology section below).

Activity 14–2: Competency Verification

Pathway of the Electrochemical Impulse of the Neuron and the Classification of Neurons

Refer to the material discussed above and to Figure 14–2 to complete this activity.

Pathway and Structures of an Electrochemical Impulse

1. _____ the two principal types of cells in the nervous system.

2. _____ the structure that conducts impulses from one part of the body to another; also called nerve cells.

3. _____ the supportive cells in the nervous system.

4. _____ the three main parts of the neuron.

5. _____ the part of the neuron that contains the cell nucleus.

6. _____ a short, thick, highly branched structure that is an extension of cytoplasm; a cell body *receives* impulses from other cells through these structures.

7. _____ a long, thin, single projection that transmits the impulse from the cell body of one neuron to the dendrites of another neuron, or to the surrounding tissue; a cell body *sends out* impulses through these structures.

8. _____ the structures that form the ends of axon terminals.

9. _____ the small space between the axon of one neuron and the dendrite, or cell body, of another.

10. _____ special chemical messengers that move impulses across the synapse.

11. _____ structures that cause the bulbs to release neurotransmitters.

12. _____ structure that has contact with up to 20 synapses.

13. _____ the fatty sheath that accelerates impulses to terminals and keeps adjacent nerves from short-circuiting.

14. _____ tissue that is made up of unmyelinated fibers, dendrites, and nerve cells.

15. _____ the cellular membrane that covers the myelin sheath of peripheral nerves.

Classification of Neurons

16. _____ three types of neurons that may be classified according to their structure or function.

17. _____ nerves that carry impulses from receptors in the skin and internal organs toward the brain and spinal cord.

18. _____ nerves that conduct messages *away from* the central nervous system; motor neurons.

19. _____ nerves that are composed of both sensory and nerve fibers; interneurons.

20. _____ four types of neuroglia.

Correct Answers _____ × 5 = _____% **Score**

Spinal Cord

The spinal cord transmits impulses to and from the brain and is protected from mechanical injury by the vertebral canal (see Chapter 12). The cord consists of bundles of nerve fibers grouped into nerve tracts. These nerve tracts are grouped according to their function. The **ascending tracts** consist of the sensory nerve fibers that carry sensory impulses to the brain. The **descending tracts** are made up of groups of motor nerves and carry impulses away from the brain to the muscles and extremities.

As stated before, the axons of the nerve fibers in the CNS are white with myelin, whereas the cell bodies and dendrites are not. A cross-section of the spinal cord reveals a butterfly-like pattern made up of the internal **gray matter** surrounded by the **white matter**.

Spinal Nerves

Label Fig 14–4 as you read the following material.

The 31 pairs of spinal nerves that emerge from the spinal cord are named according to the vertebrae from which they emanate. There are 8 cervical pairs designated as (1) **C1–C8;** 12 thoracic pairs designated as (2) **T1–T12;** 5 lumbar pairs designated as (3) **L1–L5;** 5 sacral pairs designated as (4) **S1–S5,** and 1 very small coccygeal pair designated by (5) **CO1.** Notice that each nerve in Figure 14–4 is designated by a letter and a number. The eighth cervical nerve is C8, the first thoracic nerve is T1, and so on.

In general, the cervical nerves supply the back of the head, neck, shoulders, arms, and diaphragm. The first thoracic nerve also contributes to nerves in the arms. The remaining thoracic nerves supply the trunk of the body. The lumbar and sacral nerves supply the hips, pelvic cavity, and legs. Notice that the lumbar and sacral nerves hang below the end of the spinal cord (to reach their proper openings to exit from the vertebral canal).

When a person sustains a spinal cord injury, the level of injury and the level of residual functioning is designated by these numbers. For example, a person with a T3 injury would have damage to the spinal cord at the third thoracic nerve. Injuries to the spinal cord affect people of all ages but take their greatest toll on young people. These injuries are characterized by decrease or loss of sensory and motor function below the level of the injury. Review Figure 14–4, for the graphic illustration of the spinal cord, spinal cord injuries, and the locations of the spinal nerves.

Spinal Cord Reflexes

A reflex is an automatic and involuntary response to a stimulus. Spinal cord reflexes are those that do not depend directly on the brain, although the brain may inhibit or enhance the reflexive response. There are two kinds of spinal cord reflexes: stretch and flexor reflexes. In a **stretch reflex,** a muscle that is stretched will automatically contract in response, such as the **knee-jerk reflex.** All skeletal muscles have this reflex to keep us upright without us having to consciously think about it. **Flexor reflexes** are also called *withdrawal reflexes.* An example of a flexor reflex action is that which occurs when a person touches a hot stove and the extreme heat causes an immediate withdrawal of the hand. The sensation, in this instance, is relayed at the spinal cord level, and thus, is involuntary. The body is designed this way because it would take longer for the body to react if the brain had to process the information, in which case injury (a burn) would occur.

The action that is produced by the reflex is called a **reflex action.** We have reflex actions that we learn over time and with experience, such as keeping our balance while walking or riding a bike. Other reflexes appear to be present at birth and do not need to be learned (e.g., sucking, swallowing, urination). The most common reflexes are included in Table 14–2. When reflexes are impaired it indicates that neurologic dysfunction has occurred. Therefore, checking for the presence or absence of certain reflexes is an important diagnostic procedure.

 Activity 14–3: Competency Verification
Location of the Spinal Nerves

Review Figure 14–4, and check your labeling of the designated spinal nerves in Appendix C.

Brain

The brain is the most complex organ of the body both in its structure and function. It integrates and controls every physical and mental, voluntary and involuntary, activity of the body. It is also the center for memory, emotion, thought, judgment, reasoning, and consciousness. To develop a better understanding of the structures and functions of the brain, refer to and label Figure 14–5 as you read the following material. The brain is composed of four major sections: the **brain stem, cerebellum, diencephalon,** and **cerebrum.**

Brain Stem

The (1) **brain stem** serves as a pathway for impulse conduction between the brain and the spinal cord. It also serves as the origin of the cranial nerves. It is divided into three structures. The first structure is the (2) **medulla oblongata,** which is in charge of heart rate, blood pressure, breathing rhythm, and is the reflex center for coughing, sneezing, swallowing, and vomiting. The second structure of the brain stem is the (3) **pons,** which contains another respiratory cen-

ter and some cranial nerves. The third structure of the brain stem is the (4) **midbrain** (mesencephalon). It contains motor and sensory nerve fibers as well as the

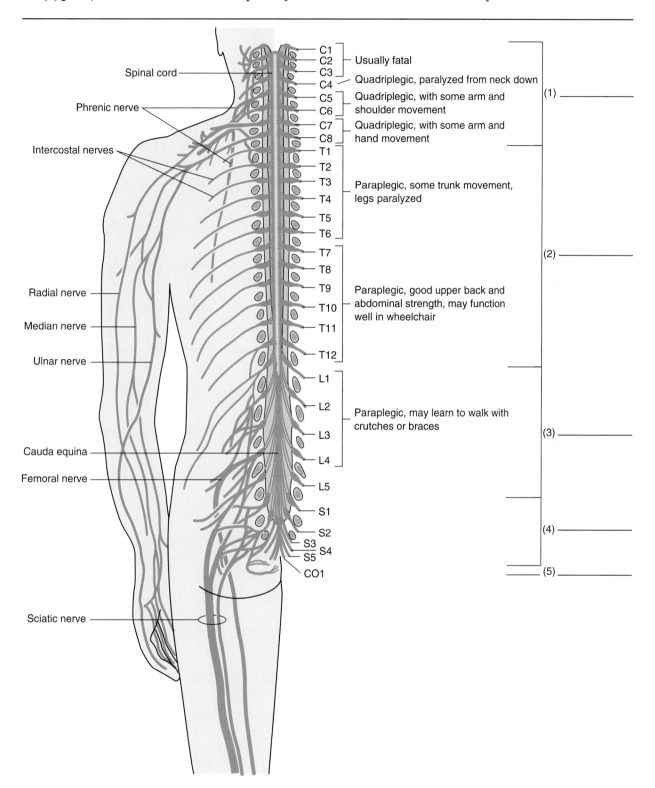

Figure 14-4 *The spinal cord, spinal cord injuries, and spinal nerves. The distribution of spinal nerves is shown on the left side. An analysis of spinal cord injuries is summarized on the right side along with the locations of the spinal nerves. (Adapted from Williams, LS, and Hopper, PD: Understanding Medical Surgical Nursing. FA Davis, Philadelphia, 1999, p 988, with permission.)*

TABLE 14–2:	Principal Reflexes	
TYPE	**STIMULUS**	**EFFECT**
Achilles tendon reflex	Sharp tap of the Achilles tendon (above the heel)	Extension of the foot
Biceps reflex	Percussion* of the tendon of the biceps (above the elbow)	Flexion† of the forearm
Knee jerk reflex	Percussion of the patellar tendon	Extension of the leg
Plantar reflex	Stroking the outer surface of the sole from heel to toes	Flexion of the toes
Pupillary reflex	Stimulation of the retina with light	Constriction of the pupil

*The technique of tapping the body surface (usually with the fingers or a small hammer) to evaluate the position, size, or density of underlying structures; used in physical examinations.

†The act of flexing or bending.

reflex centers for the head and trunk. As you can see, the brain stem houses and controls the "vital" functions of the body without which we would die.

Cerebellum

The (5) **cerebellum,** located just next to the brain stem, controls body coordination and the refinement

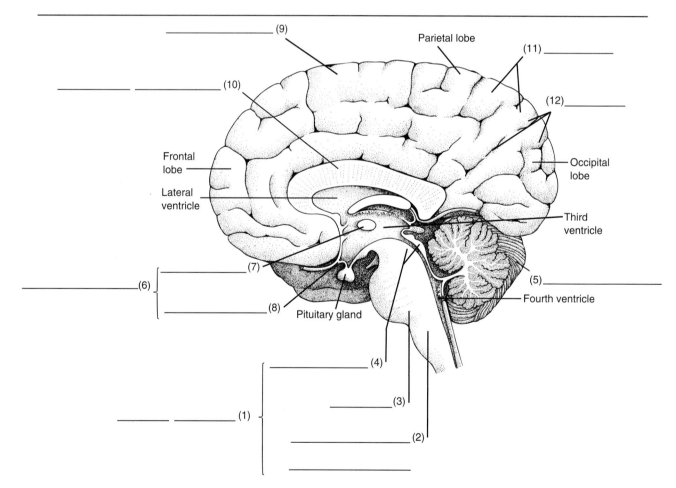

Figure 14–5 The structures of the brain. (Adapted from Williams, LS, and Hopper, PD: Understanding Medical Surgical Nursing. FA Davis, Philadelphia, 1999, p 930, with permission.)

of movement. This structure controls these functions by regulating muscle tone, determining appropriate trajectory and endpoints of movements, and by maintaining posture and equilibrium. All these functions are involuntary, making it possible to engage in complex movements, such as playing soccer, without having to think about the physical movements we are doing and allowing us to simply focus on getting the ball into the goal.

Diencephalon

The (6) **diencephalon,** or interbrain, is located directly above the brain stem. It is composed of two main structures, the (7) **thalamus** and (8) **hypothalamus.** The thalamus is a relay station for sensory information. All sensory stimuli, except olfaction (smell), are received and processed by the thalamus. The information is then transmitted to the appropriate area of the cerebrum, also known as the cerebral cortex. Impulses from the cerebral cortex are then returned to the thalamus and relayed out to the body via the efferent nerves. Beneath the thalamus is a small structure with many diverse functions called the hypothalamus. Its functions include the control and integration of the ANS, the regulation of most endocrine functions, the regulation of body temperature and food intake, and the maintenance of consciousness and sleep patterns.

Cerebrum

The largest and uppermost part of the brain is the (9) **cerebrum.** This is the structure that most people picture when they think of a brain. It consists of two hemispheres separated by a deep longitudinal fissure or groove. At the base of the groove is a structure called the (10) **corpus callosum** that joins the right and left hemispheres. The corpus callosum allows the two hemispheres of the brain to communicate with one another. In this way, various functions that may be more specialized in one hemisphere or the other can be integrated. For example, for most people, the left hemisphere is more involved in language functions and the right hemisphere is more specialized in visual-spatial relationships. However, the two sides need to communicate when a person wants to identify an object with words. In rare instances when a person's corpus callosum is severed, the person may know what an object is and be able to identify what it is by using visual-spatial means (pointing to a picture of it) but will not be able to name it. The corpus callosum is also the structure in which the nerve tracks from the body cross over to the opposite side of the cerebral hemisphere. In this way, if a focal lesion occurs in the area of the right hemisphere that controls muscle movement, only muscle functioning is impaired. Thus, if a lesion occurs in one hemi-

sphere of the brain, the opposite side of the body is affected. This crossover is known as **contralateral functioning.** This effect is often seen as a result of a stroke. A stroke may cause damage in one hemisphere and the effects are seen as weakness or paralysis on the opposite side of the body.

The surface of the cerebrum, called the **cortex,** is made up of gray matter called the cerebral cortex. The cerebral cortex is characterized by numerous folds and grooves, called convolutions. The elevated folds of the convolutions are the (11) **gyri;** the depressed grooves are the (12) **sulci.** This folding permits more surface area to fit in the skull and, therefore, allows for millions more neurons. As in the spinal cord, this gray matter is made up of the cell bodies of neurons. Again, the matter appears gray because there is no myelin surrounding that part of the cells. Internal to the gray matter is white matter, made up of myelinated axons and dendrites that connect the cerebrum to other parts of the brain and the spinal cord.

Activity 14–4: Competency Verification
Structures of the Brain

Review Figure 14–5, and check your labeling in Appendix C.

Lobes of the Brain

Label Fig 14–6 as you learn about the hemispheres of the brain.

Each hemisphere of the brain is divided into four lobes that are named for the cranial bones that lie directly above them. Therefore, each hemisphere has a (1) **frontal lobe,** (2) **parietal lobe,** (3) **temporal lobe,** and (4) **occipital lobe.** These lobes are known to contain certain areas associated with specific functions. For example, the occipital lobe is associated with visual function. Trauma or a lesion to this part of the brain can affect a person's ability to see or to process visual information. In the frontal lobe, "higher-order executive" functions appear to be concentrated. These functions are considered "higher-order" in that they are different from the basic functions of sight, smell, taste, speech, and movement. Executive functions include things like judgment and decision making, inhibition of inappropriate actions (like stopping yourself from saying something rude because it is socially inappropriate), and problem solving. An injury or lesion in this area can therefore cause personality changes and socially inappropriate behavior.

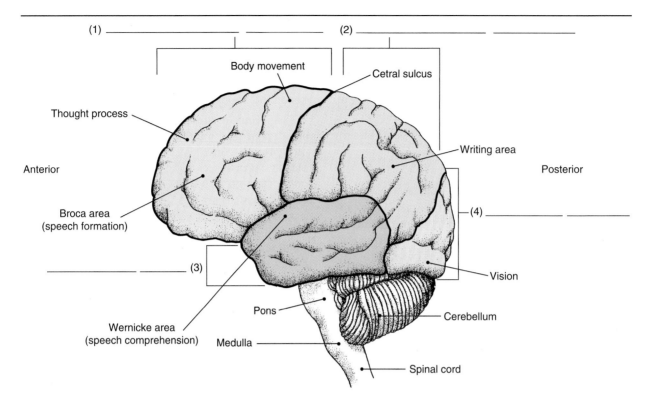

(1) _____ ____ _____ (2) _____ _____ _____

Body movement

Cetral sulcus

Thought process

Writing area

Anterior

Posterior

Broca area
(speech formation)

(4) _____ ____ _____

(3)

Vision

Wernicke area
(speech comprehension)

Pons

Cerebellum

Medulla

Spinal cord

Figure 14–6   *The lobes of the brain. (Adapted from Townsend, MC: Essentials of Psychiatric/Mental Health Nursing, ed 2. FA Davis, Philadelphia, 2001, p 48, with permission.)*

Activity 14–5: Competency Verification

Lobes of the Brain

Review Figure 14–6, and check your labeling in Appendix C.

CNS PROTECTION

Meninges and the Cerebrospinal Fluid

You have already learned that the CNS consists of the brain and spinal cord. Because of its delicate nature, the CNS is protected by a bony encasement—the cranium surrounding the brain and the vertebral column surrounding the spinal cord. Beneath these bony encasements, membranes called **meninges** (located between the bone and soft tissues of the nervous system) protect the brain and the spinal cord.

The meninges consist of three layers: the **dura mater,** the **arachnoid mater,** and the **pia mater.**

The **dura mater** is the outermost layer of the meninges that lines the skull and vertrebral canal. It is composed primarily of tough, white fibrous connective tissue and contains many blood vessels and nerves. In some regions, the dura mater extends inward between lobes of the brain and forms partitions that support and protect these parts.

The second layer, the **arachnoid** (spiderlike) **mater,** is a thin, weblike membrane that lacks bloods vessels and is located between the dura mater (first layer) and the pia mater (third layer). The arachnoid mater spreads over the brain and spinal cord but generally does not dip into the grooves and depressions on their surfaces.

Between the arachnoid mater (second layer) and the **pia mater** is a *subarachnoid space* that contains the clear, watery fluid called **cerebrospinal fluid (CSF).** The pia mater is very thin and is composed of many nerves and blood vessels that nourish underlying cells of the brain and spinal cord. This layer hugs the surfaces of these organs and follows their irregular contours, passing over high areas and dipping into depressions. The CSF protects the brain and spinal cord from shock and delivers and filters substances to and from the blood. This fluid is formed in the ventricles (interconnected cavities) of the brain. These spaces are continuous with the central canal of the spinal cord, and like it, they contain CSF. Interference with normal CSF circulation can cause serious medical problems such as hydrocephaly (see the Pathology section). Sometimes the meningeal layers can become infected by bacteria or viruses, causing inflammation (i.e., meningitis; see the Pathology section).

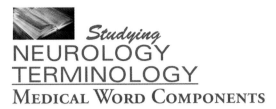

Studying
NEUROLOGY TERMINOLOGY
MEDICAL WORD COMPONENTS

Combining Forms

The major combining forms of the nervous system are summarized here. They are grouped according to the nerve cells, the central nervous system, and the peripheral nervous system.

Combining Forms: The Nerve Cells

Combining Form	Meaning	EXAMPLE Term/Pronunciation	Definition
astr/o	star	**astr**/o/glia ăs-TRŎG-lē-ă	a type of CNS supporting cell; one of the large neuroglia cells of nervous tissue *The suffix -glia means "glue," "neuroglia tissue." Glia is the non-nervous or supporting tissue of the brain and spinal cord.*
ax/o	axis, axon	**ax**/o/plasm ĂK-sō-plăzm	neuroplasm of the axon *The suffix -plasm means "formation," "growth."*
dendr/o	tree	**dendr**/itic děn-DRĬT-ĭk	pertaining to (*-itic*) a tree-like or branched form
gangli/o	ganglion	**gangl**/itis găng-LĪT-ĭs	inflammation (*-itis*) of a ganglion *The ganglion (plural, ganglia) is a mass of nervous tissue composed principally of neuron cell bodies, chiefly lying outside the brain or spinal cord.*
gli/o	glue, neuroglia tissue	**gli**/oma glī-Ō-mă	tumor composed of neuroglia tissue (supportive tissue of nervous system)
myel/o	bone marrow, spinal cord	**myel**/algia mī-ĕl-ĂL-jē-ă	pain (*-algia*) of the spinal cord or its membranes
neur/o	nerve	**neur**/o/lysis nū-RŎL-ĭs-ĭs	destruction (*-lysis*) of a nerve
olig/o	scanty	**olig**/o/cyte ŎL-ĭ-gō-sīt	cell (*-cyte*) that resembles an astrocyte but has fewer projections
synapt/o	synapsis, point of contact	**synapt**/ic sĭn-ĂP-tĭk	pertaining to (*-ic*) a synapse (the space between neurons)

Combining Forms: The Central Nervous System

Combining Form	Meaning	EXAMPLE	
		Term/Pronunciation	Definition
cephal/o	head	**cephal**/ic sĕ-FĂL-ĭk	pertaining to (-ic) the head
cerebell/o	cerebellum	**cerebell**/ar sĕr-ĕ-BĔL-ăr	pertaining to (-ar) the cerebellum
cerebr/o	cerebrum	de/**cerebr**/ate dē-SĔR-ĕ-brāt	cessation (de-) of cerebral function *The prefix* de- *means cessation; the adjective ending* -ate *means "having the form of," "possessing."*
cortic/o	cortex	**cortic**/al KOR-tĭ-kăl	pertaining to (-al) the cortex
crani/o	skull	**crani**/o/faci/al krā-nē-ō-FĀ-shăl	pertaining to (-al) the skull and face Faci/o *means "face."*
dur/o	dura mater	epi/**dur**/al ĕp-ĭ-DOO-răl	relating to (-al), upon or on the dura *The prefix* epi- *means "above," "upon."*
encephal/o	brain	**encephal**/oma ĕn-sĕf-ă-LŌ-mă	tumor (-oma) of the brain
lex/o	word, phrase	dys/**lex**/ia dĭs-LĔK-sē-ă	condition (-ia) characterized by difficulty (dys-) in reading
medull/o	medulla	**medull**/ary mĕd-ū-LĂR-ē	pertaining to (-ary) the medulla
mening/o	meninges	**mening**/itis mĕn-ĭn-JĪ-tĭs	inflammation (-itis) of the meninges
radicul/o	nerve root	**radicul**/o/pathy ră-dĭk-ū-LŎP-ă-thē	any disease (-pathy) of a spinal nerve root
spin/o	spine	**spin**/al SPĪ-năl	pertaining to (-al) the spine
thalam/o	thalamus	**thalam**/o/tomy thăl-ă-MŎT-ō-mē	destruction by incision (-tomy) of part of the thalamus to treat intractable pain or psychosis
thec/o	sheath (usually refers to the meninges)	intra/**thec**/al ĭn-tră-THĒ-kăl	pertaining to (-al) within (intra-) the meninges (as in intrathecal injection where chemotherapeutic drugs are inserted into the subarachnoid space)
ventricul/o	ventricle (of heart or brain)	**ventricul**/o/puncture vĕn-TRĬK-ū-lō-pŭnk-tūr	use of a needle to puncture a ventricle

Combining Forms: The Peripheral Nervous System

Combining Form	Meaning	EXAMPLE	
		Term/Pronunciation	Definition
clon/o	clonus	**clon**/ic KLŎN-ĭk	pertaining to (-*ic*) increased reflex; alternately contracting and relaxing the muscles
kinesi/o	movement	**kinesi**/o/therapy kĭ-nē-sē-ō-THĔR-ă-pē	treatment (-*therapy*) by movement or exercise
narc/o	stupor, numbness, sleep	**narc**/o/lepsy NĂR-kō-lĕp-sē	a disorder in which a person has sudden strong urges to sleep *The suffix* -lepsy *means "seizure."*
tax/o	order, coordination	a/**tax**/ia ă-TĂK-sē-ă	condition (-*ia*) characterized by a lack of (*a-*) coordination
ton/o	tension	**ton**/ic TŎN-ĭk	pertaining to (-*ic*) a state of continuous muscle contraction

Activity 14–6: Competency Verification
Medical Word Components

Check off the box [✓] as you complete each numbered section.

[   ] **1.** Review the components and examples in the previous section. Then pronounce each word aloud.

[   ] **2.** For the words below, first write the suffix and its meaning. Then translate the meaning of the remaining components starting with the first part of the word.

> **Example:** neur/oma
> **Answer:** *oma*=tumor; nerve

1. myel/algia   _____

2. cortic/al   _____

3. mening/itis   _____

4. encephal/oma   _____

5. medull/ary   _____

6. spin/al   _____

7. crani/o/faci/al _____

8. gangl/itis   _____

9. neur/algia   _____

10. intra/thec/al _____

Correct Answers _____ × 10 = _____ % Score

Prefixes and Suffixes
Prefixes

In this section, prefixes are listed alphabetically and highlighted, whereas key suffixes are defined in the right-hand column.

Prefixes: The Nervous System

Prefix	Meaning	EXAMPLE	
		Term/Pronunciation	**Definition**
bi-	two	**bi**/later/al *bī-LĂT-ĕr-ăl*	pertaining to (*-al*) two sides (*later/o*)
contra-	against	**contra**/later/al *kŏn-tră-LĂT-ĕr-ăl*	pertaining to (*-al*) opposite sides
para-	near, beside, beyond	**para**/lysis *pă-RĂL-ĭ-sĭs*	loss of purposeful movement, usually as a result of neurologic disease, drugs, or toxins *The suffix -lysis means "separation," "destruction," "loosening"; used to describe loss of movement on one side of the body.*
quadri-	four	**quadri**/plegia *kwŏd-rĭ-PLĒ-jē-ă*	paralysis (*-plegia*) of all four extremities
uni-	one	**uni**/later/al *ū-nĭ-LĂT-ĕr-ăl*	pertaining to (*-al*) or affecting only one side (*later/o*)

Suffixes

In this section, suffixes are listed alphabetically and highlighted, whereas prefixes are defined in the right-hand column on a need-to-know basis.

Suffixes: The Nervous System

Suffix	Meaning	EXAMPLE	
		Term/Pronunciation	**Definition**
-asthenia	weakness, debility	my/**asthenia** *mī-ăs-THĒ-nē-ă*	weakness or debility of the muscles (*my/o-*)
-esthesia	feeling	an/**esthesia** *ăn-ĕs-THĒ-zē-ă*	without (*an-*) feeling

Suffixes: The Nervous System (Continued)

Suffix	Meaning	EXAMPLE	
		Term/Pronunciation	Definition
-kinesia	movement	hyper/**kinesia** hī-pĕr-kī-NĒ-zē-ă	excessive (*hyper-*) movement
-lalia	speech, babble	echo/**lalia** ĕ-kō-LĀ-lē-ă	repetition of words *The prefix* echo- *means a "repeated sound."*
-lepsy	seizure	epi/**lepsy** ĔP-ĭ-lĕp-sē	seizure disorder *The prefix* epi- *means "above," "upon."*
-paresis	partial paralysis	hemi/**paresis** hĕm-ē-PĂR-ĕ-sĭs	paralysis of one half (*hemi-*) of the body (left half or right half) *When used by itself, the term* paresis *means "partial paralysis or motor weakness."*
-phasia	speech	a/**phasia** ă-FĀ-zē-ă	an abnormal neurologic condition in which language function is defective or absent because of an injury to certain areas of the cerebral cortex Aphasia *means "without (a-) speech."*
-plegia	paralysis	hemi/**plegia** hĕm-ē-PLĒ-jē-ă	paralysis affecting half (*hemi-*) of the body
-trophy	development, nourishment	dys/**trophy** DĬS-trō-fē	disorder caused by poor nutrition or nourishment *The prefix* dys- *means "bad," "painful," "difficult."*

Activity 14–7: Competency Verification

Prefixes and Suffixes

Check off the box [✓] as you complete each numbered section.

[   ] **1.** Review the prefixes and suffixes and their examples in the previous section. Then pronounce each word aloud.

[   ] **2.** For the words below, first write the suffix and its meaning. Then translate the meaning of the remaining components starting with the first part of the word.

> **Example:** later/al
> **Answer:** *al*=pertaining to; side

1. contra/later/al _____

2. quadri/plegia _____

3. an/esthesia   _____

4. echo/lalia   _____

5. hyper/kinesia   _____

6. a/phasia   _____

7. hemi/paresis   _____

8. my/asthenia   _____

9. dys/trophy   _____

10. epi/lepsy   _____

Correct Answers _____ **× 10 =** _____ **% Score**

PATHOLOGICAL CONDITIONS

Congenital Disorders

PATHOLOGICAL CONDITION	DESCRIPTION
hydrocephalus hī-drō-SĔF-ă-lŭs *hydro=water* *cephal=head* *us=condition*	Increased accumulation of cerebrospinal fluid within the ventricles of the brain due to interference with normal circulation and absorption. Hydrocephalic infants have an enlarged head and small face. This disorder can also occur in adults due to a tumor or infection. A shunt is used to drain the fluid from the ventricles into the peritoneal space.
neural tube defect (NTD) NŪ-răl tūb DĒ-fekt	Any of a group of congenital malformations involving defects in the skull and spinal column that are primarily caused by failure of the neural tube to close during embryonic development. Cranial fusion disorders, including anencephaly and encephalocele, or spinal fusion disorders, including spina bifida with meningocele and spina bifida with meningomyelocele (Fig. 14–7), may occur as a consequence of this failure. Prenatal folic acid (a common water-soluble B vitamin) deficiency has been implicated in NTD, but other predisposing factors may be involved as well.

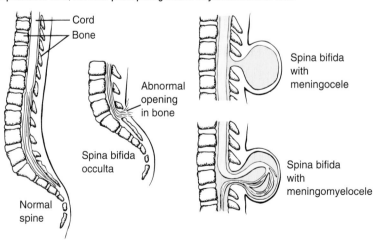

Cord

Bone

Abnormal opening in bone

Spina bifida occulta

Normal spine

Spina bifida with meningocele

Spina bifida with meningomyelocele

Figure 14–7 *Neural tube defects. (From Rothstein, JM, Roy, SH, Wolf, SL: The Rehabilitation Specialist's Handbook, ed 2. FA Davis, Philadelphia, 1998, p 704, with permission.)*

Congenital Disorders (Continued)

PATHOLOGICAL CONDITION	DESCRIPTION
spina bifida *SPĪ-nă BĬ-fĭ-dă*	A congenital malformation characterized by a defective closure of the spinal canal through which the spinal cord and meninges may or may not protrude. This condition, which usually occurs in the lumbosacral area, has several forms.
spina bifida occulta *SPĪ-nă BĬ-fĭ-dă ŭ-KŬLT-ă*	The most common and least severe form of spina bifida. This condition is marked by a defect of the bony spinal canal without protrusion of the spinal cord or meninges (see Fig. 14–7). Because the neural tube has closed, there are usually no neurologic impairments associated with this defect.
spina bifida cystica *SPĪ-nă BĬ-fĭ-dă SĬS-tĭ-kă*	A more severe form of spina bifida in which a hernial cyst containing meninges (meningocele), or both meninges and spinal cord (*meningomyelocele*) protrude through a congenital opening in the vertebral column (Fig. 14–8 and a lateral view of this defect in Fig. 14–7). The protruding sac is encased in a layer of skin or a fine membrane that readily ruptures, causing the leakage of cerebrospinal fluid and an increased risk of meningeal infection. The severity of neurologic dysfunction and associated defects depends directly on the degree of nerve involvement. Patients with large open lesions may have more severe complications such as a neurogenic bladder (which predispose to infection and renal failure) or total paralysis of the legs. *Spina bifida cystica* is frequently associated with hydrocephalus and paraplegia.

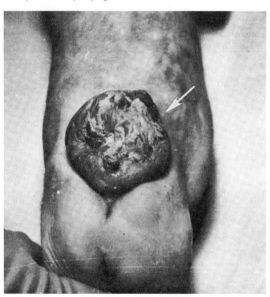

Figure 14–8 *Spina bifida cystica. Lumbar myelomeningocele in an infant with hydrocephalus and paraplegia. (From Adams, JF, and Duchen, LW: Greenfield's Neuropathy, ed 5, 1992, p 542. Reproduced with permission of Hodder Arnold.*

Tay-Sachs disease *tā săks dĭ-ZĒZ*	Genetic disorder resulting from an enzyme deficiency at birth. The lack of the enzyme causes an accumulation of lipid substances in CNS cells, which distends and destroys them. The afflicted child develops normally until the age of 4 to 8 months. After this time, a progressive deterioration is imminent. Paralysis, blindness, inability to eat, and eventually, death will follow. There is no known cure; thus, treatment is only supportive in nature. A simple blood test can identify the carriers of this gene. Primarily found in the Ashkenazi Jewish population.

Degenerative, Movement, and Seizure Disorders

PATHOLOGICAL CONDITION	DESCRIPTION
Alzheimer disease ĂLTS-hī-měr dĭ-ZĒZ	Brain disorder of unknown etiology marked by gradual, progressive deterioration of mental capacity (dementia) beginning in middle age. Symptoms include memory loss, impaired judgment, disorientation, loss of intellectual functioning, and emotional instability. Upon autopsy cerebral atrophy is evident, especially in the frontal and temporal regions. There is no effective treatment or cure. Compare the positron emission tomography (PET) scan of a normal, young patient's brain (Fig. 14–9A) with the PET scan of an Alzheimer patient's brain (Fig. 14–9B).
amyotrophic lateral sclerosis (ALS) ă-mī-ō-TRŌF-ĭk LĂT-ěr-ăl sklěr-Ō-sĭs	A fatal degenerative disease involving the cortical and spinal motor neurons and often the brain stem; manifested by progressive weakness and wasting of muscles. This condition is a sporadic disease affecting adults and usually is fatal within 2 to 5 years of onset. Also known as *Lou Gehrig disease*.

A
ANTERIOR

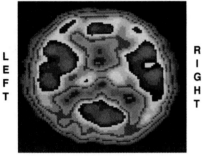

LEFT   RIGHT

POSTERIOR

B

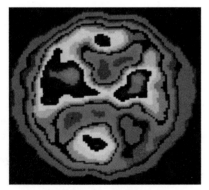

ALZHEIMER DISEASE: PET SCAN
SHOWING MARKEDLY DECREASED
METABOLISM (BLUE AND GREEN) IN
FRONTAL LOBES

C

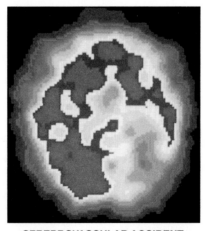

PARKINSON DISEASE
PET SCAN OF BRAIN IN PARKINSON
DEMENTIA SHOWING WIDESPREAD
REDUCED METABOLISM
(BLUE AND GREEN)

D

CEREBROVASCULAR ACCIDENT
PET SCAN OF BRAIN SHOWING
INFRACTION IN TEMPORAL LOBE (GREEN)

Figure 14–9 *Brain PET scans. (A) The brain of a healthy young patient. (From Venes, D: Taber's Cyclopedic Medical Dictionary, ed 19. FA Davis, Philadelphia, 2001, p 2203, with permission.); (B) The brain of a patient with Alzheimer disease. (From Mazziotta, JC, and Gilman, S: Clinical Brain Imaging: Principles and Applications. Oxford University Press, New York, 1992, p 310, with permission.); (C) The brain of a patient with Parkinson disease (From Mazziotta, JC, and Gilman, S: Clinical Brain Imaging: Principles and Applications. Oxford University Press, New York, 1992, p 320, with permission.); (D) The brain of a patient who experienced a cerebrovascular accident. (From Thomas, CL: Taber's Cyclopedic Medical Dictionary, ed 18. FA Davis, Philadelphia, 1997, p 350, with permission.)*

Degenerative, Movement, and Seizure Disorders (Continued)

PATHOLOGICAL CONDITION	DESCRIPTION
epilepsy ĔP-ĭ-lĕp-sē *epi=above, upon* *lepsy=seizure*	A group of neurologic disorders characterized by recurrent episodes of seizures, sensory disturbances, abnormal behavior, loss of consciousness, or all of these. Common to all types of epilepsy is an uncontrolled electrical discharge from the nerve cells of the cerebral cortex. Each attack is called a seizure, but not all seizures are caused by epilepsy. Epileptic seizures exhibit a chronic pattern, with similar characteristics at each recurrence. Various structural, chemical, or physiological disorders may cause epilepsy. These include brain injury, congenital abnormalities, metabolic disorders, brain tumors, vascular disturbances, and genetic disorders. Epilepsy can, in many instances, be effectively controlled by the use of *antiepileptic medications (anticonvulsants).*
Huntington disease HŬNT-ĭng-tŏn dĭ-ZĒZ	An inherited disease of the CNS that usually occurs in persons 30–50 years of age. This condition is characterized by quick, involuntary movements (tics), speech disturbances, and mental deterioration due to degenerative changes in the cerebral cortex and basal ganglia. Because the disease is hereditary, it is prevalent in geographic areas where affected families have lived for several generations. Although there is no cure for the disease, recent genetic studies have identified a marker for the gene linked to Huntington disease making it possible to identify those who will eventually develop the disease. Also called *Huntington chorea.*
multiple sclerosis (MS) MŬL-tĭ-pl sklĕ-RŌ-sĭs *scler=hardening, sclera* *osis=condition*	A chronic disease of the CNS in which there is destruction of myelin and nerve axons within several regions of the brain and spinal cord at different times. This condition results in temporary, repetitive, or sustained disruptions in nerve impulse conduction, causing symptoms such as muscular weakness, numbness, visual disturbances, or loss of control of bowel, bladder, and sexual functions. It is one of the leading causes of neurologic disability in persons 20 to 40 years of age. The cause of the disease is unknown, although much evidence suggests it is an autoimmune disease. There is no effective treatment, although immunosuppressive agents may produce some benefit.
myasthenia gravis mī-ăs-THĒ-nē-ă GRĂV-ĭs *my=muscle* *asthenia=weakness, debility*	Neuromuscular autoimmune disorder characterized by extreme weakness of the skeletal muscles. Antibodies block the ability of the neurotransmitter (acetylcholine) to transmit the nerve impulse to the muscles, causing failed muscle contraction. Anticholinesterase drugs, steroids, and immunosuppressive drugs are used as treatment. Thymectomy (removal of the thymus gland that produces the antibodies) may also be beneficial.
palsy PAWL-zē	Paralysis or paresis (partial or incomplete paralysis).
Bell	Paresis or paralysis, usually unilateral, of the facial muscles, caused by dysfunction of a facial nerve of unknown etiology. The person may not be able to close an eye or control salivation on the affected side. The condition often results in grotesque facial disfigurement and facial spasms, but complete recovery is possible.
cerebral sĕr-Ē-brăl *cerebr=cerebrum* *al=pertaining to*	Bilateral, symmetrical, nonprogressive motor dysfunction and partial paralysis usually caused by damage to the cerebrum during gestation or birth trauma but can be hereditary.
Parkinson disease PĂR-kĭn-sŏn dĭ-ZĒZ	Progressive neurologic disorder affecting the area of the brain responsible for the control of movement, occurring in people over 60 years of age. A degeneration of the neurons in this area and subsequent deficiency of the neurotransmitter dopamine leads to slowness of movement, a shuffling gait, tremor, stiffness of large joints, and unblinking eyes. Treatment is based on a combination of drug therapy to increase dopamine levels, physical therapy, and rehabilitation techniques. Treatment is palliative only, not curative. Compare the PET scan of a normal, young patient's brain (see Fig. 14–9A) with that of a Parkinson patient's brain (see Fig. 14–9C).

Degenerative, Movement, and Seizure Disorders (Continued)

PATHOLOGICAL CONDITION	DESCRIPTION
seizure SĒ-zhŭr	A convulsion or other clinically detectable event caused by a sudden discharge of electrical activity in the brain that may be classified as *partial* or *generalized;* characteristic symptom of epilepsy.
partial	Seizures that begin on one side of the cerebral cortex. In some cases the electrical discharge spreads to the other hemisphere and the seizure becomes generalized. Repetitive, purposeless behaviors, called *automatisms*, are the classic symptom of this type of seizures. If the person does not lose consciousness, the seizure is called a *simple partial seizure*. If consciousness is lost, it is called a *complex partial seizure* or *psychomotor seizure*.
generalized	Seizures are characterized by involvement of both cerebral hemispheres. Two types of generalized seizures are *absence seizures* and *tonic-clonic seizures*. Absence seizures (*petit mal seizures*) are considered a minor form of seizure in which there is a sudden, brief lapse of consciousness or a period of staring that lasts several seconds. There is no convulsion and the person resumes activity as if the seizure had not occurred. Tonic-clonic seizures (*grand mal seizures*) are characterized by a sudden loss of consciousness, falling down, generalized involuntary muscular contraction and cessation of respiration followed by tonic spasm (freezing of muscles) and then clonic spasms (repetitive jerking and relaxation of muscles). The teeth may be clenched, the tongue bitten, and control of the bladder or bowel lost. As this phase of the seizure passes, the person may fall asleep or experience confusion. Usually the person has no recall of the seizure on awakening. A sensory warning, or aura, can precede each tonic-clonic seizure. Anticonvulsant medications are usually prescribed to control the seizures.
Tourette syndrome too-RĔT SĬN-drōm	Neurologic disorder characterized by involuntary spasms, twitching movements (tics), uncontrollable vocal sounds, and inappropriate verbalizations. There has been some success with using antipsychotic drugs and antidepressants as treatment, even though psychosis is not present with this disorder.

Infectious Disorders

PATHOLOGICAL CONDITION	DESCRIPTION
encephalitis ĕn-sĕf-ă-LĪ-tĭs *encephal=brain* *itis=inflammation*	Inflammation of the brain as a result of the flu, measles, chickenpox, *herpesvirus*, or other disease; symptoms include changes in consciousness, signs of increased intracranial pressure such as increased restlessness, projectile vomiting, convulsions, and vital sign changes. Encephalitis may also be accompanied by behavioral changes and sleep abnormalities.
meningitis mĕn-ĭn-JĪ-tĭs *mening=meninges*	Any infection or inflammation of the membranes covering the spinal cord and brain. The most common cause in adults is bacterial infection, but aseptic meningitis may be caused by nonbacterial agents such as chemical irritants, neoplasms, or viruses. The onset is usually sudden and characterized by neck stiffness, irritability, malaise, and restlessness. Nausea, vomiting, delirium, and complete disorientation may develop quickly.
poliomyelitis (polio) pōl-ē-ō-mī-ĕl-Ī-tĭs *polio=gray, gray matter (of brain or spinal cord)* *myel=bone marrow, spinal cord* *itis=inflammation*	Inflammation of the gray matter of the spinal cord. An acute viral disease characterized by fever, sore throat, headaches, vomiting, and often stiffness of the neck and back. There may also be subsequent atrophy of groups of muscles ending in contraction and permanent deformity. Polio is rather uncommon today because of the preventable vaccinations given to children.

Infectious Disorders (Continued)

PATHOLOGICAL CONDITION	DESCRIPTION
Reye syndrome rī SĬN-drōm	A syndrome characterized by acute encephalopathy and fatty infiltration of the liver and other internal organs. The syndrome is seen in children under 15 years of age following an acute viral infection, and there appears to be an association with the administration of aspirin. Therefore aspirin is given only if prescribed by a physician for any condition in infants or children. The mortality rate can be as high as 80%.
shingles SHĬNG-lz	Eruption of acute, inflammatory vesicles in which painful blisters appear on the skin along the course of a peripheral nerve; caused by the *herpes zoster* virus, the same virus that causes chickenpox).

Neoplastic Disorders

PATHOLOGICAL CONDITION	DESCRIPTION
BRAIN TUMORS	
astrocytoma ăs-trō-sī-TŌ-mă *astro=star* *cyt=cell* *oma=tumor*	A tumor composed of astrocytes. The most malignant form of astrocytoma is *glioblastoma multiforme*. This tumor is a rapidly growing pulpy or cystic formation of the cerebrum or the spinal cord. The lesion spreads with pseudopod-like projections.
glioma glī-Ō-mă *gli=glue, neuroglial tissue* *oma=tumor*	A tumor composed of neuroglial tissue. Examples of gliomas are *astrocytoma* and *oligodendroglioma*.
meningioma mĕn-ĭn-jē-Ō-mă *meningi=meninges* *oma=tumor*	A tumor of the meninges, usually benign and encapsulated. As it grows it may then cause compression and distortion of the brain (Fig. 14–10). 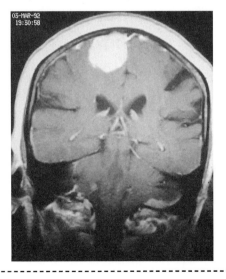 **Figure 14–10** *A meningioma. (From Williams, LS, and Hopper, PD: Understanding Medical Surgical Nursing. FA Davis, Philadelphia, 1999, p 979, with permission.)*
neuroblastoma nū-rō-blăs-TŌ-mă *neuro=nerve* *blast=embryonic cell* *oma=tumor*	A malignant hemorrhagic tumor composed primarily of cells resembling neuroblasts that give rise to cells of the sympathetic nervous system. Occurs mainly in infants and children.

Trauma Disorders

PATHOLOGICAL CONDITION	DESCRIPTION
concussion *kŏn-KŬSH-ŭn*	An injury to the brain caused by a violent jarring or shaking, such as a blow or an explosion.
cerebral *cerebr=cerebrum* *al=pertaining to*	Concussion is characterized by headache, dizziness, or nausea and vomiting. The patient may complain of amnesia of events before or after the trauma. If there is loss of consciousness, it is for 5 minutes or less. On clinical examination there is no skull or dura injury and no abnormality detected on CT or MRI. However, a severe concussion may lead to a coma.
contusion *kŏn-TOO-zhŭn*	Any mechanical injury (usually caused by a blow) resulting in hemorrhage beneath unbroken skin. Also called a *bruise.*
cerebral	Characterized by bruising of brain tissue, possibly accompanied by hemorrhage. There may be multiple areas of contusion, depending on the causative mechanism. The symptoms of a cerebral contusion depend on the area of the brain involved (e.g., brainstem contusions affect level of consciousness).
hematoma *hē-mă-TŌ-mă* *hemat=blood* *oma=tumor*	A swelling composed of a mass of extravasated blood (usually clotted) confined to an organ, tissue, or space and caused by a break in a blood vessel.
epidural *ĕp-ĭ-DŪ-răl* *epi=above, upon* *dur=dura mater, hard* *al=pertaining to*	A hematoma, usually from an arterial bleed, that forms between the skull and dura mater (see Fig. 14–11*A*).

Arterial bleeding can cause the hematoma to enlarge very quickly.

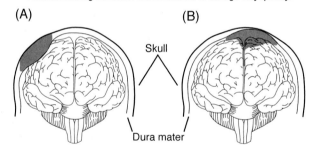

(A)   (B)

Skull

Dura mater

Epidural hematoma   Subdural hematoma

Figure 14–11 *Intracranial hemorrhage. (A) Epidural hematoma—arterial bleeding between the skull and dura mater. (B) Subdural hematoma—venous bleeding between the dura mater and brain. (From Starkey, C, and Ryan, JL. Evaluation of Orthopedic and Athletic Injuries. FA Davis, Philadelphia, 1996, p 494, with permission.)*

subdural *sŭb-DŪ-răl* *sub=under* *dur=dura mater, hard* *al=pertaining to*	A hematoma, usually from a venous bleed, that forms between the dura mater and the brain (Fig. 14–11*B*). This condition is usually the result of a head injury and is classified as acute or chronic, based on the time interval between injury and the onset of symptoms. About 24% of persons who sustain a severe brain injury develop acute subdural hematoma.
sciatica *sī-ĂT-ĭ-kă*	Severe pain in the leg along the course of the sciatic nerve felt at the back of the thigh and running down the inside of the leg. The pain may be due to compression or trauma of the nerve or its roots, especially resulting from a ruptured intervertebral disk or osteoarthritis of the lumbosacral vertebrae.

Vascular Disorders

PATHOLOGICAL CONDITION	DESCRIPTION
aneurysm ĂN-ŭ-rĭzm	A localized dilation of the wall of a blood vessel, usually an artery, due to a congenital defect or weakness in the vessel wall. Complications of an aneurysm include rupture, causing hemorrhage, and formation of thrombi or emboli. For an illustration of different types of aortic aneurysm, see Figure 9–9.
cerebrovascular accident (CVA) sĕr-ĕ-brō-VĂS-kū-lar ĂK-sĭ-dĕnt *cerebr=cerebrum* *vascul=vessel* *ar=pertaining to*	A sudden loss of neurologic function, caused by vascular injury to the brain. It is characterized by occlusion by an embolus, thrombus, or cerebrovascular hemorrhage resulting in a decrease in blood flow (ischemia) of the tissues to that area of the brain. Also called a *stroke*. Brief episodes of ischemia in the brain, causing neurologic dysfunction, are known as *transient ischemic attacks (TIAs)* or *mini strokes*. The symptoms vary with the site and the degree of occlusion (see Fig. 14–9D).
migraine MĪ-grān	A recurring, pulsating, vascular, and frequently incapacitating type of headache characterized by intense, throbbing pain often accompanied by nausea and vomiting. The exact mechanism responsible for this disorder is not known, but the head pain is related to dilation of extracranial blood vessels, which may be the result of chemical changes that cause spasms of intracranial vessels.

Other Disorders

CONDITION	DESCRIPTION
apraxia ă-PRĂK-sē-ă	Inability to perform purposeful acts or to manipulate objects although there is no sensory or motor impairment.
aura AW-ră	Subjective sensation preceding a seizure or migraine. In epilepsy the aura may precede the seizure by a few hours or by a few seconds. Epileptic aura may be of a psychic or sensory nature with olfactory, visual, auditory, or taste hallucinations. In migraines, the aura immediately precedes the attack and consists of visual sensory phenomena.
coma KŌ-mă	Abnormally deep unconsciousness with the absence of voluntary response to stimuli.
delirium dē-LĬR-ē-ŭm	State of mental confusion and excitement characterized by disorientation for time and place, often with hallucinations. Speech may be incoherent and the patient may exhibit continual aimless physical activity. There are many forms depending on the cause, which may be fever, shock, exhaustion, anxiety, drug overdose. Delirium should not be confused with dementia.
dementia dĕ-MĔN-shē-ă *de=cessation* *ment=mind* *ia=condition*	A gradual, progressive, usually irreversible impairment of cognitive and intellectual function (cognition) that interferes with normal social and occupational activities. Onset may be gradual and include memory deficits, poor judgment, and impaired abstract thinking. Primary to *Alzheimer disease*, and secondary to brain tumors, severe and prolonged alcohol abuse, or meningitis. Should not be confused with delirium.
lethargy LĔTH-ăr-jē	Condition of sluggishness, abnormal inactivity, or a lack of response to normal stimuli.

Other Disorders (Continued)

CONDITION	DESCRIPTION
paraplegia *păr-ă-PLĒ-jē-ă*	Paralysis of lower portion of the body and of both legs that may be due to maldevelopment, spinal abscess, tumor or injury, or multiple sclerosis.
pseudoseizure *soo-dō-SĒ-zhŭr*	Clinical manifestation of what appears to be a seizure but EEG is normal; usually psychogenic in origin.
quadriplegia *kwŏd-rĭ-PLĒ-jē-ă* *quadri=four* *plegia=paralysis*	Paralysis of all four extremities and usually the trunk due to an injury to the spinal cord, usually at the level of the cervical vertebrae.
Romberg sign *RŎM-bĕrg sīn*	Inability to maintain the body balance when the eyes are shut and feet are close together.
spastic *SPĂS-tĭk*	An increase in muscle tone (stiffness) associated with an increase in tendon reflexes and abnormal reflexes.
syncope *SĬN-kō-pē*	A transient loss of consciousness due to inadequate blood flow to the brain; fainting.
tinnitus *tĭn-Ī-tŭs*	Noises in the ear, such as ringing, hissing, whistling, roaring.
tonic *TŎN-ĭk* *ton=tension* *ic=pertaining to*	An involuntary, spasmodic muscular contraction most commonly involving the face, head, neck, shoulder muscles. A characteristic symptom of Tourette syndrome; characterized by tension or contraction, especially muscular.
tremor *TRĔM-or*	An involuntary quivering, shaking, or trembling; a characteristic symptom of Parkinson disease.
vertigo *VĔR-tĭ-gō*	The sensation of spinning or movement in which the world is revolving or the person is revolving in space, usually as a result of a disturbance of equilibrium in the inner ear.

Activity 14–8: Clinical Application
Pathological Conditions

Alzheimer disease	glioma	seizure
aneurysm	Huntington disease	shingles
apraxia	hydrocephalus	spina bifida
aura	meningioma	subdural
Bell palsy	meningitis	syncope
cerebral contusion	migraine	Tay-Sachs disease
coma	multiple sclerosis (MS)	TIA
CVA	myasthenia gravis	tremor
epidural	Parkinson disease	vertigo

Match the diagnoses listed above with the definitions given in the numbered list:

1. _____ a hematoma, usually from an arterial bleed, that forms between the skull and dura mater.

2. _____ progressive neurologic disorder affecting movement control that is characterized by a deficiency of the neurotransmitter dopamine that leads to slowness of movement, tremors, and a shuffling gate.

3. _____ inherited disease with tics, speech disturbances, and mental deterioration that usually occurs between 30 and 50 years of age.

4. _____ eruption of inflammatory vesicles along the course of a peripheral nerve caused by the herpes zoster virus.

5. _____ a hematoma, usually from a venous bleed, that forms between the dura mater and the brain.

6. _____ condition characterized by paralysis or paresis of the facial muscles caused by dysfunction of a facial nerve of unknown etiology.

7. _____ a severe headache usually accompanied by nausea and vomiting.

8. _____ subjective sensation preceding a seizure or migraine.

9. _____ brief episodes of ischemia in the brain causing neurologic dysfunction; synonymous with "mini strokes."

10. _____ increased accumulation of cerebrospinal fluid within the ventricles of the brain.

11. _____ any infection or inflammation of the membranes covering the brain and spinal cord.

12. _____ a congenital malformation in which there is a defective closure of the spinal canal through which the spinal cord and meninges may or may not protrude.

13. _____ bruising of brain tissue that may be accompanied by hemorrhage.

14. _____ a tumor of the meninges that is usually benign.

15. _____ localized ballooning of the wall of a blood vessel, usually an artery.

16. _____ chronic disease of the CNS with destruction of myelin and nerve axons within several regions of the brain and spinal cord.

17. _____ astrocytomas and oligodendrogliomas are examples of this type of tumor arising from neuroglial tissue.

18. _____ genetic disorder that arises from an enzyme deficiency at birth, which causes an accumulation of lipid substances in CNS cells, leading to their destruction.

19. _____ vascular injury to the brain with a sudden loss of neurologic function; characterized by occlusion by an embolus, thrombus, or hemorrhage; a stroke.

20. _____ neuromuscular, autoimmune disorder characterized by extreme weakness of the skeletal muscles.

21. _____ an involuntary quivering, shaking, or trembling; a characteristic symptom of Parkinson disease.

22. _____ abnormally deep unconsciousness with the absence of voluntary response to stimuli.

23. _____ brain disorder of unknown etiology marked by dementia with symptoms of memory loss, impaired judgment, disorientation, loss of intellectual functioning, and emotional instability.

24. _____ transient loss of consciousness due to inadequate blood flow to the brain; fainting.

25. _____ a sudden discharge of electrical activity in the brain that is clinically detectable; a convulsion.

Correct Answers_____ × 4 = _____% Score

DIAGNOSTIC PROCEDURES AND TESTS

Imaging Procedures

PROCEDURE	DESCRIPTION
cerebral angiography SĔR-ĕ-brăl ăn-jē-ŎG-ră-fē *cerebr=cerebrum* *al=pertaining to* *angio=vessel* *graphy=process of recording*	Radiographic visualization of the vascular system of the brain. A contrast medium is injected into an arterial blood vessel to detect cerebral circulation abnormalities, such as aneurysms, occlusions, vascular and nonvascular tumors, abscesses, and hematomas. Also called cerebral arteriography.
computed tomographic (CT) scan of the brain kŏm-PŪ-tĕd tō-mō-GRĂ-fĭk	Radiographic imaging modality that is more sensitive than a conventional x-ray examination. This scan provides a computerized cross-sectional view of the brain. Contrast medium may also be injected intravenously. CT scans help in differentiating intracranial pathologies such as tumors, cysts, edema, hemorrhage, blood clots, and cerebral aneurysms. Also called *computed axial tomographic (CAT) scan*.
magnetic resonance imaging (MRI) of the brain măg-NĔT-ĭk rĕz-ō-năns ĬM-ă-jĭng	Radiographic imaging procedure that uses magnetic and radio waves to produce cross-sectional, frontal, and sagittal plane views of the brain. MRI is regarded as superior to computed tomography for most CNS abnormalities, particularly those of the posterior fossa, brain stem, and spinal cord. Also called *nuclear magnetic resonance imaging (NMR)*.
positron emission tomography (PET) PŎZ-ĭ-trŏn ē-MĬSH-ŭn tō-MŎG-ră-fē	A procedure used to evaluate metabolic and physiological function of the brain. A radioactive substance is injected into a vein and travels to, and is taken up by, brain cells. A cross-sectional, color-coded image is produced on a screen that reflects the degree of metabolic activity occurring in the brain. PET scans are used to assess brain tumors, Alzheimer disease, epilepsy, and stroke (see Figure 14–9D).

Laboratory Procedures

TEST	DESCRIPTION
cerebrospinal fluid analysis *sĕr-ĕ-brō-SPĪ-năl FLOO-ĭd ă-NĂL-ĭ-sĭs*	Cerebrospinal fluid that is obtained from a lumbar puncture is evaluated for the presence of blood, bacteria, malignant cells, and the amount of protein and glucose present.

SURGICAL AND THERAPEUTIC PROCEDURES

Surgical Procedures

PROCEDURE	DESCRIPTION
craniotomy *krā-nē-ŎT-ō-mē* *cranio=cranium, skull* *tomy=incision (of)*	Surgical procedure to create an opening into the skull. This procedure is performed to gain access to the brain during neurosurgical procedures. It is also performed to relieve intracranial pressure, to control bleeding, or to remove a tumor.
thalamotomy *thăl-ă-MŎT-ō-mē* *thalamo=thalamus* *tomy=incision (of)*	Partial destruction of the thalamus to treat psychosis or intractable pain.
tractotomy *trăk-TŎT-ō-mē*	Transection (cutting made across a long axis) of a nerve fiber tract of the CNS, sometimes resorted to for the relief of intractable pain.
trephination *trĕf-ĭn-Ā-shŭn*	Excision of a circular disk of bone, especially from the skull, using a specialized saw called a trephine. Performed to reveal brain tissue during neurosurgery or to relieve intracranial pressure (ICP).

Therapeutic Procedures

PROCEDURE	DESCRIPTION
nerve block	Injection of local anesthetic along the course of a nerve or nerves to eliminate sensation to and from the area supplied by that nerve or nerves. This procedure is used to relieve chronic back pain and/or sciatica.
occupational therapy	Therapeutic use of self-care, work, and recreational activities to increase independent functioning; may include adaptation of the environment to achieve maximum independence.
physical therapy	Physical therapeutic measure to treat disability or pain and to restore functioning.
shunt placement	In the case of hydrocephalus, surgical placement of a device used to divert excess CSF in the ventricles to another cavity, such as the peritoneal cavity.
stereotactic radiosurgery *stĕr-ē-ō-TĂK-tĭk rā-dē-ō-SŬR-jĕr-ē*	A technique that uses small amounts of radiation directed at an intracranial brain tumor from different angles. A metal frame is affixed to the patient's skull, and the tumor is visualized within the framework of a CT or MRI. A computer plan is generated to direct the radiation. Because multiple small sources are used, normal brain tissue receives little radiation; most of the radiation accumulates in the tumor. This procedure is often used to treat inaccessible intracranial brain tumors and abnormal blood vessel masses.

OTHER PROCEDURES

PROCEDURE	DESCRIPTION
electroencephalog-raphy (EEG) *ē-lĕk-trō-ĕn-sĕf-ă-LŎG-ră-fē* *electro=electricity* *encephalo=brain* *graphy=process of recording*	A graphic recording of the electrical activities of the brain. Like the heart, the brain also generates weak electrical impulses that may be detected and graphically represented. For EEG, electrodes are placed on the scalp over multiple areas of the brain to detect and record brain impulses. EEGs are used to investigate epileptic states, to determine cerebral lesions or tumors, and to determine cerebral death in comatose patients.
lumbar puncture (LP) *LŬM-băr PŬNK-chŭr*	Insertion of a needle into the subarachnoid space of the spinal column at the level of the fourth intervertebral space to withdraw CSF for evaluation, to determine the pressure of the CSF, to withdraw excess CSF, or to administer intrathecal medications. Also called *spinal tap* or *spinal puncture* (Fig. 14–12).

PHARMACOLOGY

DRUG CLASSIFICATION	THERAPEUTIC ACTION
analgesics *ăn-ăl-JĒ-sĭks*	Drugs that selectively suppress pain without producing sedation.

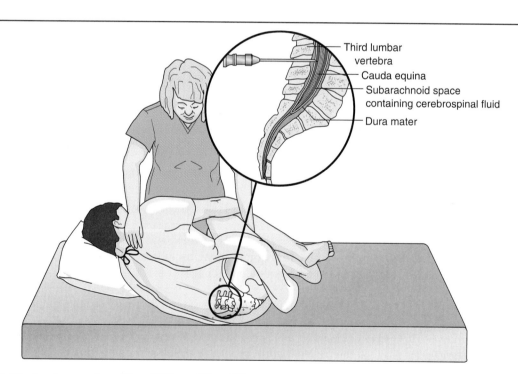

- Third lumbar vertebra
- Cauda equina
- Subarachnoid space containing cerebrospinal fluid
- Dura mater

Figure 14–12 *Lumbar puncture. (From Williams, LS, and Hopper, PD: Understanding Medical Surgical Nursing. FA Davis, Philadelphia, 1999, p 942, with permission.)*

Pharmacology (Continued)

DRUG CLASSIFICATION	THERAPEUTIC ACTION
antibiotics *ăn-tĭ-bī-ŎT-ĭks* *anti=against* *bio=life* *ic=pertaining to, relating to*	Drugs used to cure infections by killing pathogenic bacteria such as those that cause bacterial meningitis.
anticholinergics *ăn-tĭ-kōl-ĭ-NĔR-jĭks*	Drugs that block acetylcholine (cholinergic) receptors. These drugs are used to treat Parkinson disease, motion sickness, and other disorders.
anticonvulsants/ antiepileptics *ăn-tĭ-kŏn-VŬL-sănts* *ăn-tĭ-ĕp-ĭ-LĔP-tĭks*	Drugs used to suppress seizures by changing the permeability of the neuron cell membrane so that it does not depolarize so readily. Used to treat both petit mal and grand mal seizures.
antiparkinsonian agents *ăn-tĭ-păr-kĭn-SŌ-nē-ăn*	Drugs used in the treatment of Parkinson disease by increasing the amount of dopamine in the brain.
antipsychotics *ăn-tĭ-sī-KŎT-ĭks* *anti=against* *psycho=mind* *tic=pertaining to, relating to*	Drugs used to treat agitation in the elderly with dementia and schizophrenia. Also called *neuroleptics*.
barbiturates *băr-BĬT-ū-rāts*	Drugs that act by inhibiting conduction of nerve impulses to the cortex of the brain and depressing motor areas of the brain to produce sedation (sleep). Some barbiturates also possess an anticonvulsant action and are used to treat seizures.
folic acid vitamins *FŌ-lĭk*	Vitamin supplements, primarily folic acid, given to pregnant or "planning on getting pregnant" women. Folic acid has been shown to significantly reduce the risk of babies born with neural defects such as *spina bifida*. It is also used to treat certain types of anemia.
opioids *Ō-pē-oydz*	This classification includes all the natural and synthetic derivatives of opium; morphine is the prototypical opioid and is used as an analgesic for severe and intense pain such as chronic back pain.

❖ ABBREVIATIONS

ABBREVIATION	MEANING	ABBREVIATION	MEANING
AD	Alzheimer disease, right ear (auris dextra)	EEG	electroencephalogram, electroencephalography
ALS	amyotrophic lateral sclerosis (also called *Lou Gehrig disease*)	fx	fracture, frozen section
		ICP	intracranial pressure
ANS	autonomic nervous system	IV	intravenous
ASC	altered state of consciousness	LOC	loss of consciousness
BEAM	brain electrical activity mapping	LP	lumbar puncture
BP	blood pressure	mg	milligram (1/1000 gram)
cm	centimeter	MRA	magnetic resonance angiogram/angiography
CNS	central nervous system		
CO1	coccygeal vertebra	MRI	magnetic resonance imaging
CP	cerebral palsy	MS	musculoskeletal, multiple sclerosis, mental status
CSF	cerebrospinal fluid		
CT	computed tomography scan	NTD	neural tube defect
CAT	(x-ray images in a cross-sectional view)	PET	positron emission tomography
		PNS	peripheral nervous system
CVA	cerebrovascular accident	postop	postoperative
c/w	consistent with	preop	preoperative
Dx	diagnosis	SNS	sensory nervous system
		TIA	transient ischemic attack

Activity 14–9: Clinical Application
Diagnostic Tests, Treatments, and Abbreviations

CAT scan	nerve block
EEG	PET
folic acid	shunt placement
levodopa	thalamotomy
LP	tractotomy
MRI	trephination

Match the terms listed above with the definitions given in the numbered list:

1. _____ excision of a circular disk of bone from the skull to reveal brain tissue during neurosurgery or to relieve intracranial pressure.

2. _____ synthetic dopamine that is used to treat the symptoms of Parkinson disease.

3. _____ a graphic recording of the electrical activity of the brain.

4. _____ imaging procedure that produces a cross-sectional, color-coded image reflecting the metabolic and physiological function of the brain.

5. _____ transection of a nerve fiber tract of the CNS to treat pain.

6. _____ a therapeutic procedure used to divert excess CSF in the ventricles to another cavity.

7. _____ procedure performed to obtain a CSF sample for laboratory analysis.

8. _____ vitamin taken during pregnancy that helps reduce the risk of neural defects in the newborn.

9. _____ the elimination of sensation of a nerve or nerves by injection of a local anesthetic for the purpose of relieving chronic back pain.

10. _____ a partial destruction of a part of the brain in order to treat psychosis or intractable pain.

Correct Answers _____ × 10 = _____% Score

Activity 14–10: Build Medical Words
Diagnostic, Symptomatic, and Surgical Terms

Use *neur/o* (nerve) to build medical words meaning:

1. specialist in the study of the nervous system _____

2. pain in a nerve _____

3. embryonic cell of a nerve _____

Use *cerebr/o* (cerebrum) to build medical words meaning:

4. disease of the cerebrum _____

5. pertaining to the cerebrum and spinal cord _____

Use *encephal/o* (brain) to build medical words meaning:

6. inflammation of the brain _____

7. herniation of the brain _____

8. tumor of the brain _____

Use *myel/o* (spinal cord) to build medical words meaning:

9. suture (of a cut or wound) of the spinal cord _____

10. softening of the spinal cord _____

11. hardening of the spinal cord _____

Use *mening/o* (meninges) to build medical words meaning:

12. herniation of the meninges _____

13. any disease of the meninges _____

14. inflammation of the meninges _____

Use -*plegia* (paralysis) to build medical words meaning:

15. paralysis of one half (of the body) _____

16. paralysis of four (limbs) _____

Use -*trophy* (development, nourishment) to build medical words meaning:

17. without nourishment _____

18. excessive nourishment _____

Use -*phasia* (speech) to build medical words meaning:

19. difficult speech _____

20. without speech _____

Correct Answers _____ × 5 = _____ **% Score**

MEDICAL RECORDS

Larry Belcourt was treated for a neurologic disorder. A neurology consultation, MRI report, operative report, and pathology report are included in his medical chart.

The following dictionary exercise and the medical record analysis will help you develop skills to abstract information and master the terminology in the reports. Accurate interpretation is important because this type of information is used in numerous areas of the medical practice, such as initiation of treatments, evaluation of patients' progress, and completion of insurance claims.

Reading and Dictionary Exercise

Place a check mark in the box [✓] after you complete the exercise.

[ ] **1.** Underline the following words as you read the neurology consultation, the MRI report, the operative report, and the pathology report aloud. These medical records can be found at the end of the chapter.

[ ] **2.** Use a medical dictionary and Appendix F, Part 2 to define the terms below.

Note: You are not expected to fully understand all parts of the medical records. The important aspect of this exercise is to use all available resources to complete it. Eventually you will master the terminology and format of these reports.

>>> MEDICAL RECORD 14–1: NEUROLOGY CONSULTATION

Term	Pronunciation	Meaning
aphasia	ă-FĀ-zē-ă	_____

hypertension	hī-pĕr-TĔN-shŭn	_____
diabetes	dī-ă-BĒ-tēz	_____
myocardial infarction	mī-ō-KĂR-dē-ăl ĭn-FĂRK-shŭn	_____
atrial fibrillation	Ā-trē-ăl fĭ-brĭl-Ā-shŭn	_____
cholecystitis	kō-lē-sĭs-TĪ-tĭs	_____
cholecystectomy	chō-lē-sĭs-TĔK-tō-mē	_____
deep tendon reflexes	dēp TĔN-dŭn RĒ-flĕk-sĕz	_____
plantar	PLĂN-tăr	_____
flexor	FLĔKS-or	_____
bilaterally	bī-LĂT-ĕr-ăl-ē	_____
gait	gāt	_____
parietal	pă-RĪ-ĕ-tăl	_____
temporal	TĔM-pō-răl	_____
echocardiogram	ĕk-ō-KĂR-dē-ō-grăm	_____
carotid duplex study	kă-RŎT-ĭd	_____

>>> MEDICAL RECORD 14-2: MRI REPORT

Term	Pronunciation	Meaning
Circle of Willis	SĔR-kl ŏv WĬL-ĭs	_____
sagittal	SAJ-ĭ-tăl	_____
axial	ĂK-sē-ăl	_____
proton spin	PRŌ-tŏn spĭn	_____
necrotic	nĕ-KRŎT-ĭk	_____
posterior	pŏs-TĒ-rē-ŏr	_____
parietal lobe	pă-RĪ-ĕ-tăl lōb	_____
lateral	LĂT-ĕr-ăl	_____
anterior	ăn-TĬR-ē-or	_____
medial	MĒ-dē-ăl	_____

temporal	*TĔM-pōr-ăl*	_____
corpus callosum	*KOR-pŭs kă-LŌ-sŭm*	_____
peritumoral edema	*pĕr-ĭ-TOO-mor-ăl ĕ-DĒ-mă*	_____
occipital lobe	*ŏk-SĬP-ĭ-tăl lōb*	_____
fossa	*FŎS-ă*	_____
brainstem	*BRĀN-stĕm*	_____
cerebellum	*sĕr-ĕ-BĔL-ŭm*	_____
stenosis	*stĕ-NŌ-sĭs*	_____
aneurysm	*ĂN-ū-rĭzm*	_____
gliomatosis cerebri	*glī-ō-mă-TŌ-sĭs SĔR-ĕ-brī*	_____
lymphoma	*lĭm-FŌ-mă*	_____
biopsy	*BĪ-ŏp-sē*	_____

>>> MEDICAL RECORD 14-3: OPERATIVE REPORT

Term	Pronunciation	Meaning
glioblastoma	*glī-ō-blăs-TŌ-mă*	_____
stereotaxic	*stĕr-ē-ō-TĂK-zĭk*	_____
biopsy	*BĪ-ŏp-sē*	_____
endotracheal	*ĕn-dō-TRĀ-kē-ăl*	_____
hemosiderin	*hē-mō-SĬD-ĕr-ĭn*	_____
glioma	*glī-Ō-mă*	_____
glioblastoma multiforme	*glī-ō-blăs-TŌ-mă MŬL-tĭ-form*	_____

>>> MEDICAL RECORD 14-4: PATHOLOGY REPORT

Term	Pronunciation	Meaning
intracranial	*ĭn-tră-KRĀ-nē-ăl*	_____
glial	*GLĪ-ăl*	_____
neoplasm	*NĒ-ō-plăzm*	_____
undifferentiated	*ŭn-dĭf-ĕr-ĔN-shē-āt-ĕd*	_____

| endothelial | ĕn-dō-THĒ-lē-ăl | _____ |
| necrosis | nĕ-KRŌ-sĭs | _____ |

Critical Thinking: Analysis of Medical Records

This section provides experience in abstracting and analyzing information from medical records. At the same time, it reinforces the material presented in this chapter.

>>> MEDICAL RECORD 14–1: NEUROLOGY CONSULTATION

1. What was Mr. Belcourt referred for and had he experienced these symptoms previously?

_____

_____

2. Place a "+" in the space for positive findings and a "−" for negative findings in the review of systems. A positive finding indicates the patient had a history (Hx) of this condition; a negative finding indicates the patient did not have a history of this condition.

_____ aphasia   _____ high cholesterol

_____ hypertension   _____ cholecystitis

_____ cerebrovascular accident

3. How did the patient initially perform on the neurologic examination?

_____

_____

4. Did his ability to complete the neurologic examination change over time?

_____

_____

_____

5. What was the medical plan?

_____

_____

6. Why did the doctor increase the daily aspirin dosage?

_____

_____

>>> MEDICAL RECORD 14-2: MRI REPORT

7. What type of imaging procedure was performed?

_____

_____

8. Where in the brain were masses found?

_____

_____

9. What procedure was recommended to confirm the diagnosis?

_____

>>> MEDICAL RECORD 14-3: OPERATIVE REPORT

10. What kind of brain biopsy was performed?

_____

>>> MEDICAL RECORD 14-4: PATHOLOGY REPORT

11. What was the postoperative diagnosis confirmed by microscopic evaluation?

_____

12. Is the tumor malignant? What type of cells make up the tumor?

_____

_____

Audio Practice

Listen to the audio CD-ROM to practice the pronunciation of selected medical terms from this chapter.

Medical Record 14–1. Neurology Consultation

GENERAL HOSPITAL AND MEDICAL CENTER
2211 Fifth Avenue North • Healthy City, USA 12345 • (321) 123-4567

Neurology Consultation

Patient Name: Belcourt, Larry   **Patient Number:** 12-34-56
Birth Date: 11/25/xx   **Room Number:**   408

DATE OF CONSULTATION: 05-08-20xx

REASON FOR CONSULTATION: The patient is a 75-year-old, right-handed male, who was referred to our service for aphasia. Today, he went to work as usual, but at about 1:30 or 2:00 PM, he began having difficulty talking. His wife drove him to the urgent care center and he was transferred to General Hospital. On the way to the hospital, his speech worsened. He repeatedly said, "what can I do for you." He then became more fluent during the course of his admission evaluation.

For the last two months he has had two episodes of difficulty verbally expressing himself lasting for short periods. He was unable to be more specific about these episodes.

PAST MEDICAL HISTORY: There is no history of hypertension, diabetes, myocardial infarction, smoking, family or personal history of CVA, elevated cholesterol, atrial fibrillation, thyroid disease, or gastrointestinal disease. He has had cholecystitis and is scheduled for a cholecystectomy next month. No history of heart, liver, kidney, or lung disease. No previous surgeries or injuries.

MEDICATIONS: Aspirin 81 mg daily.

FAMILY MEDICAL HISTORY: His father died in his 90s. His mother died in an accidental explosion at middle-age. He has 3 brothers in good health. He has two sons in good health.

SOCIAL HISTORY: He lives with his wife, he is retired, and he walks about two miles every day. He does not smoke. He takes alcohol occasionally.

PHYSICAL EXAMINATION:

VITAL SIGNS: BP 191/84, pulse 69.

GENERAL: Patient is in no apparent distress.

Continued

Neurology Consultation, page 2
Patient Name: Belcourt, Larry

Patient Number: 12-34-56

MENTAL STATUS: Initially the patient only answered questions with the phrase "what can I do for you." He could not understand one step commands. His ability to cooperate in the neurological exam was markedly impaired. About an hour later, he was cooperative, as well as, alert and oriented. He knew the date, day of the week, months, and year, his home address and zip code. He could only name the current president and could not recall any others. He could not subtract 7 from 100 or 3 from 30, but could add 2 and 2 serially to 64, but not 128. He was able to do a 3-step command with some difficulty. He named objects. He closed his eyes on command and squeezed my hand on command. Cranial nerves and visual fields appeared intact. Pupils were equal and reactive. Sensation over his face was intact. His face was symmetrical, speech was normal. Hearing was intact to conversational speech. Tongue protruded in the midline. Motor examination revealed no arm or leg drift. Strength in both upper and lower extremities was good. The deep tendon reflexes were diminished but equal. Plantar responses were flexor bilaterally. Cerebellar testing revealed good finger-to-nose testing, gait was not tested.

ASSESSMENT: Probable left hemispheric cerebrovascular accident in the parietal temporal area. Questionable TIA.

PLAN: Echocardiogram, carotid duplex study, CT, MRI with MRA, increase aspirin to 650 mg twice daily, observation, IV fluids.

_____

Diane McDermott, M.D

DMD/gmi

D: 05/08/xx
T: 05/11/xx

Medical Record 14–2. MRI Report

GENERAL HOSPITAL AND MEDICAL CENTER
2211 Fifth Avenue North • Healthy City, USA 12345 • (321) 123-4567

MRI Report

Patient Name: Belcourt, Larry   **Patient Number:** 12-34-56
Birth Date: 11/25/xx   **Room Number:** 408

DATE OF PROCEDURE: 05-09-xx

PROCEDURE: MRI-Scan of the brain with Gadolinium with Magnetic Resonance Angiogram (MRA) of the vessels of Circle of Willis

TECHNIQUES: The imaging sequence included pre-gadolinium sagittal and axial T1 weighted images followed by axial proton spin and T2 weighted images. MRA of the vessels of the circle of Willis was also performed at the request of Dr. McDermott. The images were computer enhanced and fixtured in maximum intensity projection. 20 cc of Omniscan was then injected intravenously and axial and coronal T1 weighted images of the brain were again performed. This study is compared with the CT scan examinations of 10-25-xx and 5-8-xx.

FINDINGS: The scans demonstrated a large necrotic mass in the left posterior temporal parietal lobe. This mass extends to the ventricular surface at the level of the left lateral ventricle. In addition, there is spotty enhancement also present in the lateral more anterior aspect of the left temporal lobe and a 1 cm nodule in the medial right parietal lobe. There is a mild degree of midline shift towards the right. The mass appears to have entrapped the left temporal horn of the ventricle, which is disproportionally distended. On the T2 weighted images there is a rather extensive abnormal signal that crosses the corpus callosum. The patient also has a marked abnormal signal in the anterior right temporal lobe. There is extensive peritumoral edema in the left parietal and posterior temporal lobe. There is also edema in the left occipital lobe.

In the posterior fossa, the brainstem and cerebellum are otherwise within normal limits and there are no posterior fossa lesions. On the MRA examination, there is normal appearance of carotid arteries. There was no evidence of stenosis or aneurysm.

IMPRESSION: Multiple enhancing brain masses in the left parietal as well as the left temporal and right parietal lobes. The largest is in the left parietal region. There is also a non-enhancing abnormal signal in the anterior right temporal lobe and in the corpus callosum. The combination of findings is highly suspicious for a gliomatosis cerebri. Lymphoma could also give rise to a similar appearance. Metastatic disease could not be entirely excluded. However, it is considered less likely in view of the non-enhancing infiltrating tumor identified in the anterior right

Continued

MRI Report, page 2
Patient Name: Belcourt, Larry   **Patient Number:** 12-34-56

temporal lobe. Normal MRA of the vessels of the Circle of Willis. A brain biopsy is recommended to confirm diagnosis.

_____

Thomas R. Seline, M.D.

TRS/mmb
D: 05/09/xx
T: 05/11/xx

Medical Record 14–3. Operative Report

GENERAL HOSPITAL AND MEDICAL CENTER
2211 Fifth Avenue North • Healthy City, USA 12345 • (321) 123-4567

Operative Report

Patient Name: Belcourt, Larry   **Patient Number:** 12-34-56
Birthdate: 11/25/xx   **Room Number:** 408

DATE OF PROCEDURE: 5-10-xx

PREOPERATIVE DIAGNOSIS: Left parietal tumor

POSTOPERATIVE DIAGNOSIS: Glioblastoma

PROCEDURE PERFORMED: Stereotaxic brain biopsy.

SURGEON: Michael O. Shea, MD   **ASSISTANT:** Wendy Timmons, MD

ANESTHESIA: General endotracheal

INDICATIONS/FINDINGS: Good tissue was obtained which appeared hemosiderin laden and yellowish and tough. Specimens were sent for frozen section and the pathologist clearly indicated that this was a high-grade glioma, likely glioblastoma multiforme. They had plenty of tissue to make the diagnosis with.

_____
Micheal O. Shea, M.D.

MOS/cmc
D: 05/10/xx
T: 05/12/xx

Medical Record 14–4. Pathology Report

GENERAL HOSPITAL AND MEDICAL CENTER
2211 Fifth Avenue North • Healthy City, USA 12345 • (321) 123-4567

Pathology Report

Patient Name: Belcourt, Larry   **Patient Number:** 12-34-56
Birthdate: 11/25/xx   **Room Number:** 408

SPECIMEN: Brain tumor
            ORC MICRO: High grade glioma c/w glioblastoma multiforme

CLINICAL DATA: MRI-brain
                 PREOP/POSTOP DX: Intracranial tumor

GROSS DESCRIPTION: Received fresh for frozen section analysis in a container labeled with patient's name and "brain tumor" is a 0.6 x 0.5 x 0.1 cm aggregate of several irregular gray-white pieces of soft tissue. The frozen section residue, which is the entire specimen, is submitted in FX.

MICROSCOPIC DIAGNOSIS: GLIOBLASTOMA MULTIFORME (biopsy, brain tumor)

COMMENT: Material on the scrimp preparation, frozen section and permanents reveal a high-grade primary glial neoplasm showing undifferentiated small cells, endothelial proliferation, and areas of tissue necrosis. These features are consistent with glioblastoma multiforme.

_____
Richard W. Gisson, M.D.

RWG/edt
D: 05/11/xx
T: 05/12/xx

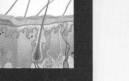

chapter

15 Hematology

Chapter Outline

Objectives

Upon completion of this chapter, you will be able to:

- Describe the type of medical treatment a hematologist provides.
- Discuss the main functions and components of blood.
- Understand the different types of blood groups and the significance of blood clotting.
- Recognize, pronounce, build, and spell correctly terms related to the blood system.
- Describe pathological conditions, diagnostic tests, and therapeutic procedures related to the blood system.
- Demonstrate your knowledge of this chapter by successfully completing the activities and the analysis of medical records.

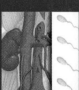

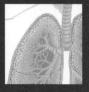
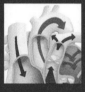
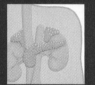
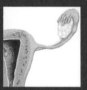
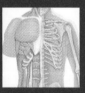

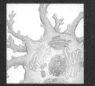
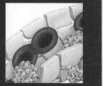

544

About Hematology

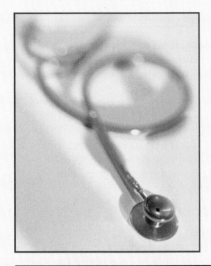

Hematology is the study of the blood, blood-forming tissues, and the diseases associated with these tissues. Physicians who specialize in the study and treatment of the blood and blood disorders are called **hematologists**. Hematologists treat both malignant (cancerous) and nonmalignant blood diseases. Historically, they were the first to use chemical therapies (chemotherapy) to treat hematologic malignancies. With time, it was discovered that these treatments could also be effective on so-called "solid tumors," such as breast, lung, and stomach cancers (previously treated only with surgery). Consequently, hematology became closely associated with another medical specialty—oncology. The medical specialty of oncology is covered in Chapter 19.

To grasp the scope of practice and the role of health-care practitioners in the medical specialty of hematology, it is important to understand the structure and function of the blood system as well as the language of medicine that is related to this medical specialty.

Selected Key Terms

erythrocyte ĕ-RĬTH-rō-cīt *erythro=red* *cyte=cell*	A mature red blood cell (RBC). The main function of the RBC is to carry oxygen.
hyperuricemia hī-pĕr-ū-rĭs-Ē-mē-ă	An abnormal amount of uric acid in the blood.
interstitial ĭn-tĕr-STĬSH-ăl	Pertaining to the space between cells, as in interstitial fluid (fluid between the cells).
leukocyte LOO-kō-sīt *leuko=white* *cyte=cell*	A white blood cell (WBC). Leukocytes are the primary effector cells against infection and tissue damage. There are five types of WBCs: *basophils*, *eosinophils*, *neutrophils*, *monocytes*, and *lymphocytes*.
osmosis ŏz-MŌ-sĭs	The passage of solvent through a semipermeable membrane that separates solutions of different concentrations. The solvent, usually water, passes through the membrane from the region of lower concentration of solute to that of a higher concentration of solute; thus the concentrations of the two solutions tend to equalize.
osmotic pressure ŏz-MŎT-ĭk	Force under which a solvent, usually water, moves from a solution of lower solute (a dissolved substance) concentration to a solution of higher solute concentration when the solutions are separated by a semipermeable membrane.
pH	Symbol for degree of acidity or alkalinity of a substance. In chemistry, the degree of acidity or alkalinity of a substance is expressed in pH values. The neutral point, at which a solution would be neither acid nor alkaline, is pH 7. Increasing acidity is expressed as a number less than 7, and increasing alkalinity is expressed as a number greater than 7. Maximum acidity is pH 0, and maximum alkalinity is pH 14.

solute
SŎL-ūt

The substance that is dissolved in a solution.

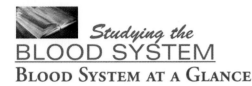

BLOOD SYSTEM

BLOOD SYSTEM AT A GLANCE

The primary function of blood is to transport nutrients throughout the body. It also prevents toxic buildup in the body by providing a transportation medium to remove waste products.

The nutrients of digested food pass through the cells that line the small intestine and are carried into the bloodstream for distribution throughout the cells of the body. Oxygen from the lungs is picked up by the blood and transported to the cells throughout the body. Wastes, such as carbon dioxide, uric acid, and urea, are carried through the bloodstream and excreted either by the lungs or the kidneys. Hormones that function as chemical messengers are picked up by the blood at their production sites and delivered to other sites to regulate activities, such as reproduction and general growth. Blood, with the help of its white blood cells (or WBCs), provides an important line of defense against pathogens. Consequently, both blood and lymph (Chapter 13) play a vital role in combating infections and work together with the body's immune system. Blood has clotting capability that prevents excessive loss of blood in cases of injury.

FUNCTIONS OF BLOOD

Blood is a complex liquid body tissue composed of a collection of similar cell types. These cells are specialized to perform a number of critical body functions, such as transportation, regulation, and protection.

The *transportation functions* of blood consist of:

- Delivering oxygen from the lungs and nutrients from the digestive tract to all body cells.

- Delivering waste products from the cells to elimination sites (to the lungs for disposal of carbon dioxide in the exhaled air, and to the kidneys for disposal of nitrogenous wastes in the urine).

- Delivering hormones from endocrine glands to their target sites.

The *regulatory functions* of blood consist of:

- Maintaining normal body temperature through the heat-absorbing and coolant properties of its water content.

- Maintaining normal pH in body tissues through buffers that prevent excessive or abrupt changes in blood pH, which could jeopardize normal cellular activities.

The *protective functions* of blood consist of:

- Prevention of blood loss through the clotting mechanism. When a blood vessel is injured, platelets and plasma proteins initiate clot formation, halting blood loss.

- Prevention of infections through antibodies, which are white blood cells, and through complement proteins. Both antibodies and complement proteins are contained in the blood and help defend the body against foreign intruders such as bacteria and viruses.

COMPONENTS OF BLOOD

Blood is composed of a straw-colored liquid portion, called **plasma,** and three types of **formed elements:** *erythrocytes, leukocytes,* and *thrombocytes (platelets).* The formed elements are living cells that are suspended and carried in plasma. Plasma is essential for transporting the cellular elements of blood throughout the circulatory system. When the formed elements are removed from the blood, the plasma remains (Fig. 15–1).

Plasma

As you read the following material, refer to Figure 15–2 for an illustration of the formed elements of the blood. This figure will help you understand the material as the discussion of the formed elements continues.

Even though blood plasma is mostly water (about 91.5%), it contains over 100 different dissolved **solutes.** These include nutrients, hormones, nitrogenous wastes, respiratory gases, and electrolytes. The most plentiful of the solutes are the **plasma proteins,** which are produced mainly by the liver. They are grouped into three major categories: albumins, globulins, and fibrinogen.

1. **Albumins,** produced by the liver, provide the required **osmotic pressure** to draw water from the surrounding tissue fluid into the capillaries. This action is needed to maintain blood volume and blood pressure. Because albumins cannot flow readily through capillary walls, they remain in the blood and attract water from the tissues into the bloodstream

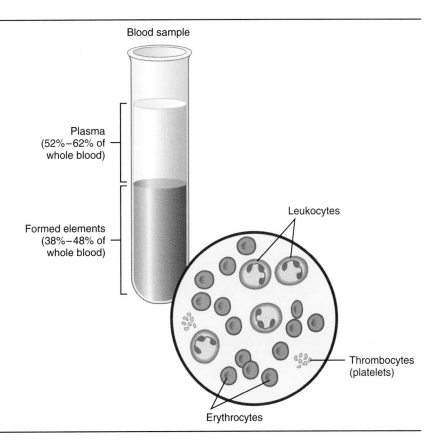

Blood sample

Plasma
(52%–62% of
whole blood)

Formed elements
(38%–48% of
whole blood)

Leukocytes

Thrombocytes
(platelets)

Erythrocytes

Figure 15–1 *Blood is composed of a liquid portion called plasma and three types of formed elements: erythrocytes, leukocytes, and thrombocytes (platelets).*

through the process of **osmosis**. They oppose the water's inclination to leave the blood and leak out into tissue spaces. This is how the balance between the fluid in the blood and the fluid in the **interstitial** tissues is maintained. If the balance of osmotic pressure is upset, the fluid from the blood vessels will leak out into surrounding tissues and cause a swelling of the tissues called **edema**. Sodium ions are the other major **solute** contributing to osmotic pressure of blood. When excessive sodium or salt is ingested, excess water is retained in the blood. Some of this excess water seeps out into surrounding tissues causing a mild form of edema.

2. **Globulins** are divided into three subtypes: alpha, beta, and gamma globulins. The **alpha** and **beta globulins** are produced by the liver and have a variety of functions, including transport of lipids and fat-soluble vitamins in the blood. Antibodies, also called *immunoglobulins (Igs)*, constitute the **gamma globulin** part of blood proteins. The **Igs** are formed in the bone marrow, spleen, and all lymphoid tissues of the body except the thymus. Human antibodies can be grouped into five Ig classes, designated by letter names: **IgA, IgD, IgE, IgG,** and **IgM.** See Table 13–1 for a summary of their locations and functions.

3. **Fibrinogens** play an important role in blood clotting, or **coagulation**. This is discussed in the following section.

Formed Elements

Although the formed elements—**erythrocytes, leukocytes,** and **thrombocytes (platelets)**—perform different functions, there are important similarities in their development. All of them arise from the same type of *primitive stem cell*, or *hemocytoblast*, which is found in the red bone marrow. The development and production of different types of blood cells (*hematopoiesis* or *hemopoiesis*) is illustrated in Figure 15–3.

Erythrocytes

The development of an erythrocyte (or red bood cell, RBC) from a stem cell is shown in Figure 15–3. Follow the *arrows* to observe how stem cells give rise to **normoblasts,** which turn into **reticulocytes.** You will note that the developing cells decrease in size, and just before maturity, the nucleus passes from the cell. It leaves behind a small fragment of nuclear material that resembles a fine, lacy net, which gives this cell its name, **reticulocyte**. In the final stage, the fragment of nuclear material disappears, and the mature erythrocyte enters the circulatory system.

Erythrocytes are the only human cells without a nucleus. They are shaped like biconcave disks—

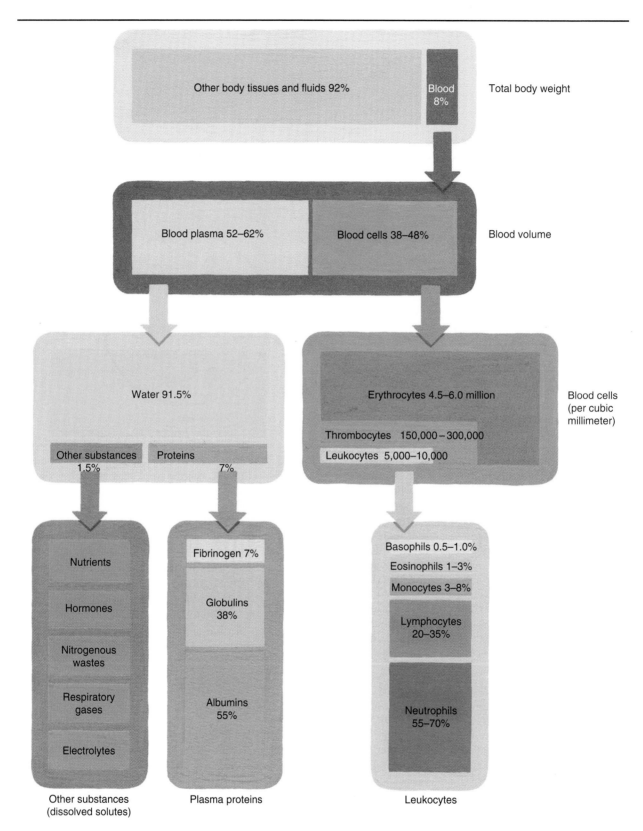

Figure 15–2 *The components of blood and the relationship of blood to other body tissues. (From Scanlon, VC, and Sanders, TS: Essentials of Anatomy and Physiology, ed 3. FA Davis, Philadelphia, 1999, p 237, with permission.)*

flattened disks with depressed centers. Consequently, erythrocytes look like mini donuts, as shown in Figure 15–3. This unique shape maximizes the surface area and makes them more efficient in their function of delivering oxygen from the lungs and releasing it to tissue cells. Erythrocytes also transport carbon dioxide released by tissue cells in the opposite direction—back to the lungs. Although erythrocytes are small cells, they vastly outnumber the other types of formed elements. They have an average life span of 120 days and are eventually destroyed by phagocytic cells in the liver, spleen, and bone marrow. Each erythrocyte contains an iron protein called **hemoglobin** (*heme=iron-containing pigment; globin= protein*). The iron group of *heme* has the ability to combine with oxygen in the lungs and in the body's cells. Hemoglobin is also responsible for the red color of erythrocytes. Lack of erythrocytes,

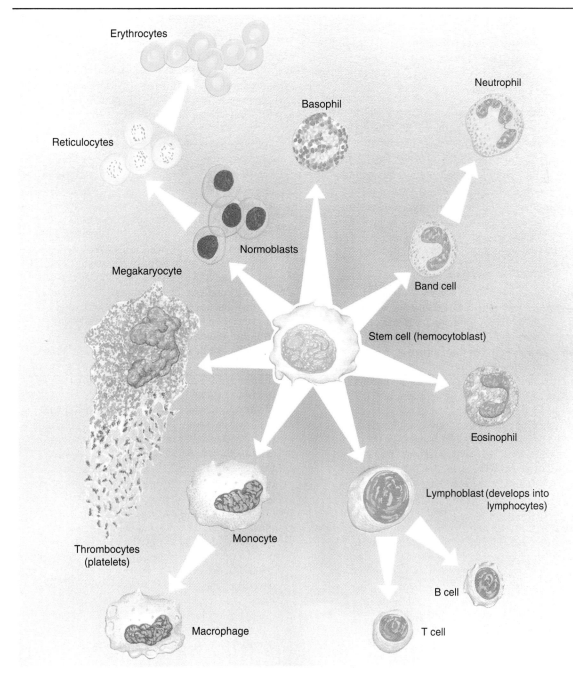

Figure 15–3   *The production of blood cells (hematopoiesis). Stem cells, or hemocytoblasts, are found in red bone marrow and in lymphatic tissue. They are the precursor cells for all the types of blood cells. (From Scanlon, VC, and Sanders, TS: Essentials of Anatomy and Physiology, ed 3. FA Davis, Philadelphia, 1999, p 239, with permission.)*

hemoglobin, or iron can result in anemia, which can produce such symptoms such as shortness of breath and general fatigue.

Leukocytes

Leukocytes (WBCs) are crucial to our defense against disease. They help protect the body from damage caused by bacteria, viruses, parasites, toxins, and tumor cells. Whereas erythrocytes are confined to the bloodstream and carry out their functions in the blood, leukocytes can slip out of capillary blood vessels. The circulatory system transports them to various areas of the body (mostly loose connective tissues or lymphoid tissues) where they are needed to mount inflammatory or immune responses. Unlike erythrocytes, leukocytes have nuclei; and they are fewer in number.

Leukocytes fall into two major groups: granulocytes and agranulocytes. The first group, the **granulocytes,** are the most abundant. Leukocytes are produced in the red bone marrow, have granules in their cytoplasm, and possess lobed nuclei. Functionally, all granulocytes are phagocytic, but each is different and has a specialized function. There are three types of granulocytes: *basophils*, *neutrophils*, *and eosinophils*. Unless they are stained, they are almost invisible under the microscope. Fortunately, their cytoplasmic granules stain quite specifically.

- **Basophils** contain large, coarse granules that stain dark purple with a basic alkaline dye (Fig. 15–4A). Basophils are believed to be involved in allergic reactions. They release *histamine*, an inflammatory chemical that acts as a vasodilator (dilates blood vessels, making them leaky) and attracts other white blood cells to the inflamed area. Basophils also release *heparin*, an anticlotting substance.
- **Neutrophils** contain very fine granules that are neutral (see Fig. 15–4B). Consequently, they do not stain dramatically with either eosin or a basic alkaline dye. The granules take up both basic (blue) and acidic (red) dyes. The combination gives the cytoplasm a very pale lilac color. Neutrophils are the most plentiful of leukocytes and are active phagocytes. They are chemically attracted to sites of inflammation. Neutrophil numbers increase explosively during acute bacterial infections such as meningitis and appendicitis. They have oddly shaped nuclei with lobes and strands, which give them an alternate name—**polymorphonuclear neutrophils (PMNs).**
- **Eosinophils** contain large, coarse granules that stain bright red with an acidic red dye (*eosin*) (Fig. 15–4C). Eosinophils perform several functions, one of which is to lead the counterattack against parasitic worms, such as flatworms (tapeworms) and roundworms

(pinworms), which are too large to be phagocytized. These worms are ingested in food, especially raw fish (sushi), or invade the body via the skin and then typically burrow into the intestinal or respiratory *mucosae*. When a parasitic worm is encountered, eosinophils gather around and release the enzymes from their cytoplasmic granules onto the parasite's surface, thus digesting it away. Eosinophils also help lessen the severity of inflammation caused by allergies.

The second major group of leukocytes, **agranulocytes,** do not contain any cytoplasmic granules. They are typically spherical or kidney shaped, contain one nucleus (**mononuclear**), and lack the dark-staining granules. There are two types of agranulocytes: lymphocytes (see Fig. 15–4B) and monocytes (see Fig. 15–4D).

- **Lymphocytes** contain large, round nuclei (*nucleus*, singular) within a thin rim of cytoplasm (see Fig. 15–4B). Although large numbers of lymphocytes are present in the body, only a small proportion of them are found in the bloodstream. Lymphocytes are so called because they are embedded in lymphoid tissues (lymph nodes, spleen, etc.), where they play an important role in immunity. The two major types of lymphocytes are the T cells and B cells. T cells circulate in the blood and provide defense against disease by attacking foreign and abnormal cells. B cells produce antibodies (immunoglobulins) in reaction to foreign antigens. Refer to Flow Chart 15–1 for a listing of the different types of leukocytes. The immune functions of B and T lymphocytes are described in greater detail in Chapter 13.
- **Monocytes** are the largest of the leukocytes and generally have an oval or kidney-shaped nucleus (see Fig. 15–4D). Like neutrophils, monocytes are phagocytic cells that ingest and destroy foreign substances. They travel from the bloodstream into tissues. Once in the tissues, monocytes develop into highly mobile *macrophages* that dispose of cellular debris by phagocytosis. The macrophages increase in number and are actively phagocytic in chronic infections, such as tuberculosis. They are also crucial in the body's defense against viruses and certain intracellular bacterial parasites. See Figure 13–4, which illustrates macrophages ingesting bacteria. As discussed in Chapter 13, macrophages are also important in activating lymphocytes to mount the immune response.

Thrombocytes

Thrombocytes, also known as platelets, are the smallest elements in blood. They initiate blood clot-

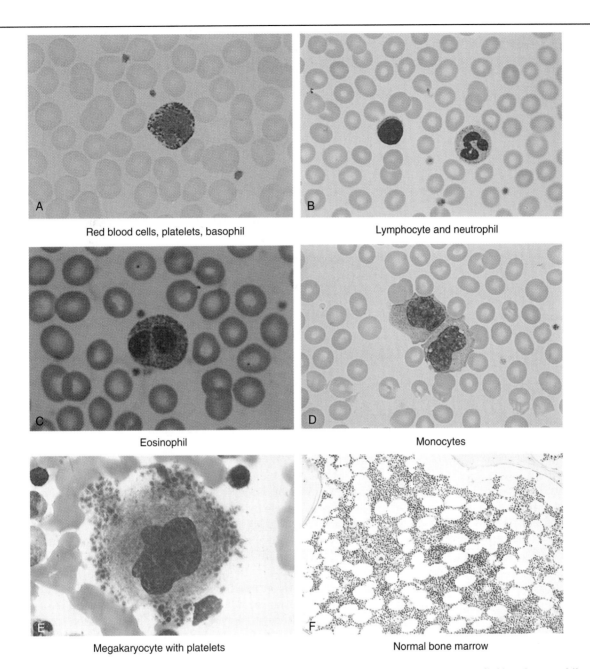

Figure 15–4 *Different types of blood cells: (A) red blood cells, platelets, and a basophil; (B) lymphocyte (left) and neutrophil (right); (C) eosinophil; (D) monocytes; (E) megakaryocyte with platelets (panels A to E: magnified × 600); (F) normal bone marrow (magnified × 200). (From Harmening, DM: Hematology and Fundamentals of Hemostatis, ed 3. FA Davis, Philadephia, 1997, pp 16, 18, 21, 26, 29, 48, with permission.)*

ting when injuries occur and help to close tears in damaged blood vessels. Platelets stem from large cells, called **megakaryocytes,** located in red bone marrow (see Fig. 15–4*E* and 15–4*F*). A megakaryocyte tends to shatter like a glass plate, releasing cytoplasm, or platelets, into the circulatory system. Platelets live for approximately 10 days. They are less than half the size of a red blood cell, and the platelet count per cubic milliliter is 130,000 to 360,000 per cubic milliliter of blood.

BLOOD CLOTTING

A number of physiological mechanisms are activated to promote **hemostasis** (cessation of bleeding) when a blood vessel is injured. The complex process of plugging a ruptured blood vessel to stop bleeding involves several plasma proteins and clotting factors—a process called **blood clotting,** or **coagulation.** Blood clotting takes place when platelets trigger a series of complex chemical reactions that result in a re-

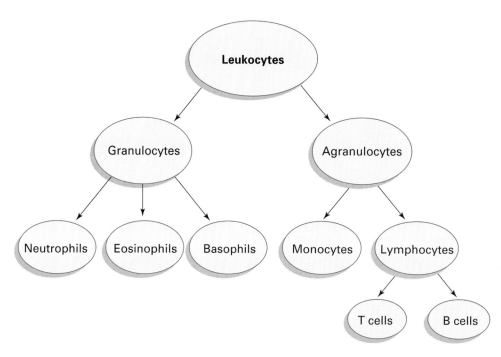

Flowchart 15–1 Types of leukocytes.

lease of protein called **thromboplastin.** Thromboplastin causes the plasma protein **prothrombin** to turn into **thrombin,** which leads to the formation of fibrin strands. The fibrin strands create a mesh at the wound site, trapping red blood cells to form a **blood clot**. The clot acts as a blockade and prevents further loss of blood from the injured area. A deficiency of one of the factors necessary for blood coagulation can be caused by a hereditary disorder called **hemophilia**.

In some instances, a blood clot may form although a blood vessel is not injured. Blood clots of this type are known as **thrombi** (singular, thrombus). A thrombus is an aggregation of platelets, fibrin, clotting factors, and the cellular elements of the blood attached to the interior wall of a vein or artery. Sometimes a thrombus occludes the lumen of the vessel. The condition of a clot dislodging and traveling through the bloodstream is called an **embolism.** The discharged circulating clot is known as an **embolus** (plural, emboli). **Emboli** are not limited to thrombi but can consist of any mass of undissolved matter present in a blood or lymphatic vessel. The emboli are transported by the blood or the lymph. Emboli may be solid, liquid, or gaseous; for example, emboli may consist of bits of tissue, tumor cells, fat globules, air bubbles, clumps of bacteria, or foreign bodies.

BLOOD TRANSFUSIONS AND BLOOD GROUPS

It is important to determine a patient's blood type before medical procedures of blood transfusions and surgery. Before blood typing was understood and conducted, blood transfusions were not always successful. Sometimes the recipient improved, but at other times, the recipient suffered a blood reaction in which the RBCs clumped (**agglutination**) and then ruptured (**hemolysis**). Agglutination obstructs vessels by hindering blood flow. A more serious consequence is that the hemoglobin of the ruptured RBCs, now called *free hemoglobin*, may clog the kidney's tubules and cause renal failure. If renal failure is complete, the recipient may die. Although some transfusion reactions are not lethal, they can cause fever, nausea, allergic responses, and general toxicity. Safe transfusions of whole blood depend on properly matching the blood types of donors and recipients. The process of **typing** and **cross-matching** of donor and recipient blood ensures that donated blood will not bring about any adverse reactions in the recipient. To explain blood types, the relationship between antigens and antibodies is briefly reviewed here.

Antigens are markers on RBCs that identify cells as being the body's own cells or as being foreign cells. Antigens of foreign substances are identified as **intruders** or **nonself**. Appearance of nonself substances stimulates the production of antibodies. **Antibodies** are proteins produced by WBCs in response to foreign antigens. The response or reaction between antigens and antibodies is known as an **immune response** or an **immune reaction**. An immune reaction is the defense function of the body that produces antibodies to destroy invading anti-

TABLE 15–1: ABO Blood Groups

BLOOD TYPE	ANTIGENS PRESENT	ANTIBODIES PRESENT IN PLASMA	BLOOD THAT CAN BE RECEIVED FOR TRANSFUSION	POPULATION WITH THIS BLOOD TYPE, %
A	A	anti-B	A, O	41
B	B	anti-A	B, O	12
AB	Both A and B	Neither anti-A nor anti-B	A, B, AB, O Universal recipient	4
O	Neither A nor B	Both anti-A and anti-B	O	45

gens. Refer to Chapter 13 for an in-depth presentation of antigens and antibodies.

Because individuals have different blood types (meaning that they have different antigen markers on their RBCs), transfusion of incompatible blood can be fatal. One individual's RBC markers may be recognized as foreign if transfused into someone with a different red blood cell type, and the transfused cells may be agglutinated and destroyed. The verification that the antigens and antibodies are compatible prevents adverse transfusion reactions.

In humans there are many naturally occurring red blood cell antigens. The absence or presence of each antigen on the RBC allows each person's blood cells to be classified into several different blood groups. The two most important groups, the *ABO blood groups* and the *Rh blood groups*, are discussed here.

ABO Blood Groups

The ABO blood groups are based on either the presence or absence of two major antigens on the RBCs: antigen A and antigen B, or no antigen (O). Depending on which of these antigens is inherited, the ABO blood group of a person will be one of the following: A, B, AB, or O. A person with the A antigen has *type A blood;* a person with the B antigen has *type B blood;* a person with both A and B antigens has *type AB* blood; and a person with neither A nor B antigens has *type O blood.*

The most common ABO blood group is *type O,* whereas the least prevalent is *type AB.* As indicated in Table 15–1, *type O blood* has neither A nor B antigens. Persons with this blood type are known as **universal donors**. If *type O blood* is given to a person with blood type A, B, or AB, it is transfused slowly so that the antibodies are diluted in the recipient's bloodstream, minimizing the chance of an adverse reaction, because it has no A or B antigens.

Also, because those with *type AB blood* are devoid of antibodies to both A and B antigens, they are theoretically **universal recipients** and can receive blood transfusions from any of the ABO types.

Rh Blood Groups

In addition to A and B antigens, many other antigens are found on the surface of RBCs, each of which is called an **Rh factor** (antigen). The **Rh blood typing** classification arose from **rhesus monkey studies** (hence, the Rh designation) in which these antigens were first discovered. People who have Rh antigens present on the red blood cells are said to be **Rh positive,** whereas those who do not have Rh antigens are **Rh negative.** The presence of Rh antigens, as with antigens A and B, is an inherited trait. Blood typing for the Rh factors is determined in the same manner as for ABO blood typing.

Activity 15–1: Competency Verification
Hematologic Components and Functions

Indicate whether the following functions of blood are true or false. If the statement is false, rewrite the statement on another sheet to make it true.

1. _____ A body fluid that transports nutrients and other substances throughout the body.

2. _____ Delivers oxygen from the lungs to all body cells.

3. _____ Depends on other body systems to halt blood loss.

4. _____ Does not have the ability to combat infections.

5. _____ Delivers waste products (i.e., carbon dioxide) to the lungs for elimination in the exhaled air.

agranulocytes	globulins	neutrophils
blood clotting	hemoglobin	plasma
embolus	Ig	platelets
erythrocyte	leukocytes	T cells and B cells
fibrin strands	megakaryocytes	universal recipient

Match the terms listed above with the definitions given in the numbered list:

6. besides albumins and fibrinogens, the third group of plasma proteins is called _____

7. another name for thrombocytes is _____

8. the only human cell without a nucleus is called _____

9. the letters used to identify the five classes of antibodies are _____

10. the liquid part of blood is called _____

11. besides erythrocytes and thrombocytes, the formed elements of blood include _____

12. leukocytes that do not have granules in their cytoplasm are called _____

13. the most abundant WBCs, which have oddly shaped nuclei and are phagocytic cells, are called _____

14. iron protein in the blood is known as _____

15. specialized groups of lymphocytes are called _____

16. large cells located in the red bone marrow are called _____

Match the blood clotting and blood groups terms listed above with the statements given in the numbered list:

17. _____ occurs when platelets trigger a series of complex chemical reactions

18. _____ create a mesh at a wound site, trapping RBCs to form a blood clot

19. _____ a discharged circulating clot

20. _____ a person who can receive a transfusion of any blood type

Correct Answers _____ × 5 = _____% Score

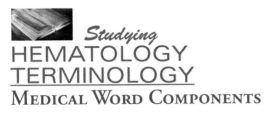

Studying
HEMATOLOGY TERMINOLOGY
MEDICAL WORD COMPONENTS
Combining Forms

Combining Forms: Hematological Components and Functions

| Combining Form | Meaning | EXAMPLE | |
		Term/Pronunciation	Definition
agglutin/o	clumping, gluing	**agglutin**/ation ă-gloo-tĭ-NĀ-shŭn	process *(-ation)* by which (foreign) cells clump. *Agglutination obstructs vessels by hindering blood flow. Transfusion with an incompatible blood type can be fatal.*
bas/o	base (alkaline, the opposite of acid)	**bas**/o/phil BĀ-sō-fĭl	a type of blood cell that attracts alkaline dyes. *The suffix* -phil *means "an attraction for."*
chrom/o	color	**chrom**/ic KRŌ-mĭk	pertaining to *(-ic)* color
eosin/o	dawn (rose colored)	**eosin**/o/phil ē-ŏ-SĬN-ō-fĭl	type of blood cell that attracts red dyes. *The suffix* -phil *means "an attraction for."*
erythr/o	red	**erythr**/o/poiesis ĕ-RĬTH-rō-poy-Ē-sĭs	the formation of erythrocytes (red blood cells). *The suffix* -poiesis *means "formation," "production."*
granul/o	granule	**granul**/o/cyte GRĂN-ū-lō-sīt	any granular blood cell *(-cyte)*
hem/o	blood	**hem**/o/philia hē-mō-FĬL-ē-ă	a group of hereditary bleeding disorders marked by deficiencies of blood-clotting proteins. *The suffix* -philia *means "attraction for."*
hemat/o		**hemat**/oma hē-mă-TŌ-mă	a localized mass of blood (usually clotted) confined to an organ, tissue, or space; caused by a break in a blood vessel. *The suffix* -oma *means "tumor."*

Combining Forms: Hematological Components and Functions (Continued)

Combining Form	Meaning	EXAMPLE	
		Term/Pronunciation	**Definition**
kary/o	nucleus	**kary**/o/cyte KĂR-ē-ō-sīt	nucleated red blood cell *(-cyte)*
leuk/o	white	**leuk**/o/cyte LOO-kō-sīt	a white blood cell *(-cyte)*
nucle/o	nucleus	mono/**nucle**/ar mŏn-ō-NŪ-klē-ăr	having one *(mono-)* nucleus, particularly a blood cell such as a monocyte or lymphocyte
lymph/o	lymph	**lymph**/o/cyte LĬM-fō-sīt	a white blood cell *(-cyte)* that arises from bone marrow and is responsible for much of the body's immune response
morph/o	form, shape, structure	**morph**/o/logy mor-FŎL-ō-jē	the study of *(-logy)* the physical shape and size of a specimen, plant, or animal
myel/o	bone marrow, spinal cord	**myel**/o/suppression mī-ě-lō-sŭ-PRĔSH-ŭn	suppression of bone marrow function
phag/o	swallowing, eating	**phag**/o/cyte FĂG-ō-sīt	a cell *(-cyte)* that can surround, engulf, and digest microorganisms and cellular debris
poikil/o	varied, irregular	**poikil**/o/cyte POY-kĭl-ō-sīt	an abnormal variation in the shape of red blood cells *(-cyte),* seen in *myelofibrosis* and certain *anemias*
reticul/o	net, mesh	**reticul**/o/cyte rě-TĬK-ū-lō-sīt	an immature erythrocyte characterized by a meshlike pattern of threads and particles at the former site of the nucleus
sider/o	iron	**sider**/o/penia sĭd-ěr-ō-PĒ-nē-ă	deficiency *(-penia)* of iron
thromb/o	blood clot	**thromb**/o/lysis thrŏm-BŎL-ĭ-sĭs	dissolution of a blood clot. *The suffix -lysis means "separation," "destruction," or "loosening."*

THERAPEUTIC PROCEDURES

PROCEDURE	DESCRIPTION
apheresis *ă-fĕr-Ē-sĭs*	A procedure in which blood is temporarily withdrawn and one or more components are removed from it by means of a continuous-flow separator; the process is similar to hemodialysis, as treated blood is reinfused into the patient. The removal of leukocytes is termed *leukapheresis*; the removal of cellular material is termed *cytapheresis*; and the removal of noncellular materials is termed *plasmapheresis*. Apheresis is used to treat various disease conditions and to harvest blood cells.
blood transfusion	Intravenous administration of blood, usually from a donor, into a patient; used to replace blood lost through surgery, trauma, or disease. Prior to transfusion, various tests are used to determine a close match of RBC or platelet type and to confirm that the specimen is free of hepatitis and the human immunodeficiency virus (HIV).
autologous *aw-TŎL-ō-gŭs*	Transfusion of blood obtained from the patient before surgery or collected from the patient during surgery. Use of the patient's own blood, rather than blood from a donor, prevents accidental exposure to the AIDS virus and other blood-borne diseases.

PHARMACOLOGY

DRUG CLASSIFICATION	THERAPEUTIC ACTION
anticoagulants *ăn-tĭ-kō-ĂG-ū-lănts*	Drugs that prevent clot formation and also decrease the risk of a stroke in patients who had transient ischemic attacks. Used to prevent clots from forming postoperatively after heart, valve, or vascular surgery, and to prevent coagulation in stored blood that is later used for transfusions.
thrombolytic enzymes *thrŏm-bō-LĬT-ĭk*	Drugs used to dissolve blood clots that have already formed in the body.

❖ ABBREVIATIONS

ABBREVIATION	MEANING	ABBREVIATION	MEANING
AB, ab	abortion, antibodies	**LDL**	low-density lipoprotein
ABO	blood groups: A, AB, B, and O	**lymphos**	lymphocytes
ACT	activated clotting time	**MCH**	mean corpuscle hemoglobin; mean cell hemoglobin (average amount of hemoglobin per cell)
AHF	antihemophilic factor (blood coagulation factor VIII)		
AHG	antihemolytic globulin	**MCHC**	mean cell hemoglobin concentration (average concentration of hemoglobin in a single red blood cell)
ANTI, anti	antibody		
Ag	antigen		
APTT	activated partial thromboplastin time	**MCV**	mean cell volume (average volume or size of a single red blood cell. High MCV= macrocytic cells; low MCV=microcytic cells)
baso	basophils		
Bx, bx	biopsy		
bid	twice a day		
CBC	complete blood count		
diff.	differential (white blood count)	**mg**	milligram (1/1000 gram)
DNA	deoxyribonucleic acid	**mono**	monocyte
DVT	deep vein thrombosis	**INR**	international normalized ratio
EBV	Epstein-Barr virus	**P&A**	percussion and auscultation
eos	eosinophils (type of white blood cell)	**PA**	posteroanterior, pernicious anemia
Epo	erythropoietin	**pH**	degree of acidity or alkalinity in a substance
ESR	erythrocyte sedimentation rate		
Hb, Hbg, Hgb	hemoglobin	**PERRLA**	pupils equal, round, and reactive to light and accommodation
HCT, Hct	hematocrit		
HDL	high-density lipoprotein	**poly, PMN, PMNL**	polymorphonuclear leukocyte
hs	at bedtime		
Igs	immunoglobulins	**PT**	prothrombin time, physical therapy
IgM	immunoglobulin M		
IgA	immunoglobulin A	**PTT**	partial thromboplastin time
IgD	immunoglobulin D	**RBC, rbc**	red blood cell(s); red blood count
IgG	immunoglobulin G		
IgE	immunoglobulin E	**qd**	every day
INR	international normalized ratio	**sed rate**	erythrocyte sedimentation rate
ITP	idiopathic thrombocytopenic purpura	**segs**	segmented neutrophils
		VLDL	very low-density lipoprotein
L1, L1, etc.	first lumbar vertebra, second lumbar vertebra, etc.	**WBC, wbc**	white blood cell(s); white blood count

Activity 15–4: Competency Verification
Diagnostic Procedures, Treatments, Pharmacology, and Abbreviations

antiglobulin test	CBC	thrombolytic enzymes
bleeding time	ESR	WBC count
blood transfusion	Hct	WBC differential
bone marrow biopsy	prothrombin time (PT)	

Match the terms listed above with the definitions given in the numbered list:

1. _____ intravenous administration of blood to a patient.

2. _____ time required for blood to stop flowing from a controlled skin puncture of the forearm.

3. _____ a routine series of tests that screens for abnormal conditions in the blood.

4. _____ used to detect the presence of antibodies that coat and damage RBCs as a result of several diseases.

5. _____ a test that measures the speed at which RBCs settle to the bottom of a narrow tube. Used in the diagnosis of inflammatory diseases, cancer, and other conditions that alter the consistency of blood.

6. _____ measures the ability of the blood to clot; used to evaluate the effectiveness of anticoagulation drug therapy, such as Coumadin.

7. _____ an agent used to dissolve blood clots that have already formed in the body.

8. _____ determination of the number of different types of WBCs in a stained blood smear viewed under a microscope.

9. _____ measures the percentage of packed RBCs in a volume of blood.

10. _____ measures the number of WBCs per cubic millimeter of blood. An increase is often noted when infection is present.

Correct Answers _____ × 10 = _____% **Score**

Activity 15–5: Build Medical Words
Diagnostic, Symptomatic, and Surgical Terms

Use *hemat/o* (blood) to build medical words meaning:

1. tumor of blood _____

2. production and development of blood cells _____

3. specialist in the study of blood _____

Use *thromb/o* (blood clot) to build medical words meaning:

4. excision or removal of a thrombus _____

5. resembling a thrombus _____

6. separation, destruction, loosening of a blood clot _____

Use *-cytes* (cells) to build medical words meaning:

7. cells that are red _____

8. cells that are white _____

9. cells that are granular _____

10. cells that swallow or eat _____

Correct Answers _____ × 10 = _____ **% Score**

MEDICAL RECORDS

An operative report, a history and physical examination, and a consultation are included in this section. The following reading and dictionary exercise and medical record analysis will help you develop skills to abstract information and master the terminology in the reports. Accurate interpretation is important, because information of this type is used in numerous areas of the medical practice, such as initiation of treatments, evaluation of patient's progress, and completion of insurance claims.

Reading and Dictionary Exercise

Check the box [✓] after you complete the exercise.

[   ] **1.** Underline the following words, as you read the operative report, the history and physical examination, and the consultation aloud. These medical records can be found at the end of the chapter.

[   ] **2.** Use a medical dictionary, Appendix A, and Appendix F, Part 2 to complete this exercise.

Note: You are not expected to fully understand all the parts of the medical records. The important aspect of this exercise is to use all available resources to complete it. Eventually you will master the terminology and format of these reports.

> > > MEDICAL RECORD 15–1: OPERATIVE REPORT

Term	Pronunciation	Meaning
bilateral	bī-LĂT-ĕr-ăl	_____
thrombosis	thrŏm-BŌ-sĭs	_____

Coumadin	KŪ-mă-dĭn	_____
hypercoagulable	hĭp-ĕr-kō-ĂG-ū-lă-bĕl	_____
embolus	ĔM-bō-lŭs	_____
infrarenal	ĭn-fră-RĒ-năl	_____
suprarenal	soo-pră-RĒ-năl	_____
mutation	mū-TĂ-shŭn	_____
polycythemia	pŏl-ē-sī-THĒ-mē-ă	_____
supine	sū-PĪN	_____
Betadine	BĀ-tă-dĭn	_____
subcutaneous	sŭb-kū-TĂ-nē-ŭs	_____
lidocaine	LĪ-dō-kān	_____
venacavogram	vē-nă-KĀ-vō-grăm	_____
hemostasis	hē-MŎS-tă-sĭs	_____

> > > MEDICAL RECORD 15–2: HISTORY AND PHYSICAL EXAMINATION

Term	Pronunciation	Meaning
sickle cell crisis	SĬK-ĕl sĕl KRĪ-sĭs	_____
aplastic	ā-PLĂS-tĭk	_____
hepatitis B	hĕp-ă-TĪ-tĭs	_____
sickle cell anemia	SĬK-ĕl sĕl ă-NĒ-mē-ă	_____
Darvocet	DĂR-vō-sĕt	_____
extraocular	ĕks-tră-ŎK-ū-lar	_____
tympanic membranes	tĭm-PĂN-ik MĔM-brānz	_____
ascites	ă-SĪ-tēz	_____
pretibial	prē-TĬB-ē-ăl	_____
deep vein thrombosis	dēp vān thrŏm-BŌ-sĭs	_____
Doppler	DŎP-lĕr	_____

> > > MEDICAL RECORD 15-3: CONSULTATION

Term	Pronunciation	Meaning
lumpectomy	*lŭm-PĔK-tō-mē*	_____
thrombosis	*thrŏm-BŌ-sĭs*	_____
tamoxifen	*tă-MŎK-sĭ-fĕn*	_____
cardiomyopathy	*kăr-dē-ō-mī-ŎP-ă-thē*	_____
hypercholesterolemia	*hī-pĕr-kō-lĕs-tĕr-ŏl-Ē-mē-ă*	_____
Prozac	*PRŌ-zăk*	_____
lymphadenopathy	*lĭm-făd-ĕ-NŎP-ă-thē*	_____
hepatosplenomegaly	*hĕp-ă-tō-splē-nō-MĔG-ă-lē*	_____

Critical Thinking: Analysis of Medical Records

This section provides experience in abstracting and analyzing information from medical records. At the same time it reinforces the material presented in this chapter.

> > > MEDICAL RECORD 15-1: OPERATIVE REPORT

1. What was the preoperative diagnosis?

_____

_____

2. What type of surgery was performed?

_____

_____

3. What type of radiograph was performed with nonionic contrast material that showed the renal veins to be without defects?

_____

_____

4. How was the defect in the internal jugular vein controlled during surgery?

_____

_____

> > > MEDICAL RECORD 15-2: HISTORY AND PHYSICAL EXAMINATION

5. How does a person acquire sickle cell anemia?

_____

6. What causes the severe pain in a sickle cell crisis?

_____

_____

7. What is the stated diagnosis?

_____

8. What diagnostic test is being performed to rule out deep vein thrombosis?

_____

> > > MEDICAL RECORD 15-3: CONSULTATION

9. What stage tumor did the patient have approximately 6 years ago?

_____

_____

10. What type of treatment did she receive at that time?

_____

_____

11. Upon physical examination, was the physician able to palpate any masses?

_____

_____

12. What cause does the doctor attribute to the present clot formation?

_____

_____

Audio Practice

Listen to the audio CD-ROM to practice the pronunciation of selected medical terms from this chapter.

Medical Record 15–1. Operative Report

GENERAL HOSPITAL AND MEDICAL CENTER
2211 Fifth Avenue North • Healthy City, USA 12345 • (321) 123-4567

Operative Report

Patient Name: Robert Duckington	**Patient Number:** 34-22-12
Birth Ddate: 08/23/xx	**Room Number:** 131

DATE OF OPERATION: 09/12/xx

PREOPERATIVE DIAGNOSIS: Bilateral deep vein thrombosis, hypercoagulable state, status post pulmonary embolus with contraindication to Coumadin anticoagulation.

POSTOPERATIVE DIAGNOSIS: Bilateral deep vein thrombosis, hypercoagulable state, status post pulmonary embolus with contraindication to Coumadin anticoagulation

OPERATION: Insertion of inferior vena cava, infrarenal, and suprarenal Greenfield filters, inferior venacavogram.

SURGEON: Nicholas Wallin, M.D.

ANESTHESIA: Local with monitored anesthesia.

INDICATIONS: This 35-year-old male was admitted with severe dehydration with known factor V Leiden mutation with hypercoagulable state and polycythemia and status post pulmonary embolus in July 2002; admitted with bilateral DVT, also status post left hemispheric cerebral infarct with noncompliance. For that reason, a contraindication to Coumadin anticoagulation.

PROCEDURE: With the patient lying supine and under sedation, the neck slightly hyper-extended and the head turned to the left, the neck, shoulder, and upper chest were prepped with Betadine, and sterile drapes were applied. The skin and subcutaneous tissue were infiltrated with 1% lidocaine. Percutaneous puncture of the internal jugular vein was not accomplished, and for that reason, a small cut-down along the space between the two sternocleidomastoid muscles was made, bleeders being electrocauterized. The internal jugular vein was exposed, found to be quite flat. A stay suture of 5-0 cardiovascular Prolene was applied, and using the Seldinger technique, the guide wire was advanced under C-arm fluoroscopy down to the level of L3-4. The introduction mechanism with dilator was then advanced along the guide wire, the dilator being removed, leaving the sleeve behind. The inferior venacavogram was performed using nonionic contrast material, which showed a patent inferior vena cava as well as the renal veins without

Continued

Operative Report, page 2

Patient Name: Robert Duckington   **Patient Number:** 34-22-12

defects. The sleeve was again irrigated with heparinized saline, and the filter was advanced under C-arm fluoroscopy and deployed at the level of L2-3. It was noted that the filter failed to open. For that reason, a different filter was deployed in a suprarenal position. This time, the filter opened well. The introduction mechanism was removed, and the defect in the internal jugular vein was controlled with a running suture of 5-0 cardiovascular Prolene. Hemostasis appeared adequate. The skin and subcutaneous layers were then closed, the subcutaneous tissues with interrupted sutures of 3-0 Dexon, the skin with Steri-Strips, and sterile gauze dressing was applied.

The patient tolerated the procedure well. The blood loss was minimal. He was taken to the intensive care unit in satisfactory condition.

_____

Nicholas Wallin, M.D.

NW/ar
D: 09/12/xx
T: 09/13/xx

Medical Record 15–2. History and Physical Examination

GENERAL HOSPITAL AND MEDICAL CENTER
2211 Fifth Avenue North • Healthy City, USA 12345 • (321) 123-4567

History and Physical Examination

Patient Name: Burt Spearman   **Patient Number:** 84-66-78
Birth Date: 06/01/xx   **Room Number:** 453

DATE OF PROCEDURE: 11/18/xx

HISTORY

CHIEF COMPLAINT: Sickle cell crisis.

HISTORY OF PRESENT ILLNESS: This 29-year-old African-American male has a history of sickle cell anemia with multiple past aplastic crises. He has been hospitalized numerous times for pain control and blood transfusions. He recently had flu-like symptoms and subsequently developed generalized pain that has now become localized and severe in his right lower leg. He presented to the Emergency Room and was admitted after being diagnosed with severe sickle cell crisis.

PAST MEDICAL HISTORY: He has a history of hepatitis B contracted from a blood transfusion approximately 8 years ago. See old medical charts for detailed previous history.

FAMILY HISTORY: Both of the patient's parents have sickle cell anemia as well as his brother.

CURRENT MEDICATIONS: None.

ALLERGIES: Patient is allergic to Darvocet.

PHYSICAL EXAMINATION

GENERAL APPEARANCE: A young African-American male looking his stated age in moderate distress complaining of generalized pain and severe pain in the right lower leg.
VITAL SIGNS: Blood pressure 130/70, pulse 124, temperature 102.5, respirations 18 and unlabored.
HEENT: PERRLA. Extraocular muscles intact. Tympanic membranes clear. Pale mucous membranes in the mouth and throat.
NECK: Supple, no masses.
CHEST: Clear to P&A in all fields.
HEART: Regular rate and rhythm.
ABDOMEN: Soft, nontender, with active bowel sounds. No masses. No ascites.

Continued

History and Physical Examination, page 2
Patient Name: Burt Spearman   **Patient Number:** 84-66-78

EXTREMITIES: Markedly tender right lower extremity in the pretibial area. This area is slightly indurated and warm. Extremities are otherwise negative without signs of trauma, ulcerations, or lesions.
NEUROLOGIC: Cranial nerves II-XII grossly intact.

IMPRESSION:
1. Sickle cell crisis.
2. Rule out right lower extremity deep vein thrombosis.

PLAN: Patient is admitted for further management for hydration with intravenous fluids, blood transfusions, and pain medication to control sickle cell crisis. Doppler studies will be performed on right lower extremity to rule out deep vein thrombosis.

_____
Fred Thomas, M.D.

FT/bab
D: 11/18/xx
T: 11/18/xx

Medical Record 15–3. Consultation

GENERAL HOSPITAL AND MEDICAL CENTER
2211 Fifth Avenue North • Healthy City, USA 12345 • (321) 123-4567

Consultation

Patient Name: Mary Poskowitz   **Patient Number**: 34-29-44
Birth Date: 10/01/xx   **Room Number**: 325

REASON FOR CONSULTATION: Possible hypercoagulable state, history of breast carcinoma.

The patient is a 68-year-old lady whom I saw approximately 6 years ago. I will be reviewing my old records to confirm this date. In any event, I believe that she had a stage II (lymph node positive) receptor-positive breast carcinoma. At that time, she received radiation therapy to the left breast after having a lumpectomy and also has been on tamoxifen. Since that time, she has been under the care of Dr. Jensen, and has been maintained on tamoxifen, which I believe is appropriate. The patient presented at this time on 02/01/xx when she had a routine follow-up and was found to have a "cramp in her leg." A Doppler study was performed which confirmed the presence of a deep vein thrombosis. She was subsequently admitted for heparin and evaluation.

Upon admission on 02/01/xx, her pro time was 11.3, INR 1.1, and on 02/03/xx, the pro time was 12.7 with an INR of 1.2. Since that time, the patient has been evaluated for the possibility of recurrent disease or an underlying carcinoma to cause her situation. CT scans of the chest and pelvis were both negative. However, a mammogram shows a speculated lesion in the 12 o'clock region of the right breast (breast without prior disease). There is also a lesion in the 2 o'clock position consistent with a possible new breast carcinoma.

As noted, the tamoxifen was discontinued since it might be correlating with her hypercoagulable state.

Past medical history is significant for multiple problems including cerebrovascular accident in the past, for which she has been taking Coumadin, a cardiomyopathy, hypertension, chronic obstructive pulmonary disease, hypercholesterolemia, and depression.

Social history reveals that she is widowed. She quit smoking about 5 years ago. Does not abuse ethanol.

Medications at the time of admission included Prozac 40 mg p.o. twice a day, Azmacort inhaler, Lipitor 20 mg at h.s., Pulmicort and Combivent inhalers, Accupril 20 mg q.d., Pepcid 20 mg b.i.d., as well as the tamoxifen which was discontinued as noted. She was taking Coumadin at the time of admission, but obviously her level was low as manifested by a normal INR.

Continued

Consultation, page 2
Patient Name: Mary Poskowitz   **Patient Number:** 34-29-44

PHYSICAL EXAMINATION: Vital signs show she is afebrile, stable vital signs. There is no palpable lymphadenopathy or hepatosplenomegaly. I can really palpate no masses in the breast as outlined on the mammogram. The left breast is without masses.

At the present time, I believe the patient does have a clot present, related possibly to tamoxifen, which can be thrombogenic. I believe she was under-coagulated at the time of admission.

From this aspect, I would suggest the patient be placed on Coumadin eventually after having had her heparin, maintaining an INR of 2.5 to 3.0. Hypercoagulable labs are pending at this time for a further workup.

At the present time, I am concerned that she may also have a new malignancy. Dr. Franklin, general surgeon, has been consulted. A bone scan has been requested as well. Until these issues have been sorted out, I believe the patient should be continued on heparin before starting onto Coumadin. I wholeheartedly agree with the discontinuation of tamoxifen.

Thank you very much for allowing us once more to participate in her care.

_____

Keith R. Rupp, M.D.

KRR/mn
D: 02/05/xx
T: 02/06/xx

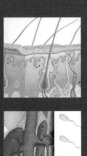
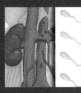

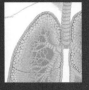
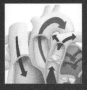
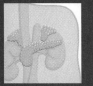
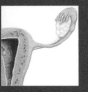
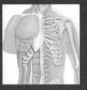

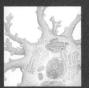
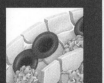

chapter

16 Ophthalmology

Objectives

Upon completion of the chapter, you will be able to:

- Describe the type of medical treatment ophthalmologists provide.
- Describe the sense of sight and explain the functions of its organs.
- Recognize, pronounce, build, and spell correctly terms related to the sense of sight.
- Describe pathological conditions, diagnostic tests, surgical procedures, and other treatments related to the sense of sight.
- Demonstrate your knowledge of this chapter by successfully completing the activities and analysis of medical records.

About Ophthalmology

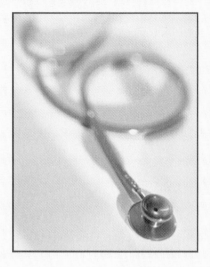

Ophthalmology is the branch of medicine concerned with the diagnosis and treatment of eye disorders. The medical specialist in ophthalmology is called an **ophthalmologist.**

Although ophthalmologists specialize only in the treatment of the eyes, it is important for them to be cognizant of other abnormalities that may be revealed during an eye examination. The importance of an eye examination cannot be underestimated, because it frequently reveals the first signs of systemic illnesses (e.g., diabetes) that may present in other parts of the body. The medical practice of ophthalmology includes prescribing corrective lenses and performing various types of corrective eye surgeries. Specialized surgeries involve techniques that are as delicate and precise as those of neurosurgery and are often performed using magnifying glasses and laser beams. Corrective eye surgeries include cornea transplantation, cataract removal, repair of ocular muscle dysfunction, glaucoma treatment, lens removal, and radial keratotomy.

Two other health-care practitioners, the **optometrist** and the **optician,** specialize in providing corrective lenses for the eyes. They are not medical doctors, but they are licensed to examine and test the eyes and to treat visual defects by prescribing corrective lenses. The optician also specializes in filling prescriptions for corrective lenses.

To grasp the scope of practice and the role of health-care practitioners in the medical specialty of ophthalmology, it is important to understand the structure and function of the eye as well as the language of medicine that is related to this medical specialty.

Selected Key Terms

aqueous humor Ā-kwē-ŭs HŪ-mor *aqueo=water* *ous=pertaining to*	Clear, watery fluid in the anterior and posterior chambers produced by the ciliary body; the tissue fluid of the eyeball that provides nutrients and oxygen to the avascular lens and cornea and aids in maintaining the shape of the front of the eye.
binocular vision bĭn-ŎK-ū-lăr	Normal vision involving the simultaneous use of both eyes.
fundus (of the eye) FŬN-dŭs	The posterior, inner part of the eye that can be directly visualized with an ophthalmoscope.
intraocular pressure (IOP) ĭn-tră-ŎK-ū-lăr *intra=in, within* *ocul=eye* *ar=pertaining to*	The internal pressure of the eye that is regulated by resistance to the flow of aqueous humor. The presence of aqueous humor in the anterior cavity of the eye creates a pressure called intraocular pressure, which helps support the eyeball internally. Early detection of glaucoma depends on measuring intraocular pressure, using an instrument called a *tonometer.*
lens	A transparent refracting medium, usually made of glass. Also, the crystalline lens of the eye.
mydriasis mĭd-RĪ-ă-sĭs *mydr=widen, enlarge* *iasis=abnormal condition* *(produced by something specified)*	A pronounced or abnormal dilation of the pupil.

optic nerve ŎP-tĭk nĕrv	The cranial nerve that transmits impulses from the retina to the cerebral cortex in the brain.
pupil PŪ-pĭl	Dark opening in the center of the iris that regulates the amount of light entering the eye by constricting when light increases, and dilating when light decreases.
refraction rĭ-FRĂK-shŭn	The bending of light rays as they pass through the various structures of the eye to bring the rays into focus on the retina.
rhodopsin rō-DŎP-sĭn	The pigment found in the rods of the retina that adapts the eye to dim light; important in night vision.
suspensory ligament sŭs-PĔN-sō-rē LĬG-ă-mĕnt	Any of a number of ligaments that help support an organ or body structure, such as the suspensory ligaments inside the eye that hold the lens in tension.
vitreous humor VĬT-rē-ŭs HŪ-mor	Clear, jellylike substance that fills the posterior chamber. Vitreous humor transmits light, contributes to intraocular pressure, helps maintain the shape of the eyeball, and keeps the retina in place.

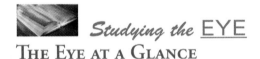

Studying the EYE

THE EYE AT A GLANCE

The eye, like the ear, is a sense organ. Both are receptors and have sensitive cells that are activated by energy from the external environment. The eyes refract (bend) and focus incoming light waves on sensitive photoreceptors located at the back of each eye. Nerve impulses from the stimulated photoreceptors are then conveyed through visual pathways within the brain to the cerebral cortex, where the sense of vision is perceived.

The eyes are located anteriorly on the skull and set apart to achieve **binocular vision** when focusing on an object. This type of focusing allows three-dimensional depth perception.

STRUCTURE AND FUNCTION

Label Figure 16–1 as you read the following material.

The eye is a sensory organ containing receptors for vision, and a refracting system that focuses light rays on the receptors in the retina. The adult eye, commonly called the (1) **eyeball,** measures about 2.5 cm (1 in). Only the anterior one-sixth of its total surface is visible. The rest is recessed into and protected by a bony depression in the skull (orbit). In addition to blood vessels, nerves, and connective tissue, a cushion of fat occupies nearly all of the orbit not occupied by the eye itself. Before discussing the eye itself, let us consider the accessory structures that protect it or aid its functioning.

Accessory Structures of the Eye

The accessory structures of the eye perform two basic functions: they protect the eyeball and provide eye movement. The protective structures consist of the eyebrows, the eyelids, the eyelashes, the conjunctiva, and the lacrimal apparatus. Eye movement is made possible by the actions of the extrinsic muscles that arise from the orbit and connect the orbit and the outer layer of the eyeball.

Eyebrows, Eyelids, and Eyelashes

Eyebrows consist of thick, short hairs and are located transversely above both eyes. Their function is to prevent perspiration and other foreign material from getting into the eyes, and also to protect the eyes from the sun.

Each (2) **eyelid** is reinforced with folds of skin that cover the eyeball, keeping its surface moist and protected from debris through their blinking motion. The (3) **levator palpebrae superioris muscle** attaches along the upper eyelid and provides it with greater movability than the lower eyelid. To avoid a blurred image, blinking usually occurs when the eyeball moves to a new fixation position. The (4) **eyelashes** are located along the edges of the eyelids to provide further protection by preventing foreign material from reaching the eyeball.

Extrinsic Eye Muscles

Six muscles known as extrinsic ocular muscles control movements of the eyeball. Each muscle originates from the bony orbit and is attached to the tough

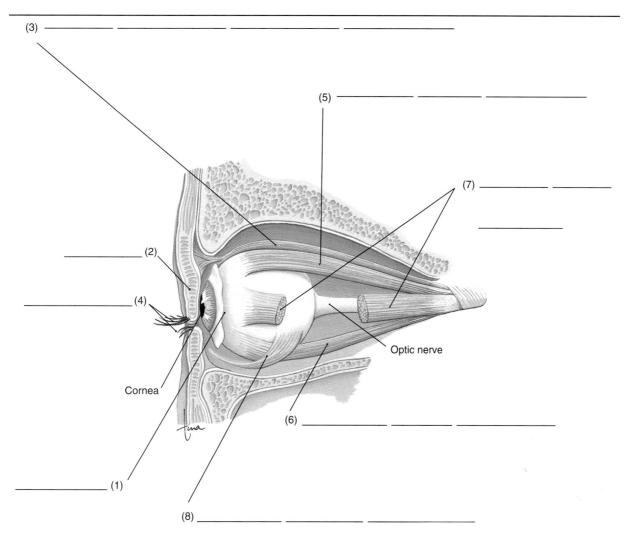

(3)

(5)

(7)

(2)

(4)

Optic nerve

Cornea

(6)

(1)

(8)

Figure 16–1 *The extrinsic muscles of the eye (the medial rectus and superior oblique are not shown). (Adapted from Scanlon, VC, and Sanders, TS: Essentials of Anatomy and Physiology, ed 3. FA Davis, Philadelphia, 1999, p 191, with permission.)*

outer surface of the eyeball. Four rectus muscles maneuver the eyeball in various directions as indicated by their names (superior, inferior, lateral, and medial). These muscles include the (5) **superior rectus muscle,** the (6) **inferior rectus muscle,** the (7) **lateral rectus muscle,** and the (8) **inferior oblique muscle.** Please note that the **medial rectus muscle** and **superior oblique muscle** are not shown. The two oblique muscles, the inferior and superior oblique muscles, rotate the eyeball on its axis.

The functioning of all these muscles in both eyes is very complex, and fortunately for us, we do not have to make any conscious effort to coordinate these movements. Weakness in the ocular muscles results in failure of the eyes to gaze in the same direction. This disorder is referred to as **strabismus,** or "cross eyes," and is discussed in the Pathological Conditions section of this chapter.

Conjunctiva

Label Fig 16–2 as you continue to learn about the associated structures of the eye.

The (1) **conjunctiva** is a thin, mucus-secreting membrane. It lines the interior surface of the eyelids and the exposed anterior surface of the eyeballs. The conjunctiva has the ability to repair itself rapidly if it is scratched. An inflammation of this membrane, called **conjunctivitis,** is often caused by allergies and is manifested by itchy, watery, red eyes.

Lacrimal Apparatus

The principal components of the lacrimal apparatus are the (2) **lacrimal gland,** which secretes the *lacrimal fluid* (tears), and a series of ducts that drain the secretion into the nasal cavity. With each blink of the eyelids, lacrimal fluid passes downward medially, and drains into two small openings. These openings are located at

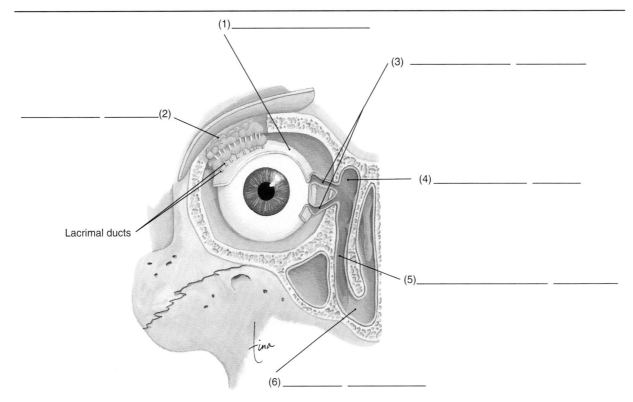

(1)_____

(3) _____ _____

(2)_____ _____

Lacrimal ducts

(4)_____ _____

(5)_____ _____

(6)_____ _____

Figure 16–2 *The lacrimal apparatus shown in an anterior view of the right eye. (Adapted from Scanlon, VC, and Sanders, TS: Essentials of Anatomy and Physiology, ed 3. FA Davis, Philadelphia, 1999, p 190, with permission.)*

the medial corner of the eyelids. From here the lacrimal fluid flows through the (3) **lacrimal canals** and the (4) **lacrimal sac** into the (5) **nasolacrimal duct,** allowing the tears to empty into the (6) **nasal cavity.**

 Activity 16–1: Competency Verification
Accessory Structures of the Eye

Review Figures 16–1 and 16–2, and check your labeling in Appendix C.

Internal Structures of the Eye

Label Figure 16–3 as you read about the internal anatomy of the eye.

The wall of the eyeball has three layers: the outer *sclera,* the middle *choroid* layer, and the inner *retina.* The (1) **sclera** is commonly known as the "white of the eye." It is a tough, fibrous membrane and performs two functions: maintaining the shape of the eyeball and providing a protective covering. Continuous with the anterior portion of the sclera is the (2) **cornea.** The cornea is transparent and convex to permit the passage and cause the refraction (bending) of incoming light waves. The transparency of the cornea is due to tightly packed, avascular (without

blood vessels) dense connective tissue. The cornea is well supplied with nerve endings, most of which are pain fibers. For this reason, some people can never adjust to wearing contact lenses.

The (3) **choroid** is a thick, highly vascular layer just beneath the sclera. It contains extensive capillaries, which provide blood and nutrients to the eye. The choroid also contains numerous pigment-producing melanocytes, which are responsible for its dark-brownish color. This coloring prevents light waves from being reflected out of the eyeball. The anterior portion of the choroid has two modified structures: the (4) **ciliary body** and the (5) **iris,** the colored portion of the eye. The ciliary body contains the smooth muscle forming an internal muscular ring toward the front of the eyeball and is connected to the (6) **lens,** or crystalline lens, by the (7) **suspensory ligament.** The ciliary body aids in changing the shape of the biconvex lens to focus images clearly on the sensitive nerve cell layer called the retina. It is the shape of the lens that determines the degree of **refraction** of the light rays that pass through the eye. The lens is thinned or flattened for distant vision, and thickened or made spherical for close vision by the ciliary body. Changes in the shape of the lens cause the bending of light rays, which allows an image to focus clearly on the retina. The refractive power of the lens is called **accommodation.** With age,

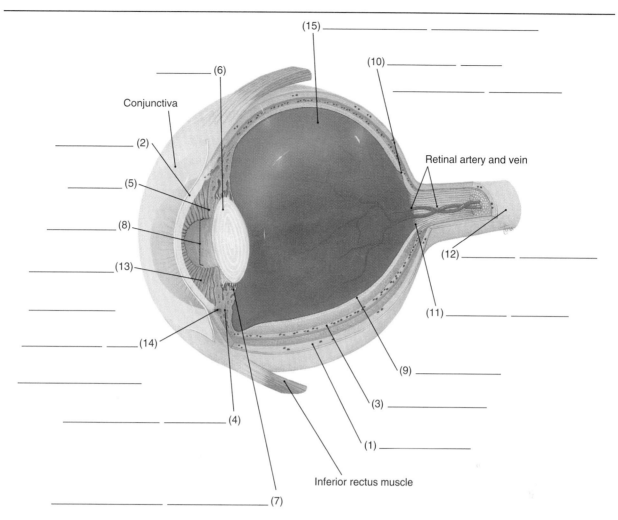

Conjunctiva

(15)

(6)

(10)

Retinal artery and vein

(2)

(5)

(8)

(13)

(14)

(4)

(7)

(12)

(11)

(9)

(3)

(1)

Inferior rectus muscle

Figure 16–3 *The internal structures of the eye. (Adapted from Scanlon, VC, and Sanders, TS: Essentials of Anatomy and Physiology, ed 3. FA Davis, Philadelphia, 1999, p 192, with permission.)*

the lens becomes less elastic and requires the aid of glasses to help compensate for its inability to thicken for close vision. This is a form of farsightedness associated with the aging process and is called *presbyopia.*

In front of the lens is the iris, the colored portion of the eye, which is continuous with the choroid. Contractions and dilations of the (8) **pupil** control the amount of light entering the eye. This dual action of the pupil is achieved by two sets of muscles within the iris. The radial muscles dilate the pupil in dim light to allow more light to enter the eye. The circular muscles tend to constrict the pupil in bright light to allow less light to enter the eye.

The (9) **retina** covers the choroid as the innermost layer of the eyeball. It lies in the posterior portion of the eye consisting of the sensitive nerve layer of the eye. The primary function of the retina is image formation. Light rays pass through the eye and are refracted by the cornea, lens, and pupil, focusing on photoreceptors

known as **rods** and **cones** (Fig. 16–4). **Rods,** over 100 million per eye, respond to small amounts of light and function better in dim light and aid in night vision. **Cones,** about 7 million per eye, are specialized to detect colors, provide sharpness of vision (visual acuity), and are used for vision in daylight or bright light. Color and sharpness of vision therefore depend on the cone cells. In Figure 16–3 the highest concentration of cones is found within the (10) **fovea in macula lutea,** an oval, yellowish spot near the center of the retina. This small area of the retina is largely composed of cones and functions as the area of sharpest vision. The retina is the only place in the body where blood vessels can be seen directly. Thus, an ophthalmologist can examine the retina and detect vascular changes associated with diabetes, hypertension, and atherosclerosis.

Ganglion neurons (see Fig. 16–4) are neurons that carry the impulses generated by the rods and cones. There is a convergence of these neurons at the (11)

optic disc. The neurons then pass through the wall of the eyeball to the (12) **optic nerve.** Because the optic disc contains no rods or cones, and is not light sensitive, it is known as the "blind spot" of the eye.

Internal Chambers and Fluids

The interior of the eyeball is composed of a large cavity divided into two smaller ones: the **anterior cavity** and the **posterior cavity.**

The (13) **anterior cavity** contains the *anterior chamber,* situated in front of the lens; and the *posterior chamber,* situated behind the lens. Both chambers are filled with a transparent watery fluid known as **aqueous humor,** which flows freely between them. Aqueous humor is constantly produced by the ciliary processes and is reabsorbed by the (14) **canal of Schlemm,** also known as the **venous sinus** (a sinus containing venous blood). The small veins from this structure carry the fluid into the bloodstream, where it is reabsorbed into the venous circulation. Both the reabsorption and the constant production of aqueous humor maintain an **intraocular pressure (IOP)** within the anterior and posterior chambers. The intraocular pressure keeps the retina smoothly applied to the choroid so the retina will form clear images. Nutrients and oxygen to the avascular lens and cornea are also provided by aqueous humor. Excessive intraocular pressure, called **glaucoma,** results in degeneration of the retina and blindness.

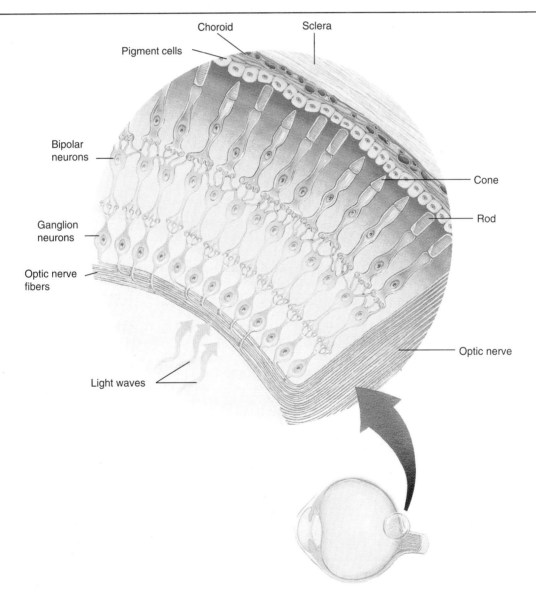

Figure 16–4 *The microscopic structure of the retina in the area of the optic disc. (From Scanlon, VC, and Sanders, TS: Essentials of Anatomy and Physiology, ed 3. FA Davis, Philadelphia, 1999, p 193, with permission.)*

The **posterior cavity,** also known as the (15) **vitreous chamber,** is situated behind the lens and is filled with a transparent, jelly-like substance called **vitreous humor.** This substance contributes to intraocular pressure, helps prevent the eyeball from collapsing, and holds the retina flush against the internal portions of the eyeball. Both the aqueous and the vitreous humors function to further refract light rays. Unlike aqueous humor, vitreous humor is not continuously produced. If there is an injury to the eye causing this fluid to escape, blindness can result.

Activity 16-2: Competency Verification
Internal Structures of the Eyeball

Review Figure 16-3, and check your labeling in Appendix C.

PROCESS OF VISION

Once light rays enter the eye, they are transmitted through the cornea, aqueous humor, pupil, lens, and the vitreous humor to the retina. The retina's sensitive nerve cells transmit the image through the optic nerve to the visual areas of the cerebral cortex in the brain. Flowchart 16–1 provides a summary of the pathway of light rays from the cornea to the cerebral cortex of the brain.

As a light ray passes through the various structures and fluids, the ray undergoes a process of bending or refraction until the image is clearly focused on the retina. When there is refraction through an irregular curvature of the cornea or lens, light rays scatter and blur the image on the retina. These are called *refraction errors*, and include *nearsightedness, farsightedness* and *astigmatism.* They are discussed in the Pathological Conditions section of the chapter.

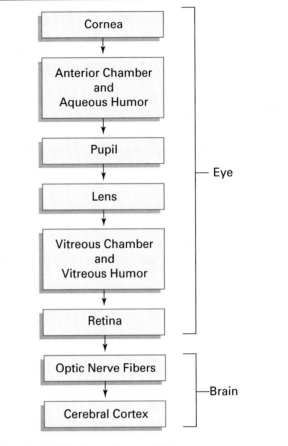

Flowchart 16–1 *The pathway of light rays.*

Activity 16-3: Competency Verification
Structures of the Eye

anterior chamber
aqueous humor
choroid
cones
conjunctiva
iris
lacrimal gland

lens
optic disc
pupil
retina
rods
sclera
vitreous humor

Match the terms listed above with the definitions given in the numbered list:

1. _____ a thin mucus-secreting membrane that lines the interior surface of the eyelids.

2. _____ secretes tears.

3. _____ the highly vascular layer that contains capillaries, which provide blood and nutrients to the eye.

4. _____ structure that dilates and contracts to control the amount of light that enters the eye.

5. _____ innermost layer of the eye the primary purpose of which is image formation.

6. _____ photoreceptor that aids in day vision and detects color.

7. _____ the colored portion of the eyeball.

8. _____ maintains the shape of the eyeball; the white of the eye.

9. _____ the structure at which neurons converge; the "blind spot" of the eye.

10. _____ the clear gel that helps maintain intraocular pressure within the chambers of the eye.

Correct Answers _____ × 10 = _____ % Score

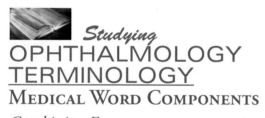

Studying
OPHTHALMOLOGY TERMINOLOGY
MEDICAL WORD COMPONENTS
Combining Forms

Combining Forms: The Eye

Combining Form	Meaning	EXAMPLE	
		Term/Pronunciation	Definition
aque/o	water	**aque**/ous Ā-kwē-ŭs	relating to (-*ous*) a watery substance
blephar/o	eyelid	**blephar**/o/spasm BLĔF-ă-rō-spăzm	twitching (-*spasm*) of the eyelid
choroid/o	choroid	**choroid**/o/pathy kō-roy-DŎP-ă-thē	any disease (-*pathy*) of the choroid
conjunctiv/o	conjunctiva	**conjunctiv**/itis kŏn-jŭnk-tĭ-VĪ-tĭs	inflammation (-*itis*) of the conjunctiva *Conjunctivitis is commonly called pinkeye.*
corne/o	cornea	**corne**/itis kor-nē-Ī-tĭs	inflammation (-*itis*) of the cornea *Corneitis is synonymous with* keratitis.

Combining Forms: The Eye (Continued)

Combining Form	Meaning	EXAMPLE	
		Term/Pronunciation	**Definition**
cycl/o	ciliary body of the eye, circular, cycle	**cycl**/o/plegia sī-klō-PLĒ-jē-ă	paralysis (-*plegia*) of the ciliary body of the eye *Cycloplegia can be a side effect of antidepressant and antipsychotic medications.*
dacry/o	tear, lacrimal sac	**dacry**/o/cele DĂK-rē-ō-sēl	protrusion of a lacrimal sac *The suffix -cele means "hernia," "swelling."*
irid/o	iris	**irid**/emia ĭr-ĭ-DĒ-mē-ă	bleeding (-*emia*) from the iris
kerat/o	horny tissue, hard, cornea	**kerat**/o/malacia kĕr-ă-tō-mă-LĀ-shē-ă	dryness with ulceration and perforation of the cornea; occurs in early childhood as a result of severe vitamin A deficiency *The suffix -malacia means "softening."*
lacrim/o	tear, lacrimal gland	**lacrim**/al LĂK-rĭ-măl	pertaining to (-*al*) tears
ophthalm/o	eye	**ophthalm**/o/logist ŏf-thăl-MŎL-ō-jĭst	a physician who specializes in the diagnosis and treatment of eye disorders *The suffix -logist means "specialist in the study of."*
ocul/o		intra/**ocul**/ar ĭn-tră-ŎK-ū-lăr	within (*intra*-) the eye *The suffix -ar means "pertaining to."*
opt/o	eye, vision	**opt**/o/metr/ist ŏp-TŎM-ĕ-trĭst	a health-care specialist (-*ist*) who examines the eyes and prescribes lenses *The combining form metr/o means "measure" or "uterus."*
optic/o		**optic**/al ŎP-tĭ-kăl	pertaining to (-*al*) the eye or vision
phac/o	lens	**phac**/o/meter făk-ŎM-ĕ-tĕr	instrument for measuring (-*meter*) the refractive power of the lens in the eye
pupill/o	pupil	**pupill**/o/metry pū-pĭl-LŎM-ĕ-trē	act of measuring (-*metry*) the diameter of the pupil

Combining Forms: The Eye (Continued)

Combining Form	Meaning	EXAMPLE	
		Term/Pronunciation	**Definition**
core/o		**core**/o/plasty KŌ-rē-ō-plăs-tē	surgical procedure to form an artificial pupil *The suffix -plasty means "surgical repair."*
retin/o	retina	**retin**/al RĔT-ĭ-năl	pertaining to (-al) the retina
scler/o	hardening, sclera	**scler**/itis sklĕ-RĪ-tĭs	inflammation (-itis) of the sclera *The sclera is the white, opaque portion of the eyeball.*
vitre/o	glassy	**vitre**/o/retin/al vĭt-rē-ō-RĔT-ĭ-năl	pertaining to (-al) the vitreous body and retina (retin/o) *The vitreous body is the clear gel that fills the area of the eyeball between the lens and retina.*

Combining Forms: Disorders of the Eye

Combining Form	Meaning	EXAMPLE	
		Term/Pronunciation	**Definition**
ambly/o	dull, dim	**ambly**/opia ăm-blē-Ō-pē-ă	dim vision (-opia) *A partial loss of sight due to the failure of the eyes to work together to focus on the same point.*
dipl/o	double	**dipl**/opia dĭp-LŌ-pē-ă	double vision (-opia)
glauc/o	gray	**glauc**/oma glaw-KŌ-mă	a condition in which increased intraocular pressure within the eye damages the retina and optic nerve causing defects in vision and often blindness *The suffix -oma means "tumor."*
mi/o	smaller, less	**mi**/o/tic mī-Ŏ-tĭk	pertaining to (-tic) drugs that cause the pupil to contract
mydr/o	widen, enlarge	**mydr**/iasis mĭd-RĪ-ă-sĭs	enlargement of the pupils *Drugs such as cocaine and atropine cause the pupils to enlarge or dilate. The suffix -iasis means an "abnormal condition (produced by something specified)."*

Combining Forms: Disorders of the Eye (Continued)

Combining Form	Meaning	EXAMPLE	
		Term/Pronunciation	**Definition**
phot/o	light	**phot**/o/sensitivity *fō-tō-sĕn-sĭ-TĬV-ĭ-tē*	unusual sensitivity to light
presby/o	old age	**presby**/opia *prĕz-bē-Ō-pē-ă*	impairment of vision (*-opia*) due to old age *Presbyopia is caused by a loss of elasticity of the crystalline lens and results in farsightedness.*
scot/o	darkness	**scot**/opia *skō-TŌ-pē-ă*	area of darkness in the visual field *The suffix -opia means "vision."*

Prefixes and Suffixes

In this section, prefixes are listed alphabetically and highlighted, whereas key suffixes are defined in the right-hand column.

Prefixes

Prefix	Meaning	EXAMPLE	
		Term/Pronunciation	**Definition**
eso-	inward	**eso**/tropia *ĕs-ō-TRŌ-pē-ă*	inward turning (*-tropia*) of an eye
exo-	outside, outward	**exo**/tropia *ĕks-ō-TRŌ-pē-ă*	outward turning (*-tropia*) of an eye
hetero-	different	**heter**/opsia *hĕt-ĕr-ŎP-sē-ă*	unequal vision in the two eyes. *The suffix -opsia means "vision."*
hyper-	excessive, above normal	**hyper**/opia *hī-pĕr-Ō-pē-ă*	farsightedness *The suffix -opia means "vision."* *Hyperopia is synonymous with hypermetropia.*

Activity 16–4: Competency Verification
Medical Word Components

Check the box [✓] as you complete each numbered section.

[   ] **1.** Review the components of the eye and the examples given in the previous section. Then pronounce each word aloud.

[   ] **2.** For the words below, first write the suffix and its meaning. Then translate the meaning of the remaining components starting with the first part of the word.

> **Example:** retin/al
> **Answer:** *al*=pertaining to, relating to; retina

1. core/o/plasty _____

2. dipl/opia _____

3. blephar/o/spasm _____

4. ambly/opia _____

5. lacrim/al _____

6. corne/itis _____

7. ophthalm/o/logist _____

8. choroid/o/pathy _____

9. cycl/o/plegia _____

10. conjunctiv/itis _____

Correct Answers _____ **× 10 =** _____ **% Score**

PATHOLOGICAL CONDITIONS
Disorders of Refraction

PATHOLOGICAL CONDITION	DESCRIPTION
astigmatism ă-STĬG-mă-tĭzm *a=without, not* *stigmat=a point* *ism=condition*	Irregular curvature of the cornea or lens in which the light rays cannot be focused clearly on the retina. Vision is typically blurred, and the eye cannot accommodate to correct the problem. Astigmatism can usually be corrected with contact lenses or with eyeglasses (Fig. 16–5).

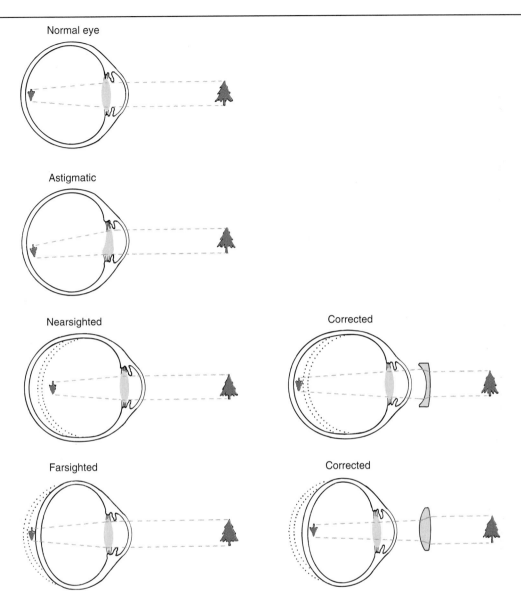

Normal eye

Astigmatic

Nearsighted   Corrected

Farsighted   Corrected

Figure 16–5 *Errors of refraction compared with a healthy eye. Corrective lenses are shown for nearsightedness and farsightedness. (From Scanlon, VC, and Sanders, TS: Essentials of Anatomy and Physiology, ed 3. FA Davis, Philadelphia, 1999, p 195, with permission.)*

Disorders of Refraction (Continued)

PATHOLOGICAL CONDITION	DESCRIPTION
hyperopia, hypermetropia hī-pĕr-Ō-pē-ă, hī-pĕr-mē-TRŌ-pē-ă *hyper=excessive, above normal* *opia=vision*	Farsightedness, or an inability of the eye to focus on nearby objects. It results from an error of refraction in which rays of light entering the eye are brought into focus behind the retina (see Fig. 16–5).

Disorders of Refraction (Continued)

PATHOLOGICAL CONDITION	DESCRIPTION
myopia *mī-Ō-pē-ă* *my=muscle* *opia=vision*	A condition of nearsightedness caused by the elongation of the eyeball or by an error of refraction so that parallel light rays are focused in front of the retina. Also called *nearsightedness, shortsightedness.* A negative (concave) lens of proper strength will correct this condition (see Fig. 16–5).
presbyopia *prĕz-bē-Ō-pē-ă* *presby=old age* *opia=vision*	A form of farsightedness associated with the aging process, which usually occurs between 40 and 45 years of age, in which the lens loses its elasticity and loses its ability to adjust for accommodation to near vision. Correction requires reading glasses that have a convex lens.

Other Conditions

CONDITION	DESCRIPTION
amblyopia *ăm-blē-Ō-pē-ă* *ambly=dull, dim* *opia=vision*	Reduction in, or dimness of, vision, especially that in which there is no apparent pathological condition of the eye.
blepharoptosis *blĕf-ă-rō-TŌ-sĭs* *blepharo=eyelid* *ptosis=prolapse, downward displacement*	A drooping of the upper eyelid causing skin to hang over the free border of the eyelid.
blindness	The inability to see. The leading causes of blindness in the United States are cataracts, glaucoma, age-related macular degeneration (ARMD), diabetes mellitus, and trauma to the eye.
cataract *KĂT-ă-răkt*	Degenerative condition of the lens of the eye characterized by loss of transparency. A gray-white opacity can be observed within the lens behind the pupil. Most cataracts are caused by degenerative changes, often occurring after 50 years of age. If cataracts are untreated, sight is eventually lost. Uncomplicated cataracts of old age (senile cataracts) are usually treated with excision of the lens and either surgical insertion of an intraocular lens (IOL) or prescription of special contact lenses or glasses (Fig. 16–6). 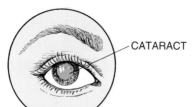CATARACT ***Figure 16–6*** *A cataract. (From Venes, D: Taber's Cyclopedic Medical Dictionary, ed 19. FA Davis, Philadelphia, 2001, p 356, with permission.)*
chalazion *kă-LĀ-zē-ōn*	A small, hard tumor on the eyelid resulting from obstruction and retained secretions of the tarsal glands (glands in the eyelid that secrete a sebaceous substance that keep the lids from adhering to each other). Chalazion is a nonmalignant condition and often requires incision and drainage (I&D).

Other Conditions (Continued)

CONDITION	DESCRIPTION
conjunctivitis kŏn-jŭnk-tĭ-VĪ-tĭs *conjunctiv=conjunctiva* *itis=inflammation*	Inflammation of the conjunctiva, caused by bacterial or viral infection, allergy, or environmental factors or disease. Red eyes, thick discharge, sticky eyelids in the morning, and inflammation without pain are characteristic results of the most common cause—bacterial infection. Choice of treatment depends on the causative agent and may include antibacterial agents, antibiotics, or corticosteroids. Also known as *pinkeye*.
corneal abrasion KOR-nē-ăl ă-BRĂ-zhŭn	The rubbing off of the outer layers of the cornea. This condition is commonly caused by a small foreign body, an eyelash, a contact lens, or a scratch from a fingernail. Treatment includes antibiotic ointment to reduce the chance of infection, and an eye bandage to reduce corneal motion against the eyelid. If treated promptly, surface abrasions usually heal quickly without complication or scarring.
glaucoma glaw-KŌ-mă *glauc=gray* *oma=tumor*	A disease of the eye characterized by increased intraocular pressure (IOP), excavation, and atrophy of the optic nerve; produces defects in the field of vision. An increase in intraocular pressure leads to an inhibited blood supply to the optic neurons that causes atrophy of the optic nerve and an eventual loss of total vision (Fig. 16–7).
chronic (open-angle or wide-angle)	The more common type of glaucoma, which is often bilateral. This condition develops slowly and is genetically determined. The obstruction is believed to occur within the *canal of Schlemm* (see Fig. 16–7B).
acute (angle-closure, closed-angle, or narrow-angle)	A condition that occurs if the pupil in an eye with a narrow angle between the iris and cornea dilates markedly, causing the folded iris to block the flow of aqueous humor from the anterior chamber (see Fig. 16–7C).
hemianopia hĕm-ē-ă-NŌ-pē-ă *hemi=one half* *an=without, not* *opia=vision*	Blindness in one-half of the visual field.
hyphema, hyphemia hī-FĒ-mă, hī-FĒ-mē-ă	A hemorrhage into the anterior chamber of the eye, usually caused by a blunt injury or trauma.
hordeolum, sty(e) hor-DĒ-ō-lŭm, stī	A localized, purulent, inflammatory infection of the sebaceous gland of an eyelash, caused by a bacterial infection. Treatment includes warm compresses and antibiotic ophthalmic preparations; incision and drainage are occasionally required.
keratitis kĕr-ă-TĪ-tĭs *kerat=cornea* *itis=inflammation*	Inflammation of the cornea, usually due to infection or other type of damage.

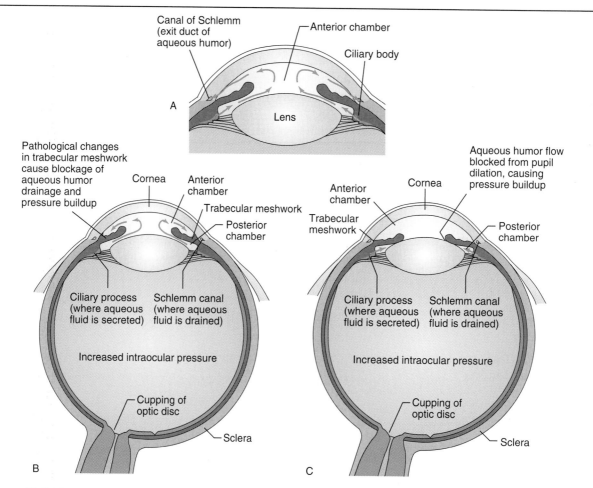

Figure 16–7 *Glaucoma. (A) Normal flow of aqueous humor; (B) open-angle glaucoma; (C) closed-angle glaucoma. (From Williams, LS, and Hopper, PD: Understanding Medical Surgical Nursing, FA Davis, Philadelphia 1999, p 1053, with permission.)*

Other Conditions (Continued)

CONDITION	DESCRIPTION
macular degeneration MĂK-ū-lăr	A progressive deterioration of the macular tissue of the retina, an area important in the visualization of fine details. The deterioration leads to loss of central vision, the vision used for reading, watching videos, and driving. Commonly affecting both eyes, macular degeneration is the leading cause of visual impairment in the United States. The most common type is age-related macular degeneration.
age-related macular degeneration (ARMD or AMD)	A type of macular degeneration that results in a severe loss of central vision. Two primary forms of ARMD are the *atrophic* (also called *involutional* or *dry*) form, which accounts for about 70% of cases, and the *exudative* (also called the *hemorrhagic* or *wet*) form of macular degeneration. No cure currently exists for the atrophic form. In patients with the exudative form, laser photocoagulation may slow the progression of severe visual loss in 5% to 10% of the cases. Approximately 10% or more of elderly Americans have irreversible central vision loss from ARMD.
monochromatism mŏn-ō-KRŌ-mă-tĭzm *mono=one* *chromat=color* *ism=condition*	Complete color blindness in which all colors are perceived shades of gray. Also called *color blindness*.

Other Conditions (Continued)

CONDITION	DESCRIPTION
nyctalopia nĭk-tă-LŌ-pē-ă *nyctal=night* *opia=vision*	Poor vision at night or in dim light resulting from decreased synthesis of *rhodopsin*, vitamin A deficiency, retinal deterioration, or a congenital defect. Also called *night blindness*.
nystagmus nĭs-TĂG-mŭs	Constant, involuntary, cyclical movement of the eyeball in any direction.
retinal detachment	A separation of the retina from the choroid in the back of the eye. The detachment usually results from a hole in the retina that allows the vitreous humor to leak between the choroid and the retina. Severe trauma to the eye, such as a contusion or penetrating wound, may be the proximate cause, but in the great majority of cases retinal detachment is the result of internal changes in the vitreous chamber associated with aging or less frequently with inflammation of the interior of the eye. Treatment to halt the detachment is required, or total blindness ultimately results.
retinoblastoma rĕt-ĭ-nō-blăs-TŌ-mă *retino=retina* *blast=embryonic cell* *oma=tumor*	Congenital, hereditary neoplasm developing from retinal germ cells. The tumor grows rapidly and may invade the brain and distant sites. Characteristic signs are diminished vision, abnormal pupillary reflex, strabismus, and retinal detachment.
retinopathy rĕt-ĭ-NŎP-ă-thē *retino=retina* *pathy=disease*	A noninflammatory eye disorder resulting from changes in the retinal blood vessels.
diabetic dī-ă-BĔT-ĭk	A disorder of retinal blood vessels. It is characterized by capillary microaneurysms, hemorrhage, exudates, and the formation of new vessels and connective tissue. The disorder occurs most frequently in patients with long-standing, poorly controlled *diabetes mellitus*. Repeated hemorrhage may cause permanent opacity of the vitreous humor, and blindness may eventually result. Photocoagulation of damaged retinal blood vessels by a laser beam may be performed to prevent hemorrhage from the vessels. Diabetic retinopathy is the leading cause of blindness in the United States.
hypertensive	Retinopathy associated with hypertension, toxemia of pregnancy, or glomerulonephritis. The changes may include blood vessel alterations, hemorrhages, exudates, and retinal edema.
strabismus stră-BĬZ-mŭs	Failure of the eyes to gaze in the same direction due to weakness in the ocular muscles. Strabismus is classified according to the direction in which the eye(s) deviates as *esotropia* or *exotropia* (Fig. 16–8). Methods of treatment include orthoptic training in which the normal eye is covered to force the use of the affected eye, corrective lenses, or surgery to restore ocular muscle balance.
esotropia ĕs-ō-TRŌ-pē-ă *eso=inward* *tropia=turning*	Inward turning of the eye(s). Esotropia usually develops in infancy or early childhood. Also known as *convergent strabismus* and "cross-eye" (see Fig. 16–8).
exotropia ĕks-ō-TRŌ-pē-ă *exo=outside, outward* *tropia=turning*	Outward turning of the eye(s). Also known as *divergent strabismus* and "wall-eye" (see Fig. 16–8).

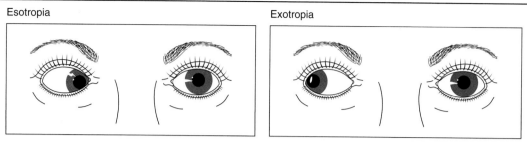

Figure 16–8 *Strabismus: (left) esotropia; (right) exotropia. (From Gylys, BA, and Masters, RM: Medical Terminology Simplified: A Programmed Learning Approach by Body Systems, FA Davis, Philadelphia, 1998, p 439, with permission.)*

Other Conditions (Continued)

CONDITION	DESCRIPTION
synechia sĭn-ĔK-ē-ă	An adhesion, especially of the iris to the cornea or lens of the eye; may develop as a complication of surgery or trauma to the eye, or from glaucoma, cataracts, uveitis, or keratitis. This condition prevents or impedes the flow of aqueous fluid between the posterior and anterior chambers, causing a rise in pressure and a rapid progression to blindness. Treatment consists of dilating the pupils with a mydriatic agent, followed by treatment of the underlying cause.
trachoma trā-KŌ-mă	A chronic, infectious disease of the eye caused by *Chlamydia trachomatis.* Initial symptoms include pain, extreme sensitivity to light (photophobia), inflammation, and lacrimation. If trachoma is left untreated, follicles form on the upper eyelid and grow larger and granulation tissue invades the cornea, eventually causing blindness.

Activity 16–5: Clinical Application
Pathological Conditions

astigmatism
cataract
esotropia
exotropia
glaucoma
hordeolum

hyperopia
hyphema
monochromatism
myopia
nyctalopia
nystagmus

Match the diagnoses listed above with the definitions given in the numbered list:

1. _____ degenerative condition of the eye characterized by clouding of the lens with gray-white opacities that commonly occurs after age 50.

2. _____ pathological condition characterized by increased intraocular pressure (IOP) caused by an excessive accumulation of aqueous humor.

3. _____ irregular curvature of the cornea or lens that causes blurred vision.

4. _____ involuntary, rhythmic eye movements.

5. _____ condition in which the affected eye(s) turns inward; also known as "cross-eye."

6. _____ complete color blindness, in which all colors are perceived as shades of gray.

7. _____ refraction error that results in farsightedness.

8. _____ localized, purulent, inflammatory infection originating in the sebaceous gland of an eyelash; also known as *sty*.

9. _____ condition in which the affected eye(s) turns outward; also known as "wall-eye."

10. _____ refraction error that results in nearsightedness.

Correct Answers _____ × 10 = _____% Score

DIAGNOSTIC PROCEDURES AND TESTS

Imaging Procedures

PROCEDURE	DESCRIPTION
fluorescein angiography *floo-ō-RĔS-ē-ĭn ăn-jē-ŎG-ră-fē*	Procedure in which fluorescein dye is injected intravenously in order to directly visualize blood flow and detect lesions in the macular area of the retina with an ophthalmoscope.
Heidelberg retinal tomogram (HRT) *RĔT-ĭ-năl TŌ-mō-grăm*	Scanning procedure using laser technology to scan the eye to detect and diagnose disorders of the eye.

Clinical Procedures

PROCEDURE	DESCRIPTION
frequency doubling technology (FDT)	A newer screening test that checks for abnormalities in particular cells of the retina that are indicators of early glaucoma.
fundoscopy *fŭn-DŎS-kō-pē*	Use of an ophthalmoscope to examine the innermost structures of the eye, particularly the blood vessels supplying the retina and the optic disc; synonymous with *ophthalmoscopy*.
gonioscopy *gō-nē-ŎS-kō-pē* *gonio=angle* *scopy=visual examination*	Examination of the angle of the anterior chamber of the eye with a gonioscope or with a contact prism lens. Used to monitor the drainage of aqueous humor from the eye in patients at risk for glaucoma. This test can differentiate between closed-angle and open-angle glaucoma.
ophthalmoscopy *ŏf-thăl-MŎS-kō-pē* *ophthalmo=eye* *scopy=visual examination*	Visual examination of the interior structures of the eye using an ophthalmoscope. The pupil is dilated, allowing the examiner to directly view the cornea, lens, and retina.

Clinical Procedures (Continued)

PROCEDURE	DESCRIPTION
perimetry test pĕr-ĬM-ĕ-trē *peri=around* *metry=act of measuring*	Any of the various types of tests that measure the peripheral visual fields (areas of sight that are on the other part of the field of vision).
slit lamp biomicroscopy bī-ō-mī-KRŎS-kō-pē *bio=life* *micro=small* *scopy=visual examination*	Use of a slit lamp (lamp emitting intense light through a small opening) and a microscope to evaluate the conjunctiva, cornea, iris, lens, and vitreous humor.
tonometry tō-NŎM-ĕ-trē *tono=tension* *metry=act of measuring*	Measurement of the intraocular pressure (IOP) of the eye. Used to detect glaucoma (Fig. 16–9).
visual acuity test ă-KŪ-ĭ-tē	Standard test of visual acuity in which a person is asked to read letters and numbers on a chart 20 feet away with the use of the Snellen chart. Also called an *E chart*. Visual acuity is expressed as a ratio. The first number is the distance at which the patient reads the chart; the second is the distance at which a person with normal vision can read the same chart. Normal vision is 20/20 (Fig. 16–10).

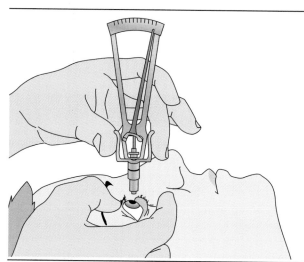

Figure 16–9 *Tonometry is used to measure intraocular eye pressure. (From Williams, LS, and Hopper, PD: Understanding Medical Surgical Nursing. FA Davis, Philadelphia, 1999, p 1047, with permission.)*

Clinical Procedures (Continued)

PROCEDURE	DESCRIPTION

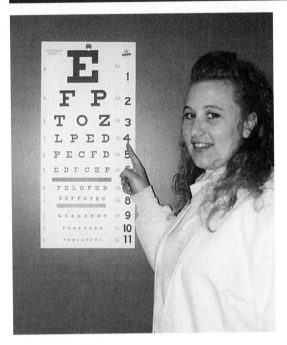

Figure 16–10   *Snellen chart examination. (From Williams, LS, and Hopper, PD: Understanding Medical Surgical Nursing. FA Davis, Philadelphia 1999, p 1025, with permission.)*

visual field examination	A test that measures the range of peripheral vision. The person keeps eyes fixed to look straight ahead while the examiner moves a pencil (or a finger) from behind the patient. The person is asked to indicate at what point the pencil is seen.

SURGICAL AND THERAPEUTIC PROCEDURES

Surgical Procedures

PROCEDURE	DESCRIPTION
cataract surgery KĂT-ă-răkt	The removal of cataracts by surgical removal of the lens. To correct the visual deficit when the eye is without a lens (*aphakic*), the insertion of an artificial lens (*intraocular lens transplant*) or the use of eyeglasses or contact lenses is needed. Several surgical techniques involving cataract removal are described below.
extracapsular surgery ĕks-tră-KĂP-sū-lăr	The removal of the majority of the lens, followed by the insertion of an intraocular lens transplant.
phacoemulsification făk-ō-ē-mŭl-sĭ-fĭ-KĀ-shŭn	Removal of the lens by ultrasonic vibrations that break the lens into tiny particles, which are then suctioned out of the eye.

Surgical Procedures (Continued)

PROCEDURE	DESCRIPTION
corneal transplant *KOR-nē-ăl TRĂNS-plănt*	The surgical transplantation of a donor cornea (from a cadaver) into the eye of a recipient. Also called *keratoplasty*.
iridectomy *ĭr-ĭ-DĔK-tō-mē* *irid=iris* *ectomy=excision, removal*	Excision of a small segment of the iris to open the anterior chamber angle and permit the flow of aqueous humor between the anterior and posterior chambers. This is performed to relieve increased IOP in the treatment of *closed-angle glaucoma*.
laser photocoagulation *fō-tō-cō-ăg-ū-LĀ-shŭn*	Surgical procedure using an *argon laser* to stimulate coagulation of tissue and blood vessels in the interior of the eye. Photocoagulation is useful to seal microaneurysms in diabetic retinopathy, to destroy ciliary body tissue in the treatment of glaucoma, to prevent abnormal growth of blood vessels in age-related macular degeneration, and to assist in forming adhesions to treat retinal detachment.
radial keratotomy (RK) *RĀ-dē-ăl kĕr-ă-TŎT-ō-mē*	Surgical procedure used to decrease nearsightedness. Radial incisions are made in the cornea with a highly precise diamond blade set to a particular depth. These incisions result in a flattening of the central portion of the cornea, which brings the focal point of the eye closer to the retina and improves one's distant vision and eliminates the need for eyeglasses.
scleral buckling *SKLĔR-ăl*	Surgical procedure to repair retinal detachment. Involves placing a silicon implant in conjunction with a beltlike device around the sclera to bring the choroid in contact with the retina (Fig. 16–11). Laser surgery or cryosurgery is also used in this procedure to assist in forming the adhesion of the retina and choroid layers.
trabeculectomy *tră-bĕk-ū-LĔK-tō-mē* *trabecul=trabecula (supporting bundles of fibers)* *ectomy=excision, removal*	Surgical removal of a section of corneoscleral tissue to increase the outflow of aqueous humor in patients with severe glaucoma. The procedure usually involves the removal of the trabecular meshwork and the *canal of Schlemm*.
trabeculoplasty *tră-BĔK-ū-lō-plăs-tē* *trabeculo=trabecula (supporting bundles of fibers)* *plasty=surgical repair*	Surgical creation of a permanent fistula that is used to drain the outflow of aqueous humor in patients with severe glaucoma.
laser trabeculoplasty	Use of an argon laser beam to blanch the trabecular meshwork, which allows an increase in the outflow of aqueous humor.
vitrectomy *vĭ-TRĔK-tō-mē* *vitr=vitreous body (of the eye)* *ectomy=excision, removal*	Procedure in which the vitreous humor is drained out of the eye chamber and replaced with saline or silicone oil. This procedure is performed when blood or scar tissue accumulates in the vitreous humor, a common complication of diabetic retinopathy.

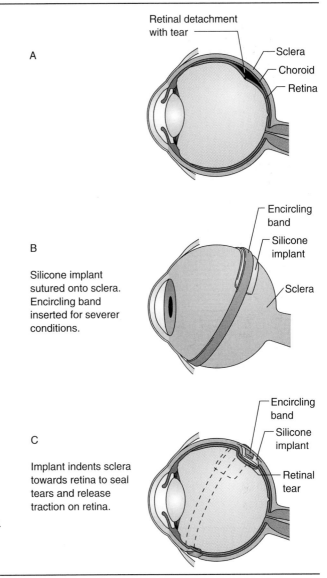

A

Retinal detachment with tear

Sclera

Choroid

Retina

B

Silicone implant sutured onto sclera. Encircling band inserted for severer conditions.

Encircling band

Silicone implant

Sclera

C

Implant indents sclera towards retina to seal tears and release traction on retina.

Encircling band

Silicone implant

Retinal tear

Figure 16–11 *Scleral buckling repair for retinal detachment. (From Williams, LS, and Hopper, PD: Understanding Medical Surgical Nursing. FA Davis, Philadelphia, 1999, p 1052, with permission.)*

Therapeutic Procedures

PROCEDURE	DESCRIPTION
orthoptic training *or-THOP-tik* *orth=straight* *optic=pertaining to the eye, vision* *ic=pertaining to*	Eye muscle exercises prescribed to correct strabismus and restore the normal coordination of the eyes.

Pharmacology

DRUG CLASSIFICATION	THERAPEUTIC ACTION
antibiotics ăn-tĭ-bī-ŎT-ĭks *anti=against* *bio=life* *tic=pertaining to*	Agents that inhibit the growth of microorganisms; ophthalmic antibiotics are dispensed as topical ointments and solutions for eye infections.
beta-adrenergics bā-tă-ăd-rĕn-ĔR-jĭks	Agents that lower intraocular pressure by reducing the production of aqueous humor; used to treat glaucoma.
carbonic anhydrase inhibitors kăr-BŎ-nĭk ăn-HĪ-drās ĭn-HĬ-bĭ-tors	Drugs that decrease the production of aqueous humor by blocking the enzyme carbonic anhydrase. Used to treat glaucoma.
corticosteroids kor-tĭ-kō-STĔR-oydz	Agents used topically to treat eye inflammation that results from allergies, trauma, surgery, or contact with chemical irritants.
cycloplegics sī-klō-PLĒ-jĭks	Agents that paralyze the ciliary muscles to dilate the pupils. Used to facilitate eye examinations.
miotics mī-ŎT-ĭks *mio=smaller, less* *tic=pertaining to*	Agents that constrict the pupils. Used to treat glaucoma.
mydriatics mĭd-rē-ĂT-ĭks	Group of topical drugs used to dilate the pupil and paralyze the muscles of accommodation of the iris. Used to prepare the eye for internal examination and treat inflammatory conditions of the iris.
nonsteroidal anti-inflammatory drugs (NSAIDs)	Drugs used topically to treat inflammation that results from eye surgery, or allergic reactions such as hay fever.

❖ ABBREVIATIONS

ABBREVIATION	MEANING	ABBREVIATION	MEANING
Acc	accommodation	**HRT**	Heidelberg retinal tomogram
ARMD, AMD	age-related macular degeneration	**I&D**	incision and drainage
		IOL	intraocular lens
Ast	astigmatism	**IOP**	intraocular pressure
D	diopter (lens strength)	**mix astig**	mixed astigmatism
Em	emmetropia	**Myop**	myopia
EOM	extraocular movement	**OD**	right eye (oculus dexter)
FDT	frequency doubling technology		

ABBREVIATION	MEANING	ABBREVIATION	MEANING
NSAIDs	nonsteroidal anti-inflammatory drugs	**RK**	radial keratotomy
		ST	esotropia
OS	left eye (oculus sinister)	**VA**	visual acuity
OU	each eye (oculus uterque); both eyes together (oculi unitas)	**VF**	visual field
		XT	exotropia
REM	rapid eye movement		

Activity 16–6: Clinical Application
Diagnostic Tests, Treatments, and Pharmacology

beta-adrenergics
cycloplegics
mydriatics
ophthalmoscopy
phacoemulsification
radial keratotomy (RK)

scleral buckling
tonometry
trabeculoplasty
visual acuity test
visual field examination
vitrectomy

Match the diagnostic test, the treatment, or pharmacological agent listed above with a definition in the numbered list:

1. _____ eye test that measures peripheral vision.

2. _____ visual examination of the interior structures of the eye.

3. _____ test that measures intraocular pressure of the eye and is used to detect glaucoma.

4. _____ standard eye test in which a person reads letters and numbers to test the clarity of vision.

5. _____ surgical creation of a permanent fistula used to drain the outflow of aqueous humor in patients with severe glaucoma.

6. _____ removal of the lens by ultrasonic vibrations that break the lens into tiny particles that are then suctioned out of the eye.

7. _____ surgical procedure used to decrease nearsightedness.

8. _____ surgical procedure to repair a detached retina.

9. _____ pharmaceutical agents that paralyze the ciliary muscles to dilate the pupils; used to facilitate eye examinations.

10. _____ pharmaceutical agents that lower IOP by reducing the production of aqueous humor; used to treat glaucoma.

Correct Answers _____ × 10 = _____ % Score

Activity 16–7: Build Medical Words
Diagnostic, Symptomatic, and Surgical Terms

Use *ophthalm/o* (eye) to build medical words meaning:

1. instrument to examine the eye _____

2. study of the eye _____

Use *blephar/o* (eyelid) to build medical words meaning:

3. paralysis of the eyelid _____

4. involuntary contraction or twitching of the eyelid _____

Use *kerat/o* (cornea) to build medical words meaning:

5. any disease of the cornea _____

6. surgical repair of the cornea _____

7. instrument to incise the cornea _____

Use *pupill/o* (pupil) to build medical words meaning:

8. measurement of the pupil _____

9. visual examination of the pupil _____

Use *scler/o* (sclera) to build medical words meaning:

10. softening of the sclera _____

11. inflammation of the sclera and choroid _____

Use *-opia* (vision) to build medical words meaning:

12. dim or dull vision _____

13. double vision _____

Use *-tropia* (turning) to build medical words meaning:

14. turning inward _____

15. turning outward _____

> **Correct Answers** _____ × 6.67 = _____% **Score**

MEDICAL RECORDS

Authentic reports from a medical record of two operative reports and a consultation letter are included in this section.

The following reading and dictionary exercise and medical record analysis will help you to develop skills abstracting information and mastering the terminology in the reports. Accurate interpretation is important because information of this type is used in numerous areas of the medical practice, such as initiation of treatments, evaluation of patients' progress, and completion of insurance claims.

Reading and Dictionary Exercise

Place a check mark [✓] after you complete the exercise.

[   ] **1.** Underline the following words in the reports as you read both operative reports and the consultation letter aloud.

[   ] **2.** Use a medical dictionary, and Appendix F, Part 2, to define the terms below.

Note: You are not expected to fully understand all the parts of medical reports. The important aspect of this exercise is to use all available resources to complete it. Eventually you will master the terminology and format of these reports.

>>> MEDICAL RECORD 16–1: OPERATIVE REPORT

Term	Pronunciation	Meaning
cataract	KĂT-ă-răkt	_____
phacoemulsification	făk-ō-ē-mŭl-sĭ-fĭ-KĀ-shŭn	_____
posterior chamber	pŏs-TĒ-rē-or CHĂM-bĕr	_____
intraocular lens	ĭn-tră-ŎK-ū-lăr lĕnz	_____
intravenous	ĭn-tră-VĒ-nŭs	_____
sedation	sĕ-DĀ-shŭn	_____
nuclear	NŪ-klē-ăr	_____
sclerotic	sklĕ-RŎT-ĭk	_____
Honan balloon	HŌ-năn bă-loon	_____
topical anesthesia	TŎP-ĭ-kăl ăn-ĕs-THĒ-zē-ă	_____
Marcaine	MĂR-kān	_____
scleral	SKLĔR-ăl	_____
cornea	KOR-nē-ă	_____

paracentesis	*păr-ă-sĕn-TĒ-sĭs*	_____
Xylocaine	*ZĪ-lō-kān*	_____
anterior capsulorrhexis	*ăn-TĬR-ē-or kăp-sū-lō-RĔK-sĭs*	_____
viscoelastic	*vĭs-kō-ē-LĂS-tĭk*	_____
hydrodissected	*hī-drō-dī-SĔK-tĕd*	_____
emulsified	*ē-MŬL-sĭ-fīd*	_____
phacofracture	*făk-ō-FRĂK-chūr*	_____
cortical	*KOR-tĭ-kăl*	_____
diopter	*dī-ŎP-tĕr*	_____
silicone	*SĬL-ĭ-kōn*	_____
capsular	*KĂP-sū-lăr*	_____
anterior chamber	*ăn-TĬR-ē-or CHĀM-bĕr*	_____
normotensive	*nor-mō-TĔN-sĭv*	_____
Ocuflox	*Ŏ-kū-floks*	_____
Maxitrol	*MĂK-sĭ-trŏl*	_____

>>> MEDICAL RECORD 16-2: OPERATIVE REPORT

Term	Pronunciation	Meaning
glaucoma	*glaw-KŌ-mă*	_____
trabeculectomy	*tră-bĕk-ū-LĔK-tō-mē*	_____
5-fluorouracil	*fīv-floor-ō-ŪR-ă-sĭl*	_____
cup-to-disk ratio	*KŬP-too-dĭsk RĀ-shē-ō*	_____
conjunctival	*kŏn-jŭnk-TĪ-văl*	_____
limbus-based	*LĬM-bŭs-bāsd*	_____
microcautery	*mī-krō-KAW-tĕr-ē*	_____
sclera	*SKLĔR-ă*	_____
gentian violet	*JĔN-shŭn VĪ-ō-lĕt*	_____
scleral	*SKLĔR-ăl*	_____
apex	*Ā-pĕks*	_____

corneoscleral	*kor-nē-ō-SKLĔR-ăl*	_____
iridectomy	*ĭr-ĭ-DĔK-tō-mē*	_____
nylon sutures	*SŪ-chŭrs*	_____
Vicryl suture	*VĬK-rĭl sū-chūr*	_____
Solu-Medrol	*sŏl-ū-MĔD-rŏl*	_____
Ancef	*AN-sĕf*	_____
inferior cul-de-sac	*ĭn-FĒ-rē-or KŬL-dĕ-săk*	_____

>>> MEDICAL RECORD 16-3: CONSULTATION LETTER

Term	Pronunciation	Meaning
amblyopic	*ăm-blē-Ō-pĭk*	_____
visual acuity	*VĬZH-ū-ăl ă-KŪ-ĭ-tē*	_____
intraocular pressure	*ĭn-tră-ŎK-ū-lăr PRĔSH-ŭr*	_____
afferent	*ĂF-ĕr-ĕnt*	_____
pupillary	*PŪ-pĭ-lĕr-ē*	_____
slit lamp exam		_____
conjunctiva	*kŏn-jŭnk-TĪ-vă*	_____
cornea	*KŌR-nē-ă*	_____
rubeosis	*roo-bē-Ō-sĭs*	_____
iris	*Ī-rĭs*	_____
nuclear	*NŪ-klē-ăr*	_____
sclerotic	*sklĕ-RŎT-ĭk*	_____
cortical	*KOR-tĭ-kăl*	_____
funduscopic	*fŭn-dŭs-KŎP-ĭk*	_____
macula	*MĂK-ū-lă*	_____
dot-and-blot	*DŎT-ănd-BLŎT*	_____
hemorrhage	*HĔM-ĕ-rĭj*	_____
optic nerve	*ŎP-tĭk nĕrv*	_____

fluorescein angiogram	*floo-ō-RĔS-ē-ĭn* *ĂN-jē-ō-grăm*	_____
disc edema	*dĭsk ě-DĒ-mă*	_____
ischemia	*ĭs-KĒ-mē-ă*	_____
rubeotic glaucoma	*roo-bē-ŎT-ĭk* *glaw-KŌ-mă*	_____

Critical Thinking: Analysis of Medical Records

This section provides experience in abstracting and analyzing information from the medical records. At the same time, it reinforces the material presented in this chapter.

>>> MEDICAL RECORD 16–1: OPERATIVE REPORT

1. What problems was the patient having that indicated a need for cataract surgery?

_____

_____

2. What was the patient's vision in the left eye prior to surgery?

_____

3. What type of anesthesia was used during the surgery?

_____

4. Why does the physician use the expressions "12 o'clock position" and "1 o'clock position"?

_____

_____

_____

_____

>>> MEDICAL RECORD 16–2: OPERATIVE REPORT

5. What is the patient's diagnosis?

_____

6. What are the possible complications of uncontrolled glaucoma?

_____

_____

7. How was bleeding controlled during the surgery?

_____

8. What medications were given at the end of the surgery just before moving the patient to the recovery room?

_____

>>> MEDICAL RECORD 16-3: CONSULTATION LETTER

9. What is significant in the patient's past medical history?

_____

10. What type of examination was done to view the conjunctiva and cornea?

_____

11. Did the fundoscopic examination reveal any abnormalities in the right eye?

_____

12. What did the intravenous fluorescein angiogram reveal?

_____

Audio Practice

Listen to the audio CD-ROM to practice the pronunciation of selected medical terms from this chapter.

Medical Record 16–1. Operative Report

GENERAL HOSPITAL AND MEDICAL CENTER
2211 Fifth Avenue North • Healthy City, USA 12345 • (321) 123-4567

Operative Report

Patient Name: Maria Andrews   **Patient Number:** 33-33-67
Birth Date: 04/12/xx   **Room Number:** OP

DATE OF OPERATION: 03/24/xx

PREOPERATIVE DIAGNOSIS: Cataract, left eye.

POSTOPERATIVE DIAGNOSIS: Cataract, left eye.

OPERATION: Phacoemulsification and posterior chamber intraocular lens implant, left eye.

SURGEON: Ronald Jason, M.D.

ANESTHESIA: Topical with intravenous sedation.

INDICATIONS: This lady has had progressive decrease in visual acuity in the left eye due to a nuclear sclerotic cataract. Her best corrected vision in this eye is 20/60. She is having difficulty seeing at a distance and reading, and cataract extraction with implant is indicated.

PROCEDURE: Honan balloon was applied for 20 minutes. Topical anesthesia was achieved with 0.75% Marcaine topical, one drop, and the eye was prepped and draped in the sterile fashion including the lashes and lid margins and adhesive drape. Scleral tunnel incision was developed into clear cornea at the 12 o'clock position. Paracentesis tract was put at the 1 o'clock position, and 1% preservative-free Xylocaine was irrigated over the iris. Continuous anterior capsulorrhexis was performed under viscoelastic, and nucleus was hydrodissected and emulsified using the phacofracture technique. All cortical material was aspirated. A +26 diopter silicone foldable lens was deposited into the capsular bag. Viscoelastic was aspirated out of the posterior and anterior chambers and was replaced with balanced salt solution to normotensive level. Ocuflox ophthalmic drops and Maxitrol ophthalmic drops were put in the eye, and the patient was returned to the recovery room in satisfactory condition, and later on discharged home, to be followed up in the office the next morning.

_____
Ronald Jason, M.D.

RJ/alm
D&T: 03/24/xx

Medical Record 16–2. Operative Report

GENERAL HOSPITAL AND MEDICAL CENTER
2211 Fifth Avenue North • Healthy City, USA 12345 • (321) 123-4567

Operative Report

Patient Name: Jane Richards
Birth Date: 01/03/xx

Patient Number: 09-94-00
Room Number: OP

DATE OF OPERATION: 02/17/xx

PREOPERATIVE DIAGNOSIS: Uncontrolled glaucoma.

POSTOPERATIVE DIAGNOSIS: Uncontrolled glaucoma.

OPERATION: Left trabeculectomy with 5-fluorouracil.

ANESTHESIA: Monitored.

INDICATION: Patient has questionable compliance, is on maximal medical therapy for her in view of allergic problems with some of the drops. She has a cup-to-disk ratio of 0.9 and shows definite field loss. In view of the above reasons, a trabeculectomy with 5-fluorouracil was advised.

PROCEDURE: After satisfactory preparations were completed, a conjunctival limbus-based flap was formed from the 12 o'clock to the 3 o'clock position, left eye. Bleeding was carefully controlled with microcautery. When a clear sclera with gentian violet was developed, a 4 x 4 x 4 mm triangle was made. A preset metal knife 0.4 mm in depth was then used to dissect a scleral flap. This was done without complication. At this point, a cellule sponge soaked in 5-fluorouracil was placed over the scleral flap and beneath the conjunctival flap for 5 minutes. This was removed, and the area was copiously irrigated. A #10-0 nylon suture was then placed at the apex of the flap. A stab incision was made into the anterior chamber at the 3 o'clock position, and the same diamond knife was used to enter the anterior chamber at the base of the triangle. A 1 x 3 mm bite was taken of corneoscleral tissue. An iridectomy was then performed. The flap was then closed with three #10-0 nylon sutures. The conjunctival flap was then closed with a running Vicryl suture. At the termination of the procedure, filtration was taking place, there were no leaks detected in the conjunctival closure. Then 40 mg of Solu-Medrol and 100 mg of Ancef were placed in the inferior cul-de-sac. A double eye pad was positioned, and the patient was sent to the recovery room in good condition.

_____
Rodney Torch, M.D.

RT/ajh
D&T: 02/17/xx

Medical Record 16–3. Consultation Letter

GENERAL HOSPITAL AND MEDICAL CENTER
2211 Fifth Avenue North • Healthy City, USA 12345 • (321) 123-4567

Consultation

November 21, 20xx

Maurine Euline, MD
3392 Main St.
Healthy City, USA 12345

RE: Joseph Lither

Dear Dr. Euline:

This patient was seen on September 20 for a possible vein occlusion in the left eye. He states that the left eye has been amblyopic since early childhood without any worsening. There is no other outstanding medical history.

On examination, visual acuity is 20/60 in the left eye and 20/20 in the right eye, with current prescription glasses. Intraocular pressure is 16 in both eyes. Motility is straight with full versions. The pupils are normal and there is no definite afferent pupillary defect noted. Slit lamp exam reveals a white conjunctiva with a clear cornea. The anterior chamber is 2+ deep, and there is no rubeosis of the iris noted. The lenses have nuclear sclerotic and cortical cataracts, 2+ in nature. Dilated fundoscopic exam reveals a 0.3 cup-to-disc ratio. The macula and periphery are normal on the left eye. The right eye has dot-and-blot hemorrhage of the optic nerve, 1+ in nature.

An intravenous fluorescein angiogram was performed. This revealed disc edema on the left eye and some ischemia. I feel, however, it is best that we just watch him for now. He could develop rubeotic glaucoma at any time. As this can progress quite rapidly, I recommended he return in four weeks, unless he notices problems sooner.

I would like to thank you for this interesting referral. I will keep you apprised of this patient's progress.

Sincerely,

_____

Lawrence Barron, MD

LB/ajh
D: 11/20/xx
T: 11/21/xx

olfactory ŏl-FĂK-tō-rē	Relating to the sense of smell.
ossicles ŎS-ĭ-klz	The small bones of the middle ear: the incus, the malleus, and the stapes.
patent PĂT-ĕnt	Open and unblocked.
turbinates TŬR-bĭ-nāts	Conchae bones; three S-shaped bones located in the nasal cavity.
utricle Ū-trĭk-l	Saclike structure in the inner ear that is associated with maintaining balance.

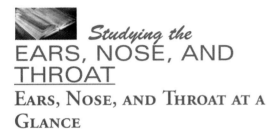

Studying the
EARS, NOSE, AND THROAT

Ears, Nose, and Throat at a Glance

The organs that contain receptors for hearing and smelling are located in the ears and nose, respectively. The sense of hearing occurs through the mechanical action of the ear and its three anatomic divisions: the external, middle, and inner ear. The external ear funnels sound waves to the middle ear and directs them through the auditory canal to strike the tympanic membrane, or eardrum. The central area of the tympanic membrane is connected to a tiny bone called the malleus (hammer), which also begins to vibrate. The vibrations are then picked up by two other small bones, the incus and the stapes. As the stapes moves, it touches a membrane called the oval window, which separates the middle from the inner ear. The movement of the oval window sets up waves in the special auditory fluids of the cochlea. Within the cochlea, a sensitive auditory receptor area, known as the *organ of Corti*, receives and relays the sound waves to the auditory nerve fibers and transmits them to the auditory area of the cerebral cortex. This is where the impulses terminate and are interpreted.

The nose contains the receptor cells for smell and serves as a resonating chamber for speech. It also provides an airway for respiration and moistens, warms, and filters inspired air, and cleanses it of foreign matter. Continuous with the nasal (nose) cavity is the uppermost portion of the pharynx (throat), the nasopharynx, which serves solely as an air passage. Anatomically, the nasopharynx is linked to the middle ear cavity with the auditory (eustachian) tube. Normally, this tube is flattened and closed; however, swallowing or yawning opens it briefly to equalize pressure. The eardrum does not vibrate freely unless the pressure on both of its surfaces is the same so that the pressure in the middle ear cavity is equal with the external air pressure.

STRUCTURE AND FUNCTION

Ear

As you read the following material, label Figure 17–1 to understand the structure of the ear.

The ears are organs of both hearing and balance. Each ear is divided into three parts: the outer ear, the middle ear, and the inner ear. The structures of the outer and middle ear are involved with hearing only and are rather simply designed. However, the structures of the inner ear are extremely complex and function in both hearing and equilibrium.

Outer Ear

The outer ear is structurally designed to collect sound waves and to direct them inward. It consists of the (1) **auricle,** or pinna, the (2) **external auditory canal,** and the (3) **tympanic membrane,** also known as the *eardrum.*

The auricle is a trumpet-shaped flap of elastic cartilage covered with thick skin. In cats, the auricle moves to funnel the sound waves more efficiently. In people, it is stationary. The auditory canal is lined with skin that contains **ceruminous glands.** These glands emit a yellowish-brown substance called **cerumen,** which protects and lubricates the ear. Cerumen is what is commonly referred to as earwax.

Middle Ear

Sound waves that travel through the external auditory canal strike the eardrum, which moves back and forth

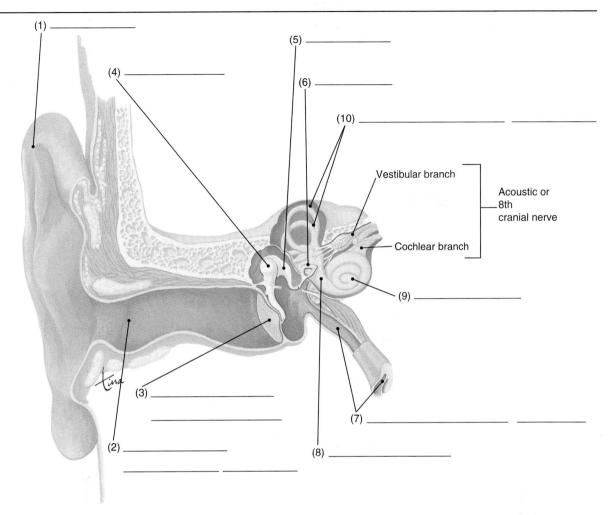

(1) _____

(4) _____

(5) _____

(6) _____

(10) _____ _____

Vestibular branch

Acoustic or
8th
cranial nerve

Cochlear branch

(9) _____

(7) _____ _____

(3) _____

_____ _____

(2) _____

_____ _____

(8) _____

Figure 17–1 *The outer, middle, and inner ear structures as shown in a frontal section through the right temporal bone. (Adapted from Scanlon, VC, and Sanders, TS: Essentials of Anatomy and Physiology, ed 3. FA Davis, Philadelphia, 1999, p 198, with permission.)*

in response and vibrates. The energy caused by the vibrating eardrum is transferred to the three tiny movable bones or **ossicles** of the middle ear. The bones are named for their characteristic shapes. The (4) **malleus** resembles a hammer; the (5) **incus** resembles an anvil; and the (6) **stapes** resembles a tiny stirrup. The three bones bridge the eardrum and the inner ear, which allows the transmission of vibrations between these structures.

An auditory tube, also known as the (7) **eustachian tube,** connects the middle ear to the nasopharynx. This tube conducts air between the tympanic cavity and the outside of the body by way of the nasopharynx and the mouth. The eustachian tube helps maintain equal air pressure on both sides of the eardrum, which is necessary for normal hearing. The eustachian tube is usually closed and opens only when one swallows or yawns. For the eardrum to vibrate properly, the air pressure in the middle ear must be equal to the exter-

nal pressure. It is not uncommon for airplane passengers to experience a "popping" sensation in their ears upon ascent or descent when the pressure within the cabin changes. The "pop" sensation is created when the eustachian tubes open up to equalize air pressure between the outside and middle ear. Swallowing or yawning allows the air from the middle ear to leave and enter the throat until the atmospheric and middle ear air pressures are equalized. If the air pressure between the middle ear and the outside is not eventually balanced, there is a danger of an eardrum rupture. With equalized air pressure, the eardrum tends to remain in a relaxed state. The middle ear is separated from the inner ear by the **oval window.**

Inner Ear

Continue to label Figure 17–1.

The inner ear, also called the **labyrinth** ("maze"), is a complex system of communicating chambers and tubes that contain receptors for hearing and balance. Each ear has two labyrinths: the *osseous (bony) labyrinth* and the *membranous labyrinth.* The osseous labyrinth is a bony canal in the temporal bone. The membranous labyrinth is a tube that lies within the osseous labyrinth. The **osseous labyrinth** consists of the (8) **vestibule,** (9) **cochlea** (snail-shaped structure), and the (10) **semicircular canals.**

Label Figure 17–2 to understand the position and anatomic structures of the membranous labyrinth.

The **membranous labyrinth** consists of the (1) **utricle,** and the (2) **saccule** (inside the vestibule). The smaller saccule is continuous with the membranous labyrinth extending anteriorly into the (3) **cochlear duct,** whereas the utricle is continuous with the ducts extending into the (4) **semicircular canals** posteriorly. The semicircular canals, the utricle, and the saccule house the receptors of equilibrium (see Fig. 17–1 and Fig.17–2). The three structures are filled with endolymph and perilymph fluids and have hairlike receptors that are sensitive to the body's rotational movement and the angular acceleration and deceleration of the head. These movements stimulate the nerve fibers that lead to the **cerebellum** in the brain; from here messages are then sent to the body to maintain body position and equilibrium. As stated earlier, the (5) **oval window** separates the middle and inner ear. Next to the oval window is the snail-shaped (6) **cochlea,** which contains a basilar membrane (see Fig.17–3) that forms the floor of the cochlear duct and provides a fibrous base for the spiral organ of Corti. The special auditory fluids, endolymph and perilymph, in the cochlea aid the transmission of sound vibrations. As the fluids fluctuate, they transmit the stimulus to the tiny hair cells of the organ of Corti.

Review the organ of Corti as you label the structures in Figure 17–3.

With the bending of the (1) **hair cells,** impulses are generated and transmitted via the (2) **auditory fibers of the cranial nerve VIII** (vestibulocochlear nerve) to the **cerebral cortex** of the brain. It is here that the impulses are interpreted and you hear sounds.

In summary, hearing involves the transmission of vibrations and the generation of nerve impulses. As

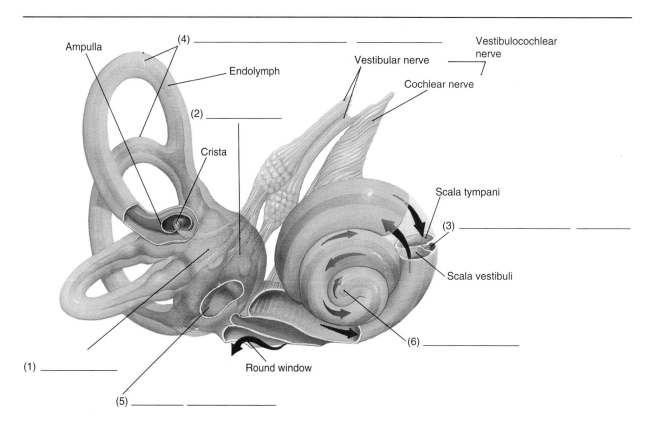

Figure 17–2 *The inner ear structures. The arrows show the transmission of vibrations during hearing (Adapted from Scanlon, VC, and Sanders, TS: Essentials of Anatomy and Physiology, ed 3. FA Davis, Philadelphia, 1999, p 199, with permission.)*

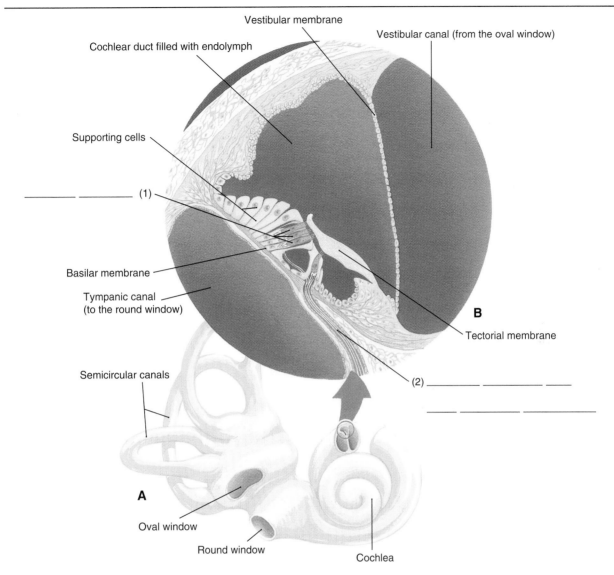

Vestibular membrane

Vestibular canal (from the oval window)

Cochlear duct filled with endolymph

Supporting cells

(1) _____ _____

Basilar membrane

Tympanic canal
(to the round window)

B

Tectorial membrane

Semicircular canals

(2) _____ _____ ___

_____ _____ _____ _____

A

Oval window

Round window

Cochlea

Figure 17–3 *The organ of Corti. (A) The inner ear structures. (B) Magnification of the organ of Corti within the cochlea (Adapted from Scanlon, VC, and Sanders, TS: Essentials of Anatomy and Physiology, ed 3. FA Davis, Philadelphia, 1999, p 200, with permission.)*

sound waves enter the external auditory canal, vibrations are transmitted by the following sequence of structures: the tympanic membrane or eardrum, the malleus, the incus, the stapes, the oval window, the perilymph and the endolymph within the cochlea, and the hair cells of the organ of Corti. The tiny hair cells stimulate nearby neurons that give rise to impulses that travel to the brain, which interprets them as sound.

Review the pathway summary of the transmission of sound waves from the outer ear to the brain in Flowchart 17–1.

Activity 17–1: Competency Verification
Structures of the Ear

Review Figure 17–1, and check your labeling in Appendix C.

Activity 17–2: Competency Verification
Structures of the Inner Ear

Review Figures 17–2 and 17–3, and check your labeling in Appendix C.

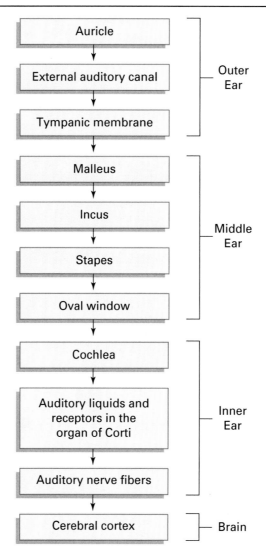

Flowchart 17–1 *Pathway summary of the transmission of sound waves from the outer ear to the brain.*

Activity 17–3: Competency Verification

Tracing the Sequence of Hearing

auricle	vestibulocochlear nerve	organ of Corti
basilar membrane	incus	oval window
cerumen	malleus	stapes
cochlea	uricle	tympanic membrane

From the list above, place in sequential order the organs that are involved in the hearing process:

1. _____ the structure that funnels sound waves from the environment.

2. _____ protects and lubricates the ear.

3. _____ the eardrum.

4. _____ the auditory bone that resembles a hammer.

5. _____ the auditory bone that resembles an anvil.

6. _____ the auditory bone that resembles a tiny stirrup.

7. _____ the structure that separates the middle ear from the inner ear.

8. _____ the snail-shaped structure of the osseous labyrinth.

9. _____ the structure within the cochlea that houses the hair cell receptors of hearing.

10. _____ neurons that transmit impulses to the cerebral cortex for interpretation of sound.

Correct Answers _____ × 10 = _____ % Score

Nose, Throat, and Larynx
Nose

As you read the following material, label Figure 17–4 to understand the structure of the nose.

Air enters and leaves the body through the (1) **nose,** which is made up of bone and cartilage covered with skin. The entrance to the nose is known as the (2) **nostril** (naris). As air enters the nose, it passes into the **nasal cavity,** which is divided into a right and left chamber by a dividing wall called the *septum.* The nasal cavity is lined with *ciliated epithelium* and is highly vascular. The nasal mucosa, or mucous membrane, warms and moistens the inhaled air, where the hairs (**cilia**) help prevent the entry of dust and other foreign bodies. Protruding into the nasal cavity are three (3) **conchae** (turbinates). These scroll-like bones—superior, middle, and inferior conchae—increase the surface area of the nasal cavity.

The (4) **olfactory receptors** transmit the sensation of *olfaction* (smelling) directly to the cerebral cortex for interpretation. The cells are located high in the nasal cavity and within a specialized area of mucous membrane known as the *olfactory epithelium.* Fibers of these cells pass through the (5) **ethmoid bone** and extend up into the *olfactory bulb,* which links with the *olfactory areas of the brain.* These areas of the brain are associated with the sense of smell.

To sum up, the mechanism of smell allows perception of odors through the stimulation of the olfactory nerves. Odor molecules dissolve in nasal mucus and stimulate the hairlike endings, or *cilia,* of the receptor cells, generating a nerve impulse. The sensory impulse travels along the fibers of the cells that pass through holes in the plate of the ethmoid bone into the olfactory bulb. From the olfactory bulb, the sensory impulses are conveyed into the cerebral cortex, where they are interpreted as odor and cause the perception of smell.

Adjacent to the nasal cavity, connected by small ducts, are four pairs of **paranasal sinuses,** which are small cavities in the skull bones. The sinuses are named in relation to the bones in which they are located: the (6) **frontal sinus** is located above the eyes; the (7) **ethmoid sinuses** are located on both sides of the nasal cavities between each eye; the (8) **sphenoid sinus** is located above and behind the nose, and the **maxillary sinus** is located above the jaw. Review Figure 17–5 for anterior and left lateral views of the paranasal sinuses.

All of the sinuses are lined by a continuation of the mucous membranes from the nasal cavity, which continues to warm and moisten the air passing through them. The sinuses add resonance to the voice. The change in voice sound often associated with a head cold is a result of sinus cavity blockage.

Throat

The throat, or the **pharynx,** is posterior to the nasal and oral cavities and functions as an air passage. It is divided into three parts: the nasopharynx, oropharynx, and laryngopharynx. The (9) **nasopharynx** is located behind the nasal cavities and is above the (10) **soft palate.** Recall from Chapter 7, Gastroenterology, that the pharynx serves as a dual passageway for both air and food. Thus it has both respiratory and digestive functions.

The (11) **uvula** is the small cone-shaped process suspended from the middle of the posterior border of the soft palate. During swallowing, the soft palate and its pendulous uvula close off the nasopharynx to prevent food from entering the nasal cavity. A col-

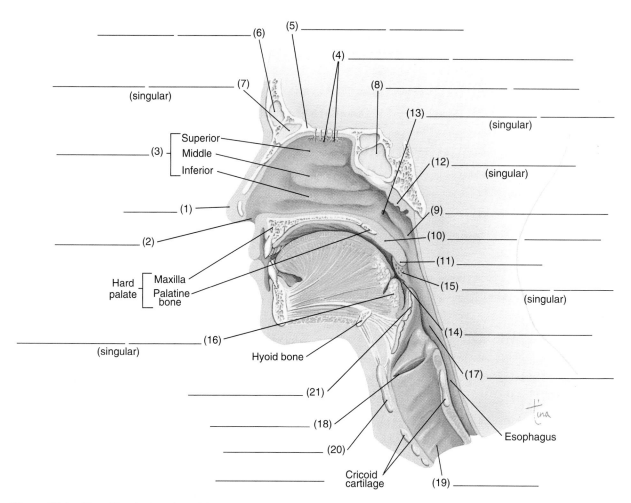

Figure 17–4 *The midsagittal section of the head and neck showing the structures of the upper respiratory tract. (Adapted from Scanlon, VC, and Sanders, TS: Essentials of Anatomy and Physiology, ed 3. FA Davis, Philadelphia, 1999, p 327, with permission.)*

lection of lymphatic tissue, the (12) **adenoids** (pharyngeal tonsils), is found on the posterior wall of the nasopharynx. The two (13) **eustachian tubes** connect the nasopharynx to the middle ear. They extend to the middle ear cavities. Eustachian tubes permit air to leave or enter the middle ear to maintain equal pressure that allows proper vibration of the eardrum.

Although the nasopharynx is designed for air passage only, the (14) **oropharynx,** which lies behind the oral cavity, is both a food and air passage. The (15) **palatine tonsils,** more commonly known as the tonsils, are located in the oropharynx. Together with the (16) **lingual tonsils,** the palatine tonsils and the adenoids form a ring of lymphatic tissue around the pharynx that functions to destroy pathogens that penetrate the mucosa.

As mentioned earlier, the (17) **laryngopharynx** is both a food and air passageway. It opens anteriorly into the larynx and posteriorly into the esophagus. Muscular wall contraction of the oropharynx and laryngopharynx is part of the swallowing reflex.

Larynx

The (18) **larynx,** also known as the voice box, is responsible for sound production. It also functions as an air passageway between the pharynx and the (19) **trachea.** It is made up of nine pieces of cartilage, all connected with ligaments. Although the esophagus is a collapsible muscular tube, the pharynx is a firm, flexible tissue that is **patent** at all times.

The (20) **thyroid cartilage,** more commonly called the Adam's apple, is the largest of the individual carti-

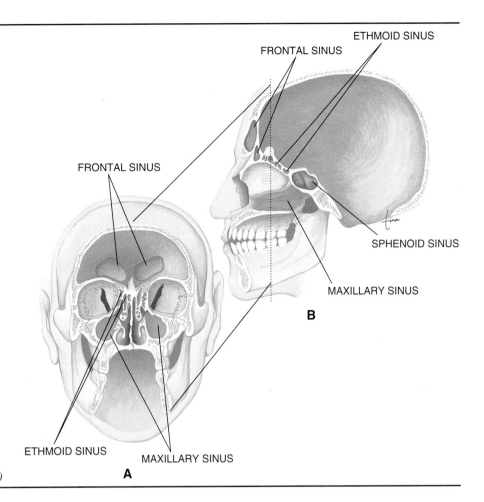

Figure 17–5 *The paranasal sinuses: (A) anterior; (B) left lateral. (From Venes, D: Taber's Cyclopedic Medical Dictionary, ed 19. FA Davis, Philadelphia, 2001, p 1981, with permission.)*

lages. The (21) **epiglottis** is a cartilaginous structure that overhangs the larynx like a lid and prevents food from entering the larynx and the trachea during the swallowing process.

 Activity 17–4: Competency Verification
Structures of the Nose, Pharynx, and Larynx

Review Figure 17–4, and check your labeling in Appendix C.

Review Figure 17–6, which shows the larynx, and label the (1) **thyroid cartilage** and (2) **epiglottis.**

The (3) **vocal cords** are found on either side of the **glottis,** or the airway (Fig. 17–7).

During the process of speaking, the muscles of the larynx pull the vocal cords across the glottis and are vibrated by exhaled air, producing sound. Even though the sound originates with the vocal cords, other structures such as the mouth, pharynx, nasal cavity, and paranasal sinuses are all necessary for converting the sound into recognizable speech.

 Activity 17–5: Competency Verification
Structures of the Larynx

Review Figure 17–6, and check your labeling in Appendix C.

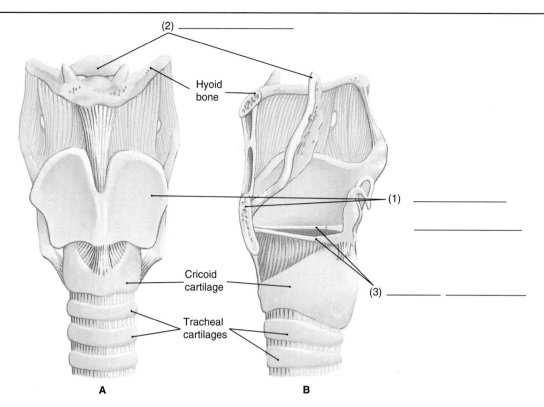

(2)

Hyoid
bone

(1)

Cricoid
cartilage

(3)

Tracheal
cartilages

A   B

Figure 17–6   *The larynx: (A) anterior view; (B) midsagittal section through the larynx viewed from the left side. (Adapted from Scanlon, VC, and Sanders, TS: Essentials of Anatomy and Physiology, ed 3. FA Davis, Philadelphia, 1999, p 328, with permission.)*

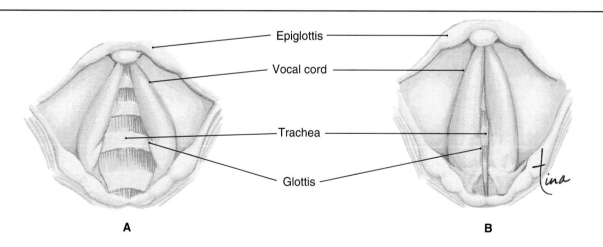

Epiglottis

Vocal cord

Trachea

Glottis

A   B

Figure 17–7   *The superior view of the vocal cords: (A) position of the vocal cords during breathing; (B) position of the vocal cords during speaking. (From Scanlon, VC, and Sanders, TS: Essentials of Anatomy and Physiology, ed 3. FA Davis, Philadelphia, 1999, p 329, with permission.)*

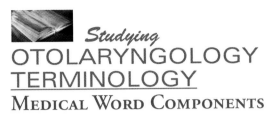

Studying
OTOLARYNGOLOGY
TERMINOLOGY
MEDICAL WORD COMPONENTS
Combining Forms

Combining Forms: Ear, Nose, and Throat

Combining Form	Meaning	EXAMPLE	
		Term/Pronunciation	Definition
EAR			
acous/o	hearing	**acous**/tic ă-KOOS-tĭk	pertaining to (*-tic*) sound or the sense of hearing
audi/o		**audi**/o/meter aw-dē-ŎM-ĕ-tĕr	instrument for testing hearing *The suffix -meter literally means "instrument for measuring."*
audit/o		**audit**/ory ĂW-dĭ-tō-rē	pertaining to (*-ory*) the sense of hearing
cochle/o	cochlea	**cochle**/ar KŎK-lē-ăr	pertaining to (*-ar*) the cochlea
labyrinth/o	labyrinth, inner ear	**labyrinth**/itis lăb-ĭ-rĭn-THĪ-tĭs	inflammation (*-itis*) of the labyrinth *Labyrinthitis is synonymous with otitis interna.*
mastoid/o	mastoid process	**mastoid**/ectomy măs-toyd-ĔK-tō-mē	excision (*-ectomy*) of the bony partitions forming the mastoid cells *The mastoid process is a projection of the temporal bone.*
ot/o	ear	**ot**/o/dynia ō-tō-DĬN-ē-ă	pain (*-dynia*) in the ear *Otodynia is synonymous with otalgia and means "earache."*
aur/o		**aur**/al AW-răl	pertaining to (*-al*) the ear
auricul/o		**auricul**/ar aw-RĬK-ū-lăr	pertaining to (*-ar*) the ear
salping/o	tubes (usually fallopian or eustachian [auditory] tubes)	**salping**/o/scope săl-PĬNG-gō-skōp	instrument used to examine (*-scope*) the nasopharynx and eustachian tube
staped/o	stapes	**staped**/ectomy stā-pē-DĔK-tō-mē	excision of the stapes *This procedure is often done to improve hearing, especially in cases of otosclerosis. The stapes is then replaced by a prosthesis.*

Combining Forms: Ear, Nose, and Throat (Continued)

Combining Form	Meaning	EXAMPLE	
		Term/Pronunciation	Definition
tympan/o	tympanic membrane, eardrum	**tympan**/o/centesis *tĭm-păn-ō-sĕn-TĒ-sĭs*	surgical puncture (-*centesis*) of the eardrum to drain fluid *The excess fluid is usually a result of infection.*
myring/o		**myring**/o/tome *mĭ-RĬN-gō-tōm*	surgical knife used for incising the tympanic membrane *The suffix -tome means "instrument to cut."*
NOSE AND THROAT			
adenoid/o	adenoid	**adenoid**/ectomy *ăd-ĕ-noyd-ĔK-tō-mē*	removal (-*ectomy*) of the adenoids
epiglott/o	epiglottis	**epiglott**/itis *ĕp-ĭ-glŏt-Ī-tĭs*	inflammation of the epiglottis *This condition is most common in young children and can cause airway obstruction and become life threatening.*
laryng/o	larynx (voice box)	**laryng**/o/edema *lăr-ĭn-gō-ĕ-DĒ-mă*	swelling (-*edema*) of the larynx that is usually caused by an allergic reaction
nas/o	nose	**nas**/al *NĀ-zl*	pertaining to (-*al*) the nose
rhin/o		**rhin**/o/plasty *RĪ-nō-plăs-tē*	surgical repair (-*plasty*) of the nose to correct an anatomic defect or for cosmetic purposes
pharyng/o	pharynx (throat)	**pharyng**/o/scopy *făr-ĭn-GŎS-kō-pē*	visual examination (-*scopy*) of the throat
sinus/o	sinus cavity	**sinus**/itis *sī-nŭs-Ī-tĭs*	inflammation (-*itis*) of a sinus cavity due to an allergy, virus, or bacteria *Inadequate drainage of mucus often results in chronic sinusitis.*
tonsill/o	tonsils	**tonsill**/o/tome *tŏn-SĬL-ō-tōm*	surgical instrument (-*tome*) used to remove the tonsils (*tonsillectomy*)
trache/o	trachea	**trache**/o/stomy *trā-kē-ŎS-tō-mē*	forming an opening (-*stomy*) by incising the skin over the trachea to permit an open airway *This procedure is performed as an emergency procedure when the airway is blocked.*

Suffixes

In this section, suffixes are listed alphabetically and highlighted, whereas, key prefixes are defined in the right-hand column.

Suffixes

| Suffix | Meaning | EXAMPLE | |
		Term/Pronunciation	Definition
-acusis	hearing	**an**/acusis ăn-ă-KŪ-sĭs	total loss of hearing the prefix -an means "without," "not."
-cusis		**presby**/cusis prĕz-bĭ-KŪ-sĭs	loss of hearing due to the natural aging process
-rrhea	discharge, flow	**ot/o**/rrhea ō-tō-RĒ-ă	any discharge from the external ear; usually associated with inflammation of the ear Otorrhea may be serous, sanguineous, or purulent.

Activity 17–6: Competency Verification
Medical Word Components

Check the box [✓] as you complete each numbered section.

[   ] **1.** Review the word components for the ear, the nose, and the throat. Then pronounce each word aloud.

[   ] **2.** For each of the following words, first write the suffix and its meaning. Then translate the meaning of the remaining components starting with the first part of the word.

Example: nas/al
Answer: al=pertaining to, relating to; nose

1. pharyng/o/scopy _____
2. epiglott/itis _____
3. trache/o/stomy _____
4. sinus/itis _____
5. tonsill/o/tome _____
6. rhin/o/plasty _____
7. staped/ectomy _____
8. acous/tic _____

9. mastoid/ectomy _____

10. tympan/o/centesis _____

Correct Answers _____ × 10 = _____% Score

PATHOLOGICAL CONDITIONS

Disorders of the Ear

PATHOLOGICAL CONDITION	DESCRIPTION
anacusis *ăn-ă-KŪ-sĭs* *an=without, not* *acusis=hearing*	Total deafness.
acoustic neuroma *ă-KOOS-tĭk nū-RŌ-mă* *acous=hearing* *tic=pertaining to*	Benign tumor of the 8th cranial nerve (vestibulocochlear nerve) in the brain. Tinnitus, vertigo, and impaired hearing are the initial symptoms.
cholesteatoma *kō-lē-stē-ă-TŌ-mă* *chole=bile, gall* *steat=fat* *oma=tumor*	Cystlike sac containing epithelial cells and cholesterol in the middle ear and mastoid area. Occurs as a congenital defect or as a result of chronic otitis media. If not removed or drained, conductive hearing loss and erosion of the middle ear may result.
hearing loss	The most common disability in the United States, it ranges from difficulty understanding words or hearing sounds to total deafness. Various types of hearing losses and their causes are illustrated in Figure 17–8.
conductive *kŏn-DŬK-tĭv*	Hearing loss caused by a breakdown in the transmission of sound waves through the external ear and the middle ear. (See Fig. 17–8*A* and *B.*)
presbycusis *prĕz-bĭ-KŪ-sĭs* *presby=old age* *cusis=hearing*	Normal loss of hearing acuity associated with aging.
sensorineural *sĕn-sō-rē-NŪ-răl*	Hearing loss caused by disease or trauma to the sensory or neural components of the inner ear. (See Fig. 17–8*C.*). Sensory hearing loss originates in the cochlea and involves the hair cells and nerve endings. Neural hearing loss originates in the nerve or brain stem. Also known as *noise-induced hearing loss* (NIHL).
labyrinthitis *lăb-ĭ-rĭn-THĪ-tĭs* *labyrinth=labyrinth, inner ear* *itis=inflammation*	Inflammation of the inner ear that may be viral or bacterial in nature. The primary symptom is vertigo with altered balance, fever, and nausea or vomiting.

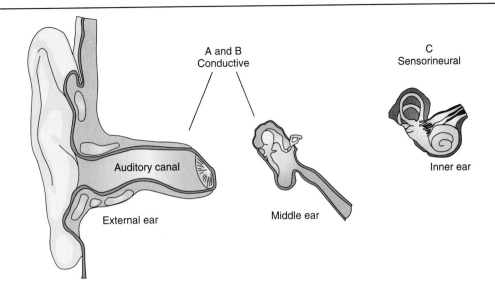

A and B
Conductive

C
Sensorineural

Auditory canal

Inner ear

External ear

Middle ear

A. External Ear
   impacted cerumen
   foreign body
   external otitis
   perforated eardrum

B. Middle Ear
   otitis media
   dislocation of
      ossicles
   otosclerosis

C. Inner Ear
   noise trauma
   drug toxicity
   presbycusis
   congenital defect
   syphilis
   Ménière disease

Figure 17–8 *Types of hearing losses and their causes. (From Williams, LS, and Hopper, PD: Understanding Medical Surgical Nursing. FA Davis, Philadelphia 1999, p 1059, with permission.)*

Disorders of the Ear (Continued)

PATHOLOGICAL CONDITION	DESCRIPTION
mastoiditis *măs-toyd-Ī-tĭs* *mastoid=mastoid* *itis=inflammation*	Infection of the mastoid area that usually results from the spreading of a middle ear infection. Symptoms include throbbing pain, tenderness and swelling over the mastoid process, and possible fever and tinnitus.
Ménière disease *măn-ē-ĀRZ dĭ-ZĒZ*	Chronic inner ear disease in which there is an overaccumulation of fluid in the labyrinth. Recurrent episodes of vertigo, tinnitus, and ear pressure with progressive hearing loss occur. Initially one ear is involved; however, over time both may become affected. Etiology is unknown.
otitis externa *ō-TĪ-tĭs ĕks-TĔR-nă* *ot=ear* *itis=inflammation*	Infection of the external auditory canal from the growth of bacteria or fungi. Swimming, humid climates, and other factors leading to maceration (softening by water) of the external canal skin, predisposes one to these infections. Also known as *"swimmer's ear."*
otitis media *ō-TĪ-tĭs MĒ-dē-ă* *ot=ear* *itis=inflammation*	Infection or inflammation of the middle ear. There are two types, serous and suppurative.

Disorders of the Ear (Continued)

PATHOLOGICAL CONDITION	DESCRIPTION
serous sē-rŭs *ser=serum* *ous=pertaining to*	Noninfectious inflammation of the middle ear with accumulation of serum (clear fluid). Treatment may include myringotomy to aspirate fluid and the surgical insertion of tubes in the eardrum to allow ventilation of the middle ear.
suppurative SŬP-ū-rā-tĭv	Inflammation of the middle ear with pus formation. This is a common affliction in infants and young children due to the horizontal orientation and the small diameter of the eustachian tube, which predisposes them to infection. It is often preceded by an upper respiratory infection and is usually bacterial in nature. Symptoms include otalgia, fever, a sense of fullness in the ear, and diminished hearing. Initial treatment consists of antibiotic therapy and analgesics. If no improvement is shown after 48 hours, myringotomy to drain the abscess is performed. If left untreated, complications include rupture of the eardrum, mastoiditis, labyrinthitis, hearing loss, meningitis, and brain abscess.
otosclerosis ō-tō-sklĕ-RŌ-sĭs *oto=ear* *scler=hardening, sclera* *osis=abnormal condition*	Hereditary disorder of bone metabolism where abnormal bone develops at the anterior end of the oval window, resulting in fixation of the stapes and a conductive hearing loss. A recent technique has been developed to treat this disorder. A small opening (*fenestra*) is created in the footplate with a laser and a Teflon piston prosthesis is inserted to restore normal hearing. A *stapedectomy* (Fig. 17–9) is performed to treat otosclerosis.
tinnitus tĭn-Ī-tŭs	Subjective, chronic ringing or other distressing noise in the ears or head. The cause may be unknown or related to other medical problems such as acoustic trauma, Ménière disease, otosclerosis, presbycusis, labyrinthitis, high blood pressure, or an underactive thyroid.
tympanic membrane perforation tĭm-PĂN-ĭk MĔM-brăn pĕr-fō-RĀ-shŭn	Rupture of the eardrum caused by severe middle ear infection, direct trauma, or increased environmental pressure or barotrauma, as with deep sea diving.
vertigo VĔR-tĭ-gō	Sensation of spinning of oneself or of external objects spinning around oneself; balance and equilibrium are affected and nausea is often present. Causes usually stem from an abnormality in the labyrinth or inner ear.

Disorders of the Nose, Throat, and Associated Structures

PATHOLOGICAL CONDITION	DESCRIPTION
allergic rhinitis ă-LĔR-jĭk rī-NĪ-tĭs *rhin=nose* *itis=inflammation*	Inflammation of the mucous membranes of the nose caused by inhaled allergens. Symptoms include sneezing, rhinorrhea, nasal pruritus, congestion, and ophthalmorrhea.
anosmia ăn-ŎZ-mē-ă *an=without, not* *osmia=smell*	Loss of the sense of smell; the ability to taste food and liquids is also impaired or lost.
coryza kŏ-RĪ-ză	Inflammation of the nasal mucous membranes; synonymous with *rhinitis* and *head cold*.

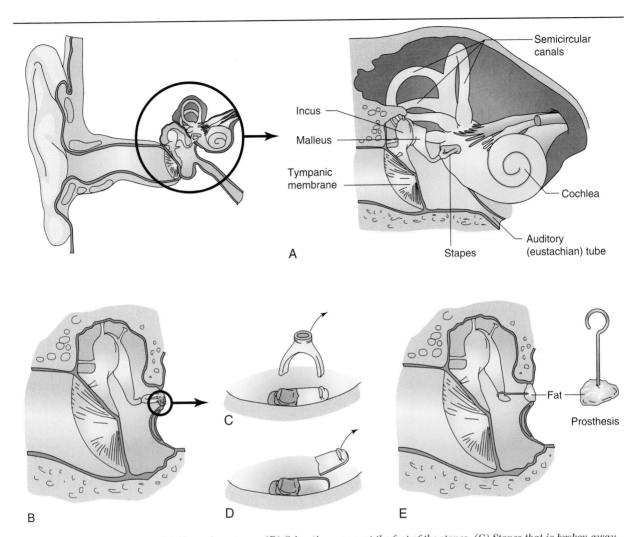

Figure 17–9 *Stapedectomy. (A) Normal anatomy. (B) Sclerotic process at the foot of the stapes. (C) Stapes that is broken away surgically. (D) The footplate is removed. (E) The prosthesis is implanted. (From Williams, LS, and Hopper, PD: Understanding Medical Surgical Nursing. FA Davis, Philadelphia 1999, p 1069, with permission.)*

Disorders of the Nose, Throat, and Associated Structures (Continued)

PATHOLOGICAL CONDITION	DESCRIPTION
croup, acute laryngotracheo-bronchitis KROOP, ă-KŪT lăr-ĭn-gō-trā-kē-ō-brŏng-KĪ-tĭs *laryngo=larynx* *tracheo=trachea* *bronch=bronchus* *itis=inflammation*	Acute respiratory syndrome of childhood characterized by a barking cough, suffocative and difficult breathing, stridor, and laryngeal spasm. This condition results from obstruction of the larynx caused by an allergen, infection, or foreign body.
deviated septum DĒ-vē-ā-tĕd SĔP-tŭm	A shift of the nasal septum away from the midline; may be either traumatic or congenital. This condition is asymptomatic unless the deviation is severe enough to cause obstruction of air through the nasal passages. The condition can be corrected with rhinoplasty.

Disorders of the Nose, Throat, and Associated Structures (Continued)

PATHOLOGICAL CONDITION	DESCRIPTION
diphtheria dĭf-THĒ-rē-ă	Acute, contagious infection marked by the formation of a pseudomembrane in the pharynx and respiratory tract. Injecting infants with the DPT (diphtheria, pertussis, tetanus) vaccine provides immunity to these diseases.
epiglottitis (acute) ĕp-ĭ-glŏt-Ī-tĭs *epi=above, upon* *glott=glottis* *itis=inflammation*	Severe, life-threatening infection of the epiglottis and surrounding area that occurs most often in children between 2 and 12 years of age. Symptoms include fever, inspiratory stridor, respiratory distress, and dysphagia. Intubation or tracheostomy may be required to open the airway.
epistaxis ĕp-ĭ-STĂK-sĭs	Nasal hemorrhage; nosebleed. This condition results from traumatic or spontaneous rupture of blood vessels in the nasal mucosa.
influenza ĭn-floo-ĔN-ză	Acute, contagious respiratory infection characterized by the sudden onset of fever, chills, headache, and myalgia; a self-limited disease that usually lasts 2 to 7 days.
laryngitis lăr-ĭn-JĪ-tĭs *laryng=larynx* *itis=inflammation*	Inflammation of the mucous membranes lining the larynx and edema of the vocal cord with resulting hoarseness (dysphonia) or loss of voice (aphonia), cough, and dysphagia. Causes include excessive use of the voice, exposure to irritating fumes or other environmental irritants, and viral or bacterial respiratory infection.
nasal polyposis NĀ-zl pŏl-ē-PŌ-sĭs *nas=nose* *al=pertaining to* *polyp=small growth* *osis=abnormal condition*	Condition of multiple polyps (tumor on a stalk) in the nose.
peritonsillar abscess pĕr-ĭ-TŎN-sĭ-lăr ĂB-sĕs *peri=around* *tonsill=tonsils* *ar=pertaining to*	An infection of tissue between the tonsil and the pharynx, usually associated with tonsillitis. Symptoms include difficulty swallowing (dysphagia), fever, and pain radiating to the ear. Treatment includes antibiotics, incision and drainage (I&D) of the abscess, and sometimes tonsillectomy.
pertussis pĕr-TŬS-ĭs	Acute bacterial infection characterized by a "whoop"-sounding cough that affects the pharynx, larynx, and trachea. Injecting infants with the DPT vaccine provides immunity to these diseases. Pertussis is also called *whooping cough*.
sinusitis sī-nŭs-Ī-tĭs *sinus=sinus* *itis=inflammation*	Inflammation of one or more paranasal sinuses caused by a virus, bacteria, or allergy. Predisposing factors include inadequate drainage that may be a result of the presence of polyps, enlarged turbinates, a deviated septum, or chronic rhinitis.

Disorders of the Nose, the Throat, and Associated Structures (Continued)

PATHOLOGICAL CONDITION	DESCRIPTION
sleep apnea *slēp ăp-NĒ-ă* *a=without, no* *pnea=breathing*	Intermittent short period of cessation of breathing (apnea) followed by snorting and gasping during sleep. This condition occurs more frequently in males and may be associated with airway obstruction, obesity, and hypertension. The condition may be treated with uvulectomy, uvulopalatopharyngoplasty, or continuous positive airway pressure (CPAP).
thrush *thrŭsh*	Yeast infection caused by *Candida albicans.* A whitish coating in the oral cavity is present; commonly seen in immunocompromised patients.
tonsillitis *tŏn-sĭl-Ī-tĭs* *tonsill=tonsil* *itis=inflammation*	Infection or inflammation of a tonsil Acute tonsillitis, frequently caused by *Streptococcus*, is characterized by fever, sore throat, headache, malaise, dysphagia, and enlarged, tender lymph nodes in the neck. Treatment includes antibiotics and analgesics. In cases of recurrent tonsillitis, a tonsillectomy is performed.
tracheoesophageal fistula *trā-kē-ō-ē-sŏf-ă-JĒ-ăl FĬS-tū-lă* *tracheo=trachea* *esophag=esophagus* *eal=pertaining to*	Congenital defect in which there is an abnormal tubelike passage between the trachea and esophagus resulting in the passage of food from the esophagus into the respiratory tract.
upper respiratory infection (URI)	Almost any infectious disease process involving the nasal passages, pharynx, and bronchi. Etiologic agent may be viral or bacterial.

Activity 17-7: Clinical Application
Pathological Conditions

anosmia
conductive
croup
deviated septum
epistaxis
influenza
labyrinthitis
Ménière disease
nasal polyposis
otitis externa

pertussis
presbycusis
sensorineural
serous
sinusitis
suppurative
thrush
tinnitus
tonsillitis
vertigo

Match the terms listed above with the definitions given in the numbered list:

1. _____ inflammation of the inner ear with a primary symptom of vertigo and altered balance, fever, and nausea or vomiting.

2. _____ normal loss of hearing acuity associated with aging.

3. _____ a type of hearing loss caused by the breakdown in the transmission of sound waves through the external and middle ear.

4. _____ the type of otitis media that presents with an accumulation of serum in the middle ear.

5. _____ nosebleed or nasal hemorrhage.

6. _____ inflammation of the tonsil(s).

7. _____ loss of the sense of smell.

8. _____ chronic inner ear disease characterized by an overaccumulation of fluid in the labyrinth that results in progressive hearing loss.

9. _____ inflammation of one or more of the paranasal sinuses.

10. _____ a type of hearing loss caused by a malfunction in the neural or sensory components of the inner ear.

11. _____ acute, contagious respiratory infection with fever, headache, and myalgia that usually lasts no longer than a week.

12. _____ yeast infection of the oral cavity caused by _Candida albicans._

13. _____ a shift of the nasal septum away from the midline.

14. _____ the type of otitis media that presents with pus in the middle ear.

15. _____ also known as whooping cough.

16. _____ condition of multiple polyps in the nose.

17. _____ acute respiratory syndrome of childhood characterized by a barking cough, dyspnea, stridor, and laryngeal spasm that results from obstruction of the larynx.

18. _____ infection of the external auditory canal known as "swimmer's ear."

19. _____ chronic ringing or other distressing noise in either one or both ears.

20. _____ sensation of spinning or of the environment spinning around one's self.

Correct Answers _____ × 5 = _____ % Score

DIAGNOSTIC PROCEDURES AND TESTS
Clinical Procedures

PROCEDURE	DESCRIPTION
audiometry _aw-dē-ŎM-ĕ-trē_ _audio=hearing_ _metry=act of measuring_	Test that measures hearing acuity of various sound frequencies. An instrument called an _audiometer_ delivers acoustic stimuli at different frequencies and the results are plotted on a graph called an _audiogram._

Clinical Procedures (Continued)

PROCEDURE	DESCRIPTION
laryngoscopy *lăr-ĭn-GŎS-kō-pē* *laryngo=larynx (voice box)* *scopy=visual examination*	Visual examination of the interior of the larynx to diagnose abnormalities of the vocal cords and surrounding structures.
nasopharyngoscopy *nā-zō-făr-ĭn-GŎS-kō-pē* *naso=nose* *pharyngo=pharynx (throat)* *scopy=visual examination*	Visual examination of the nasal cavity and pharynx using a flexible endoscope to diagnose structural abnormalities.
otoscopy *ō-TŎS-kō-pē* *oto=ear* *scopy=visual examination*	Visual examination of the external auditory canal and the tympanic membrane using an otoscope (Fig. 17–10).

pneumatic
   nū-MĂT-ĭk
   pneum=air, lung
   tic=pertaining to
	Procedure that assesses the ability of the tympanic membrane to move in response to a change in air pressure.
	
	By increasing and decreasing the pressure, the healthy tympanic membrane moves in and out. Lack of movement indicates either increased impedance or eardrum perforation.

polysomnography *pŏl-ē-sŏm-NŎG-rō-fē* *poly=many, much* *somno=sleep* *graphy=process of recording*	Continuous measurement and recording of physiological activity during sleep. This is the recommended test to determine a sleep apnea diagnosis.
rapid group A strep test	Immunologic test performed on a throat culture swab to detect the presence of group A streptococci in the throat.

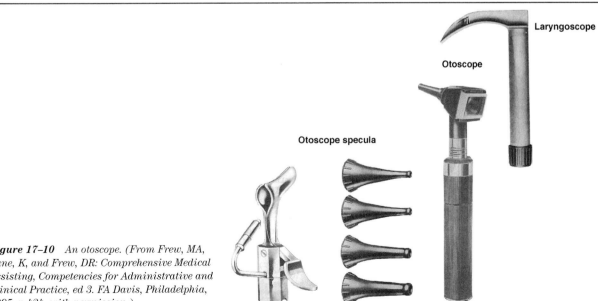

Figure 17–10 An otoscope. (From Frew, MA, Lane, K, and Frew, DR: Comprehensive Medical Assisting, Competencies for Administrative and Clinical Practice, ed 3. FA Davis, Philadelphia, 1995, p 424, with permission.)

Clinical Procedures (Continued)

PROCEDURE	DESCRIPTION
rhinoscopy *rī-NŎS-kō-pē* *rhino=nose* *scopy=visual examination*	Examination of the nasal passages using a rhinoscope.
Rinne test *RĬN-nē tĕst*	Hearing acuity test that is performed with a vibrating tuning fork placed on the mastoid process (Fig. 17–11A) and then in front of the external auditory canal to test bone and air conduction (see Fig. 17–11B). **This test is useful for differentiating between conductive and sensorineural hearing loss.**
throat culture	Test used to determine the presence of pathogenic bacteria, such as streptococci in the throat.
tympanometry *tĭm-pă-NŎM-ĕ-trē* *tympano=tympanic* *membrane, eardrum* *metry=act of measuring*	Test that measures the compliance of the tympanic membrane and differentiates problems in the middle ear. **Varying amounts of pressure are applied to the eardrum and the results are recorded on a graph called a *tympanogram*.**

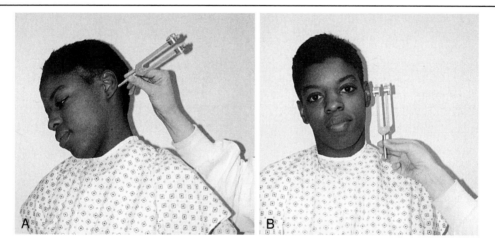

Figure 17–11 *Rinne test. (From Williams, LS, and Hopper, PD: Understanding Medical Surgical Nursing. FA Davis, Philadelphia, 1999, p 1034, with permission.)*

Clinical Procedures (Continued)

PROCEDURE	DESCRIPTION
Weber test WĔB-ĕr tĕst	Hearing acuity test that is performed with a vibrating tuning fork placed on the center of the forehead. This test compares bone conduction in the two ears and evaluates whether hearing is the same in both ears (Fig. 17–12).

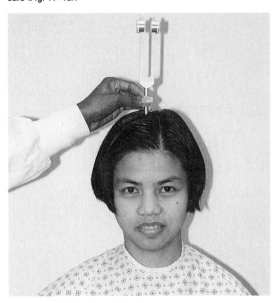

Figure 17–12 Weber test. (From Williams, LS, and Hopper, PD: Understanding Medical Surgical Nursing. FA Davis, Philadelphia, 1999, p 1035, with permission.)

SURGICAL AND THERAPEUTIC PROCEDURES

Surgical Procedures

PROCEDURE	DESCRIPTION
laryngectomy lăr-ĭn-JĔK-tō-mē *laryng=larynx* *ectomy=excision, removal*	Excision of the larynx. This procedure is performed to treat cancer of the larynx. The patient is referred to a speech pathologist before surgery to discuss esophageal speech and prostheses. A partial laryngectomy consists only of vocal cord removal.
myringotomy, tympanotomy mĭr-ĭn-GŎT-ō-mē, tĭm-păn-ŎT-ō-mē *myringo=tympanic membrane, eardrum* *tympano=tympanic membrane, eardrum* *tomy=incision*	Incision of the eardrum to relieve pressure and release pus or serous fluid from the middle ear, or to surgically insert tympanostomy tubes in the eardrum. These small tubes provide ventilation and drainage of the middle ear when repeated ear infections do not respond to antibiotic treatment and are also used when persistent severely negative middle ear pressure is present.

Surgical Procedures (Continued)

PROCEDURE	DESCRIPTION
myringoplasty, tympanoplasty mĭr-ĬN-gō-plăs-tē, tĭm-păn-ō-PLĂS-tē *myringo=tympanic membrane, eardrum* *tympano=tympanic membrane, eardrum* *plasty=surgical repair*	Surgical repair of a perforated eardrum with a tissue graft, performed to correct hearing loss.
otoplasty Ō-tō-plăs-tē *oto=ear* *plasty=surgical repair*	Reconstructive plastic surgery during which some of the cartilage in the ears is removed to bring the auricle closer to the head. This procedure is done for cosmetic purposes.
rhinoplasty RĪ-nō-plăs-tē *rhino=nose* *plasty=surgical repair*	Plastic surgery of the nose to correct a deviated septum or for cosmetic purposes.
stapedectomy stā-pē-DĔK-tō-mē	Excision of the stapes to improve hearing. This surgery is performed to correct otosclerosis. The stapes is removed and replaced with a prosthesis. (See Fig. 17–9.)
tonsillectomy and adenoidectomy (T&A) tŏn-sĭl-ĔK-tō-mē, ăd-ĕ-noyd-ĔK-tō-mē *tonsill=tonsils* *ectomy=excision, removal* *adenoid=adenoid* *ectomy=excision, removal*	Surgical removal of the tonsils and adenoids, usually performed because of chronic infection or inflammation.
uvulectomy ū-vū-LĔK-tō-mē *uvul=uvula* *ectomy=excision, removal*	Surgical removal of the uvula to improve symptoms of snoring (see Fig. 17–4, No. 11).
uvulopalatopharyngo-plasty (UPPP) ū-vū-lō-păl-ă-tō-făr-ĬN-gō-plăs-tē *uvulo=uvula* *palato=palate (roof of the mouth)* *pharyngo=pharynx* *plasty=surgical repair*	Operation to improve certain sleep disorders and relieve symptoms such as obstructive sleep apnea and snoring.

Therapeutic Procedures

PROCEDURE	DESCRIPTION
continuous positive airway pressure (CPAP) SĒ-păp	A method of noninvasive ventilation assisted by a flow of air delivered at a constant pressure throughout the respiratory cycle. This procedure is performed for patients who can initiate their own respirations but who are not able to maintain adequate arterial oxygen levels without assistance. CPAP may be given through a ventilator and endotracheal tube, through a nasal cannula, or into a hood over the patient's head. Severe sleep apnea and respiratory distress syndrome in the newborn are often treated with CPAP.
ear lavage ēr lă-VĂZH	Irrigation of the external auditory canal, commonly performed to remove excessive cerumen buildup or to remove a foreign object.
hearing aid	A small device that amplifies sound to provide more precise perception and interpretation of words communicated to the individual with a hearing loss. The device is designed to be worn behind or inside of the ear (Fig. 17–13).

PHARMACOLOGY

DRUG CLASSIFICATION	THERAPEUTIC ACTION
antibiotics ăn-tĭ-bī-ŎT-ĭks *anti=against* *bio=life* *tic=pertaining to*	Substances that inhibit the growth of microorganisms; various classes include those effective against *gram-negative* and *gram-positive* bacteria that infect the ears, nose, and throat.
antiemetics ăn-tĭ-ē-MĔT-ĭks	Agents that control nausea and vomiting related to vertigo and motion sickness by reducing the sensitivity of the inner ear to motion or by inhibiting the increased inner ear stimuli from reaching the center in the brain that triggers vomiting.

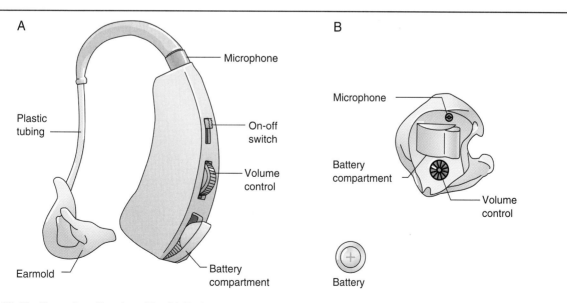

Figure 17–13 *Examples of hearing aids. (A) Behind-the-ear hearing aid. (B) In-the-ear hearing aid. (From Williams, LS, and Hopper, PD: Understanding Medical Surgical Nursing. FA Davis, Philadelphia, 1999, p 1061, with permission.)*

PHARMACOLOGY (Continued)

DRUG CLASSIFICATION	THERAPEUTIC ACTION
antifungals *ăn-tĭ-FŬNG-găls*	Agents that are effective against yeast infections caused by *Candida albicans* that occur in the oral cavity and pharynx.
antihistamines *ăn-tĭ-HĬS-tă-mēnz*	Drugs that block histamine (H_1) receptors in the nose and throat and dry up secretions, decrease itching, and reduce swelling of edematous mucous membranes. Histamine is released by the antibody–antigen complex that occurs during allergic reactions.
corticosteroids *kor-tĭ-kō-STĒR-oydz*	Substances that decrease the body's inflammatory response and is administered intranasally to treat nonallergic rhinitis and nasal polyps.
decongestants *dē-kŏn-JĔST-ănts*	Agents that decrease swelling of mucous membranes, alleviate nasal stuffiness, allow secretions to drain, and help to unclog the eustachian tubes. These drugs are often combined with an antihistamine and are commonly prescribed for allergies and colds. These can be administered in drop, spray, or tablet form.
mydriatics *mĭ-drī-ĂT-ĭks*	Drugs that dilate the pupil and paralyze the muscles of accommodation (cycloplegia) of the iris; used to prepare the eye for internal examination and to treat inflammatory conditions of the iris.

❖ ABBREVIATIONS

ABBREVIATION	MEANING	ABBREVIATION	MEANING
AC	air conduction	**ET**	endotracheal
AD	right ear (*auris dextra*)	**ETF**	eustachian tube function
ARD	acute respiratory disease	**HD**	hemodialysis, hip disarticulation, hearing distance
AS	aortic stenosis; left ear (*auris sinistra*)	**NIHL**	noise-induced hearing loss
AU	both ears (*aures unitas*)	**PE tube**	polyethylene ventilating tube (placed in the eardrum)
BC	bone conduction		
CPAP	continuous positive airway pressure	**T&A**	tonsillectomy and adenoidectomy
DPT	diphtheria, pertussis, tetanus (vaccine)	**UPPP**	uvulopalatopharyngoplasty
ENT	ear, nose, and throat	**URI**	upper respiratory infection

Activity 17–8: Clinical Application
Diagnostic Tests and Treatments

antiemetic	rhinoplasty
decongestant	Rinne test
ear lavage	stapedectomy
hearing aid	tonsillectomy and adenoidectomy (T&A)
myringotomy	uvulopalatopharyngoplasty (UPPP)
polysomnography	Weber test

Match the terms listed above with the definitions given in the numbered list:

1. _____ a drug that controls nausea and vomiting related to vertigo and motion sickness.

2. _____ test in which a vibrating tuning fork is placed on the center of the forehead to compare bone conduction in both ears, and to evaluate whether hearing is the same in both ears.

3. _____ small device to amplify sound and aid individuals with hearing loss.

4. _____ test in which a vibrating tuning fork is placed on the mastoid process, and then in front of the ear to test bone and air conduction, and is useful in differentiating between conductive and sensorineural hearing loss.

5. _____ a drug that decreases swelling of mucous membranes, alleviates nasal stuffiness, and allows drainage of secretions.

6. _____ irrigation of the external auditory canal to remove a foreign object or cerumen buildup.

7. _____ surgical procedure performed to correct otosclerosis.

8. _____ operation to improve obstructive sleep apnea and snoring.

9. _____ plastic surgery of the nose to correct a deviated septum or for cosmetic purposes.

10. _____ surgical removal of the tonsils and adenoids.

Correct Answers _____ × 10 = _____% **Score**

Activity 17-9: Build Medical Words
Diagnostic, Symptomatic, and Surgical Terms

Use *tympan/o* (tympanic membrane, eardrum) to build words meaning:

1. surgical repair of the tympanic membrane _____

2. condition of tympanic membrane hardening _____

Use *ot/o* (ear) to build words meaning:

3. pain in the ear _____

4. surgical repair of the ear _____

Use *audi/o* (hearing) to build words meaning:

5. instrument for measuring hearing _____

6. a writing or record of hearing _____

Use *laryng/o* (larynx) to build words meaning:

7. narrowing of the larynx _____

8. inflammation of the larynx and trachea _____

Use *sinus/o* (sinus cavity) to build words meaning:

9. inflammation of a sinus _____

10. resembling a sinus _____

Use *labyrinth/o* (labyrinth, inner ear) to build words meaning:

11. inflammation of the labyrinth _____

12. incision of the labyrinth _____

Use *rhin/o* (nose) to build words meaning:

13. discharge, or flow, from the nose _____

14. any disease of the nose _____

Use the suffix *-scopy* (visual examination) to build a word meaning:

15. visual examination of the ears _____

Correct Answers _____ × 6.67 = _____ % Score

Medical Records

Authentic reports of a SOAP note and operative reports are included in this section.

The following reading and dictionary exercise and the medical record analysis will help you develop skills to abstract information and master the terminology in the reports. Accurate interpretation is important because this type of information is used in numerous areas of the medical practice, such as in initiating treatments, evaluating patients' progress, and completing insurance claims.

Reading and Dictionary Exercise

Place a check mark [✓] after you complete the exercise.

[   ] **1.** Underline the following words in the reports as you read the SOAP note and the operative reports aloud. These medical reports can be found at the end of the chapter.

[   ] **2.** Use a medical dictionary and Appendix F, Part 2 to complete this exercise.

> *Note: You are not expected to fully understand all the parts of the medical records. The important aspect of this exercise is to use all available resources to complete it. Eventually you will master the terminology and format of these reports.*

>>> MEDICAL RECORD 17-1: SOAP NOTE

Term	Pronunciation	Meaning
sinusitis	sī-nŭs-Ī-tĭs	_____
maxillary	MĂK-sĭ-lĕr-ē	_____
nonpurulent	nŏn-PŪR-ū-lĕnt	_____
erythematous	ĕr-ĭ-THĔM-ă-tŭs	_____
nasal	NĀ-zl	_____
mucosa	mū-KŌ-să	_____
tympanic membranes	tĭm-PĂN-ĭk MĔM-brānz	_____
benign	bē-NĪN	_____
oropharynx	or-ō-FĂR-ĭnks	_____
exudates	ĔKS-ū-dāts	_____
supple	SŬ-pĕl	_____
lymphadenopathy	lĭm-făd-ĕ-NŎP-ă-thē	_____
auscultation	aws-kŭl-TĀ-shŭn	_____
bilaterally	bī-LĂT-ĕr-ăl-ē	_____

amoxicillin	*ă-mŏks-ĭ-SĬL-ĭn*	_____
penicillin	*pĕn-ĕ-SĬL-ĭn*	_____
Nasonex	*NĀ-zō-nĕks*	_____
Relafen	*RĔL-ă-fĕn*	_____
Naprosyn	*NĂP-rō-sĭn*	_____

>>> MEDICAL RECORD 17–2: OPERATIVE REPORT

Term	Pronunciation	Meaning
otitis media	*ō-TĪ-tĭs MĒ-dē-ă*	_____
effusion	*ĕ-FŪ-zhŭn*	_____
subacute	*sŭb-ă-KŪT*	_____
bilateral	*bī-LĂT-ĕr-ăl*	_____
myringotomy	*mĭr-ĭn-GŎT-ō-mē*	_____
fluoroplastic bobbin tubes	*floor-ō-PLĂS-tĭk BŎB-ĭn tūbz*	_____
mucus	*MŪ-kŭs*	_____
aerobes	*ĔR-ōbz*	_____
anaerobes	*ĂN-ĕr-ōbz*	_____
polypoid	*PŎL-ē-poyd*	_____
Vasocidin	*vā-sō-SĬ-dĭn*	_____

>>> MEDICAL RECORD 17–3: OPERATIVE REPORT

Term	Pronunciation	Meaning
adenotonsillitis	*ăd-ĕ-nō-tŏn-sĭl-Ī-tĭs*	_____
oral	*OR-ăl*	_____
endotracheal	*ĕn-dō-TRĀ-kē-ăl*	_____
Marcaine	*MĂR-kān*	_____
tonsillar fossae	*TŎN-sĭl-ăr FŎS-ā*	_____
catheter	*KĂTH-ĕ-tĕr*	_____
adenoid	*ĂD-ĕ-noyd*	_____
curet	*kū-RĔT*	_____

dissection	*dĭ-SĔK-shŭn*	_____
cauterized	*KAW-tĕr-īzd*	_____
hemostasis	*hē-MŎS-tă-sĭs*	_____
amoxicillin	*ă-mŏks-ĭ-SĬL-ĭn*	_____
hydrocodone	*hī-drō-KŌ-dōn*	_____

Critical Thinking: Analysis of Medical Records

This section provides experience in abstracting and analyzing information from medical records. At the same time, it reinforces the material presented in this chapter.

>>> MEDICAL RECORD 17–1: SOAP NOTE

1. What objective findings led to the diagnosis of sinusitis?

_____

2. What are the possible causes of this patient's sinusitis?

_____

>>> MEDICAL RECORD 17–2: OPERATIVE REPORT

3. Why was the surgery performed?

_____

_____

4. What surgical procedure was performed on the patient?

_____

5. What type of residue was cleaned from the left ear?

_____

6. What tests were done on the mucus cultures?

_____

7. State and describe the changes seen in the middle ear spaces.

_____

_____

8. What instrument was used to keep the oral cavity open and the tongue retracted during surgery?

_____

9. How was the bleeding controlled during surgery?

_____

_____

10. Did the patient lose any blood during the surgery? If so, what was the estimated blood loss?

_____

 Audio Practice

Listen to the audio CD-ROM to practice the pronunciation of selected medical terms from this chapter.

Medical Record 17–1. SOAP Note

GENERAL HOSPITAL AND MEDICAL CENTER
2211 Fifth Avenue North • Healthy City, USA 12345 • (321) 123-4567

SOAP Note

Patient Name: Jillian Edwards
Age: 33 yrs.

Patient Number: 02-32-53
Room Number: Clinic

DATE OF VISIT: February 26, 20xx

SUBJECTIVE:
She has a history of recurrent sinusitis. She presents with two weeks of upper respiratory symptoms. She has had increasing maxillary headache with throbbing discomfort that occasionally radiates into her teeth. She has had no fevers but occasionally feels chilled. Her drainage is mucous and nonpurulent in appearance. She has a dry cough, scratchy throat, and some watery eyes. No new allergen exposures. She says the worst part is the maxillary headache.

OBJECTIVE:
Physical exam shows her to be well developed, well nourished, and in no acute distress. She has moderate maxillary sinus tenderness with erythematous nasal mucosa. The tympanic membranes are benign. Oropharynx shows slight erythema, but there are no exudates or enlargement of the tonsils. The neck is supple without lymphadenopathy. The lungs are clear to auscultation bilaterally.

ASSESSMENT:
Sinusitis.

PLAN:
She says amoxicillin has worked the best for her in the past. She actually would prefer plain penicillin if that would work better. We will start her on amoxicillin 500 mg three times a day. I have given her prescription for Nasonex and sample, two sprays each nostril once a day and given her 9 days of Relafen samples, 1000 mg once a day. She was offered Naprosyn but says this never works for her aches and pains. Additionally, she was counseled that her blood pressure is mildly elevated today at 140/70. She will have this rechecked in 2 weeks after improving from her sinus infection. She will follow up, if not improving in 2-3 days, and not better in 7-10 days.

_____
Robert Scottsdale, M.D.

RS/dw
d&t: 02/26/xx

Medical Record 17–2. Operative Report

GENERAL HOSPITAL AND MEDICAL CENTER
2211 Fifth Avenue North • Healthy City, USA 12345 • (321) 123-4567

Operative Report

Patient Name: Jana Moraldo   **Patient Number:** 11-11-88
Age: 3 yrs.   **Room Number:** OP

DATE OF OPERATION: 06/01/xx

PREOPERATIVE DIAGNOSIS: Chronic otitis media with effusions.

POSTOPERATIVE DIAGNOSIS: Chronic otitis media with effusions. Possible subacute infection, left worse than right.

OPERATION: Bilateral myringotomy and placement of fluoroplastic bobbin tubes.

SURGEON: Mark David, M.D.

ANESTHESIA: General mask inhalation.

INDICATIONS: Recurrent ear infections with persistent fluid despite prolonged appropriate medical management.

PROCEDURE: The patient was brought to the operating room and placed under general anesthesia with mask inhalation technique. The ear canals were cleaned of dry wax and crust, particularly on the left side. Anterior inferior myringotomies were placed bilaterally. On the left side, the mucus seemed to be under some pressure, and cultures were taken for aerobes and anaerobes. Fluoroplastic bobbin tubes were placed in the myringotomy sites bilaterally. It was noted that there were some polypoid changes in the middle ear spaces. Vasocidin drops and cotton balls were placed in the ear canal. The patient tolerated the procedure well and was awakened and taken to the recovery room in satisfactory condition, having had no complications at the end of the surgical procedure.

The plans will be for discharge home as an outpatient, and 7 days of Vasocidin drops, and to return to my office in 2-3 weeks for follow up. I will see Jana back in 6-month intervals until the tubes extrude and the eardrums are healed and hearing checked.

_____

Mark David, M.D.

MD/uml
D&T: 06/02/xx

Medical Record 17–3. Operative Report

GENERAL HOSPITAL AND MEDICAL CENTER
2211 Fifth Avenue North • Healthy City, USA 12345 • (321) 123-4567

Operative Report

Patient Name: John Jackson

Age: 13 yrs.

Patient Number: 01-03-44

Room Number: 520-1

DATE OF OPERATION: 11/16/xx

PREOPERATIVE DIAGNOSIS: Chronic recurrent adenotonsillitis.

POSTOPERATIVE DIAGNOSIS: Chronic recurrent adenotonsillitis.

SURGEON: Mark David, M.D.

ANESTHESIA: General with oral endotracheal tube supplemented with 4.5 cc of 0.5% Marcaine plain placed at the end of the case into the tonsillar fossae.

INDICATIONS: Recurrent adenotonsillitis despite prolonged appropriate medical management.

PROCEDURE: The patient was brought to the operating room and placed under general anesthesia with an oral endotracheal tube. The table was turned 90 degrees, and the patient was monitored, and IV had been started. The hemi-Crowe-Davis mouth gag was used for anterior tongue retraction, and the palate was retracted with the red rubber catheter. The adenoid pad was removed by a combination of adenoid curet and adenoid punch. The tonsils were moderately enlarged and removed by a combination of sharp and blunt dissection with wire snare of the inferior pole. Prominent bleeding sites were cauterized for hemostasis, and tonsil sponges were used as well. Estimated blood loss was 40 to 50 cc. Then 4.5 cc of 0.5% Marcaine plain was infiltrated into the tonsillar fossae. The patient was awakened and taken to the recovery room in satisfactory condition, having had no complications at the end of the surgical procedure.

The plans will be for short stay observation, discharge home, on amoxicillin suspension and cough syrup with hydrocodone. To return to my office in 2–3 weeks for a follow up visit. Postoperative instructions were given to the mother.

_____

Mark David, M.D.

MD/jrs

D&T: 11/16/xx

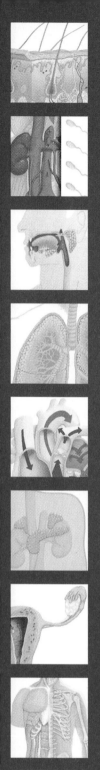

chapter

18 Radiology and Nuclear Medicine

Chapter Outline

Objectives

Upon completion of this chapter, you will be able to:

- Differentiate among the radiologist, nuclear physician, and radiation oncologist.
- Explain the role and importance of other health-care practitioners who assist the radiologist in the administration of diagnostic radiographic procedures.
- Differentiate between radiologic diagnostic imaging procedures and therapeutic procedures to treat cancer patients.
- Recognize diagnostic and therapeutic procedures used by radiologists and radiation oncologists.
- Recognize, pronounce, and spell correctly terms related to the field of radiology and nuclear medicine.
- Demonstrate your knowledge of this chapter by successfully completing the activities and analysis of medical records.

About Radiology

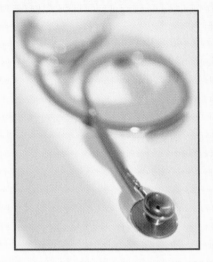

The **x-ray,** also known as the **roentgen ray,** is named after the German physicist Wilhelm K. Roentgen, who accidentally discovered the x-ray in 1895. He experimented with electrical discharges in a vacuum glass tube called a Crookes tube. Those discharges were electromagnetic energy rays that had the capability of penetrating a person's hand and leaving an outline image of the bones on a chemically coated fluorescent screen located behind the hand. Because he did not know what the rays were, Roentgen labeled them "x-rays." Eventually he replaced the fluorescent screen with photographic film, which produced a permanent impression of the image. Today, radiology involves not only the use of x-rays but also the application of advanced technologic imaging procedures, such as high-strength magnetic fields (magnetic resonance imaging), high-frequency sound waves (ultrasound), and numerous radioactive compounds (nuclear medicine).

Radiology, the branch of medicine concerned with the study of x-rays, uses various techniques of visualization to diagnose and treat disease. The three main branches of radiology are (1) **diagnostic radiology,** which concerns itself with imaging using external sources of radiation; physicians who specialize in diagnostic radiology are called **radiologists;** (2) **nuclear medicine,** which is involved with radioactive substances in the diagnosis and treatment of disease; physicians who specialize in **nuclear medicine** are called **nuclear physicians;** (3) **therapeutic radiology,** which is concerned with the treatment of cancer using radiation; physicians who specialize in **radiation therapy** are called **radiation oncologists.** Types of therapeutic radiology, such as **radiation therapy** (also called **radiotherapy** or **radiation oncology**), involve treatment of diseases by implantation of radioactive substances or by the administration of external sources of high-energy rays.

Usually physicians do not administer these tests or treatments but depend on **radiologic technologists** to administer diagnostic procedures and radiation treatments. Generally there are three types of radiologic technologists: the **radiographer,** the **nuclear medicine technologist,** and the **radiation therapy technologist.** All of these technologists administer diagnostic x-ray procedures. In addition, nuclear medicine and radiation therapy technologists help to treat patients, as ordered by the physician.

Selected Key Terms

angiography ăn-jē-ŎG-ră-fē *angio=vessel* *graphy=process of recording*	Radiography of vessels after the injection of a radiopaque contrast medium. The contrast may be injected into an artery or vein or introduced into a catheter inserted in a peripheral artery and threaded into the appropriate blood vessel or heart chamber.
coronary KOR-ō-nă-rē	Angiography of the coronary arteries to determine any pathological obstructions of the arteries that supply blood to the heart.
angiogram ĂN-jē-ō-grăm *angio=vessel* *gram=record, writing*	A radiographic image of the heart and blood vessels obtained after the injection of a contrast medium.
barium sulfate BĂ-rē-ŭm	A contrast medium used in diagnostic contrast studies of the gastrointestinal (GI) system.

catheter KĂTH-ĕ-tĕr	A hollow, flexible tube that can be inserted into a vessel or cavity of the body to inject or remove fluids.
cineradiography sĭn-ĕ-rā-dē-ŎG-ră-fē *cine=movement* *radio=radiation, x-ray, radius* *(lower arm bone on thumb side)* *graphy=process of recording*	The filming with a movie camera of the images that appear on a fluorescent screen, especially those images of body structures that have been injected with a nontoxic radiopaque medium; used for diagnostic purposes.
coldspot	Light shades of gray on a scan that indicate a decreased uptake of a radiopharmaceutical substance.
contrast medium	In radiology, a substance that is injected into the body, introduced via catheter, or swallowed, to facilitate radiographic imaging of internal structures that otherwise are difficult to visualize on x-ray films. The substance can be radiopaque and positive (e.g., barium sulfate) or radiolucent and negative (e.g., air). Barium sulfate is a commonly used contrast agent for the gastrointestinal tract. Barium can be administered alone or in combination with air. The gas-enhanced study is referred to as an "air contrast" study.
gamma camera GĂ-mă	A device that uses the emission of light from a crystal struck by gamma rays to produce an image of the distribution of radioactive material in a body organ. The gamma camera is a workhorse of nuclear medicine departments, where it is used to produce scans of patients who have been injected with small amounts of radioactive materials.
gamma rays	High-energy waves emitted by radioactive substances.
half-life	The time required for a radioactive substance to lose 50% of its activity through decay.
hotspot	Darker shades of gray on a scan that indicate an increased uptake of a radiopharmaceutical substance.
in vitro ĭn VĒ-trō	A biologic reaction occurring in laboratory apparatus, such as in a test tube or culture medium.
isotope Ī-sō-tōp	One of two or more forms of a chemical element having almost identical properties. Many hundreds of radioactive isotopes are used in diagnostic and therapeutic procedures.
lumen LŪ-mĕn	A tubular cavity or the channel within any organ or structure of the body.
myelogram MĪ-ĕ-lō-grăm *myelo=bone marrow, spinal cord* *gram= record, writing*	Radiograph of the spinal canal after injection of a contrast medium.

percutaneous approach pĕr-kū-TĀ-nē-ŭs *per=through* *cutane=skin* *ous=pertaining to*	Technique in which a catheter is introduced through the skin into an organ, body cavity, or vessel to perform an interventional procedure such as fluid drainage or stone removal.
radiation rā-dē-Ā-shŭn	Emission of x-rays from a common source; used for diagnostic and therapeutic purposes.
radioactive rā-dē-ō-ĂK-tĭv	Pertaining to a substance capable of emitting radiant energy.
radioisotope rā-dē-ō-Ī-sō-tōp	A radioactive isotope of an element; used for therapeutic and diagnostic purposes.
radiopharmaceutical rā-dē-ō-fărm-ă-SŪ-tĭ-kăl *radio=x-ray, radiation* *pharmaceutic=drug, medicine* *al=relating to*	Radioactive chemical occurring either as an individual element or as an element attached to another substance called a *carrier*. It is used in testing the location, size, outline, or function of tissues, organs, vessels, or body fluids.
shield	A protective device, usually containing lead, to block radiation absorption by the body.
tracer study	Study in which radionuclides are used as tags, attached to a chemical, and followed as they move through the body.
ultrasound tests, ultrasonography, sonography	Studies in which ultrasound images of the internal structures of the body are produced using sound waves. Ultrasonic echoes are recorded as they strike tissues of different densities.
uptake	Absorption of a radiopharmaceutical into tissues or organs of the body.

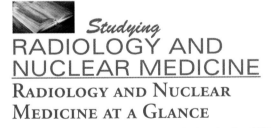

Studying
RADIOLOGY AND NUCLEAR MEDICINE

Radiology and Nuclear Medicine at a Glance

Until the advent of nuclear medicine in the 1950s, the x-ray was the only noninvasive radiographic procedure to detect pathological conditions in the internal organs of the body.

With the implementation of nuclear medicine, other noninvasive scanning techniques were developed, such as computed tomography (CT), positron-emission tomography (PET), and magnetic resonance imaging (MRI). All of these imaging procedures view the body's internal organs for evidence of disease without subjecting the person to the invasiveness of exploratory surgery. In addition, these procedures are reliable diagnostic tools, with CT and PET scans accounting for about 25 percent of imaging procedures performed today. Nevertheless, the x-ray, or radiograph, which is essentially a shadowy negative of the internal structures of the body, remains the workhorse of diagnostic imaging techniques and accounts for over half of all imaging currently done.

The purpose of this chapter is to provide information about the medical specialty of radiology. It focuses on the field of diagnostic radiology and does not include therapeutic radiology or radiation oncology (covered in Chapter 19).

Radiography

Radiography is the process of obtaining an image for diagnosis using a radiological modality.

A **radiograph** is the film on which an image is produced through exposure to x-rays. Radiographs are an important diagnostic tool used to identify or confirm an existing condition within the body (e.g., to identify a tumor, to diagnose the extent of a fracture, to establish the shape, size, and functioning of an organ).

For a body part to be seen on a radiograph, it must display a contrasting shade of black or white compared with the structures surrounding it. The overall shade of the radiographic image depends on whether or not the substance or body structure is radiopaque (substance does not permit x-rays to pass through it), or radiolucent (substance permits x-rays to pass through it).

The various structures and substances of the body (e.g., bones, tissues, organs, gases) are composed of different densities and are either radiopaque or radiolucent. **Radiopaque substances,** such as bone tissue, absorb or block the x-rays and appear white on a radiograph (Fig. 18–1). **Barium sulfate,** undissolved medications, calcium deposits, and metals are also radiopaque substances that appear white on a radiograph. **Radiolucent substances,** such as body fat and lymph, allow most x-rays to pass through them quickly, and appear very dark or black on the radiograph. The soft body tissues in the gastrointestinal tract are also radiolucent and appear black on the radiograph. Because of this phenomenon, barium sulfate (a radiopaque contrast medium) may be used to increase the density of the area under study (lower gastrointestinal system). The increased density outlines the boundaries of the specific area or of the specific organ and produces a precise image. Unless a patient is adequately prepared for an x-ray, the radiographic image may not be accurate and becomes an ineffective diagnostic tool (Fig. 18–2).

X-Ray Machines and Radiographic Projections

A variety of x-ray machines are found in diagnostic centers and hospitals. They are complex machines, designed to produce distinctive types of radiographs and diagnostic studies.

Basically, the x-ray machine has four basic parts: (1) x-ray tube, (2) table, (3) high-voltage generator, and (4) control panel. The x-ray tube, above the table, produces and transmits the x-ray beam. The table is usually adjustable, so that the patient can be placed in various positions at various angles to the x-ray beam. The control panel operates and controls x-ray emissions.

To obtain a clear and accurate picture of a body part that is to be **radiographed** or x-rayed, the patient, film, and x-ray tube must be positioned in the most favorable alignment. Whereas radiographic positioning refers to specific patient body positions (e.g., *recumbent,* lying down; *supine,* lying on the back, face up; *prone,* lying on the belly, face down), radiographic projections refer to the portion of the body in which the x-ray beam first enters the body. It is important to understand the difference between patient positioning (see Fig. 4–4) and radiographic projections (Fig. 18–3). Listed below are examples of radiographic projections. They are listed in the same order as those illustrated in Figure 18–3.

A. **Anteroposterior (AP):** The beam enters anteriorly and exits posteriorly.

B. **Posteroanterior (PA):** The beam enters posteriorly and exits anteriorly.

C. **Oblique:** The beam enters at an oblique (diagonal) point and exits at the opposite oblique point.

D. **Lateral (lat.):** The beam crosses the side plane (either through the left or right side).

Safety Procedures

Excessive exposure to radiation causes damage to the tissues of the body. Because radiation exposure is **cu-**

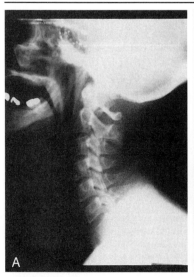
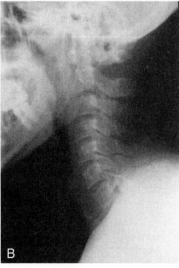

Figure 18–1 *(A) Dense, healthy bones display high contrast. (B) Demineralized bones display low contrast. (From Wallace, JE: Radiographic Exposure: Principles and Practice. FA Davis, Philadelphia, 1995, p 79, with permission.)*

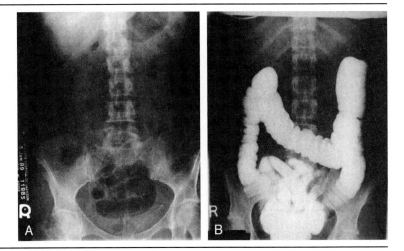

Figure 18–2 *(A) An image of a patient who was poorly prepared for a barium enema. (B) An image of a patient who was adequately prepared for a barium enema. (From Williams, LS, and Hopper, PD: Understanding Medical Surgical Nursing. FA Davis, Philadelphia 1999, p 630, with permission.)*

mulative (accumulation of previous exposures), there are both long-term as well as short-term damaging effects. Long-term overexposure may cause cancer, damage to the ovaries and testes, and/or produce genetic defects in offspring. Short-term overexposure may cause lowered red and white blood cell counts due to alteration of the bone marrow and the blood-forming organs.

Lead, a radiopaque substance, is known to be an effective barrier against exposure to x-rays. Healthcare practitioners working with x-ray equipment commonly wear lead aprons, vests, and/or gloves.

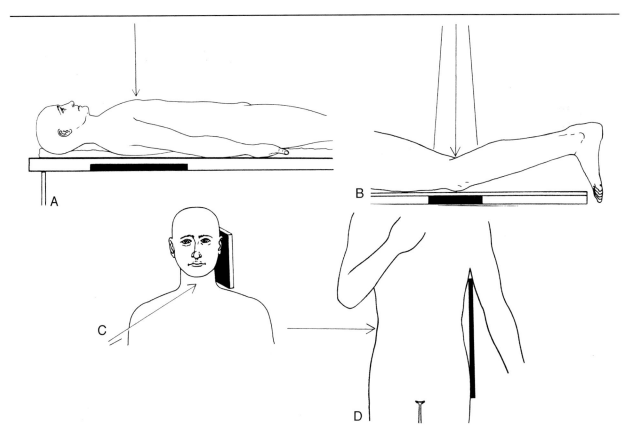

Figure 18–3 *Radiographic projections. (From Frew, MA, Lane, K, and Frew, DR: Comprehensive Medical Assisting, Competencies for Administrative and Clinical Practice, ed 3. FA Davis, Philadelphia, 1995, p 868, with permission.)*

Rooms containing x-ray equipment are usually lined with lead or some type of metal to prevent the escape of radiation into adjacent surroundings. Lead aprons, or **shields,** are also used to cover parts of the patient's body that are not being x-rayed.

Exposure to radiation can be primary or secondary. **Primary radiation** is the radiation emitted directly to the patient from the x-ray source. **Secondary radiation** is the radiation that results from the scattering of primary x-rays. It "bounces" off the patient and its strength is proportionate to the distance from the patient receiving radiation. Therefore, x-ray technologists do not remain next to the patient during the x-ray process. They either stand behind a lead shield divider or leave the room. Some facilities have a red light that flashes when x-ray equipment is being used to warn others not to enter.

Further safety precautions include wearing a radiation **film badge,** also called a **dosimeter badge.** The badges are used to detect and measure cumulative radiation exposure. The radiation exposure is measured in **rads** (radiation absorbed dose). A pencil-sized ionization chamber with a self-reading electrometer is used to monitor exposure to personnel.

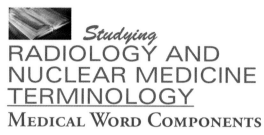

Studying
RADIOLOGY AND NUCLEAR MEDICINE TERMINOLOGY
MEDICAL WORD COMPONENTS
Combining Forms

Combining Forms: Radiology and Nuclear Medicine

Combining Form	Meaning	EXAMPLE	
		Term/Pronunciation	Definition
anter/o	anterior, front	**anter**/o/posterior *ăn-tĕr-ō-pŏs-TĒ-rē-or*	from the front to the back (*poster/o*) of the body
fluor/o	luminous, fluorescence	**fluor**/o/scope *FLOO-or-ō-skōp*	an instrument used for immediate projection of a radiographic image on a fluorescent screen for visual examination. *The suffix -scope means an "instrument to view or examine."*
later/o	side, to one side	**later**/al *LĂT-ĕr-ăl*	pertaining to (*-al*) one side of the body
medi/o	middle	**medi**/o/later/al *mē-dē-ō-LĂT-ĕr-ăl*	pertaining to (*-al*) the middle and the side (*later/o*) of the body
poster/o	back (of body), behind, posterior	**poster**/o/later/al *pŏs-tĕr-ō-LĂT-ĕr-ăl*	pertaining to (*-al*) the back and side (*later/o*) of the body
proxim/o	near, nearest	**proxim**/al *PRŎK-sĭ-măl*	pertaining (*-al*) nearer to a point of reference, usually the trunk of the body, when compared with another part of the body
radi/o	radiation, x-ray, radius (lower arm bone on thumb side)	**radi**/o/graphy *rā-dē-ŎG-ră-fē*	the process of recording (*-graphy*) an x-ray

Combining Forms: Radiology and Nuclear Medicine (Continued)

Combining Form	Meaning	EXAMPLE	
		Term/Pronunciation	Definition
son/o	sound	**son**/o/gram SŌ-nō-grăm	an image of the internal structures of the body obtained through the use of high-frequency sound waves. Also called ultrasonogram. *The suffix* -gram *means "record," "writing."*
therapeut/o	treatment	**therapeut**/ic thĕr-ă-PŪ-tĭk	pertaining to (*-ic*) a treatment that is beneficial to the body
tom/o	to cut	**tom**/o/graphy tō-MŎG-ră-fē	radiographic technique that produces a film representing a detailed cross-section of tissue (*hist/o*) structure. *The suffix* -graphy *means "process of recording."*
ventr/o	belly, belly-side	**ventr**/al VĔN-trăl	pertaining to (*-al*) the front side of the body

Prefixes and Suffixes
Prefixes

In this section, prefixes are listed alphabetically and highlighted, whereas key suffixes are defined in the right-hand column.

Prefixes: Radiology and Nuclear Medicine

Prefix	Meaning	EXAMPLE	
		Term/Pronunciation	Definition
ab-	from, away from	**ab**/duction ăb-DŬK-shŭn	lateral movement of a limb away from the body *The suffix* -duction *refers to "the act of leading, bringing, conducting."*
ad-	toward	**ad**/duction ă-DŬK-shŭn	lateral movement of a limb toward the body
cine-	movement	**cine**/radi/o/graphy sĭn-ĕ-rā-dē-ŎG-ră-fē	a motion picture record of images produced during fluoroscopic examination *The suffix* -graphy, *means "process of recording."*
echo-	a repeated sound	**echo**/gram ĔK-ō-grăm	radiographic image produced when ultrasound echo patterns reflect off tissues (*hist/o*) of different densities *The suffix* -gram *means "record," "writing."*

Prefixes (Continued)

Prefix	Meaning	EXAMPLE	
		Term/Pronunciation	**Definition**
epi-	above, upon	**epi**/gastr/ic *ĕp-ĭ-GĂS-trĭk*	pertaining to (-*ic*) the region of the abdomen above the stomach (*gastr/o*)
hypo-	under, below	**hypo**/gastr/ic *hī-pō-GĂS-trĭk*	pertaining to (-*ic*) the region of the abdomen below the stomach (*gastr/o*)
infra-		**infra**/cost/al *ĭn-fră-KŎS-tăl*	pertaining to (-*al*) the area below the ribs (*cost/o*)
inter-	between	**inter**/cost/al *ĭn-tĕr-KŎS-tăl*	pertaining to (-*al*) the area between the ribs (*cost/o*)
intra-	in, within	**intra**/ven/ous *ĭn-tră-VĒ-nŭs*	pertaining to (-*ous*) within a vein (*ven/o*)
iso-	same, equal	**iso**/therm/al *ī-sō-THĔR-măl*	having equal temperature *The combining form* therm/o *means "heat."*
peri-	around	**peri**/metry *pĕr-ĬM-ĕ-trē*	act of measuring (-*metry*) a border or edge of the body
retro-	backward, behind	**retro**/pharynx *rĕ-trō-FĂR-ĭnks*	the posterior portion of the throat (*pharyng/o*)
sub-	below	**sub**/stern/al *sŭb-STĔR-năl*	pertaining to (-*al*) the area below the sternum, or breastbone (*stern/o*)
trans-	across, through	**trans**/abdomin/al *trănz-ăb-DŎM-ĭ-năl*	pertaining to (-*al*) across or through the abdominal (*abdomin/o*) wall
ultra-	excess, beyond	**ultra**/sound *ŬL-tră-sownd*	diagnostic test that uses high-frequency sound waves to produce images of the internal structures of the body

Suffixes

In this section, suffixes are listed alphabetically and highlighted, whereas key prefixes are defined in the right-hand column.

Suffixes: Radiology and Nuclear Medicine

| Suffix | Meaning | EXAMPLE | |
		Term/Pronunciation	Definition
-gram	record, writing	arteri/o/**gram** ăr-TĒ-rē-ō-grăm	a radiograph of an artery (*arteri/o*) after the injection of a radiopaque contrast medium
-graph	instrument for recording	cardi/o/**graph** KĂR-dē-ō-grăf	an instrument for recording the electrical activity of the heart (*cardi/o*) muscle. Also called *electrocardiograph* (*EKG* or *ECG*).
-graphy	process of recording	arthr/o/**graphy** ăr-THRŎG-ră-fē	radiography of a joint (*arthr/o*) after the injection of a contrast medium
-lucent	to shine, clear	radi/o/**lucent** rā-dē-ō-LŪ-sĕnt	substances that allow x-rays (*radi/o*) to penetrate with a minimum of absorption *The combining form* radi/o *means "radiation, x-ray, radius (lower arm bone on thumb side)."*
-opaque	obscure	radi/**opaque** RĂ-dē-ō-pāk	substances that do not permit the passage of x-rays (*radi/o*) or other radiant energy

Activity 18–1: Competency Verification
Medical Word Components

Check the box [✓] as you complete each numbered section.

[   ] **1.** Review the word components related to radiology. Then pronounce each word aloud.

[   ] **2.** For the words below, first write the suffix and its meaning. Then translate the meaning of the remaining components, starting with the first part of the word.

> **Example:** albumin/oid
> **Answer:** *oid* = resembling; albumin (protein)

1. son/o/gram   _____

2. ventr/al   _____

3. arteri/o/gram _____

4. sub/stern/al _____

5. proxim/al _____

6. radi/o/graphy _____

7. later/al _____

8. fluor/o/scopy _____

9. epi/gastr/ic _____

10. intra/ven/ous _____

11. iso/therm/al _____

12. peri/metry _____

13. therapeut/ic _____

14. medi/al _____

15. echo/gram _____

Correct Answers _____ **× 6.67 =** _____ **% Score**

Activity 18–2: Competency Verification
Build Medical Words

arteri/o	-al	ab-
later/o	-gram	ad-
medi/o	-graphy	inter-
son/o	-ist	intra-
therapeut/o	-ous	trans-
ven/o	-scope	
	-scopy	

Use the word components listed above to form medical words. Some components may be used more than once:

1. area between the ribs: _____/cost/al

2. images produced from sound waves: _____/gram

3. specialist in the study of x-rays: radi/o/log/_____

4. instrument used for fluoroscopy: fluor/o/_____

5. across the abdomen: _____/abdomin/al

6. pertaining to treatment: _____/ic

7. lateral movement of a limb toward the body: ____/duction

8. pertaining to the middle and the side: _____

9. pertaining to within a vein: _____

10. pertaining to an artery: _____

Correct Answers _____ **× 10 =** _____ **% Score**

DIAGNOSTIC IMAGING PROCEDURES

Contrast Media

The clarity of radiographs can be enhanced by the use of a **contrast medium** (plural, media). As you have already learned, a contrast medium is a radiopaque substance that shows up as white on the x-ray film, and increases the density of selected tissue to provide better visualization of internal structures. Because the contrast medium accentuates the boundaries of the area that is being filmed, it produces a clearer image. Contrast media can be administered orally, intravenously, or rectally.

The most commonly used contrast media are **iodine** and barium sulfate. Iodine compounds are used for vessel studies of the arteries and veins, urinary system studies, **myelograms,** and many other radiographic studies. Barium sulfate is usually prescribed for radiographic visualization of the gastrointestinal tract (see Fig. 18–2). In addition to radiation hazards, the use of intravenous contrast media poses additional risk of allergic reactions to the patient that may range from mild to life threatening. The allergic reaction may include nausea and vomiting, rash, dizziness, cardiac arrest, laryngospasm, central nervous system depression, and anaphylactic shock (a severe and sometimes fatal hypersensitivity reaction that is commonly marked by respiratory distress and vascular collapse).

Contrast media are also used in fluoroscopy, computed tomography (CT), **angiography,** and magnetic resonance imaging (MRI).

Tomography

Tomography, or body section radiography, allows an organ or body structure to be imaged as a detailed cross-section or "slice." It produces detailed cross-sectional images that provide extensive anatomic and diagnostic information. Tomography is a valuable diagnostic tool for discovering and identifying space-occupying lesions, such as tumors and calcifications, which may not be evident on conventional radiographs.

Computed tomography (CT), also called **computerized tomography,** or **computerized axial tomography (CAT),** makes use of a computer and a radiation beam to create cross-sectional and three-dimensional reconstructions of body structures. The x-ray beam passes through successive horizontal layers of tissues. A computer then detects variation of tissue density in each layer and the amount of radiation absorbed. An image in varying shades of gray is produced based on this information. The images are displayed on a television monitor and stored on magnetic optical disc, film, or both.

During this procedure, the patient lies supine on a motorized couch that moves in a cylinder-shaped frame called a **gantry.** The patient is instructed to remain still as a series of images is taken while the x-ray tubes within the gantry move around the patient.

CT scanners are highly sensitive in detecting diseases in bony structures and can provide images of internal organs that cannot be visualized with standard x-ray procedures. CT scans can detect brain tumors, hematomas, spinal cord lesions, as well as masses in the chest, liver, kidney, and pancreas. To further enhance a contrast for the CT scan, an iodinated dye may be injected intravenously.

Fluoroscopy

Fluoroscopy is a radiographic procedure that uses a fluorescent screen instead of a photographic plate to produce an image of tissues and deep structures of the body. During fluoroscopy, the patient is placed into position so that the organ or body structure to be viewed is between the x-ray tube and a fluorescent screen. X-rays from the tube pass through the body and project a visual image of organs and bones on the fluorescent screen.

A major advantage of fluoroscopy is the ability to view the motion of organs such as the digestive tract, the heart, and the joints. This radiographic procedure is also used during biopsy surgery, nasogastric tube placement, and catheter insertion during angiography. Fluoroscopy is also performed in combination with other applications, such as the use of motion in **cine-radiography** (*cine=motion*), which is motion picture recording of images produced during fluoroscopic examination. This diagnostic procedure permits a radiologist to view a sequence of images and to observe organs in motion (i.e., the heart, the gastrointestinal tract).

Interventional Radiology

In the 1960s, the branch of radiology known as cardiovascular angiography expanded to include not only diagnostic procedures, but also therapeutic interventions to treat heart abnormalities and diseases. Hence, this new branch of radiology is identified in a number of different ways: interventional angiography, special procedures, invasive vascular procedures, vascular interventional angiography, and interventional radiography, to name a few.

Interventional radiology includes therapeutic procedures performed in conjunction with fluoroscopy. Interventional radiology can be further classified into *vascular interventional procedures* and *nonvascular interventional procedures*. Both are considered therapeutic interventions.

- **Vascular interventional procedures** are used to treat vascular and heart abnormalities. The cardiac surgeon is able to identify and correct obstruction in the coronary vessels with the use of a fluoroscope. Refer to Chapter 9 for a discussion of the vascular procedures known as **angiogram** and **angioplasty.**
- **Nonvascular interventional procedures** are used for placement of **catheters** that may be used to remove fluids or drain abscesses, or to instill antibiotics or chemotherapy. *Percutaneous nephrostomy* is an example of a nonvascular interventional procedure in which a catheter is introduced into the target area of the kidney or ureter to remove a stone(s).

Magnetic Resonance Imaging

Magnetic resonance imaging (MRI), a noninvasive scanning procedure, uses magnetic waves to produce multi-planar cross-sectional images. Instead of **radiation,** it uses a powerful magnet, radio-frequency energy, and a special computer to create images of the body. Although an MRI does not require a contrast medium, it may be used to enhance visualization of the internal structures of the body. The image is created when hydrogen atoms, present in most tissues, interact with the MRI magnet. The magnet and radio waves cause hydrogen atoms in the scan area to move in predictable patterns. This movement produces the signals that create the MRI image.

MRI is not prescribed for patients with implanted metal devices, such as pacemakers, joint or bone pins,

or vascular clips because the powerful magnetic conduction may dislodge the metal devices and/or interfere with their functioning. The patient is asked to remove all other metallic objects (hearing aids, hairpins, jewelry, and watches) because these objects may also cause interference with magnetic conduction.

During the MRI procedure, the patient is placed in a long, cylindrical, tube-shaped chamber and instructed to lie still. Although the procedure is painless, it can be upsetting to patients who suffer from claustrophobia. To reduce anxiety and promote relaxation, a sedative may be administered. Some recent MRI machines are open and do not have the closed, cylindrical, tube-shaped chamber, which helps to reduce the patient's claustrophobia.

Once the patient is fully prepared for the MRI study, the technologist conducts the scan from an adjoining room and can communicate with the patient through an intercom. The examination time for an MRI varies from 20 minutes to 2 hours, depending on the number of body structures to be scanned. Figure 18–4 shows a technologist performing MRI.

Magnetic resonance images show subtle differences in soft tissue, making it very useful for diagnosing anomalies of the brain (Fig.18–5). Any soft tissue that contains fat and water is viewed most clearly through an MRI. This imaging modality can also yield more detailed views of the spine and the interior of joints that are not visible in CT imaging. It also identifies tumors in the chest and abdomen, detects edema in the brain, projects a direct image of the spinal cord, and visualizes the cardiac chambers.

Review Table 18–1, which lists different types of MRI studies.

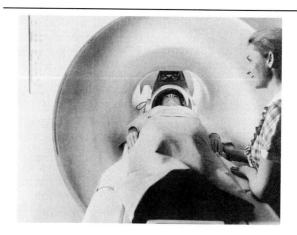

Figure 18–4 *A technician with a patient about to proceed with MRI. (From Frew, MA, Lane, K, and Frew, DR: Comprehensive Medical Assisting: Competencies for Administrative and Clinical Practice, ed 3. FA Davis, Philadelphia, 1995, p 865, with permission.)*

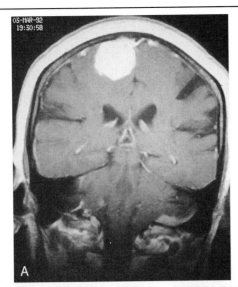

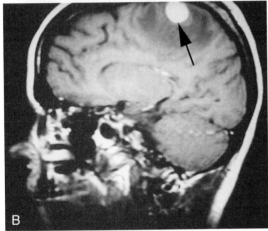

Figure 18–5 An MRI of the brain: (A) meningioma; (B) metastatic brain tumor. This patient's primary cancer was in the lung. (From Williams, LS, and Hopper, PD: Understanding Medical Surgical Nursing. FA Davis, Philadelphia, 1999, p 979, with permission.)

Mammography

Mammography is the radiographic imaging of the breast to screen for (and detect) breast cancer. The actual radiograph of the breast is called a **mammogram.**

Patient preparation includes instructing the patient not to apply deodorant, perfume, or powder on the day of examination because these substances could adversely affect image clarity. The radiographer directs the patient where to place her arms and hands and how to position her body while the x-rays are taken. During the entire procedure the patient stands in front of the x-ray machine as each breast (one at a time) is placed on the plate and compressed (Fig. 18–6) to allow better visualization of the soft tissue.

Normally, the procedure is painless. Nevertheless, some patients may feel discomfort from the pressure during the breast compression, which lasts less than a minute. Taking an x-ray of each view of the breast lasts only a few seconds, but the entire procedure may last half an hour. A routine mammogram consists of two views of each breast. The American Cancer Society (ACS) recommends a baseline mammogram for women between the ages of 35 and 40, and a mammogram every 2 years after the age of 40. If the patient is identified to be in a risk group, the ACS recommends a mammogram every year. After the age of 50, ACS recommends yearly mammograms for all women.

Ultrasonography

A diagnostic procedure that uses ultrasound (US), that is high-frequency, inaudible sound waves, to image internal structures of the body. It consists of emitting a beam of ultrasound waves rather than x-rays into the body. The body tissues, composed of structures with different acoustic properties, reflect sound waves with varying degrees of intensity. The various reflected waves, or **echoes,** are electronically processed and displayed as a visual picture.

During an ultrasound procedure, conduction material such as jelly or oil is placed on the outer surface of the body part that is to be recorded. An instrument called a **transducer,** which contains a conduction head, is placed on or near the skin. As the sound waves pass through the skin, ultrasonic echoes of the body over which the conduction head has passed are recorded on an instrument called an **oscilloscope.** The images produced through the application of ultrasound are called **sonograms** or **echograms.** US is painless and fairly quick, a few minutes to an hour, and requires little or no patient preparation. Many medical specialties rely on ultrasound as a diagnostic tool. It is especially effective for imaging the thyroid gland, heart, liver, gallbladder and biliary tract, pancreas, kidney, male reproductive organs, and female reproductive organs. It is also used to view a developing fetus (see Fig. 11–7).

Two specialized ultrasound techniques, the **Doppler** ultrasound and the **Doppler color flow,** produce detailed visualization of the anatomy of blood vessels and the blood flow through them. Detection of perfusion disturbances and blood flow direction and velocity aid the cardiologist in diagnosing heart valve and blood vessel disorders.

NUCLEAR MEDICINE

Diagnostic nuclear medicine is a medical specialty that uses **radioactive** substances (**radionuclides** and **radioisotopes**) in the diagnosis and treatment of disease. In contrast to conventional radiography in which radiation passes through the body from an

TABLE 18–1: Types of Magnetic Resonance Imaging (MRI) Studies

STUDY	DESCRIPTION
Body	Chest, abdomen, spinal cord, pelvis, and extremities; any area of the body other than the head
Angiography	Arteries and veins of the neck, thorax, abdomen, extremities, and intracranial contents
Abdominal	Abdominal and pelvic organs
Head and intracranial	Brain and face
Heart and chest	Cardiovascular and pulmonary structures and circulation
Musculoskeletal	Bones and joints and surrounding soft tissue structures of cartilage, synovium, ligaments and tendons

external source, nuclear medicine detects radiation produced by radioactive substances that are deliberately placed inside of the body. These substances are used to diagnose and treat disease.

In nuclear imaging studies, minute amounts of radioisotopes, also known as **radiopharmaceuticals** (radionuclide plus a chemical), are administered to the patient by injection, mouth, or nose (through inhalation) before imaging. The radiopharmaceutical travels throughout the tissues and organs of the body and disintegrates. As disintegration occurs, it emits radiation in the form of alpha, beta, or **gamma rays** (the most common). Each radionuclide has a unique **half-life,** which is the time required for a radioactive substance to lose 50 percent of its activity through decay.

When the distribution is complete, measurement of changing levels of the disintegrated radiopharmaceuti-

cal is detected by scanning the body with a **gamma camera.** The gamma camera detects the location and energy of gamma rays emitted from the radiopharmaceutical and inputs the readings into a computer, converting them into an image for viewing. The procedure

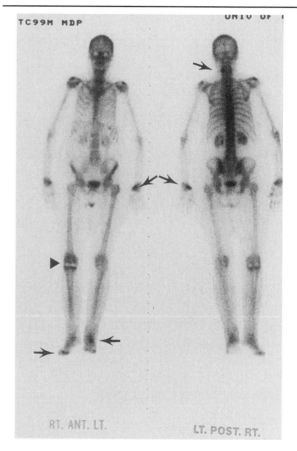

Figure 18–7 *A bone scan of entire skeleton in patient with degenerative joint disease. Arrows show abnormal areas with increased uptake. Total knee prosthesis is shown at arrowhead. (From Williams, LS, and Hopper, PD: Understanding Medical Surgical Nursing. FA Davis, Philadelphia, 1999, p 881, with permission.)*

Figure 18–6 *A mammography screening of a woman's breast. (From Tortorici, MR, and Apfel, PJ: Advanced Radiographic and Angiographic Procedures with an Introduction to Specialized Imaging. FA Davis, Philadelphia, 1995, p 300, with permission.)*

of producing an image to follow the distribution of radioactive substances in the body is called **scanning.** The image produced by the gamma camera is called a **scan.** Figure 18–7 is a bone scan of a whole skeleton with varying shades of gray and black. The appearance of gray and black identifies the **uptake,** (i.e., the absorption of a radiopharmaceutical into the bone tissue). Areas of uptake indicate potential abnormalities. A darker shade on a scan indicates a **hotspot,** an increased area of uptake. A light shade on a scan indicates a **coldspot,** an area of decreased uptake. Images can also be recorded in color (see Fig. 14–9, PET scans) or in **cine mode,** which displays sequential pictures of the movement or flow of the radiopharmaceutical in the body.

Because radionuclides have a short half-life, there are very few side effects for the patient and less chance of an allergic reaction. The short half-life also results in exposure to much lower doses of radiation than other radiographic techniques.

Nuclear Imaging Studies

There are a variety of scans used in nuclear imaging studies. All **scans** produce an image of the area being studied by recording the concentration of a radioactive substance specifically drawn to that area. Scans provide information about the structure as well as the function of an organ or system.

Positron-emission tomography (PET) combines computed tomography with the use of radiopharmaceuticals (see Fig. 14–9, PET scans). The PET scan produces a cross-sectional image of the dispersement of radioactivity in a section of the body. The hotspots and coldspots indicate those areas where the radionuclide is being metabolized and where there is a deficiency in metabolism. PET scans are used to diagnose disorders that involve metabolism abnormalities such as schizophrenia, in which glucose is unequally metabolized in the brain. PET can pinpoint the degree and intensity of the metabolic process. Therefore it can aid in the diagnosis of neurologic disorders such as brain tumors, epilepsy, stroke, Alzheimer disease, and abdominal, cardiac, and pulmonary disorders. See Figure 14–9B for an illustration of a PET scan showing Alzheimer disease.

Single photon emission computed tomography (SPECT) is another type of nuclear imaging study to scan organs. It is similar to PET but uses a more advanced **gamma camera** that has the capability of producing a three-dimensional image from the composite of numerous views. SPECT provides more sensitive and specific diagnostic information than PET does. Organs commonly studied by SPECT include the brain, heart, lungs, liver, spleen, bones, and in some cases, joints.

Radionuclide Laboratory Studies

In radionuclide laboratory studies, also known as **in vitro** (in the test tube) procedures, the administration of small amounts of radioactive substances is followed by the detection of radioactivity in the blood, the urine, or other body fluids. These tests determine the ability of the body to absorb the radionuclide that was administered by measuring the concentration of radioactivity in the designated body fluid. Some of the laboratory studies include scanning in combination with laboratory analysis.

The in vitro (in the test tube) procedure, which is called **radioimmunoassay (RIA),** combines the use of antibodies with radioactive chemicals to detect a wide variety of substances, especially hormones, in a patient's blood. In newborns, it may be used to detect *hypothyroidism.* Other substances that can be detected are immunoglobulins, proteins, vitamins, carcinogens, and drugs.

❖ ABBREVIATIONS

ABBREVIATION	MEANING	ABBREVIATION	MEANING
ACS	American Cancer Society	ECHO	echocardiogram, echoencephalogram
Angio	angiography		
AP	anteroposterior	ED	emergency department, erectile dysfunction
BaE, BE	barium enema		
CNS	central nervous system	ER	emergency room, estrogen receptor
CT	computed tomography		
CV	cardiovascular	EU	excretory urogram, same as IVP
CXR	chest x-ray		

ABBREVIATION	MEANING	ABBREVIATION	MEANING
IVP	intravenous pyelogram, same as EU	rad	radiation absorbed dose
		sono	sonogram
lat	lateral	SPECT	single photon emission computed tomography
LGI	lower gastrointestinal		
MRI	magnetic resonance imaging	UGI	upper gastrointestinal
PET	positron-emission tomography	US	ultrasound
PA	posteroanterior, pernicious anemia	W/O	without

Activity 18–3: Clinical Application

Diagnostic Imaging Procedures

angiography
cineradiography
Doppler
interventional radiology
magnetic resonance imaging (MRI)

mammogram
positron-emission tomography (PET)
radioimmunoassay (RIA)
single-photon emission computed tomography (SPECT)
ultrasonography

Match the terms listed above with the definitions given in the numbered list:

1. _____ used to diagnose disorders that involve metabolism abnormalities, such as schizophrenia; combines CT with the use of radiopharmaceuticals.

2. _____ an in vitro procedure that combines the use of antibodies with radioactive chemicals to measure a wide variety of substances in the blood (e.g., immunoglobulins, proteins, hormones).

3. _____ uses magnetic energy without ionizing x-rays to produce cross-sectional images.

4. _____ employs high-frequency sound waves to image internal structures of the body.

5. _____ production of film images on a fluorescent screen with a movie camera. This diagnostic procedure allows the radiologist to view the functions of an organ.

6. _____ a specialized ultrasound technique that produces detailed visualization of the anatomy of blood vessels and the blood flow through them.

7. _____ radiograph of the breast.

8. _____ therapeutic intervention performed in conjunction with fluoroscopy.

9. _____ nuclear imaging study that is more sensitive and specific than PET; a more sophisticated gamma camera is used to scan organs.

10. _____ radiography of the heart and blood vessels after the injection of a
    contrast medium.

Correct Answers _____ × 10 = _____% Score

Activity 18–4: Clinical Application
Radiologic Terminology

coldspot	myelogram
gamma rays	nonvascular interventional procedure (NIP)
half-life	oscilloscope
head and intracranial	rad
hotspot	radiopaque
in vitro	radiopharmaceutical
intravenous pyelogram	scan
iodine	uptake

Match the terms listed above with definitions given in the numbered list:

1. _____ a biologic reaction occurring in laboratory apparatus,
   such as in a test tube or culture medium.

2. _____ an MRI study of the brain and face.

3. _____ the presence of lighter shades on a scan that indicate
   a decreased area of radioisotope absorption.

4. _____ conduction head that records ultrasonic echoes of an
   organ to produce an image; also used to provide
   images of a developing embryo.

5. _____ the absorption of a radioisotope into an organ or tissue.

6. _____ time required for a radioactive substance to lose 50
   percent of its activity through decay.

7. _____ radionuclide plus a chemical.

8. _____ darker shade on a scan that indicates an increased
   area of uptake (absorption of the radioisotope).

9. _____ image produced by the gamma camera.

10. _____ a unit of absorbed radiation by the body.

11. _____ referring to substances that do not permit the passage
    of x-rays or other radiant energy, and, therefore,
    appear as a light area on the radiograph.

12. _____ the meaning of IVP.

13. _____ radiograph of the spinal column after injection of a
    contrast medium.

14. _____ a contrast medium used for vessel studies, urinary system studies, and myelograms.

15. _____ a fluoroscopic procedure for placement of a drainage catheter.

Correct Answers _____ × 6.67 = _____ % Score

Medical Records

Timon Andrews was brought to the emergency room after an auto accident. A CT scan of the head was taken to rule out injury to the brain. Radiographs of both legs were taken to rule out any fractures. Another radiograph was taken of his jaw (mandible), to find the cause of his right, lower face pain, and a chest radiograph was taken to rule out injury to the lungs and chest. His discharge summary is also included.

The following reading and dictionary exercise and the medical record analysis will help you develop skills to abstract information and master the terminology in the reports. Accurate interpretation is important because this type of information is used in numerous areas of the medical practice, such as initiation of treatments, evaluation of patients' progress, and completion of insurance claims.

 Reading and Dictionary Exercise

Place a check mark [✓] after you complete the exercise.

[   ] **1.** Underline the following words in the reports as you read the radiology reports and the discharge summary aloud. These medical reports can be found at the end of the chapter.

[   ] **2.** Use a medical dictionary and Appendix F, Part 2 to complete this exercise.

> *Note: You are not expected to fully understand all the parts of the medical records. The important aspect of this exercise is to use all available resources to complete it. Eventually you will master the terminology and format of these records.*

>>> MEDICAL RECORD 18-1: RADIOLOGY REPORT: BRAIN CT WITHOUT CONTRAST

Term	Pronunciation	Meaning
axial	ĂK-sē-ăl	_____
vertex	VĔR-tĕks	_____
ventricle	VĔN-trĭ-kl	_____
cistern	SĬS-tĕrn	_____
sulci	SŬL-kī	_____
punctate	PŬNK-tāt	_____
attenuation	ă-tĕn-ū-Ā-shŭn	_____

bilaterally	*bī-LĂT-ĕr-ăl-ē*	_____
shearing	*SHĒR-ĭng*	_____
diffuse	*dĭ-FŪS*	_____
axonal	*ĂK-sŏn-ăl*	_____

>>> MEDICAL RECORD 18-2: RADIOLOGY REPORT: RULE OUT
      FRACTURE, KNEES AND LEGS

Term	Pronunciation	Meaning
fracture	*FRĂK-chŭr*	_____
dislocation	*dĭs-lō-KĀ-shŭn*	_____
subluxation	*sŭb-lŭk-SĀ-shŭn*	_____
tibia	*TĬB-ē-ă*	_____
fibula	*FĬB-ū-lă*	_____
mortise	*MOR-tĭs*	_____

>>> MEDICAL RECORD 18-3: RADIOLOGY REPORT: RULE OUT
      FRACTURE, RIGHT LOWER JAW

Term	Pronunciation	Meaning
radiolucent	*rā-dē-ō-LŪ-sĕnt*	_____
mentum	*MĔN-tŭm*	_____
foramen	*for-Ā-mĕn*	_____

>>> MEDICAL RECORD 18-4: RADIOLOGY REPORT: CHEST X-RAY

Term	Pronunciation	Meaning
mediastinum	*mē-dē-ăs-TĪ-nŭm*	_____
pneumothorax	*nū-mō-THŌ-răks*	_____
aerated	*ĀR-ā-tĕd*	_____
trachea	*TRĀ-kē-ă*	_____
midline	*MĬD-līn*	_____

>>> MEDICAL RECORD 18-5: DISCHARGE SUMMARY

Term	Pronunciation	Meaning
paresthesia	păr-ĕs-THĒ-zē-ă	_____
occipital	ŏk-SĬP-ĭ-tăl	_____
laceration	lă-sĕ-RĀ-shŭn	_____
tympanic membrane	tĭm-PĂN-ĭk MĔM-brān	_____
cerumen	sĕ-ROO-mĕn	_____
bicarb	BĪ-kărb	_____
alk phos	ălk fŏs	_____
occult blood	ŭ-KŬLT	_____
atelectasis	ăt-ĕ-LĔK-tă-sĭs	_____
lumbar	LŬM-băr	_____
C-collar	sē KŎL-ăr	_____
lumbosacral	lŭm-bō-SĀ-krăl	_____
oblique	ō-BLĒK	_____
tibial	TĬB-ē-ăl	_____

Critical Thinking: Analysis of Radiology Reports

This section provides experience in abstracting and analyzing information from medical records. At the same time, it reinforces the material presented in this chapter.

>>> MEDICAL RECORD 18-1: RADIOLOGY REPORT: BRAIN CT WITHOUT CONTRAST

1. Why was a CT scan ordered on this patient's brain instead of a normal x-ray?

_____

_____

_____

2. What view was taken using CT?

_____

_____

3. What abnormal findings were reported?

_____

_____

> >> MEDICAL RECORD 18-2: RADIOLOGY REPORT: RULE OUT FRACTURE, KNEES AND
>   LEGS

4. What abnormalities are cited in this report?

_____

> >> MEDICAL RECORD 18-3: RADIOLOGY REPORT: RULE OUT FRACTURE, RIGHT
>   LOWER JAW

5. What is the recommended follow-up treatment if the patient is experiencing jaw pain? What might this indicate?

_____

_____

> >> MEDICAL RECORD 18-4: RADIOLOGY REPORT: CHEST X-RAY

6. Why was a chest x-ray performed on this patient?

_____

> >> MEDICAL RECORD 18-5: DISCHARGE SUMMARY

7. Why was this patient seen in the ER?

_____

8. What treatment was given to repair the mandibular fracture?

_____

9. Why was outpatient evaluation of cognitive language by a speech therapist suggested?

_____

_____

10. What are the discharge diagnoses?

_____

_____

Audio Practice

Listen to the audio CD-ROM to practice the pronunciation of selected medical terms from this chapter.

Medical Record 18–1. Radiology Report

GENERAL HOSPITAL AND MEDICAL CENTER
2211 Fifth Avenue North • Healthy City, USA 12345 • (321) 123-4567

Radiology Report

Patient Name: Timon Andrews   **Patient Number**: 55-77-34
Birth Date: 06/06/xx   **Room Number**: ER

DATE: 09/12/xx

REQUESTING PHYSICIAN: Thomas Bloan, MD

REASON FOR EXAM: Motor vehicle accident with head injury, rule out bleed.

BRAIN CT WITHOUT CONTRAST: Axial images were obtained from the skull base
to the vertex and displayed in both brain and bone windows.

There is normal appearance to the ventricles, cisterns, and sulci. No midline shift is
noted. Good gray/white differentiation is identified. There are several small punctate
areas of increased attenuation seen in the deep matter bilaterally which may represent
areas of bleeding from a shearing injury. No gross bleed with mass effect is noted.

Images displayed in bone window show no evidence of fracture or air-fluid level.

IMPRESSION: SEVERAL BILATERAL PUNCTATE AREAS OF INCREASED
ATTENTUATION SUGGESTING SMALL BLEED FROM SHEARING INJURY.
FOLLOW-UP CT SCAN TO EVALUATE FOR DIFFUSE AXONAL INJURY IS
RECOMMENDED.

_____

Ray A. Reknirb, MD

RAR/pb
D: 09/12/xx
T: 09/13/xx

Medical Record 18–4. Radiology Report

GENERAL HOSPITAL AND MEDICAL CENTER
2211 Fifth Avenue North • Healthy City, USA 12345 • (321) 123-4567

Radiology Report

Patient Name: Timon Andrews   **Patient Number**: 55-77-34
Birth Date: 06/06/xx   **Room Number**: 415-3

DATE: 09/12/xx

REQUESTING PHYSICIAN: Thomas Bloan, MD

REASON FOR EXAM: Restrained driver in motor vehicle accident, rule out injury.

CHEST: The heart and mediastinum appear normal. There is no pneumothorax, effusions, or displaced rib fracture. The lungs are well aerated and clear. The trachea is midline.

IMPRESSION: NO RADIOGRAPHIC EVIDENCE OF WIDE MEDIASTINUM, PNEUMOTHORAX, OR ACUTE CHEST INJURY.

_____

Ray A. Reknirb, MD

RAR/js
D: 09/12/xx
T: 09/12/xx

Medical Record 18–5. Discharge Summary

GENERAL HOSPITAL AND MEDICAL CENTER
2211 Fifth Avenue North • Healthy City, USA 12345 • (321) 123-4567

Discharge Summary

Patient Name: Timon Andrews
Birth Date: 06/06/xx

Patient Number: 55-77-34
Room Number: 415-3

ADMISSION DATE: September 12, xx   **DISCHARGE DATE**: September 14, xx

ADMITTING DIAGNOSES:
1. Status post motor vehicle accident with positive loss of consciousness.
2. Right paresthesia at the knee and caudal.
3. Left occipital laceration.
4. Right mandibular fracture.

DISCHARGE DIAGNOSES:
1. Status post motor vehicle accident with positive loss of consciousness.
2. Mandibular fracture.
3. Left occipital laceration.
4. Right paresthesia at the knee and extending inferior.

HISTORY OF PRESENT ILLNESS: The patient is a 16-year-old white male who was the restrained driver in a side impact accident by a truck. The patient had positive loss of consciousness and no memory of the accident. The passenger of the vehicle was taken to another hospital. No headache and no visual changes were noted by the patient. The patient was complaining of right leg numbness at the knee and inferior jaw pain.

PAST MEDICAL HISTORY: None.

PAST SURGICAL HISTORY: None.

FAMILY HISTORY: Noncontributory.

SOCIAL HISTORY: No tobacco. No alcohol.

MEDICATIONS: None.

ALLERGIES: No known drug allergies.

PHYSICAL EXAMINATION: Generally, the patient was alert and oriented x 3 and in no acute distress. **Vital signs** are blood pressure 135/65, pulse 100, respirations 20.

Tympanic membrane is clear on the right; cerumen occluded the left. The mouth had a right lower small vertical laceration. Neck was nontender. The trachea at the midline. Neuro: Sensation was decreased of the right leg and knee. Strength 5/5 on all extremities. Reflexes were 2+ at each joint bilaterally.

Continued

Discharge Summary, page 2
Patient Name: Timon Andrews

Patient Number: 55-77-34

LABORATORY: Na 138, K 3.6, chloride 106, bicarb 23, blood urea nitrogen 15, creatinine 0.9, glucose 139, white blood cell count 11.2, hemoglobin 17.8, hematocrit 41.1. Platelets were 359,000. Total protein was 6.6, albumin 2.9, lactate 1.7, total bilirubin 0.7, AST 55, alk phos 138, lipase 22. Urinalysis showed specific gravity 1.026, small occult blood in the urine. White blood cell count is 1 per high power field, red blood cells 2 per high power field.

TESTS: Radiographs showed a right mandibular hairline fracture. Cervical spine showed no fractures and no subluxations on three views. Chest radiograph showed no pneumothorax or atelectasis. Pelvis showed no fractures. Magnetic resonance imaging of the lumbar spine was negative for any subluxations or compressions of the spinal cord.

HOSPITAL COURSE: The patient was admitted and was placed on 4CD. His C-collar was cleared the next day. As stated above, the patient received a lumbar magnetic resonance imaging secondary to his paresthesia of his right lower extremity. Magnetic resonance imaging was negative. Neurosurgery was consulted, and it was felt that he had a lumbosacral stretch. ENT was also consulted for his mandibular fracture. The patient was taken to the dental clinic and received panoramic views of his mandible, and it was found that he had a nondisplaced, oblique partial fracture in the right mandible. It was decided at this point that it will heal on its own and the patient would have a soft diet for 2-4 weeks. The dental service was consulted to apply a dental alveolar splint to the mandible and teeth.

It was decided at this point that the ENT would see the patient in one month. Orthopedics was also consulted for the patient's right lower extremity numbness, and orthopedic surgery felt that there was no fracture with specific attention to the patient's anterior tibial region. The patient was started on a soft diet, he tolerated it well and did not have any abdominal pain or any other complaints and was discharged on 9/14/xx. The patient saw the speech pathologist and scored lower than average on the cognitive test. He was scheduled for an outpatient evaluation of cognitive language by the speech pathologist.

DISPOSITION: The patient was stable to go home.

INSTRUCTIONS: The patient was told to restrict activity for at least one week and to have a soft diet. Given Tylenol #3 for pain. Follow-up will be in one week in Dr. Dona's clinic.

_____

Thomas Bloan, MD

TB/bab
d&t: 09/14/xx

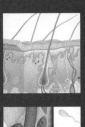

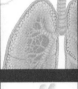

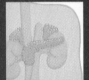

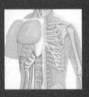

chapter

19 Oncology

Chapter Outline

Objectives

Upon completion of this chapter, you will be able to:

- Describe the types of treatment an oncologist provides.
- Explain the difference between benign and malignant tumors.
- Describe the characteristics, histogenesis, and staging systems of neoplasms.
- Recognize, pronounce, and spell correctly terms related to oncology.
- Describe pathological conditions, diagnostic tests, surgical procedures, and other treatments related to oncology.
- Demonstrate your knowledge of this chapter by successfully completing the activities and analysis of medical records.

About Oncology

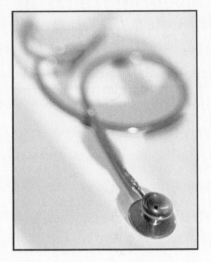

Oncology is the branch of medicine concerned with the study, development, treatment, and prevention of cancer. **Oncologists** are internal medicine physicians who treat both **solid tumors** (e.g., carcinomas, sarcomas) and **liquid tumors** (e.g., hematologic malignancies such as leukemias). Because of the historical association between hematology and oncology, these specialties are often housed as one division (hematology/oncology) in a department of medicine. However, even with this association, there are hematologists who specialize only in nonmalignant blood disorders and oncologists who specialize only in certain solid tumors.

Because there are several types of cancer treatments, oncologists often specialize in one area. **Surgical oncologists** specialize in the surgical resection of cancers. **Radiation oncologists** specialize in the treatment of cancer using radiation therapy. **Medical oncologists** specialize in the use of chemotherapy in the treatment of cancer. Other oncologists specialize in the treatment of cancers related to certain body systems, such as the female reproductive system. These oncologists are called **gynecologic oncologists**. **Pediatric oncologists** specialize in treating cancers that affect children.

A considerable amount of cancer research has taken place in recent decades, and much has been learned about the various types of this disease. Cancer was once a terminal (or fatal) disease. Now it is often a treatable and sometimes a curable disease. As this field of medicine has expanded, specialized and technical terminology has been developed to describe the various cancer diseases and the diagnostic and therapeutic procedures involved in the field of oncology.

To grasp the scope of practice and the role of health-care practitioners in the medical specialty of oncology, it is important to understand the language of medicine that is related to this medical specialty.

Selected Key Terms

DNA (deoxyribonucleic acid) *dē-ŏk-sē-rī-bō-nū-KLĒ-ĭk Ă-sĭd*	A nucleic acid found in all living cells; carries the genetic information of an organism.
human immunodeficiency virus (HIV) *HŪ-măn ĭm-ū-nō-dē-FĬSH-ĕn-sē VĪ-rŭs*	A retrovirus that causes acquired immunodeficiency syndrome (AIDS).
metastasis	The process by which tumor cells spread to different parts of the body.
mutation *mū-TĀ-shŭn*	An unusual change in genetic material occurring spontaneously or by induction. The alteration changes the original expression of the gene. Genes are stable units, but when a mutation occurs, it often is transmitted to later generations.
precursor *PRĒ-kŭr-sor*	One that precedes and indicates the approach of something else. For example, a *polyp* may be a precursor of a cancerous tumor of the colon.
RNA (ribonucleic acid) *rī-bō-nū-KLĒ-ĭk Ă-sĭd*	A nucleic acid found in both the nucleus and cytoplasm of cells that transmits genetic instructions from the nucleus to the cytoplasm. In the cytoplasm, RNA functions in the assembly of proteins. RNA is also found in many viruses, as in the genetic material of AIDS.
RNA virus	Any group of viruses with the core of RNA.

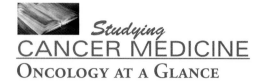

Studying CANCER MEDICINE
ONCOLOGY AT A GLANCE

Oncology is the study of tumors, or **neoplasms,** that develop when cells reproduce at an abnormally high rate. Neoplasms may form in any part of the body. Some of these masses may develop into **malignant** (cancerous) tumors, whereas others may remain **benign** (noncancerous). The beginning or formation of cancer is called **carcinogenesis.** This term designates the process whereby a normal cell develops into a cancerous cell. Cancer is not one disease but many diseases with different causes, manifestations, treatments, and prognoses. There are over 100 different types of this disease caused by the **mutation** of cellular genes. Cancer also occurs when the growth-regulating signals in the cell's environment are ignored, and the growth rate of abnormal cells increases. The growth pattern of normal cells is quite different from that of malignant cells. Normal cells develop in a highly organized pattern. They have specialized structures and functions. This means they are **differentiated** and align themselves in a very orderly arrangement. In contrast, malignant cells multiply in very disorganized ways. They resemble primitive cells that do not have the ability to perform mature cellular functions. Thus, malignant cells are **undifferentiated** or **dedifferentiated** and are characteristic of **anaplasia** (*ana*=without, *plasia*=formation). Whereas normal cells usually experience about 50 to 60 divisions before they die, cancer cells have no division limits and, in a sense, are considered immortal. The transformation of a normal cell to a cancerous cell is still not fully understood. It is certain that the key to malignant transformation results from damage encountered to the genetic material, or **deoxyribonucleic acid (DNA),** of the cell.

Although the incidence of cancer is higher in individuals 60 to 69 years of age, it may occur at any age in any body tissue. Cancer is the leading cause of death in children between the ages of 3 and 15 years. Approximately 25 percent of all Americans alive today will develop cancer during their lifetimes. The American Cancer Society (ACS) reports that approximately 10 million Americans alive today have a history of cancer. The most common site for cancer in women is the breast whereas for men, it is the prostate gland. Prognosis for cancer patients depends on many factors, including but not limited to: age, the stage of the disease, the type of cancer, the state of one's health, and treatment response. See Figure 19–1 for the leading sites of new cancer cases and deaths.

CAUSES OF CANCER

Because all cells reproduce according to instructions contained within the DNA, if something happens to change the deoxyribonucleic acid (DNA) of a cell, the cell will develop, grow, and reproduce according to the new instructions. Let us assume that a genetic change, or mutation, causes a normal cell to become malignant. When this happens, the malignant cell reproduces and passes the malignant trait to its daughter cells, which in turn grow and reproduce as malignant cells. Because malignant cells are **anaplastic,** their DNA stops producing codes that allow the cells to carry out their normal functions. The altered DNA and the altered cellular codes or programs in the anaplastic, mutated cells send new signals that lead to invasion of adjacent tissue, or **metastasis** (Fig. 19–2). Thus, malignant tumors result from the adoption of mutated cellular blueprints. Nevertheless, only some **mutations** lead to cancer. Other mutations lead to other types of diseases that may be relatively harmless. Anything that has the ability to cause mutations, whether cancer-causing or not, is referred to as a *mutagen.* Mutagens that have the ability to cause cancer are referred to as **carcinogens.** Tobacco, asbestos, ultraviolet rays, industrial chemicals, and soot are examples of carcinogens.

Malignant cell transformation is considered to be at least a two-step cellular process. The first, or the *initiation step,* takes place when initiators, such as radiation, viruses, chemicals, and biologic agents, cause alterations in the genetic structure of DNA. Although these alterations are irreversible, they usually are not of significance to body cells until the promotion step of carcinogenesis occurs. During the promotion step, repeated exposure to carcinogenic agents causes the production of mutant cells rather than the normal cells that were originally produced. Mutations are changes in the cell's genetic material (DNA) that may occur spontaneously or may be caused by exposure to carcinogenic agents, genetics, familial factors, diet, and hormone imbalance.

The World Health Organization (WHO) believes that carcinogens may be associated with 60 to 90 percent of all human cancer. The most common carcinogenic agent is the hydrocarbon found in cigarette tar. Over 90 percent of all lung cancer patients are smokers or ex-smokers (Fig. 19–3). Automobile exhaust, fungicides, insecticides, dyes, insulation, industrial chemicals, and certain hormones are examples of the other major chemical carcinogens. Exposure to these carcinogenic agents can be controlled to some degree. Unfortunately, the uncontrollable factor that influences one's susceptibility to developing cancer is

Leading Sites of New Cancer Cases and Deaths ▬ 2000 Estimates

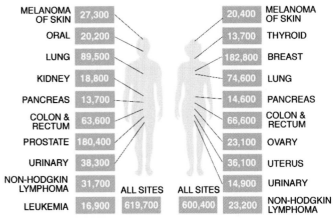

CANCER CASES BY SITE AND SEX

	MEN			WOMEN
MELANOMA OF SKIN	27,300		20,400	MELANOMA OF SKIN
ORAL	20,200		13,700	THYROID
LUNG	89,500		182,800	BREAST
KIDNEY	18,800		74,600	LUNG
PANCREAS	13,700		14,600	PANCREAS
COLON & RECTUM	63,600		66,600	COLON & RECTUM
PROSTATE	180,400		23,100	OVARY
URINARY	38,300		36,100	UTERUS
NON-HODGKIN LYMPHOMA	31,700	ALL SITES / ALL SITES	14,900	URINARY
LEUKEMIA	16,900	619,700 / 600,400	23,200	NON-HODGKIN LYMPHOMA

Excluding basal and squamous cell skin cancers and in situ carcinoma except bladder.

CANCER DEATHS BY SITE AND SEX

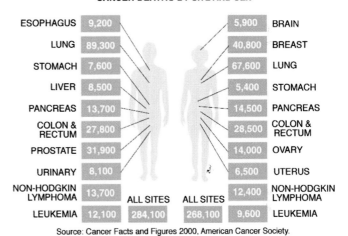

	MEN			WOMEN
ESOPHAGUS	9,200		5,900	BRAIN
LUNG	89,300		40,800	BREAST
STOMACH	7,600		67,600	LUNG
LIVER	8,500		5,400	STOMACH
PANCREAS	13,700		14,500	PANCREAS
COLON & RECTUM	27,800		28,500	COLON & RECTUM
PROSTATE	31,900		14,000	OVARY
URINARY	8,100		6,500	UTERUS
NON-HODGKIN LYMPHOMA	13,700	ALL SITES / ALL SITES	12,400	NON-HODGKIN LYMPHOMA
LEUKEMIA	12,100	284,100 / 268,100	9,600	LEUKEMIA

Figure 19–1 Leading sites of new cancer cases and deaths. (From Cancer Facts and Figures 2000, American Cancer Society.)

Source: Cancer Facts and Figures 2000, American Cancer Society.

heredity. Research indicates that approximately 25 percent of cancer cases are related to a genetic factor.

Radiation

Any kind of radiation such as that from nuclear fission, radioactive substances, sunlight, or x-rays pose an increased risk of cancer. Radiation is the energy given off from a radioactive substance or some other matter. X-rays and radioactive substances emit *ionizing radiation*. This form of radiation releases tiny particles in the cells, which then damage the DNA. Not surprisingly, leukemia can be caused by ionizing radiation and is a serious hazard for radiologists or for anyone who is exposed to radiation around x-ray equipment. Individuals exposed to radioactive materials in large doses at atomic bomb test sites or nuclear power plants are at risk for leukemia, breast, bone, lung, and thyroid cancer. Controlled radiation therapy is used to treat cancer patients by destroying rapidly dividing cells. Radiation can also damage normal cells. The de-

cision to use radiation is made after careful evaluation of the location and tumor vulnerability to other treatments.

Viruses

Although viruses in human cancers are very difficult to ascertain, certain viruses, such as **retroviruses,** are known to be linked to cancer. These cancer-causing viruses belong to the family of *retroviridae*. They are very simple viruses that carry their genetic material in the form of **ribonucleic acid (RNA)** rather than DNA. Retroviruses are transmitted by sexual contact with an infected person, through exposure to infected blood products, and perinatally from an infected mother to the child. Human immunodeficiency virus (HIV), which causes AIDS, is a good illustration of a retrovirus. There are other retroviruses that are associated with *leukemias* and *lymphomas*.

The Epstein-Barr virus (EBV), which causes infectious mononucleosis, is highly suspect as a causative

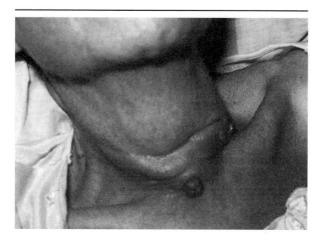

Figure 19–2 *Lesions on the neck that depict an example of cancer metastasis. (From Williams, LS, and Hopper, PD: Understanding Medical Surgical Nursing. FA Davis, Philadelphia 1999, p 157, with permission.)*

agent in Burkitt lymphoma, nasopharyngeal cancers, and Hodgkin disease. The herpes simplex type-2 virus, the causative agent of genital herpes, has been associated with cancer of the cervix uteri. The papillomavirus, a virus that causes genital warts, has been linked with cancer of the cervix uteri and colon cancer, and the hepatitis B virus (HBV) has been associated with liver cancer.

Chemicals

Approximately 80 percent of all cancers are believed to be environmentally related. Because chemicals are present in air, water, soil, food, drugs, and tobacco smoke, these chemical carcinogens are implicated as triggering mechanisms in malignant tumor development. Individuals are at greater risk for can-

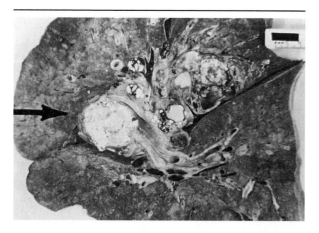

Figure 19–3 *Lung cancer. The black arrow marks the tumor site. (From Williams, LS, and Hopper, PD: Understanding Medical Surgical Nursing. FA Davis, Philadelphia, 1999, p 155, with permission.)*

cer development as their length of exposure time and degree of exposure intensity increase. Most hazardous chemicals produce their toxic effects by altering DNA structure in body sites that are distant from chemical exposure. The most frequently affected sites are the kidneys and liver, most likely owing to their roles in detoxification of chemicals. Other proven environmental carcinogens, some of which are found in the workplace, include asbestos (mesothelioma of the lung); vinyl chloride (angiosarcoma of the liver); airborne aromatic hydrocarbons and benzpyrene (lung cancer); alkylating agents (leukemia); and tobacco (lung, mouth, upper airways, esophagus, pancreas, kidneys, bladder).

Genetic Factors

Genetics plays a part in cancer formation. If DNA damage occurs in cell populations in which chromosomal patterns are abnormal, mutant cell populations may develop. Abnormal chromosomal patterns and cancer have been associated with extra chromosomes, too few chromosomes, or translocated chromosomes. Specific cancers with underlying genetic abnormalities include Burkitt lymphoma, chronic myelogenous leukemias, meningiomas, acute leukemias, and retinoblastomas.

Familial dispositions are evident in some adult and childhood cancers. Usually these cancers occur at multiple sites in one organ or pair of organs in the patient's early years. Cancers linked with familial inheritance include retinoblastomas, nephroblastomas, pheochromocytomas, malignant neurofibromatosis, leukemias, and breast, endometrial, colorectal, stomach, prostate, and lung cancers.

Diet

Especially in the development of gastrointestinal cancer, diet has been implicated as a carcinogen linked with high-protein and high-fat diets. Food additives, such as nitrates, and certain food preparation methods, particularly charbroiling, may also induce carcinogenesis. Diets high in fiber tend to reduce the risk of colon cancer. A diet low in vitamins A, C, and E is associated with cancers of the lungs, esophagus, mouth, larynx, cervix, and breast.

Hormones

Hormonal agents that cause a disturbance in the balance of the body may also promote cancer. Long-term use of the female hormone estrogen can be associated with cancer of the breast, uterus, ovaries, cervix, and vagina. Daughters of women who were treated with diethylstilbestrol (DES) during pregnancy have an increased incidence of developing vaginal cancer. DES is a synthetic hormone with estrogenlike properties used in the past to prevent miscarriage. The role of hormones in carcinogenesis remains controversial.

Immune Factors

The development of cancer may also be linked to failure of the normal immune system. A healthy immune system can often destroy cancer cells before they replicate and become cancerous. It is important to remember that any substance that weakens or alters the immune system puts the individual at risk for cell mutation. Medical research supports the theory that cancer is a symptom of a weakened immune system. An individual with altered immunity is more susceptible to cancer formation when exposed to small amounts of carcinogens compared with someone with a healthy immune system. Immune system suppression allows malignant cells to develop in large numbers. Refer to Chapter 13 for a discussion of immunity.

CHARACTERISTICS OF NEOPLASMS

Neoplasms, also called *tumors*, can develop in any body tissue. They can be either benign (noncancerous) or malignant (cancerous).

Benign neoplasms are new growths that develop in body tissues. They are composed of the same type of cells as the tissue in which they are growing. For example, a benign glandular tumor is composed of the glandular tissue from which it is developing. Benign neoplasms are contained within a capsule (encapsulated) and do not invade the surrounding tissue. They harm the individual only insofar as they place pressure on surrounding structures. If the benign neoplasm remains small and places no pressure on adjacent structures, it often is not removed. When it becomes excessively large, causes pain, or places pressure on other organs or structures, excision is necessary. Benign brain tumors are always very serious because the cranial cavity is enclosed and pressure on other parts of the brain inevitably results. As a general rule, benign tumors are not life threatening. Once they are removed, they usually do not regrow.

Malignant neoplasms are composed of cells that do not necessarily resemble the tissue in which they are growing. They are nonencapsulated masses that grow and spread more relentlessly and may become life threatening. Their cells, which usually resemble immature (undifferentiated or dedifferentiated) cells, invade the surrounding tissue. Malignant cells can also break away from the *primary tumor* and travel via blood or lymph to other body organs, where they form *secondary cancer masses*. This capability of invasiveness, known as **metastasis,** distinguishes cancer cells from the cells of benign neoplasms. See Figure 19–2 for an illustration of invasive metastasis.

Cancer cells consume an exceptional amount of the body's nutrients and lead to weight loss and tissue wasting that eventually contribute to death. They are poorly constructed, loosely formed, and without organization. Cancer cells resemble embryonic, or primitive, cells that do not have the capacities of mature, normal cells. During a person's life, various body tissues normally experience periods of rapid proliferation or growth that must be distinguished from malignant growth activity. To distinguish between normal and abnormal proliferations, the following patterns of cell growth are discussed: *hyperplasia*, *metaplasia*, *dysplasia*, *anaplasia*, and *neoplasia*.

- **Hyperplasia** is an increase in the number of cells of a body part that results from an increased rate of cellular division. Hyperplasia can be *compensatory*, *hormonal*, or *pathological*. Hyperplasia is a common proliferative process during periods of rapid body growth (e.g., fetal and adolescent growth and development) and during epithelial and bone marrow regeneration. It is a normal cellular response when a physiological demand exists. It becomes an abnormal response when growth exceeds the physiological demand.
- **Metaplasia** is an abnormal transformation of a mature, fully differentiated tissue of one kind into a differentiated tissue of another kind. This conversion occurs because of an outside stimulus that affects the parent stem cell. Chronic irritation or inflammation, vitamin deficiency, and chemical exposure may be factors leading to metaplasia. Metaplastic changes may be reversible or may progress to dysplasia.
- **Dysplasia** is any abnormal development of tissues or organs. An alteration in cell growth results in cells that differ in size, shape, and appearance and is often caused by some chronic irritation. Dysplasia can occur from chemicals, radiation, or chronic inflammation or irritation. A common site for dysplasia is the respiratory tract in smokers. Dysplasia can be reversible or can precede irreversible neoplastic change.
- **Anaplasia** is a change in the structure and orientation of cells characterized by a loss of differentiation and reversion to a more primitive form (blasts). Anaplastic cells are poorly differentiated, irregularly shaped, or disorganized with respect to growth and arrangement. They lack normal cellular characteristics and are nearly always malignant.
- **Neoplasia** is the pathological process that results in the formation and growth of a neoplasm.

The characteristics of neoplasms ultimately determine their malignant potential. Benign and malignant cells differ in many cellular growth characteristics.

Some neoplasms are not injurious to a person's health; others may result in death unless the growth can be eliminated or controlled. A comparison of the characteristics of neoplasms is found in Table 19–1.

HISTOGENESIS OF NEOPLASMS

Cancers are identified by the tissue affected, speed of cell growth, cell appearance, and location. Neoplasms occurring in the epithelial cells are termed *carcinoma.* Carcinoma (a solid tumor) is the most common type of cancer and includes cells of the skin, gastrointestinal system, and lungs (Fig. 19–4). Cancer cells affecting connective tissue—including fat, the sheath that contains nerves, cartilage, muscle, and bone—are called *sarcomas.*

To distinguish among the various types of tumors, four major groups are classified according to the type of body tissue in which they originate. This classification is based on the **histogenesis** (*histo=tissue; genesis=forming, producing origin*) of neoplasms and is presented in Table 19–2.

STAGING AND GRADING SYSTEMS

Staging is used to determine the size of a tumor and the existence of metastasis. Pathologists also use a **tumor grading** system which refers to the degree of abnormality of cancer cells compared with normal cells. Treatment options and prognosis for an individual cancer patient are determined on the basis of staging and grading. This approach facilitates the exchange of information about similar types of cancer and their associated survival and response rates.

Ultimately, these classifications can assist in ongoing cancer research. The most common system used for staging tumors is the **TNM staging system.** The

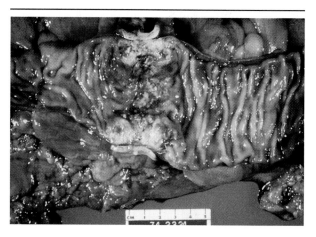

Figure 19–4 *Cancer of the gastrointestinal system: colon cancer. (With permission from the late Dr. W. R. Spence.)*

TNM (tumor, node, metastasis) system stages tumors according to three basic criteria: *T* refers to the size and extent of the primary tumor, *N* indicates the number of area lymph nodes involved, and *M* refers to any metastasis of the primary tumor. A *subscript number* is used to indicate the size or spread of the tumor. For example, the designation of a small tumor (T_2) with no lymph node involvement (N_0) and no evidence of metastasis (M_0) would be designated in a medical report T_2, N_0, M_0. The TNM staging system is presented in Table 19–3.

Along with the TNM staging system, which identifies the tumor size and whether there is evidence of metastasis, a grading system is also used to determine the degree of abnormal cancer cells compared with normal cells. Based on the microscopic appearance of cancer cells, pathologists commonly de-

TABLE 19–1:	**Characteristics of Neoplasms**	
CHARACTERISTICS	**BENIGN**	**MALIGNANT**
Cellular characteristics	Cells resemble normal cells of the tissue from which the tumor originated	Cells often bear little resemblance to the normal cells of the tissue from which they arose
Growth rate	Expands slowly, pushing aside surrounding tissues but not infiltrating	Usually infiltrates surrounding tissues rapidly, expanding in all directions
Metastasis	Does not spread by metastasis; remains localized at original site	Metastasis by way of blood or lymph system, or both, with establishment of secondary tumors
Recurrence	Seldom recurs after surgical removal	Recurrence can be seen after surgical removal and following radiation and chemotherapy
Tissue damage	Does not cause tissue damage unless location interferes with blood flow	Often causes necrosis and ulceration of tissue
Prognosis	Not injurious unless location causes pressure or obstruction to vital organs	Causes death unless growth can be controlled or eliminated

TABLE 19–2: Histogenesis of Neoplasms		
TISSUE TYPE	**BENIGN**	**MALIGNANT**
Epithelial Tumors		
Surface	Papilloma	Papillocarcinoma
Glandular	Adenoma	Adenocarcinoma
Basal cell layer of epidermis		Basal cell carcinoma
Melanocytes of basal layer	Nevus (mole)	Malignant melanoma
Connective Tissue Tumors		
Adipose tissue (fat)	Lipoma	Liposarcoma
Bone	Osteoma	Osteosarcoma
Cartilage	Chondroma	Chondrosarcoma
Fibrous tissue	Fibroma	Fibrosarcoma
Smooth muscle	Leiomyoma	Leiomyosarcoma
Striated muscle	Rhabdomyoma	Rhabdomyosarcoma
Blood vessel tissue	Hemangioma	Hemangiosarcoma
Lymph vessel tissue	Lymphangioma	Lymphangiosarcoma
Nerve Cell Tumors		
Glial tissue	Neuroglioma, glioma	Neurogliosarcoma
Nerve sheaths	Neurilemoma	Neurolemic sarcoma
Meninges	Meningioma	Meningeal sarcoma
Neuroectoderm	Neurocytoma	Neuroblastoma
Hematopoietic Tissue		
White blood cells		Leukemias
Plasma cells		Multiple myeloma
Lymphoid tissue		Lymphoma

scribe tumor grade by four degrees of severity: grades 1, 2, 3, and 4. The cells of grade 1 tumors are often well differentiated; low-grade tumors are generally considered the least aggressive in behavior. Conversely, the cells of grade 4 tumors are undifferentiated; these high-grade tumors are generally the most aggressive in behavior. Patients with grade 1 tumors have the best prognosis, whereas those with grade 4 tumors have the worst prognosis.

Although grade describes most types of cancer, its importance in planning treatment and estimating the future course and outcome of disease (prognosis) is greater for certain types of cancers, such as soft tissue sarcomas, primary brain tumors, lymphomas, and breast and prostate cancers. In addition, specific grading systems are used with some cancers. For example, pathologists use the Gleason system to describe the degree of differentiation of prostate cancer cells. The

TABLE 19–3: The TNM Staging System		
CLASSIFICATION	**STAGING**	**TISSUE INVOLVEMENT**
Tumor		
T_0		No evidence of primary tumor
T_{is}	Stage I	Tumor in situ, indicates no invasion of other tissues
T_1, T_2, T_3, T_4*	Stage II	Progressive increase in tumor size with local metastasis
Nodes		
N_0		Regional lymph nodes not considered to contain tumor
N_1, N_2, N_3, N_4†	Stage III	Metastasis to regional lymph nodes
Metastasis		
M_0		No evidence of metastasis
M_1‡	Stage IV	Distant metastasis

*T_1–T_4 indicate progressive increase in tumor size with local metastasis, T_1 being smallest and T_4 being largest.

†N_1–N_4 designate increasing degree and distant location of spread to regional lymph nodes, N_1 being the smallest and N_4 being largest (number and distance) of lymph node.

‡M designates the absence or presence of metastasis or tumor cells.

American Joint Commission on Cancer has recommended the following guidelines for grading tumors:

Grade 1: Well differentiated, closely resembling normal tissue cells (low grade)

Grade 2: Moderately well differentiated (intermediate grade)

Grade 3: Poorly differentiated (high grade)

Grade 4: Undifferentiated or anaplastic (high grade)

Activity 19-1: Competency Verification
Oncology

carcinogenesis	grade 4	mutation
differentiated cells	histogenesis	T_0
DNA (deoxyribonucleic acid)	M_0	TNM staging
grade 1	malignancy	undifferentiated cells

Match the terms or abbreviations listed above with the definitions in the numbered list:

1. _____ the cell's genetic material.

2. _____ a system used to determine the size of a tumor and existence of metastasis.

3. _____ for no evidence of a primary tumor.

4. _____ notation for no evidence of metastasis in the medical report.

5. _____ normal cells that develop in a highly organized pattern.

6. _____ tumor grade for patients with the best prognoses.

7. _____ tumor grade for the patients with the worst prognoses.

8. _____ literally means beginning or formation of cancer.

9. _____ change in the cell's genetic material (DNA). It may occur spontaneously or be caused by chemicals, viruses, or radiation.

10. _____ cells that multiply in a very disorganized pattern; also called *anaplastic cells.*

Correct Answers _____ **× 10 =** _____ **% Score**

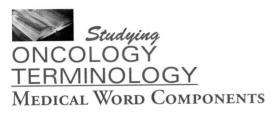

Studying
ONCOLOGY
TERMINOLOGY
MEDICAL WORD COMPONENTS

Combining Forms

Combining Forms: Neoplasms

Combining Form	Meaning	EXAMPLE	
		Term/Pronunciation	Definition
aden/o	gland	**aden**/o/carcin/oma ăd-ĕ-nō-kăr-sĭn-Ō-mă	a malignant tumor (-*oma*) of glandular epithelium
blast/o	embryonic cell	neur/o/**blast**/oma nū-rō-blăs-TŌ-mă	a malignant neoplasm characterized by immature, only slightly differentiated nerve cells of embryonic type *The combining form* neur/o *means "nerve"; the suffix* -oma *means "tumor."*
carcin/o	cancer	**carcin**/o/genesis kăr-sĭ-nō-JĔN-ĕ-sĭs	forming, producing, or origin (-*genesis*)
cauter/o	heat, burn	**cauter**/ization kaw-tĕr-ĭ-ZĀ-shŭn	process of (-*ization*) burning a part of the body by cautery
chem/o	chemical, drug	**chem**/o/therapy kē-mō-THĔR-ă-pē	treatment (-*therapy*) of disease by means of chemical substances or drugs; usually used in reference to neoplastic disease of cancer
cry/o	cold	**cry**/o/surgery krī-ō-SĔR-jĕr-ē	use of subfreezing temperature to destroy tissue
hist/o	tissue	**hist**/o/path/o/logy hĭs-tō-pă-THŎL-ō-jē	the study of (-*logy*) diseases (*path/o*) involving the tissue cells
immun/o	immune, immunity	**immun**/o/therapy ĭm-ū-nō-THĔR-ă-pē	the application of immunologic knowledge and techniques to prevent and treat (-*therapy*) disease
leiomy/o	smooth muscle (visceral)	**leiomy**/o/sarc/oma lī-ō-mī-ō-săr-KŌ-mă	a malignant neoplasm composed of smooth (visceral) muscle *The combining form* sarc/o *means "flesh" (connective tissue); the suffix* -oma *means "tumor." The suffix* -sarcoma *refers to a malignant tumor of connective tissue.*

Combining Forms: Neoplasms (Continued)

Combining Form	Meaning	EXAMPLE	
		Term/Pronunciation	**Definition**
leuk/o	white	**leuk**/emia *loo-KĒ-mē-ă*	hematologic malignancies (liquid tumors) in which immature blood cells multiply at the expense of normal blood cells *As normal cells are depleted from the body, anemia, infection, hemorrhage, or death may result. Leukemia literally means "white blood."*
mut/a	genetic change	**mut**/a/gen *MŪ-tă-jĕn*	any agent that promotes or produces (*-gen*) a mutation or causes an increase in the rate of mutational events *Examples of mutagens are radioactive substances, x-rays, and certain chemicals.*
myel/o	bone marrow, spinal cord	**myel**/oma *mī-ĕ-LŌ-mă*	tumor (*-oma*) composed of cells derived from hemopoietic tissues of the bone marrow *Hemopoietic means "pertaining to or related to the formation of blood cells."*
onc/o	tumor	**onc**/o/logy *ŏng-KŎL-ō-jē*	study of tumors
rhabdomy/o	striated (skeletal) muscle	**rhabdomy**/oma *răb-dō-mī-Ō-mă*	a striated muscular tissue tumor (*-oma*)
sarc/o	flesh (connective tissue)	**sarc**/oma *săr-KŌ-mă*	a malignant tumor (*-oma*) of connective tissue

Prefixes and Suffixes

In this section, prefixes are listed alphabetically and highlighted, whereas key suffixes are defined in the right-hand column.

Prefixes

Prefix	Meaning	EXAMPLE	
		Term/Pronunciation	**Definition**
ana-	without, not	**ana**/plasia *ăn-ă-PLĀ-zē-ă*	loss of cellular differentiation, characteristic of most malignancies *The suffix -plasia means "formation," "growth."*
dys-	bad, painful, difficult	**dys**/plasia *dĭs-PLĀ-zē-ă*	any abnormal development of tissues or organs *The suffix -plasia means "formation," "growth."*
hyper-	excessive, above normal	**hyper**/plasia *hī-pĕr-PLĀ-zē-ă*	excessive proliferation of normal cells in the normal tissue arrangement of an organ *The suffix -plasia means "formation," "growth."*
hypo-	under, below normal	**hypo**/chrom/ia *hī-pō-KRŌ-mē-ă*	a condition (*-ia*) of the blood in which the red blood cells have a reduced hemoglobin content *The combining form chrom/o means "color."*
meta-	change, beyond	**meta**/stasis *mĕ-TĂS-tă-sĭs*	the process by which tumor cells spread to distant parts of the body *The suffix -stasis means "standing still."*
neo-	new	**neo**/plasm *NĒ-ō-plăzm*	new formation or growth (*-plasm*)

Activity 19–2: Competency Verification
Medical Word Components

Check the box [✓] as you complete each numbered section.

[   ] **1.** Review the medical word components in the previous section. Then pronounce each word aloud.

[   ] **2.** For the following words, first write the suffix and its meaning. Then translate the meaning of the remaining components starting with the first part of the word.

> **Example:** mono/nucle/ar
> **Answer:** *ar*=pertaining to, relating to; one; nucleus

1. hemat/oma _____

2. carcin/o/genesis _____

3. chem/o/therapy _____

4. myel/oma _____

5. neo/plasm _____

6. mut/a/gen _____

7. ana/plasia _____

8. sarc/oma _____

9. onc/o/logy _____

10. neur/o/blast _____

11. cauter/ization _____

12. leiomy/o/sarc/oma _____

13. hyper/plasia _____

14. meta/stasis _____

15. oste/o/sarc/oma _____

Correct Answers _____ **× 6.67 =** _____ **% Score**

PATHOLOGICAL CONDITIONS

PATHOLOGICAL CONDITION	DESCRIPTION
choriocarcinoma kō-rē-ō-kăr-sĭ-NŌ-mă *chorio=chorion* *carcin=cancer* *oma=tumor*	An epithelial malignancy of fetal origin that develops from the chorionic portion of the products of conception. The primary tumor usually appears in the uterus as a soft, dark red, crumbling mass that may invade and destroy the uterine wall. It may metastasize through lymph or blood vessels, forming secondary hemorrhagic and necrotic tumors in the vaginal wall, vulva, lymph nodes, lungs, liver, and brain. The urine often contains much more chorionic gonadotropin than is expected in pregnancy.
leukemia loo-KĒ-mē-ă *leuk=white* *emia=blood*	A malignant disease of white blood cells, which affects all age groups. The immature white blood cells (blast cells) generate in an explosive fashion in the bone marrow, the lymph tissue, and the spleen. As the disease progresses, the bone marrow continues to produce large numbers of useless cells. The peripheral circulation is filled with the abnormal cells, and the bone marrow is packed with the blast cells; production of most other normal cells is impossible. Leukemias are classified as either *acute* or *chronic*, and either *lymphoid* or *myeloid*. Symptoms of acute leukemias begin very suddenly with an onset of stormy symptoms; chronic leukemias develop very slowly. Lymphoid leukemias affect the lymphocytes; myeloid leukemias originate in the bone marrow.
acute lymphocytic leukemia (ALL) ă-KŪT lĭm-fō-SĬT-ĭk loo-KĒ-mē-ă	A type of leukemia that involves abnormal growth of the lymphocyte precursors (lymphoblasts); commonly affects children under the age of 15 years.
acute myelocytic leukemia (AML) ă-KŪT mī-ĕ-lō-SĬT-ĭk loo-KĒ-mē-ă	A leukemia of uncontrolled proliferation of immature granulocytes (myeloblasts); also called *acute myelogenous leukemia.*
chronic lymphocytic leukemia (CLL) KRŎ-nĭk lĭm-fō-SĬT-ĭk loo-KĒ-mē-ă	A leukemia characterized by an excessive number of lymphocytes found in the marrow, spleen, and lymph nodes; usually affects adults over age 40. CLL follows a slow, progressive course.
chronic myelocytic leukemia (CML) KRŎ-nĭk mī-ĕ-lō-SĬT-ĭk loo-KĒ-mē-ă *myelo=bone marrow,* *spinal cord* *gen=forming, producing,* *origin*	A leukemia characterized by a proliferation of granular leukocytes and, often, of megakaryocytes in the marrow and bloodstream. The disease occurs most frequently in mature adults; also called chronic myelogenous leukemia and chronic granulocytic leukemia (CGL).
meningioma měn-ĭn-jē-Ō-mă *meningi=meninges* *oma=tumor*	Slow-growing tumor of the membranes enveloping the brain and spinal cord. Meningiomas usually occur in adults.
mesothelioma měs-ō-thē-lē-Ō-mă	A rare malignant tumor of the mesothelium of the pleura, pericardium, or peritoneum.

Pathological Conditions (Continued)

PATHOLOGICAL CONDITION	DESCRIPTION
myeloma mī-ĕl-Ō-mă *myelo=bone marrow, spinal cord* *oma=tumor*	Neoplasm consisting of a profusion of cells typical of the bone marrow; these cells may develop in many sites and cause extensive destruction of the bone.
multiple	A neoplastic disease characterized by the infiltration of bone and bone marrow by myeloma cells, forming multiple tumor masses that lead to pathological fractures. The condition is usually progressive and generally fatal.
retinoblastoma rĕt-ĭ-nō-blăs-TŌ-mă *retino=retina* *blast=embryonic cell* *oma=tumors*	A malignant *glioma* of the retina, usually unilateral, that occurs in young children and usually is hereditary. Characteristic signs are diminished vision, *strabismus*, retinal detachment, and an abnormal pupillary reflex. The rapidly growing tumor may invade the brain and metastasize to distant sites. Treatment includes removal of the eye and as much of the optic nerve as possible, followed by radiation and chemotherapy.

Clinical Procedures and Laboratory Tests

Clinical Procedures

PROCEDURE	DESCRIPTION
apheresis ă-fĕr-Ē-sĭs	A procedure in which blood is temporarily withdrawn and one or more components are removed from it by means of a continuous-flow separator; the process is similar to hemodialysis, because treated blood is reinfused into the patient. The removal of leukocytes is called *leukapheresis;* the removal of cellular material is called *cytapheresis;* and the removal of noncellular materials is called *plasmapheresis.* Apheresis is used to treat various disease conditions and to harvest blood cells.
biopsy BĪ-ŏp-sē *bi=life* *opsy=view of*	Obtaining a representative tissue sample for microscopic examination, usually to establish a diagnosis. The tissue may be obtained surgically or through a syringe and needle. The procedure can be guided by computed tomography, ultrasonography, magnetic resonance imaging, or radiography. The three most common biopsy methods are the excisional, incisional, and needle methods. These biopsy methods are discussed in the Diagnostic Surgery section.
bone marrow biopsy	The extraction of a small amount of bone marrow tissue from the bone marrow cavity through a needle. This procedure is used for microscopic examination and evaluation and for assessing and diagnosing blood disorders such as anemias, leukemias, and cytopenias.
exfoliative cytology ĕks-FŌ-lē-ă-tĭv sī-TŎL-ō-jē	Microscopic examination of cells for diagnostic purposes. The cells are obtained from lesions, sputum, secretions, or urine, or from the region of suspected disease by aspiration, scraping, a smear, or washing of the tissue. An example of exfoliative cytology is the *Pap test.* It is used in routine examinations to detect carcinoma of the cervix or vagina.

Laboratory Tests

TEST	DESCRIPTION
acid phosphatase Ă-sĭd FŎS-fă-tās	Detects enzyme concentration in the blood; an elevated level is found in men with prostate cancer.
alpha-fetoprotein (AFP) ĂL-fă fē-tō-PRŌ-tēn	Elevated levels of AFP are found in the serum of patients with testicular and liver cancer.
beta-HCG	Specific test to detect the presence of *human chorionic gonadotropin.* HCG is present in the serum of patients with testicular cancer and trophoblastic disorders.
CA-125	Blood test to detect the presence of cell surface protein produced by ovarian cancer cells; used to confirm a diagnosis of recurrence of cancer.
carcinoembryonic antigen (CEA) kăr-sĭn-ō-ĕm-brē-ŎN-ĭk ĂN-tĭ-jĕn	Blood test to measure carcinoma-associated embryonic proteins. CEA concentration in the blood is used to evaluate recurrent or disseminated disease and in monitoring treatment effectiveness. Elevated levels of CEA are found in the blood of patients with gastrointestinal, lung, and breast carcinomas.
human chorionic gonadotropin (HCG, hCG) HŪ-măn kor-ē-ŎN-ĭk gŏn-ă-dō-TRŌ-pĭn	Specific test to detect the presence of *human chorionic gonadotropin.* HCG is present in the serum of patients with testicular cancer and trophoblastic disorders.
prostate-specific antigen (PSA) test PRŎS-tāt spĕ-SĬF-ĭk ĂN-tĭ-jĕn	Blood test to screen for prostate cancer; an elevated level of a protein produced by the prostate indicates the possibility of a tumor or other disease of the prostate.

Activity 19–3: Clinical Application

Pathological Conditions, Clinical Procedures, and Laboratory Tests

acid phosphatase
alpha-fetoprotein (AFP)
apheresis
CA-125

carcinoembryonic antigen (CEA)
exfoliative cytology
human chorionic gonadotropin (HCG)
leukemia
meningioma

mesothelioma
multiple myeloma
prostate-specific antigen (PSA)
retinoblastoma

Match the terms listed above with the definitions given in the numbered list:

1. _____ a slow-growing tumor of the membranes enveloping the brain and spinal cord; usually occurs in adults.

2. _____ removal of unwanted or pathological components from a patient's blood by means of a continuous-flow separator; the process is similar to hemodialysis, because treated blood is reinfused into the patient.

3. _____ blood test to screen for prostate cancer or other diseases of the prostate.

4. _____ elevated levels are found in patients with gastrointestinal, lung, and breast carcinomas.

5. _____ blood test to detect the presence of cell surface protein produced by ovarian cancer cells; used to confirm a diagnosis of recurrence of cancer.

6. _____ a malignant disease of the WBCs; affects all age groups.

7. _____ a malignant *glioma* of the retina that occurs in young children.

8. _____ a neoplastic disease characterized by numerous tumor masses in the bone marrow, causing bones to fracture.

9. _____ microscopic examination of cells for diagnostic purposes.

10. _____ elevated levels of this protein, which are found in the serum of patients with testicular and liver cancer.

Correct Answers _____ **× 10 =** _____ **% Score**

Cancer Treatments

As new technology develops, the treatment of cancer undergoes continuous changes. Each patient's treatment plan depends on the type, stage, localization, and responsiveness of the tumor, as well as the patient's limitations.

Surgery

Once the principal method of cancer treatment, surgery is now regularly combined with chemotherapy, radiation therapy, and immunotherapy. Surgery removes the bulk of the tumor, whereas the other treatments discourage residual cell proliferation. Today surgery is more precise because of improved diagnostic equipment, operating procedures, and advances in preoperative and postoperative care. Cancer surgery may be diagnostic, palliative, preventive, or specific.

Diagnostic Surgery

This type of surgery is usually performed to obtain a biopsy from a suspicious growth to analyze the tissues and cells of the suspected malignancy and establish a diagnosis. The three most common methods are excisional, incisional, and needle biopsies.

- **Excisional biopsy** is most frequently used for biopsies of the skin, the upper respiratory tract, and the upper and lower portions of the gastrointestinal tract in which removal of the entire tumor is often possible. This procedure may cure small neoplasms.

- **Incisional biopsy** is used if the tumor mass is too large to be removed. It is important that the biopsy specimen be representative of the tumor mass so that the pathologist can provide an accurate diagnosis. Both excisional and incisional approaches are often endoscopic procedures. Surgical incision is often required to determine the anatomic extent or the stage of the tumor. The remaining tumor may be treated with other forms of extensive surgical procedures such as chemotherapy and/or radiation therapy.

- **Needle biopsy** is used to sample suspicious masses that are difficult to access, such as some growths in the breast, lung, liver, and kidney. The procedure is fast, relatively inexpensive, and relatively easy to perform. Usually the patient experiences minimal and temporary physical discomfort. In addition, the degree to which the surrounding tissue is disturbed is kept to a minimum, thus decreasing the likelihood of cancer cell dissemination (seeding). However, there is a chance that even the most skilled physician will obtain too small of a tissue sample. In this case, a full description of the cellular types is not possible.

Palliative Surgery

This type of surgery is used when cure of the cancer is not possible. The goal of this type of surgery is to reduce the manifestations and difficulties related to the cancer and to prolong life. Palliative surgery is performed in an attempt to relieve complications of cancer, such as ulcerations, obstructions, hemorrhage, pain, or infection. It includes tumor resection for relief of bowel obstruction and simple mastectomies for ulcerative breast disease. In advanced cancers, palliative surgery may be performed to sever nerves and to alleviate pain. If warranted, surgical removal of hormone-producing glands that might enhance tumor growth may be performed. These glands include the pituitary glands, the adrenals, the ovaries, and the testes.

Preventive Surgery

This type of surgery may be performed to prevent the development of cancer. For example, polyps of the colon are removed because they are thought to be precancerous tumors. Recently, more aggressive surgeries are being performed as preventive measures in persons who are at a significantly high risk for cancer because of personal and family history. The more common preventive surgeries are *colectomies* and *mastectomies*.

Specific Surgeries

These types of surgery are performed to remove cancerous tissue and hopefully cure the patient. They include, but are not limited to, the *en-bloc resection, cryosurgery, electrocauterization,* and *exenteration.*

- **En-bloc resection** may be performed during a radical mastectomy, colectomy, or gastrectomy. It includes the removal of a tumor and a large area of surrounding tissue that contains lymph nodes.
- **Cryosurgery** involves the use of subfreezing temperatures to destroy tissue. This procedure is used to treat bladder, brain, prostate tumors, and papillomas by freezing the malignant tissue.
- **Electrocauterization** is the application of a needle or snare heated by electric current for the destruction of tissue. This procedure is used to burn off and destroy diseased tissue. It is the preferred method of treating tumors of the rectum and colon when surgical removal is not possible.
- **Exenteration** is a wide resection that includes the excision of an organ(s) and surrounding tissue. It is performed to treat large primary tumors. For example, a carcinoma of the fallopian tubes would include excision of fallopian tubes and ovaries as well as the adjacent tissue surrounding these structures.

Chemotherapy

Chemotherapy involves the use of chemical agents (drugs) designed to exert actions against rapidly dividing cells, such as cancer cells. However, in our bodies, there are many normal cells that tend to divide at a fast rate, such as blood cells, hair cells, and cells lining the gastrointestinal (GI) tract. As a result, chemotherapy also tends to affect these cells, causing decreased red and white blood cell counts, hair loss, gingivitis, and inflammation of the GI tract.

The *cytotoxic agents* used in cancer treatments generally function in the same manner as ionizing radiation. They do not kill the cancer cells directly but instead impair their ability to replicate. Most of the commonly used anticancer drugs act by interfering with DNA and RNA activities associated with cell division. Useful for controlling residual disease or as an adjunct to surgery or radiation therapy, chemotherapy can induce long remissions and possibly cures, especially in patients with childhood leukemia, Hodgkin disease (discussed in Chapter 13), choriocarcinoma, and testicular cancer. The aim of chemotherapy as a palliative treatment is to improve the patient's quality of life by relieving pain and other symptoms. Chemotherapy drugs are often used in combination with radiation treatments for their *synergistic* (acting or working together) effect. For example, a cytotoxic agent may be used to render a tumor cell more sensitive to the effects of ionizing radiation. This allows the cancer to be controlled with smaller doses of radiation.

Most chemotherapeutic agents are used alone or in combination for the treatment of cancer. They may also be used in combination with other cancer treatments. Toxicity from most chemotherapeutic agents includes adverse side effects on the GI tract, skin, and bone marrow, as well as long-standing fatigue. Five selected groups of chemotherapy drugs are discussed next.

- **Alkylating drugs:** These agents inhibit cell growth and their division by reacting with DNA. The reaction causes the DNA strand to break apart or to bind together incorrectly. The cell is then unable to divide properly and loses its ability to replicate. Toxic side effects include diarrhea, nausea, vomiting, hematuria, alopecia, tiredness, loss of appetite, and cardiac damage. With suspension of treatment, most side effects disappear.
- **Antibiotics:** A special class of antibiotics is used as chemotherapy drugs. All chemotherapeutic antibiotics act on DNA to inhibit synthesis of it or to break or bind DNA strands so that cell division cannot be completed. Chemotherapeutic antibiotics are never used to treat bacterial infection. Toxic side effects include nausea, vomiting, tiredness, stomatitis, alopecia, vomiting, red urine, dizziness, drowsiness, and tissue necrosis.
- **Antimetabolites:** These drugs prevent cell growth by either blocking the replication of DNA or by inhibiting the production of substances that are the necessary components of DNA. Once cell metabolism is disrupted, the cell dies. Toxic side effects include diarrhea, nausea, vomiting, loss of appetite, sores in the mouth, fever, and chills.
- **Hormonal agents:** Certain tumors, specifically those arising from tissue influenced by the

hormones estrogen, progesterone, and androgen, show regression when treated with a drug that produces the opposite hormonal effect. For example, estrogen given to a patient with testicular cancer changes the favorable hormonal environment provided by endogenous androgens (male hormones) and causes the tumor cells to die. The hormonal drugs used to treat breast, ovarian, or endometrial cancer include androgens/progestin and estrogen-blocking drugs. Toxic side effects are hot flashes, weight gain, nausea, and bone pain.

- **Antimitotics:** These drugs act during a very specific point in cell division (mitosis) known as metaphase that occurs just before the chromosomes divide and migrate to each end of the cell. Antimitotics stop metaphase and prevent any of the subsequent steps of cell division. They are often used in combination with other chemotherapy drugs. Common side effects include nerve damage, alopecia, and myelosuppression.

Radiation Therapy

The goal of radiation therapy (also called *radiotherapy* or *irradiation*) is to destroy the rapidly dividing cancer cells and at the same time avoid damage to normal cells as much as possible. Unfortunately, some cancers are situated in a place where radiation might cause serious harm to surrounding tissues. Moreover, some cancers are *radioresistant*, that is, they are not affected by radiation within the safe dosage range. As with other types of cancer therapy, radiation may be used alone or in combination with other forms of treatment. Radiation treatment approaches include *external beam radiation* (also called *teletherapy*), in which the source of radiation is external to the patient's body, and *brachytherapy*, in which radioactive "seeds" are temporarily implanted in the patient. More than half of all cancer patients receive some type of radiation therapy. The decision to use radiation is often based on cancer site and size. Radiation treatment may be curative if the disease is localized. The effects of irradiation of the body include cell death because ionizing radiation disrupts DNA and interferes with cell replication and growth. Recovery from radiation damage to normal tissue does occur, but the degree varies, depending on the radiosensitivity of the normal tissue. The radiation dose is determined by the size, type, and location of the tumor. Generally, the adverse effects of radiation occur in the skin, mucous membranes, and bone marrow. Hair begins to fall out, and eating may be difficult because of the nausea, vomiting, and mucosal damage to the mouth and stomach. Many effects, such as fatigue and, in some cases, sterility, extend beyond the course of treatment. Fortunately, new developments in cancer radiology are continually appearing for both curative and palliative purposes.

Immunotherapy

Immunotherapy, also known as *biotherapy*, is a recent approach in the treatment of tumors that stimulates the body's own immune defenses. When combined with surgery, chemotherapy, or radiation, immunotherapy may be most effective in early cancer stages. Some tumors overwhelm the body's immune system. Radiation therapy and chemotherapy may also suppress the immune system. Thus, treatment to enhance the immune system's response may be indicated. Because much immunotherapy remains investigational, its availability may depend on the treatment facility. Many adverse effects remain unpredictable.

Stem Cell Transplantation

Stem cells are immature cells destined to develop into white blood cells, red blood cells, and platelets. Most stem cells are found in the bone marrow, the spongy tissue found inside the bones. Some stem cells are also found in the bloodstream, in *peripheral blood*, and in the umbilical cord. Both bone marrow transplantation (BMT) and peripheral blood stem cell transplantation (PBSCT) are **stem cell transplantation procedures.** These procedures are used to restore stem cells that were destroyed by diseases, such as leukemia and lymphoma. The cells may also be destroyed because of the administration of high doses of chemotherapy or radiation necessary to eradicate certain cancers, such as breast cancer. High-dose chemotherapy and radiation therapies necessary to fight refractory cancer not only destroy rapidly dividing cancer cells but can also damage a patient's stem cells. Without these cells, patients with cancer are likely to die, because they cannot produce the new blood cells that are needed to carry oxygen, fight disease, and prevent bleeding. Thus stem cells gathered from healthy bone marrow, peripheral blood, or an umbilical cord can restore the patient's ability to produce the blood cells he or she needs. The healthy stem cells can be gathered either from the patient before treatment (**autologous transplant**) or from a donor (**allogeneic transplant**).

For a **bone marrow transplant,** 400 to 700 mL (500 mL is a little more than half a quart) of marrow is harvested (removed) by aspiration with a special needle, usually from the iliac crest of the pelvic bone of the patient or from a compatible donor. After the aspiration is performed on the donor, the marrow is filtered and transplanted intravenously (IV) into the recipient to repopulate the recipient's marrow. Utmost care is given to match the tissue and blood cells of the donor and the recipient to ensure compatibility. (See Chapter 15.)

For **peripheral blood stem cell transplantation,** the blood cells are removed from the circulating blood rather than the bone marrow. The patient or donor is given a medication for 4 or 5 days to increase the number of stem cells being released in the bloodstream. Next, the blood is removed through a catheter and filtered through a machine that removes the stem cells, and the remaining blood is returned to the patient. This process is called **apheresis,** and it usually takes 4 to 5 hours to complete. The stem cells are frozen until ready to be given to the patient intravenously when needed.

Prior to stem cell transplantation, total body irradiation may be performed on the recipient to destroy any remaining malignant cells. Immunosuppressants may be used to allow a better acceptance of the donor graft. Once infused into the bloodstream, the new marrow cells travel to the bone marrow where they belong. It takes 2 to 4 weeks for the implanted marrow cells to mature in the recipient.

Generally, patients who receive autologous transplants experience a quicker, easier recovery period because their own cells are being returned to their body. However, the risk of relapse of the original disease may be greater than with an allogeneic transplant. With allogeneic transplants, there is the possibility of the body's rejecting the donated tissue cells (graft). Nevertheless, the graft itself can produce an immune response against the recipient's body (host body), most often the liver, the skin, and the digestive tract. This can cause an acute or chronic condition called **graft-versus-host disease (GVHD).** It can be mild or very severe and can occur any time after the transplantation, even years later. Approximately 40 to 50 percent of allogeneic transplant patients develop moderate to severe GVHD.

In addition to leukemia and lymphoma, stem cell transplantation may also be effective in treating patients with other hematologic malignancies (e.g., aplastic anemia, multiple myeloma), solid-tumor cancers, and certain immunodeficiency diseases.

PHARMACOLOGY

Selected chemotherapy drugs are discussed earlier in the Chemotherapy section of this chapter.

DRUG CLASSIFICATION	THERAPEUTIC ACTION
anticoagulants *ăn-tĭ-kō-ĂG-ū-lănts*	Drugs that prevent clot formation and also decrease the risk of a stroke in patients who had transient ischemic attacks; used to prevent clots from forming postoperatively after heart, valve, or vascular surgery, and to prevent coagulation in stored blood that is later used for transfusions.
antiemetics *ăn-tĭ-ē-MĔT-ĭks*	Drugs used to control nausea and vomiting associated with chemotherapy and radiation therapy.
thrombolytic enzymes *thrŏm-bō-LĬT-ĭk ĔN-zimz*	Drugs used to dissolve blood clots that have already formed in the body.

❖ ABBREVIATIONS

ABBREVIATION	MEANING	ABBREVIATION	MEANING
ALL	acute lymphocytic leukemia	**CML**	chronic myelogenous leukemia
AML	acute myelogenous leukemia	**CR**	complete response, complete
ANA	antinuclear antibody		remission
BMT	bone marrow transplant	**DES**	diethylstilbestrol
CEA	carcinoembryonic antigen	**diff.**	differential (white blood count)
CGL	chronic granulocytic leukemia	**DNA**	deoxyribonucleic acid
chem, chemo	chemotherapy	**ER**	estrogen receptor
CLL	chronic lymphocytic leukemia;	**GVHD**	graft-versus-host disease
	cholesterol-lowering lipid	**HCG**	human chorionic gonadotropin

ABBREVIATION	MEANING	ABBREVIATION	MEANING
NED	no evidence of disease	PSA	prostate-specific antigen
NHL	non-Hodgkin lymphoma	RNA	ribonucleic acid
PD	progression of a disease	TNM	tumor, nodes, metastases
poly, PMN,	polymorphonuclear leukocyte	WHO	World Health Organization
PMNL		XRT	radiation therapy
PR	partial response, partial remission	V_4, V_5	fourth chest (lead), fifth chest (lead)

Activity 19–4: Clinical Application
Diagnostic Tests, Treatments, and Pharmacology

allogeneic transplant   chemotherapy   immunotherapy
antiemetics   cryosurgery   needle biopsy
antimetabolites   exenteration   palliative surgery
autologous transplant   hormonal agents   radiation

Match the terms listed above with the definitions in the numbered list:

1. _____ a wide resection that includes the excision of a(n) organ(s) and surrounding tissue.

2. _____ the use of chemicals to destroy cancer cells.

3. _____ drugs that control nausea and vomiting.

4. _____ surgery that does not cure cancer but is performed in an attempt to relieve complications of cancer, such as obstructions, ulcerations, or pain.

5. _____ use of subfreezing temperature to destroy tissue.

6. _____ a recent approach in treatment of tumors that stimulates the body's own immune defenses; also called *biotherapy*.

7. _____ transplant from a donor who is a relative or unrelated person with compatible blood cells.

8. _____ drugs that prevent cell growth by either blocking replication of DNA or by inhibiting the production of substances that are the necessary components of DNA.

9. _____ the use of estrogen, progesterone, and androgen to shrink tumor cells.

10. _____ treatment to destroy cancer cells; also known as *radiotherapy*.

Correct Answers _____ × 10 = _____ **% Score**

Activity 19–5: Build Medical Words

Diagnostic, Symptomatic, and Surgical Terms

Use *onc/o* (tumor) to build medical words meaning:

1. study of tumors _____

2. specialist in the study of tumors _____

3. forming, producing, origin of a tumor _____

4. separation, destruction, loosening of a tumor (cells) _____

Use *carcin/o* (cancer) to build medical words meaning:

5. cancerous tumor _____

6. forming, producing, or origin of cancer _____

7. morbid fear of cancer _____

Use *-oma* (tumor) to build medical words meaning:

8. tumor composed of fat (benign) _____

9. tumor of glandular tissue (benign) _____

10. tumor composed of smooth muscle (benign) _____

11. tumor composed of nerve cells (benign) _____

Use *-sarcoma* (malignant tumor of connective tissue) to build medical words meaning:

12. sarcoma of bone _____

13. sarcoma of smooth muscle _____

14. sarcoma of cartilage _____

15. sarcoma of striated (skeletal) muscle _____

> **Correct Answers** _____ × 6.67 = _____ % Score

MEDICAL RECORDS

Authentic documents of an operative report and a discharge summary are included in this section.

The following dictionary and reading exercise and the medical record analysis will help you develop skills to abstract information and master the terminology in the reports. Accurate interpretation is important because this type of information is used in numerous areas of the medical practice, such as initiation of treatments, evaluation of patients' progress, and completion of insurance claims.

Reading and Dictionary Exercise

Place a check mark [✓] after you complete the exercise.

[   ] **1.** Underline the following words in the reports as you read the operative report and the discharge summary aloud. These medical records can be found at the end of the chapter.

[   ] **2.** Use a medical dictionary and Appendix F, Part 2 to complete this exercise.

Note: You are not expected to fully understand all parts of the medical records. The important aspect of this exercise is to use all available resources to complete it. Eventually you will master the terminology and format of these reports.

>>> MEDICAL RECORD 19–1: OPERATIVE REPORT

Term	Pronunciation	Meaning
adenocarcinoma	ă-dĕ-nō-kăr-sĭn-Ō-mă	_____
intubated	ĬN-tū-bā-tĕd	_____
apex	Ā-pĕks	_____
cystoscopy	sĭs-TŎS-kō-pē	_____
panendoscopy	păn-ĕn-DŎS-kō-pē	_____
Flomax	FLŌ-măks	_____
Detrol	DĔT-rŏl	_____
Levaquin	LĔV-ă-kwĭn	_____

>>> MEDICAL RECORD 19–2: DISCHARGE SUMMARY

Term	Pronunciation	Meaning
anorexia	ăn-ō-RĔK-sē-ă	_____
cerebral	sĕ-RĒ-brăl	_____
atrophy	ĂT-rō-fē	_____
needle biopsy	NĒ-dl BĪ-ŏp-sē	_____
malignant	mă-LĬG-nănt	_____
adenocarcinoma	ăd-ĕ-nō-kăr-sĭn-Ō-mă	_____
echocardiogram	ĕk-ō-KĂR-dē-ō-grăm	_____
ventricular	vĕn-TRĬK-ū-lăr	_____

hypertrophy	hī-PĔR-trō-fē	_____
hemoglobin	hē-mō-GLŌ-bĭn	_____
hematocrit	hē-MĂT-ō-krĭt	_____
neutrophils	NŪ-trō-fĭls	_____
sedimentation rate	sĕd-ĭ-mĕn-TĀ-shŭn rāt	_____
electrolytes	ē-LĔK-trō-līts	_____
urinalysis	ū-rĭ-NĂL-ĭ-sĭs	_____
titer	TĪ-tĕr	_____
antibody	ĂN-tĭ-bŏd-ē	_____
chemotherapy	chē-mō-THĔR-ă-pē	_____

Critical Thinking: Analysis of Medical Records

This section provides experience in abstracting and analyzing information from medical records. At the same time it reinforces the material presented in this chapter.

>>> MEDICAL RECORD 19–1: OPERATIVE REPORT

1. What laboratory test indicated that the patient had adenocarcinoma of the prostate?

_____

2. What is a "prostatic seed implant"?

_____

_____

3. Why was fluoroscopy used during the operation?

_____

_____

4. What did the panendoscopy reveal?

_____

_____

>>> MEDICAL RECORD 19-2: DISCHARGE SUMMARY

5. What did the chest x-ray reveal?

_____

6. What diagnostic test confirmed the findings on the chest x-ray? What were the specific findings of this test?

_____

_____

7. What type of biopsy was performed? What is the advantage of this type of biopsy?

_____

8. What were the biopsy findings?

_____

_____

9. What do the findings above suggest?

_____

10. What type of treatment options are available to the patient?

_____

_____

 Audio Practice

Listen to the audio CD-ROM to practice the pronunciation of selected medical terms from this chapter.

Medical Record 19–1. Operative Report

GENERAL HOSPITAL AND MEDICAL CENTER
2211 Fifth Avenue North • Healthy City, USA 12345 • (321) 123-4567

Operative Report

Patient Name: John Turkington   **Patient Number:** 34-22-78
Birth Date: 01/03/xx   **Room Number:** 453

DATE OF PROCEDURE: 01/18/xx

PREOPERATIVE DIAGNOSIS: Adenocarcinoma of the prostate.

POSTOPERATIVE DIAGNOSIS: Adenocarcinoma of the prostate.

OPERATION: Prostatic ultrasound, prostate seed implant, cystoscopy, and removal of foreign body from the bladder.

SURGEONS: Thomas Seaman, M.D., and James Zucker, M.D.

ANESTHESIA: General.

COMPLICATIONS: None.

INDICATIONS: The patient is a 75-year-old white male who was diagnosed in October with adenocarcinoma of the prostate with a PSA of 9.7. There is a Gleason 8 on the right side of the gland; the left side was spared. We discussed treatment options with the patient, and he elected to have prostatic seed implant.

PROCEDURE: After preoperative evaluation, the patient was brought to the operating room. He was given a general anesthetic and intubated without difficulty. He was then placed in the extended dorsal lithotomy position with a bump under the pelvis. The area was prepped and draped in the usual fashion. A Foley catheter was inserted, and 150 cc of fluid was placed in the bladder, and a sludge of lubricant and air bubbles was then injected into the patient's rectum. The prostatic ultrasound probe was then passed into the patient's rectum, and the prostate was scanned from the seminal vesicles to the apex. After appropriate positioning, the needle implant then began. He had a total of 45 needles placed into the prostate gland in the outline predetermined by the nuclear physicist and the radiation therapist. There appeared to be excellent distribution of the seeds. There were 2 additional seeds placed at the end of the procedure, one of which was removed from the bladder. Fluoroscopy was used throughout the procedure to assure proper positioning. At the end of the procedure, cystoscopy was performed. Panendoscopy revealed a normal anterior and prostatic urethra with no evidence of needles seen coming from the urethra. The bladder was investigated, and one seed was identified. It was grasped and recovered. The bladder was emptied, and he was left without a Foley catheter. The total needle implants numbered 46. The patient was taken to the recovery room in satisfactory

Continued

Operative Report, page 2
Patient Name: John Turkington   **Patient Number:** 34-22-78

condition without complication. He is on Flomax and will be continued on Flomax and Detrol. He will also be given Levaquin. He will be seen back in our office and the radiation therapist's office in a month.

_____

Thomas Seaman, M.D.

TS/bab
D&T: 01/18/xx

Body System Connections
Psychiatry

THE CARDIOVASCULAR SYSTEM
◆ Psychiatric conditions such as anxiety can affect blood flow and blood pressure.

THE LYMPHATIC AND IMMUNE SYSTEMS
◆ Immune responses may be weakened by chronic stress, depression, and anxiety.

THE DIGESTIVE SYSTEM
◆ The rate of digestion and elimination can be affected by stress and mental health disorders.

THE MUSCULOSKELETAL SYSTEM
◆ Psychiatric conditions, such as tic disorders, depression, and dementia can affect movement, coordination, and motor functioning.

THE ENDOCRINE SYSTEM
◆ Endocrine abnormalities, such as those of the thyroid, can cause symptoms of anxiety or depression.

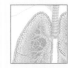

THE RESPIRATORY SYSTEM
◆ Mental state and mental disorders, such as anxiety, can affect rate and depth of breathing.

THE FEMALE REPRODUCTIVE SYSTEM
◆ Certain psychiatric disorders can affect menses, sexual arousal, and sexual functioning.

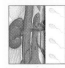

THE URINARY AND MALE REPRODUCTIVE SYSTEMS
◆ Urine retention and elimination can be affected by anxiety disorders. ◆ Reproductive activities can be affected by erectile dysfunction and sexual desire disorders, both possible psychiatric conditions.

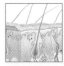

THE INTEGUMENTARY SYSTEM
◆ Changes in skin temperature and moisture may point to a psychiatric symptom.

THE NERVOUS SYSTEM
◆ Chemical imbalances in the nervous system may cause psychiatric disorders.

Figure 20–1 *The interrelationship of the mind and mental health to other body systems.*

(over long periods of time). As a result, an individual's ability to work and to engage in interpersonal relationships can become impaired. When this disturbance is severe enough to interfere with daily functioning over a period of time, it is considered a **psychiatric disorder** or **mental illness.** Mental illness is the term that refers collectively to all diagnosable mental or psychiatric disorders. Mental disorders are health conditions that are characterized by alteration in thinking, mood, and/or behavior accompanied by distress and/or impaired functioning.

The diagnosis of mental disorders is considered to be more difficult than the diagnosis of general medical disorders because mental illnesses cannot be identified by any laboratory test or imaging technique. Instead, the diagnosis of mental disorders depends on the patient's report of the intensity and duration of their symptoms, information from the mental status examination, and clinical observations of behavior. The information from these various sources is evaluated by the practitioner, who identifies a pattern or **syndrome.** When the syndrome meets all the criteria for the diagnosis, it constitutes a mental disorder. The term "disorder" is used more often in psychiatry than the term "disease." This is because "disorders" are based on clinically diagnosed clusters of symptoms and signs associated with distress and impairment, whereas "diseases" refer to conditions with known pathology.

Psychiatric disorders are classified into 16 different categories, which are described in the *Diagnostic and*

Statistical Manual of Mental Disorders, 4th edition: DSM-IV (American Psychiatric Association, 1998). For each disorder, the criteria required for diagnosis are listed and described. These are summarized in Table 20–1. As you examine the *DSM-IV* table, keep in mind that it is important to distinguish symptoms from disorders. All people who experience physical symptoms such as headaches and stomachaches do not necessarily have a medical illness. Similarly, all individuals who experience mental health problems such as sadness or anxious feelings do not typically suffer from psychiatric disorders. For example, it is normal for an individual to feel anxious before a big test or extremely sad after the death of a loved one. There is a continuum of symptoms from mild and normal to severe and pathological as illustrated in Figure 20–2. The *DSM-IV* has very specific criteria related to the severity, intensity, and duration of the symptoms before a diagnosis can be made. Generally speaking, if the symptoms are severe, longer lasting, and are interfering with activities of daily living, they are more likely to be considered a mental disorder.

TABLE 20–1: Diagnostic Categories of Mental Disorders (DSM-IV)

DIAGNOSTIC CATEGORY	EXAMPLES OF SPECIFIC DISORDERS OF THE CLASS
Disorders usually first diagnosed in infancy, childhood, or adolescence	Autistic disorder Learning, language, and speech disorders Attention deficit disorder Separation anxiety disorder
Delirium, dementia and amnestic and other cognitive disorders	Dementia of the Alzheimer type
Substance-related disorders	Substance abuse Substance dependence
Schizophrenia and other psychotic disorders	Schizophrenia Schizophreniform disorder
Mood disorders	Major depressive disorder Bipolar disorder Seasonal affective disorder
Anxiety disorders	Phobic disorders Obsessive-compulsive disorder Posttraumatic stress disorder
Somatoform disorders	Somatization disorder Conversion disorder Hypochondriasis
Factitious disorders	Munchausen syndrome
Dissociative disorders	Dissociative identity disorder Dissociative fugue Depersonalization disorder
Sexual and gender identity disorders	Paraphilias Sexual dysfunction Gender identity disorder
Eating disorders	Anorexia nervosa Bulimia nervosa
Sleep disorders	Insomnia Night terrors
Impulse-control disorders	Kleptomania Pyromania
Adjustment disorders	Adjustment disorder with anxiety
Personality disorders	Antisocial, borderline, histrionic, narcissistic, paranoid, schizoid
Mental disorders due to a general medical condition	Almost any of the above

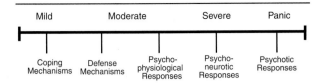

Figure 20–2 *The adaptation of responses on a continuum of anxiety. (From Townsend, MC: Essentials of Psychiatric/Mental Health Nursing. FA Davis, Philadelphia, 1999, p 11, with permission.)*

CLASSIFICATION SYSTEM OF PSYCHIATRIC DISORDERS

The *DSM-IV* defines a mental disorder in the following way: a clinically significant behavioral or psychological syndrome or pattern that is associated with current distress or disability (impairment in one or more important areas of functioning). This syndrome or pattern must be more than what would be an expected response to an event, such as grief over the death of a loved one. To add diagnostic detail and information to the medical diagnosis, the *DSM-IV* uses a *multiaxial approach*. Specifically, the multiaxial approach is designed to make note of all factors that may be contributing to the mental disorder, as well as to note the person's current level of functioning. This level of detail can be of significant help with the formulation of a treatment plan and the prediction of treatment outcome. The multiaxial approach may be difficult to understand the first time one is introduced to it. Nevertheless, a general understanding of this information is useful because it may be a documented section of the psychiatric report. That is why you may find it particularly helpful to review the five elements of the multiaxial approach again before analyzing the medical records that are presented at the end of this chapter.

There are five axes or domains on which each patient is evaluated:

- **Axis I: Clinical Disorder(s)**—usually the presenting problem(s).
- **Axis II: Personality Disorders and/or Mental Retardation**—a description of a concurrent personality or intellectual problem is included, if applicable.
- **Axis III: General Medical Conditions**—a description of any concurrent medical condition or disorder.
- **Axis IV: Psychosocial and Environmental Problems**—a description of psychosocial or environmental stressors that may be contributing to the problem.
- **Axis V: Global Assessment of Functioning (GAF) Scale**—an indicator of the level of overall psychological, social, and occupational

functioning using a rating scale of 1 to 100. A low score indicates serious impairment to functioning or heightened threat of harm to self or others. A high score indicates absent or minimal symptoms, a high level of functioning, and no threat of harm to self or others. The time period that the score refers to is included in parentheses after the score. For example, the score could refer to current functioning, functioning at time of discharge from the hospital, or highest functioning in the last year.

The first three axes are the official medical diagnoses. Axis IV documents the effect of psychosocial and environmental stressors on the patient including marital, familial, interpersonal, occupational, domestic, financial, legal, developmental, and medical concerns, as well as environmental factors and natural disasters. Axis V is used to indicate how well the patient has functioned over the past year and/or to indicate the current level of functioning. Axes IV and V simply add important information to the medical diagnoses listed in the first three axes.

Here is an example of a diagnosis after a patient's evaluation on these five axes:

Axis I:	Major depressive disorder
Axis II:	Borderline personality
Axis III:	Fibromyalgia
Axis IV:	Recent divorce; death of mother
Axis V:	GAF = 65 (current)

CATEGORIES OF MENTAL DISORDERS

As stated previously, the mind is housed in the brain, and the brain is the organ that integrates cognitive, emotional, and behavioral functioning. However, as you will see later, only a few psychiatric disorders are the direct result of lesions or biochemical processes. The vast majority is the result of a combination of biopsychosocial processes. Although psychiatric disorders share the same somatic origins as neurologic disorders, they are differentiated from the latter, which are considered general medical conditions. However, it would be useful to review Chapter 14, which examines the central nervous system in general and in particular—the structure, function, and biochemical properties of the brain.

Unlike the preceding chapters, which discuss the structure and function of a body system, this chapter gives a brief overview of the 16 types of psychiatric disorders, presenting the essential features of each type of disorder. Descriptions of specific pathological symptoms and conditions are also included. You will find that they are the same 16 categories of *DSM-IV* mental disorders as those listed in Table 20–1.

Disorders of Infancy, Childhood, and Adolescence

This section includes a group of disorders that are usually first diagnosed in the early years of life. Some of these disorders may be present in an individual but not diagnosed until adulthood. Other categories of disorders, such as anxiety disorders, do occur in children, but are more often diagnosed in adults. Thus, the disorders in this category are those that most typically are diagnosed in infancy, childhood, and adolescence.

Many of the disorders in this category relate to problems with developing basic cognitive and social skills. **Developmental disorders** include problems associated with one area of development such as intelligence (mental retardation), learning (reading disability), or communication (stuttering disorders). **Tic disorders** are those in which a child develops tics, which are sudden, rapid, recurrent, involuntary, stereotyped movements or vocalizations. **Pervasive developmental disorders** are characterized by severe deficits in multiple areas of development. These include impairment in social interaction, communication, and the presence of stereotyped (repetitive) behavior, interests, and activities. People with pervasive developmental disorders such as **autism** may be severely withdrawn from others, have a great deal of difficulty communicating even on a very basic level, and may engage in repetitive behavior such as rocking or repeating words.

In addition, several disorders in this category are related to behavioral problems, and not cognitive or social skills, for example, *attention deficit hyperactivity disorder* and *disruptive behavior.* **Attention deficit disorder (ADD)** is characterized by a persistent pattern of inattention and/or hyperactivity-impulsivity, which is more pronounced than is typical of children at a comparable level of development. Severe disruptive behavior disorders include **conduct disorder** and **oppositional defiant disorder,** characterized by behaviors that violate the basic rights of others, and negativistic, hostile, and defiant behavior, respectively. Other disorders in this category relate to feeding and eating problems, elimination problems, and attachment and separation issues. To be considered psychiatric disorders, these behaviors must be severe enough and of long enough duration to significantly interfere with adaptive functioning.

Delirium, Dementia, Amnesia, and Other Cognitive Disorders

In this category, the predominant disturbance is a deficit in cognition or memory that represents a significant change from a previous level of functioning. For these disorders, the cause is either a medical condition or a substance (drug of abuse, medication, or toxin). This is the reason why some of these disorders also were included in Chapter 14. Please review that chapter for details on etiology, diagnosis, and treatment.

Delirium is an acute impairment of consciousness and cognitive functioning. Memory dysfunction occurs in association with reduced ability to focus, sustain, or shift attention. **Dementia** is characterized by a progressive deterioration of memory and of multiple other cognitive functions, including information processing, verbal functioning, and the execution of complex tasks. Alzheimer disease and Parkinson disease are examples of dementia. **Amnesia,** or amnestic disorder, is characterized by memory impairment only (the ability to learn new information or recall previously learned information) with no other cognitive impairments. It is most like delirium, except that it does not include the disorientation and the impairment in consciousness.

Delirium and amnesia are caused by general medical conditions, such as head trauma, hypoglycemia, electrolyte imbalances, or drug intoxication. Generally the conditions are short-lived and reversible. By contrast, dementia usually results from the deterioration of brain tissue that occurs in progressive and often irreversible conditions such as Alzheimer, Parkinson, and Huntington diseases as well as brain tumors or strokes.

Substance-Related Disorders

These disorders result from side effects of medications, exposure to toxins, and use of substances of abuse. Substances of abuse include the following: amphetamines (e.g., crystal methylene or speed) and cocaine (e.g., crack); alcohol, sedatives, hypnotics, and anxiolytics (e.g., Valium or Xanax); caffeine; cannabis (e.g., marijuana or pot); hallucinogens (e.g., acid or mushrooms); inhalants; nicotine; opioids (e.g., heroin); and phencyclidine (e.g., PCP or Angel Dust).

Substance-related disorders are divided into two groups: the **substance use disorders** (substance dependence and substance abuse) and the **substance-induced disorders** (substance intoxication, substance withdrawal, and other substance-induced disorders). Substance dependence is a cluster of cognitive, behavioral, and physiological symptoms indicating that the person continues to use the substance despite substance-related problems. It may or may not include symptoms of tolerance or withdrawal, but must include maladaptive behaviors to continue the drug use despite the impairment to functioning (e.g., stealing to buy more drugs). By contrast, substance abuse focuses on recurrent use of a substance resulting in situations that cause physical, social, interpersonal, or legal problems (e.g., a drunk-driving charge). Substance-induced disorders are characterized by the development of a reversible, substance-specific, maladaptive behavioral or psychological change because of the recent ingestion of, or withdrawal of, a substance.

Schizophrenia and Other Psychotic Disorders

The defining feature of these disorders is the presence of psychotic symptoms. These symptoms may occur in other disorders but not as their defining feature. The disorder that refers to disturbances of perception and thought, specifically the experience of delusions and/or hallucinations is called **psychosis.** **Hallucinations** occur when an individual has a sensory experience that has no basis in reality. Hallucinations may be auditory (e.g., hearing voices that are not there), olfactory, gustatory, kinesthetic, tactile, or visual. A **delusion,** on the other hand, is a false belief that an individual holds despite evidence to the contrary. A common example is paranoia, in which a person has delusional beliefs that others are trying to harm him or her. Attempts to persuade that person that these beliefs are unfounded usually fail and may result in the further entrenchment of the beliefs.

One of the primary psychotic disorders is **schizophrenia.** For a diagnosis of schizophrenia to be made, a symptom other than hallucinations and delusions must also be present for a significant period of time. These symptoms are divided into two broad classes: **positive symptoms** and **negative symptoms.** Positive symptoms involve the experience of something in consciousness that should not normally be present. For example, hallucinations and delusions represent perceptions or beliefs that should not normally be experienced and are, therefore, positive symptoms. In addition to hallucinations and delusions, patients with psychotic disorders frequently have marked disturbances in the logical process of their thoughts. This means that their thought processes are loose, disorganized, illogical, or odd, a situation that can result in bizarre behavior.

In addition to positive symptoms, patients with schizophrenia and other psychotic disorders have negative symptoms as well. These reflect the absence of thoughts and behaviors that would otherwise be present. These symptoms include major deficits in affect or emotional expression, motivation, the ability to think abstractly and to be spontaneous. Although the positive symptoms of hallucination and delusions are responsible for much of the acute distress associated with this disorder, the negative symptoms contribute to the long-term disability often associated with this disorder. The common symptoms seen in schizophrenia are listed in Table 20–2.

Mood Disorders

The predominant feature of mood disorders is a disturbance in mood. Most of us have an intuitive understanding of the notion of mood. We can easily understand what it means to feel sad or happy. However, disturbances of mood are characterized by a sustained or prolonged feeling of sadness (depression) or euphoria (mania) which dominates a person's life and interferes with normal functioning. As with **anxiety** and **psychosis,** disturbances in mood may occur in a variety of patterns associated with different mental disorders. The disorder most closely associated with persistent sadness is **major depression,** whereas that associated with sustained elevation or fluctuation of mood is **bipolar disorder,** also known as manic depression. The most common signs of these mood disorders are listed in Table 20–3. Along with the prevailing feelings of sadness or elation, disorders of mood are associated with a host of related symptoms that include disturbances in appetite, sleep patterns, energy level, concentration, and memory.

Anxiety Disorders

The predominant feature of anxiety disorders is anxiety. **Anxiety** includes feelings of fear or dread accompanied by heart palpitations, sweating, trembling, and dizziness. Each of us encounters anxiety through the course of our daily lives, whether in response to concrete, threatening events such as narrowly avoiding a traffic accident or to dangers that are remote or abstract such as public speaking. In fact, anxiety has evolved as a critical, physiological, protective mechanism to signal danger and help us prepare for a response (see Fight or Flight Response, Chapter 14). However, the mechanisms that regulate anxiety may break down, leading to excessive or inappropriate ex-

TABLE 20–2: Common Symptoms of Schizophrenia	
POSITIVE SYMPTOMS	**NEGATIVE SYMPTOMS**
Hallucinations	Lack of emotional expression
Delusions	Inability to think abstractly
Disorganized thoughts and behaviors	Inability to experience pleasure (anhedonia)
Agitation	Poor motivation, spontaneity, and initiative

TABLE 20–3: Common Symptoms of Mood Disorders	
SYMPTOMS COMMONLY ASSOCIATED WITH DEPRESSION	**SYMPTOMS COMMONLY ASSOCIATED WITH MANIA**
Persistent sadness or despair	Persistently elevated or euphoric mood
Insomnia (sometimes hypersomnia)	Grandiosity (inappropriately high self-esteem)
Decreased appetite	Psychomotor agitation
Anhedonia (inability to experience pleasure)	Decreased sleep
Irritability	Racing thoughts and distractibility
Apathy, poor motivation, social withdrawal	Poor judgment and impaired impulse control
Hopelessness	Rapid or pressured speech
Poor self-esteem, feelings of helplessness	
Suicidal ideation	
Decreased attention and concentration	

pression of anxiety such as with **phobic disorder** or **phobia, panic disorder,** and **generalized anxiety disorder.** In a phobia, a high level of anxiety is triggered by a specific situation or object. The phobia may or may not be accompanied by panic attacks, which are brief and very intense episodes of anxiety, which can occur without a precipitating event or stimulus. Generalized anxiety disorder is a more diffuse and nonspecific kind of anxiety that is most often experienced as a chronic pattern of excessive worrying, restlessness, and tension. In each case, an anxiety disorder is said to exist if the anxiety experienced is disproportionate to the circumstance, is difficult for the individual to control, or interferes with normal functioning.

Obsessive-compulsive disorder (OCD) and **posttraumatic stress disorder (PTSD)** are thought to be related to the anxiety disorders. Obsessive-compulsive disorder (OCD) involves recurrent thoughts (**obsessions**) and/or repetitive acts (**compulsions**), which dominate an individual's behavior. These individuals experience intense anxiety if they are unable to carry out the acts or rituals, which seem to allay their fears. Often the compulsions consume an enormous amount of time, and, thus, significantly interfere with social or occupational functioning. Posttraumatic stress disorder is produced by an intense, extreme, and often life-threatening external event. A cluster of symptoms develops from exposure to such a traumatic event, including a persistent reexperiencing of the event in dreams and memories; persistent avoidance of anything associated with the event, including thoughts or feelings about it; and increased arousal such as difficulty sleeping, irritability, and an exaggerated startle response.

Somatoform Disorders

The common feature of somatoform (*somat/o=body*) disorders is the presence of physical symptoms that suggest or look like a general medical condition but for which there are no organic findings, physiological mechanisms, or substance exposure to explain the findings. The physical symptoms are not intentional (i.e., not under voluntary control). Some of the disorders in this category refer to physical symptoms or deficits for which no physiological cause can be found. Instead, psychological factors appear to play a role in the onset, severity, exacerbation, or maintenance of the symptoms. An example would be a **conversion disorder,** characterized by paralysis of an arm with no known physiological cause. Another somatoform disorder is **hypochondriasis.** This disorder is characterized by a preoccupation with disease or deficit for which there are no objective findings of actual disease. A hypochondriac would be, for instance, convinced that he or she has cancer although there are no symptoms and no objective evidence to support that fact.

Factitious Disorders

Like somatoform disorders, factitious disorders are also characterized by physical symptoms. Unlike somatoform disorders, these symptoms are intentionally produced or feigned by one bent on assuming the role of a sick person. The presentation of a factitious disorder may include fabrication of subjective complaints (e.g., acute abdominal pain), self-inflicted conditions (e.g., the production of abscesses by injection of saliva into the skin), and/or exaggeration or exacerbation of pre-existing general medical conditions (e.g., feigning a grand mal seizure by an individual with a previous history of seizures). The motivation for this behavior is gaining the attention usually enjoyed by sick people. An example of a factitious disorder is the *Munchausen syndrome*, an unusual condition characterized by habitual presentation for hospital treatment for an apparent acute illness with the patient reporting a plausible and dramatic history, which is, however, false. Individuals affected with this syndrome are fully aware that they have no physical illness; nevertheless, they will go to great lengths to present the symptoms and history of a real disease because their only goal is to appear sick. Factitious disorders are never motivated by external incentives, such as economic gain or avoiding legal responsibility.

Dissociative Disorders

The essential feature of dissociative disorders is a disturbance in identity, memory, consciousness, or perception of the environment. This disturbance is not caused by the direct effect of brain injury or drug abuse. Symptoms may hide the pain or anxiety associated with traumatic or stressful events or with internal psychological conflicts. The four main types of dissociative disorders are discussed below.

Dissociative identity disorder (formerly known as **multiple personality disorder**): This disorder is characterized by the coexistence of two or more distinct personalities that take hold of the individual's behavior.

Dissociative amnesia: This disorder is characterized by an inability to recall important personal information, usually of a traumatic or stressful nature.

Dissociative fugue (*fugue=flight, running away*): This is a condition in which an individual suddenly abandons a present activity or lifestyle and starts a new and different one for a period of time, often in a different city. Afterward, the individual no recollection of the events having occurred during the fugue period, although the individual remembers earlier events. His or her habits and skills are usually unaffected by the dissociative fugue.

Depersonalization disorder: This disorder is characterized by a recurrent feeling of detachment from one's mental processes or body, whereas reality testing remains intact.

Sexual and Gender Identity Disorders

Sexual disorders are disturbances related to sexual function and are also called **sexual dysfunction disorders.** They affect the ability to experience and sustain sexual desire, and to experience sexual pleasure, arousal, and orgasm. Some sexual disorders are characterized by recurrent sexually arousing fantasies, urges, or behavior involving (1) nonhuman objects, (2) oneself or one's partner, or (3) children or other nonconsenting persons. The latter two varieties of paraphilia usually entail infliction of suffering and humiliation. Such disorders are called **paraphilias.**

Gender identity disorders refer to a strong and persistent cross-gender identification, which consists of the desire to be, or the insistence that one is, of the other sex. There must also be evidence of persistent discomfort about one's assigned sex, a situation that causes clinical, significant distress or impairment in functioning.

Eating Disorders

Eating disorders are characterized by severe disturbances in eating behavior and include one of two specific diagnoses, **anorexia nervosa** or **bulimia nervosa.**

Anorexia nervosa is characterized by a refusal to maintain a minimally normal body weight. An individual is intensely afraid of gaining weight and has a disturbance in the perception of the shape or size of his or her body. (The term *anorexia*, which means "lack of appetite," is a misnomer because lack of appetite is rare.) Anorexia usually occurs in young women and often results in life-threatening weight loss, disturbance in body image, hyperactivity, and amenorrhea (absence or abnormal cessation of menses).

Bulimia nervosa is characterized by repeated and secretive uncontrolled rapid ingestions of large quantities of food (binge eating), followed by self-induced vomiting or by the use of laxatives or diuretics (purging) to prevent weight gain. Individuals with this disorder generally maintain normal weight. This disorder, which may be hidden from others for long periods of time, is usually accompanied by feelings of guilt, depression, and shame.

Sleep Disorders

Sleep disorders are thought to arise from abnormalities in sleep-wake generating and timing mechanisms in the brain and are often complicated by conditioning factors. For example, a person may have a sleep difficulty because of a biologic cause, but the difficulty may persist or worsen because the person develops anxiety that they will not be able to fall asleep. Primary sleep disorders (those not related to other mental disorders, general medical conditions, or substance use) are subdivided into two categories, **dyssomnias** and **parasomnias.**

Dyssomnias are characterized by abnormalities in the amount, quality, or timing of sleep. Examples include **primary insomnia** (difficulty initiating or maintaining sleep), **primary hypersomnia** (prolonged sleep episodes), **narcolepsy** (sudden attacks of deep sleep), and disorders related to disruption of sleep (**breathing-related sleep disorder** and **circadian rhythm sleep disorder**).

Parasomnias are characterized by abnormal behavioral or physiological events occurring during the sleep cycle as well as by the activation of physiological systems at inappropriate times during the sleep-wake cycle. Specifically, they occur when the autonomic nervous system, motor system, or cognitive processes are inappropriately active during sleep. Examples include **nightmare disorder, sleep terror disorder,** and **sleepwalking disorder.**

Impulse-Control Disorders

The essential feature of **impulse-control disorders** is the failure to resist an impulse, drive, or temptation to perform an act that is harmful to the individual or to others. For most of these disorders, the person feels an increasing sense of tension or arousal before committing the act and then experiences pleasure, gratification, or relief at the time of committing the act. The impulses include the following: aggressive tendencies that result in serious assault or destruction of property (**intermittent-explosive disorder**); stealing objects not needed for personal use or monetary value (**kleptomania**); fire setting (**pyromania**); pathological gambling; and recurrent pulling out of one's hair resulting in noticeable hair loss (**trichotillomania**).

Adjustment Disorders

An adjustment disorder is a temporary condition that occurs as a reaction to some stressful life event such as a divorce, death of a loved one, or loss of a job. The reaction is considered to be an adjustment disorder if the symptoms go beyond what would be expected given the stressful situation or if the effects last considerably longer than expected and significantly interfere with normal functioning. Adjustment disorders differ from acute anxiety disorders such as posttraumatic stress disorder in that the stressor is not extreme or life-threatening, and the symptoms are wide ranging and do not fit a particular pattern. Symptoms may include anxiety, depression, crying spells, irritability, behavior problems, sleep difficulties, and loss of appetite.

Personality Disorders

Personality traits are established patterns of thinking and ways of relating to and perceiving other people, the environment, and one's self. However, when these traits become inflexible and rigid, causing impairment of functioning, extreme distress, and consistent conflict with others, they constitute personality disorders. Examples include **antisocial, borderline, histrionic, narcissistic, paranoid,** and **schizoid personality disorders.**

Mental Disorders Due to a Medical Condition

Most of the categories already mentioned include mental disorders that can occur solely as a result of a medical condition. Delirium, dementia, and amnestic disorder are conditions that are *always* a result of a medical condition or substance intoxication. However, many of the other disorders listed in the *DSM-IV* and discussed previously (e.g., mood and anxiety disorders, psychotic disorders, sexual dysfunction and sleep disorders, and personality changes) can occur exclusively as a result of a medical condition or substance intoxication. When they do, they are considered to be a part of this category. Otherwise it is assumed that a general medical cause has been ruled out. The medical conditions could be neurologic (e.g., head traumas, brain tumors, cerebrovascular disease, encephalitis), metabolic (e.g., hepatic encephalopathy, diabetic ketoacidosis), endocrinal (hyperthyroidism), or autoimmune (AIDS, system lupus erythematosus). These conditions would be listed in Axis III (see the Classification System of Psychiatric Disorders discussed earlier in this chapter).

Activity 20–1: Competency Verification
The Types of Psychiatric Disorders

adjustment disorders	impulse-control disorders
anxiety disorders	mood disorders
delirium	personality disorders
delusion	schizophrenia
dementia	sexual and gender identity disorders
eating disorders	sleep disorders
factitious disorder	somatoform disorders
hallucinations	substance-related disorders

Match the terms listed above with the definitions given in the numbered list:

1. _____disorders characterized by feelings of fear or dread accompanied by heart palpations, sweating, and dizziness.

2. _____progressive deterioration of cognitive function as seen in Alzheimer and Parkinson patients.

3. _____disorders involving abuse of, or dependence on, alcohol and drugs.

4. _____psychotic illness with positive and negative symptoms; characteristic symptoms of this disorder include delusions, hallucinations, and disturbances of the logical process of the patient's thoughts.

5. _____disorders related to sexual functioning and one's assigned sex.

6. _____sensory perceptions that do not result from an external stimulus and that occur in the waking state, as in hearing voices when none is present.

7. _____disorders of body image and food intake.

8. _____a false belief or incorrect judgment that cannot be changed by logical reasoning or evidence to the contrary.

9. _____any group of neurotic disorders characterized by symptoms for which there are no demonstrable organic causes or physiological dysfunctions (e.g., *conversion disorder,* characterized by paralysis of an arm with no known physiological cause).

10. _____disorders characterized by extreme sadness and/or euphoria.

11. _____inflexible and rigid traits causing impairment of functioning and consistent conflict with others; inability to relate to people.

12. _____disorders marked by an inability to refrain from engaging in harmful behaviors such as stealing or fire setting.

13. _____temporary disorders of varying severity that occur as a reaction to some stressful life event (e.g., loss of job, forced retirement, death of a loved one, divorce). Symptoms usually recede and eventually disappear, as stress diminishes.

14. _____disturbances in the amount, quality, timing, or autonomic nervous system during the sleep cycle.

15. _____intentionally producing physical symptoms to gain attention by assuming the sick role, as seen in Munchausen syndrome.

Correct Answers _____ × **6.67** = _____ **% Score**

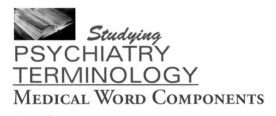

Studying
PSYCHIATRY
TERMINOLOGY
MEDICAL WORD COMPONENTS

Combining Forms

Combining Forms: Psychiatric Disorders

Combining Form	Meaning	EXAMPLE Term/Pronunciation	EXAMPLE Definition
hallucin/o	hallucination	**hallucin**/o/gen *hă-LOO-sĭ-nō-jĕn*	an agent that produces hallucinations *The suffix -gen means "forming, producing, origin."*
hypn/o	sleep	**hypn**/osis *hĭp-NŌ-sĭs*	an induced, trancelike state during which perception and memory are altered, resulting in increased responsiveness to suggestion Hypnosis has been used to treat phobias and anxiety, and to manage pain. *The suffix -osis means "abnormal condition, increase" (used primarily in reference to blood cells).*
iatr/o	physician, medicine, treatment	psych/**iatr**/ist *sī-kī-ă-trĭst*	a specialist (-ist) who treats mental disorders *The combining form psych/o means "mind."*
ment/o	mind	**ment**/al *MĔN-tăl*	pertaining to (-al) the mind
neur/o	nerve	**neur**/osis *nū-RŌ-sĭs*	a disease of the nerves, a mental disorder *In traditional (e.g., Freudian) psychiatry, this term designates an unconscious conflict that produces anxiety and other symptoms and leads to maladaptive use of defense mechanisms.*
phren/o	diaphragm, mind	schiz/o/**phren**/ia *skĭz-ō-FRĔN-ē-ă*	psychiatric disorder characterized by psychoses *The combining form schiz/o means "split."*
psych/o	mind	**psych**/o/logy *sī-KŎL-ō-jē*	the study (-logy) of the mind

Combining Forms: Psychiatric Disorders (Continued)

Combining Form	Meaning	EXAMPLE Term/Pronunciation	EXAMPLE Definition
schiz/o	split	**schiz**/oid SKĬZ-oyd	characteristic of or resembling (-oid) schizophrenia; a person, not necessarily a schizophrenic, who exhibits the traits of a schizoid personality
somat/o	body	psych/o/**somat**/ic sī-kō-sō-MĂT-ĭk	the expression of an emotional conflict through physical symptoms *The combining form* somat/o *means "body."*

Suffixes and Prefixes

In this section, suffixes are listed alphabetically and highlighted, whereas key prefixes are defined in the right-hand column.

Suffixes: Psychiatric Disorders

Suffix	Meaning	EXAMPLE Term/Pronunciation	EXAMPLE Definition
-mania	state of mental disorder, frenzy	klept/o/**mania** klĕp-tō-MĀ-nē-ă	a disorder of impulse control characterized by a morbid tendency to steal *The combining form* klept/o *means "to steal."*
-philia	attraction for	ped/o/**philia** pē-dō-FĬL-ē-ă	an abnormal attraction to children by an adult for sexual purposes *The combining form* ped/o *means "foot," "child."*
-phobia	fear	xen/o/**phobia** zĕn-ō-FŌ-bē-ă	fear of strangers *The combining form* xen/o *means "foreign," "strange." Phobias are irrational and often disabling. Refer to Table 20–4 for a list of specific phobias.*
-phoria	feeling (mental state)	eu/**phoria** ū-FOR-ē-ă	good (eu-) feeling
-thymia	mind, emotion	dys/**thymia** dĭs-THĪ-mē-ă	chronic depressed mood *The prefix* dys- *means "bad, painful, difficult."*

TABLE 20–4: Specific Phobias

MEDICAL TERM FOR PHOBIA	REPRESENTS FEAR OF:
Aerophobia	Air
Ailurophobia	Cats
Apiphobia, melissophobia	Bees
Arachnophobia	Spiders
Belonephobia	Needles
Claustrophobia	Enclosed spaces
Coitophobia, cypridophobia	Sexual intercourse
Cynophobia	Dogs
Emetophobia	Vomiting
Entomophobia	Insects
Gamophobia	Marriage
Gynophobia	Women
Hodophobia	Traveling
Hypnophobia	Sleep
Necrophobia	Corpses
Nyctophobia, scotophobia	Darkness
Ophidiophobia	Snakes
Phagophobia	Eating
Pharmacophobia	Drugs
Photophobia	Light
Thanatophobia	Death
Zoophobia	Animals

Activity 20–2: Competency Verification
Medical Word Components

Check the box [✓] as you complete each numbered section.

[   ] **1.** Review the components and their examples in the previous section. Then pronounce each word aloud.

[   ] **2.** For the following words, first write the suffix and its meaning. Then translate the meaning of the remaining components, starting with the first part of the word.

> **Example:** psych/ic
> **Answer:** *ic*=pertaining to, relating to; mind

1. hallucin/o/gen _____

2. hypn/osis _____

3. psych/iatr/ist _____

4. ment/al _____

5. schiz/o/phren/oid _____

6. neur/osis _____

7. ped/o/philia _____

8. klept/o/mania _____

9. xen/o/phobia _____

10. eu/phoria _____

Correct Answers _____ × 10 = _____% Score

Psychiatric Disorders

DISORDERS	DESCRIPTION
agoraphobia *ăg-ō-ră-FŌ-bē-ă* *agora=marketplace* *phobia=fear*	An anxiety disorder characterized by fear of being alone, of leaving the familiar setting of home, or of being in open, crowded public places from which escape would be difficult or where help would be unavailable. Causes avoidance or limitation in activities conducive to anxiety.
amnestic disorder, amnesia *ăm-NĔS-tĭk dĭs-OR-dĕr,* *ăm-NĒ-zē-ă*	A cognitive disorder marked by a loss of long-term memory. May be a result of trauma, brain injury, or disease.
anhedonia *ăn-hē-DŌ-nē-ă* *an=without, not* *hedon=pleasure* *ia=condition*	Absence of pleasure from acts that would ordinarily be pleasurable; often a symptom of depression.
anorexia nervosa *ăn-ō-RĔK-sē-ă nĕr-VŌ-să* *an=without, not* *orexia=appetite*	An eating disorder characterized by extreme fear of becoming obese and an aversion to food. Usually occurs in young women and can result in life-threatening weight loss and amenorrhea.
antisocial personality disorder *anti=against* *social=society*	A personality disorder characterized by little concern for others and no moral standards. A person suffering from this disorder acts only in response to personal desires and impulses; synonymous with *psychopathic, sociopathic* personality.

Psychiatric Disorders (Continued)

DISORDERS	DESCRIPTION
Asperger syndrome ĂS-pĕr-gĕr	A pervasive developmental disorder marked by severe, enduring impairment in social skills, and restrictive and repetitive behaviors or interests causing impaired social and occupational functioning but without significant delays in language development.
attention deficit disorder (ADD)	A disorder usually diagnosed in childhood and characterized by decreased attention span, poor concentration, increased impulsivity, and hyperactivity manifested at home, school, and in social situations. There is no known cure, and symptoms often subside with time. Medication is available to control the symptoms. Sometimes this disorder persists into adulthood.
autistic disorder aw-TĬS-tĭk	A pervasive developmental disorder characterized by a severe lack of response to other people. Symptoms include withdrawal, inability to interact, and retarded language development.
bipolar disorder bī-PŌL-ăr bi=two	A mood disorder marked by the occurrence of alternating periods of mania and depression. Also known as manic-depressive disorder.
body dysmorphic disorder dĭs-MOR-fĭk	A somatoform disorder characterized by a preoccupation with some imagined defect in appearance in a normal-looking person.
borderline personality disorder	A personality disorder characterized by impulsivity and unpredictability, unstable interpersonal relationships, inappropriate or uncontrolled affect, identity disturbances, rapid shifts of mood, suicidal gestures, self-mutilations, job and marital instability, and feelings of emptiness, and intolerance of being alone.
bulimia nervosa bŭ-LĬM-ē-ă nĕr-VŌ-să	An eating disorder involving repeated, secretive episodes of binge eating followed by purging behavior (self-induced vomiting, use of laxatives or diuretics) to prevent weight gain; often accompanied by feelings of guilt, depression, and shame.
catatonia kăt-ă-TŌ-nē-ă	Syndrome of psychomotor disturbance, characterized by periods of physical rigidity or stupor that may occur in schizophrenia, mood disorders, or organic mental disorders.
compulsion cŏm-PŬL-shŭn	Uncontrollable thoughts or impulse to perform an act repeatedly; typically an unconscious way to avoid unacceptable ideas or desires that arouse anxiety.
conduct disorder	A disorder of childhood or adolescence characterized by a persistent pattern of violating societal norms and the rights of others; may include physical aggression, cruelty to animals, vandalism, robbery, truancy, cheating, and lying; may develop into antisocial personality disorder.
conversion disorder	A somatoform disorder in which an unconscious emotional conflict is expressed as an alteration of loss of physical functioning; formerly called *hysteria*.

PSYCHIATRIC DISORDERS (CONTINUED)

DISORDERS	DESCRIPTION
cyclothymia *sī-klō-THĪ-mē-ă* *cyclo=ciliary body of eye,* *circular, cycle* *thymia=mind, motion*	An affective disorder characterized by marked mood swings from depression to hypomania but not to the degree that occurs in bipolar disorder.
defense mechanisms	Unconscious psychological mechanisms used to control anxiety; include rationalization, projection, denial, repression. Specific examples are given in Table 20–5.
delirium *dē-LĬR-ē-ŭm*	An altered state of consciousness characterized by confusion, distractibility, disorientation, disordered thinking and memory, and irrational behavior. Delirium is caused by a disturbance in cerebral function that may result from a wide range of causes including metabolic disorders, ingestion of various toxic substances such as drugs and alcohol, and other causes of physical and mental shock or exhaustion.

TABLE 20–5: Defense Mechanisms

DEFENSE MECHANISM	EXAMPLE
Denial Refusing to acknowledge the existence of a real situation or the feelings associated with it	A woman drinks alcohol every day and cannot stop, failing to acknowledge that she has a problem.
Displacement The transfer of feelings from one target to another that is considered less threatening or that is neutral	A patient is angry at the doctor, does not express it, but becomes verbally abusive with the nurse.
Intellectualization An attempt to avoid expressing actual emotions associated with a stressful situation by using the intellectual processes of logic, reasoning, and analysis	Kay's husband is being transferred with his job to a city far away from her parents. She hides anxiety by explaining to her parents the advantages associated with the move.
Suppression The voluntary blocking of unpleasant feelings and experiences from one's awareness	Scarlett O'Hara says, "I don't want to think about that now. I'll think about that tomorrow."
Projection Attributing to 8another person feelings or impulses unacceptable to one's self	Sue feels a strong sexual attraction to her track coach and tells her friend, "He's coming on to me!"
Rationalization Attempting to make excuses or formulate logical reasons to justify unacceptable feelings or behaviors	John tells the rehab nurse, "I drink because it's the only way I can deal with my bad marriage and my tough job."
Regression Retreating in response to stress to an earlier level of development and the comfort measures associated with that level of functioning	When 2-year old Jay is hospitalized for tonsillitis he will drink only from a bottle, even though his mom states he has been drinking from a cup for 6 months.
Repression Involuntary blocking of unpleasant feeling and experiences from one's awareness	An accident victim can remember nothing about an accident.

Source: Adapted from Townsend, M: Essentials of Psychiatric/Mental Health Nursing. FA Davis, Philadelphia, 1999, p 12, with permission.

Psychiatric Disorders (Continued)

DISORDERS	DESCRIPTION
delirium tremens (DT) *dē-LĬR-ē-ŭm TRĔM-ĕnz*	A severe and sometimes fatal form of delirium caused by alcoholic withdrawal after a period of excessive alcohol intake over a long period of time.
dementia *dē-MĔN-shē-ă*	A progressive organic mental disorder characterized by decreased intellectual capacity and function, confusion, and changes in personality. Dementia can be caused by infection or toxins but is most commonly associated with structural brain disease, such as Alzheimer disease.
dependent personality disorder	A personality disorder characterized by an excessive need to be taken care of that leads to submissive and clinging behaviors and fear of separation.
depersonalization disorder	A dissociative disorder characterized by recurrent experiences of detachment from one's mental thoughts or body but with intact reality testing; often accompanied by significant distress.
dissociative amnesia *dĭs-SŌ-sē-ă-tĭv ăm-NĒ-sē-ă*	A dissociative disorder marked by an inability to recall important personal information, usually of a stressful or traumatic nature.
dissociative fugue *dĭs-SŌ-sē-ă-tĭv fūg*	A dissociative disorder characterized by sudden, unexpected travel away from home or work with an inability to recall one's past and personal identity.
dissociative identity *dĭs-SŌ-sē-ă-tĭv ĭ-DĔN-tĭ-tē*	A dissociative disorder marked by the presence of two or more distinct identities or personalities; formerly known as *multiple personality disorder.*
dysthymic disorder *dĭs-THĪ-mĭk*	An affective disorder characterized by a chronic disturbance of mood such as mild depression or loss of interest in usual activities.
enuresis *ĕn-ū-RĒ-sĭs*	Childhood elimination disorder of repeated passage of urine in inappropriate places for at least 3 months after the age of 5.
encopresis *ĕn-kō-PRĒ-sĭs*	Childhood elimination disorder of repeated passage of feces in inappropriate places for at least 3 months after the age of 4.
euphoria *ū-FOR-ē-ă* *eu=good, normal* *phoria=feeling (mental state)*	Elevated mood; a feeling of well-being, commonly exaggerated and not necessarily well-founded.
exhibitionism *ĕg-zĭ-BĬSH-ŭn-ĭzm*	A paraphilia characterized by the compulsive need to expose a part of the body, especially the genitals, to an unsuspecting stranger.
female sexual arousal disorder	A sexual dysfunction marked by recurrent inability to attain or maintain an adequate lubrication-swelling response to sexual excitement until the completion of the sexual activity. This disorder causes marked distress or interpersonal difficulty; formerly known as *frigidity.*
fetishism *FĔ-tĭsh-ĭzm*	A paraphilia characterized by the act of using an inanimate object or non-sexual body part for sexual arousal and gratification.

PSYCHIATRIC DISORDERS (CONTINUED)

DISORDERS	DESCRIPTION
frotteurism *frŏ-TOOR-ĭzm* *frotter=to rub* *ism=condition*	A paraphilia characterized by a compulsive need for, and attainment of, sexual gratification from touching or rubbing against a nonconsenting person.
gender identity disorder	Characterized by a strong, enduring cross-gender identification, belief, or desire to be the other sex; involves persistent discomfort with one's sex or the gender roles of one's sex, such that there is distress or impairment in functioning.
hypochondriasis *hī-pō-kŏn-DRĪ-ă-sĭs*	A somatoform disorder in which a person believes that he or she is suffering from a serious disease for which no physical basis exists.
hypomania *hī-pō-MĀ-nē-ă* *hypo=under, below* *mania=state of mental disorder, frenzy*	A mild degree of mania.
histrionic personality disorder *hĭs-trē-ŏ-nĭk*	A personality disorder in which the person is emotional, attention-seeking, immature, dependent, and theatrical, and exhibits irrational outbursts and tantrums.
intermittent explosive disorder	An impulse control disorder characterized by repeated acts of violent and agressive behavior in an otherwise normal person; may begin in early childhood or after a head injury at any age.
kleptomania *klĕp-tō-MĀ-nē-ă* *klepto=to steal* *mania=state of mental disorder, frenzy*	An impulse control disorder characterized by failure to resist impulses to steal even though the items are not needed.
labile *LĀ-bīl*	Emotionally unstable; exhibiting rapid shifts from one emotion to another.
major depressive disorder	A mood disorder with chronic sadness, loss of energy, hopelessness, worry, and often, suicidal thoughts or impulses.
male erectile disorder *māl ě-RĔK-tĭl*	A sexual dysfunction characterized by the recurrent inability to attain or maintain an adequate erection until the completion of the sexual activity. This disorder causes marked distress or interpersonal difficulty.
mania *MĀ-nē-ă*	A mood characterized by an unstable, expansive emotional state, extreme excitement, excessive elation, hyperactivity, inflated self-esteem, and agitation.

Psychiatric Disorders (Continued)

DISORDERS	DESCRIPTION
mental retardation MĚN-tăl rē-tăr-DĀ-shŭn	A disorder usually diagnosed in childhood characterized by significantly subaverage intellectual functioning with deficits or impairments in adaptive functioning such as self-care, social and interpersonal skills, academic skills, and safety.
Munchausen syndrome měn-CHOW-zěn	A factitious disorder characterized by repeated fabrication of clinically convincing simulations of disease for the purpose of gaining medical attention.
Munchausen syndrome by proxy	A factitious disorder characterized by a form of child abuse inflicted by a caretaker with fabrications of symptoms and/or induction of signs of disease leading to unnecessary investigation and interventions. It can have serious health consequences including death of the child and is exhibited by the caretaker for the purpose of gaining attention.
narcissistic personality disorder năr-sĭ-SĬST-ĭk	A personality disorder marked by a grandiose sense of self-importance or uniqueness and preoccupation with fantasies of success and power coupled with a lack of empathy for others.
obsessive-compulsive disorder ŏb-SĔS-ĭv cŏm-PŬL-sĭv	A type of anxiety disorder with the essential feature of recurrent obsessions, persistent and intrusive ideas, thoughts, impulses, or compulsions (repetitive, purposeful, and intentional behaviors performed in response to an obsession) that dominate behavior.
oppositional defiant disorder	A disorder of childhood or adolescence marked by a recurrent pattern of hostile and disobedient behavior toward authority figures.
panic attack	A period of intense fear and rapid development of accelerated heart rate, shaking, shortness of breath, tightness in the chest, and dizziness. Often related to the fear of losing control or dying.
panic disorder	An anxiety disorder marked by recurrent panic attacks accompanied by either worry about having additional attacks or a change in behavior related to the attacks.
paranoid personality disorder PĂR-ă-noyd	A personality disorder in which a person is continually suspicious and mistrustful of others to the degree of blaming others for his or her own mistakes and failures and goes to abnormal lengths to validate biases, prejudices, and attitudes.
paraphilia păr-ă-FĬL-ē-ă *para=abnormal* *philia=attraction for*	A sexual disorder characterized by recurrent intense sexual urge, fantasy, or behavior that involves unusual objects, activities, or situations.
pathological gambling păth-ō-LŎJ-ĭ-kăl *patho=disease* *log=study of* *ical=pertaining to*	An impulse-control disorder marked by recurrent maladaptive gambling behavior that disrupts personal, family, or work pursuits.

PSYCHIATRIC DISORDERS (CONTINUED)

DISORDERS	DESCRIPTION
pedophilia *pē-dō-FĬL-ē-ă* *pedo=foot, child* *philia=attraction for*	A paraphilia characterized by the sexual urges and fantasies of someone who is at least 16 years old that involve sexual activity with a prepubescent child (age 13 or younger).
post-traumatic stress disorder (PTSD)	An anxiety disorder marked by the development of symptoms after exposure to an extreme traumatic, life-threatening event.
premature ejaculation *PRĒ-mă-chŭr ē-jăk-ū-LĀ-shŭn*	A sexual dysfunction marked by recurrent onset of orgasm and ejaculation with minimal sexual stimulation.
primary insomnia *ĭn-SŎM-nē-ă*	Sleep disorder marked by difficulty initiating sleep.
pyromania *pī-rō-MĀ-nē-ă* *pyro=fire* *mania=state of mental disorder, frenzy*	An impulse-control disorder characterized by multiple episodes of purposeful fire setting. It is usually preceded by tension or emotional arousal before the act and pleasure or relief afterward.
schizoaffective disorder *skĭz-ō-ă-FĔK-tĭv* *schizo=split* *affect=mood* *ive=pertaining to, relating to*	A psychotic disorder characterized by a period of illness during which a person concurrently exhibits a mood disorder and the primary symptoms of schizophrenia.
schizoid personality disorder *SKĬZ-oyd* *schiz=split* *oid=resembling*	A personality disorder marked by being emotionally cold and aloof, indifferent to praise, criticism, or the feelings of others, having few friendships, and rarely experiencing strong emotions.
schizophrenia *skĭz-ō-FRĔN-ē-ă* *schizo=split* *phren=mind* *ia=condition*	A severe psychotic disorder characterized by delusions, hallucinations, disorganized speech and behavior, flat affect, and impaired ability to initiate activities.
catatonic *kăt-ă-TŎN-ĭk*	Predominant features include marked psychomotor disturbance that may involve immobility, mutism, and stupor.
disorganized type	Predominant features include disorganized speech and behavior, and flat or inappropriate affect.
paranoid type *PĂR-ă-noyd*	Predominant features include preoccupation with one or more *delusions* or *hallucinations* with little evidence of disorganized speech or behavior, or inappropriate affect.

PSYCHIATRIC DISORDERS (CONTINUED)

DISORDERS	DESCRIPTION
schizophreniform disorder *skĭz-ō-FRĔN-ĭ-form*	A psychotic disorder with features identical to schizophrenia except with a shorter duration (less than 6 months).
seasonal affective disorder (SAD)	A depressive mood disorder that occurs approximately the same time year after year and spontaneously remits at the same time each year. Most common type is winter depression and is characterized by morning hypersomnia, low energy, increased appetite, weight gain, and carbohydrate craving that disappear in the spring.
separation anxiety disorder	Childhood disorder characterized by extreme fear concerning separation from home or from those to whom the child is attached.
sexual masochism *MĂS-ō-kĭzm*	A paraphilia characterized by the sexual gratification gained by being humiliated, beaten, bound, and made to suffer by another person.
sexual sadism *SĀ-dĭzm*	A paraphilia characterized by the sexual gratification gained by inflicting physical or psychological pain or humiliation on another.
sleep terror disorder	A sleep disorder characterized by repeated occurrence of abrupt awakenings from sleep with a panicky cry, intense fear, and unresponsiveness to efforts of others to provide comfort.
sleepwalking	A sleep disorder marked by repeated episodes of complex motor behavior initiated during sleep, including rising from bed and walking. On awakening, the person has amnesia about the episode.
social phobia *FŌ-bē-ă*	An anxiety disorder marked by fear of social or performance situations in which embarrassment may occur; formerly called *social anxiety disorder*.
specific phobia	An anxiety disorder marked by persistent, excessive, unreasonable fear cued by the presence or anticipation of an object or situation. (See Table 20–4, which lists some of the different phobias.)
transference *trăns-FĔR-ĕns*	In the situation of psychodynamic therapy, it is generally applied to the projection of feelings, thoughts, and wishes onto the therapist, who has come to symbolically represent an important person from the patient's past.
transvestic fetishism *trăns-VĔS-tĭk FĒ-tĭsh-ĭzm* *trans=across* *vest=clothes* *ic=pertaining to*	A paraphilia characterized by sexually arousing fantasies or behaviors involving wearing clothes of the opposite sex.
trichotillomania *trĭk-ō-tĭl-ō-MĀ-nē-ă* *tricho=hair* *tillo=to pull* *mania=state of mental disorder, frenzy*	An impulse-control disorder characterized by recurrent pulling out of one's hair resulting in noticeable hair loss and accompanied by increasing tension before, and pleasure or relief after the act.

Psychiatric Disorders (Continued)

DISORDERS	DESCRIPTION
voyeurism VOY-yĕr-ĭzm *voyeur=to see* *ism=condition*	A paraphilia characterized by the sexual excitement achieved by observing unsuspecting people who are naked, undressing, or engaging in sexual activity.

Activity 20–3: Clinical Application
Pathological Conditions

anhedonia
anorexia nervosa
bipolar disorder
conduct disorder
delirium tremens (DT)
encopresis
euphoria
fetishism
hypochondriasis
kleptomania

Munchausen syndrome
narcissistic personality disorder
panic attack
pedophilia
primary insomnia
seasonal affective disorder (SAD)
separation anxiety disorder
sleepwalking
social phobia
trichotillomania

Match the terms listed above with the definitions given in the numbered list:

1. _____ elevated mood; a feeling of well-being.

2. _____ repeated fabrication of clinically convincing medical symptoms for the purpose of gaining medical attention.

3. _____ sleep disorder marked by difficulty initiating sleep.

4. _____ an eating disorder characterized by extreme fear of gaining weight with a serious disturbance in body image and an aversion to food.

5. _____ mood disorder that occurs the same time each year.

6. _____ a paraphilia characterized by the act of using an inanimate object for sexual arousal and gratification.

7. _____ a mood disorder marked by alternating periods of mania and depression.

8. _____ anxiety disorder marked by fear of social embarrassment.

9. _____ a personality disorder marked by a grandiose sense of self-importance.

10. _____ sexual urges toward a prepubescent child.

11. _____ a childhood disorder marked by a pattern of violated societal norms and the rights of others; may include physical aggressiveness and cruelty to animals.

12. _____ an impulse control disorder marked by pulling out one's hair.

13. _____ an impulse control disorder marked by inability to refrain from stealing.

14. _____ a severe form of delirium caused by alcoholic withdrawal.

15. _____ childhood disorder marked by extreme fear of separation from parent.

16. _____ childhood elimination disorder of repeated passage of feces in inappropriate places.

17. _____ period of intense fear with rapid development of shortness of breath, accelerated heart rate, and the fear of losing control or dying.

18. _____ loss of pleasure or interest in previously pleasurable activities; often a sign of depression.

19. _____ sleep disorder characterized by complex motor behavior during sleep.

20. _____ a somatoform disorder characterized by the belief that one is suffering from a serious medical disease for which there is no physical evidence.

Correct Answers _____ × 5 = _____ **% Score**

DIAGNOSTIC PROCEDURES AND TESTS

Psychological Testing

TEST	DESCRIPTION
clinical interview	Clinical diagnostic tool used when laboratory tests or imaging scans cannot be used to diagnose a mental disorder. Also used as a critical diagnostic tool. The clinical interview contains information about the chief complaint, history of the present illness, intensity and duration or current symptoms; psychiatric and medical histories including medications; demographic and socioeconomic data; and information about cultural and religious beliefs which may provide information about current stressors, life situations, and the patient's view of the current illness.
intelligence tests	Tests used by psychologists to assess an individual's general aptitude or level of potential competence (as opposed to achievement) by using well-researched questions and a systematic method of administration and scoring. Several such tests exist, but the most common include the Wechsler Adult Intelligence Scale and the Wechsler Intelligence Scale for Children. These tests consist of several subscales and include both verbal and nonverbal aptitudes, which together form the *intelligence quotient* (*IQ*); used to diagnose mental retardation, learning disabilities (by comparing with achievement tests), neuropsychological testing, and after trauma or toxicity to determine the level of cognitive impairment and rehabilitative progress.
mental status examination (MSE)	Examination based on observations and answers to structured questions regarding patient appearance, behavior, mood, thought processes, cognitive function, coping mechanisms, and potential for self-destructive behavior. The components of the MSE are listed in Table 20–6.
personality tests	Tests used by psychologists to assess personality traits, emotions, psychological strengths, coping strategies, gender identification, self-esteem, inner conflicts and fears, and defenses; types of personality tests include objective and projective tests (See Table 20–7).

☐ TABLE 20–6: Components of the Mental Status Examination

☐ Appearance, behavior, and attitude
☐ Attention
☐ Orientation
☐ Language function and characteristics of speech
☐ General intellectual evaluation and memory
☐ Cortical and cognitive functions
☐ Mood and affect—emotional state
☐ Thought content—preoccupations and experiences
☐ Insight

Source: Glod, CA: Contemporary Psychiatric-Mental Health Nursing. FA Davis, Philadelphia, 1998, p. 32, with permission.

☐ TABLE 20–7: Personality Tests

Objective Personality Tests	Consist of "objective" questions, true-false, forced-choice statements	**Projective Personality Tests**	Patient must interpret or "project" meaning onto abstract or ambiguous pictures, or create own pictures.
Minnesota Multiphasic Personality Inventory	Most widely used. Designed to measure psychopathology, but contains additional scales to measure personality traits. Over 500 self-report, true or false questions.	**Rorschach**	Most widely known. Patient is asked to say what a series of ink blots looks like; particularly useful for detecting the types of disordered thought patterns seen in schizophrenia.
Myers-Briggs Trait Inventory	Useful for personality in the normal range and particularly helpful for career counseling	**Thematic Apperception Test (TAT)**	Patient is asked to tell stories from pictures of people in ambiguous situations. Provides information about themes in a person's life, particularly interpersonal ones.
		Draw-a-Person	Patient is asked to draw a person and various aspects of the drawing are interpreted by the clinician.

Imaging Procedures

PROCEDURE	DESCRIPTION
computed tomography (CT) *kŏm-PŪ-tĕd tō-MŎG-ră-fē*	Radiological and computer analysis of tissue density. Used for detecting brain contusions or calcifications, cerebral atrophy, hydrocephalus, inflammation, space-occupying lesions, and vascular abnormalities.
electroencephalography (EEG) *ē-lĕk-trō-ĕn-sĕf-ă-LŎG-ră-fē*	The process of recording brain wave activity. Abnormal results may indicate seizure activity, organic disease, psychotropic drug use, or certain psychological and sleep disorders.
magnetic resonance imaging (MRI) *măg-NĚT-ĭk RĔZ-ō-năns ĬM-ă-jĭng*	A noninvasive scanning procedure that uses magnetic waves to produce multiplanar cross-sectional images of the brain, blood vessels, heart, and soft tissue.
polysomnography *pŏl-ē-sŏm-NŎG-ră-fē* *poly=many* *somno=sleep* *graphy=recording*	An EEG performed during sleep.

Imaging Procedures (Continued)

PROCEDURE	DESCRIPTION
positron emission tomography (PET) PŎZ-ĭ-trŏn ē-MĬ-shŭn tō-MŎG-ră-fē	A tomography that provides colorimetric information about the brain's metabolic activity by detecting how quickly tissues consume radioactive isotopes. This procedure helps diagnose neuropsychiatric problems, such as Alzheimer disease, and some mental illness (see Fig. 14–9B).
single photon emission computed tomography (SPECT) SĬN-gl FŌ-tŏn ē-MĬ-shŭn kŏm-PŪ-tĕd tō-MŎG-ră-fē (spĕkt)	A tomography that uses radiopharmaceuticals to visualize and measure the density of neuroreceptors in the brain (Fig. 20–3).

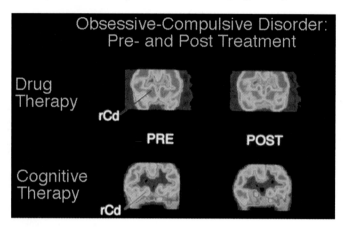

Figure 20–3 *The PET scans of two patients with obsessive-compulsive disorder (OCD) before and after treatment. (From Jeffrey Schwartz, MD, UCLA School of Medicine, copyright American Medical Association, Arch Gen Psychiatry, 53:109–113, 1996, with permission.)*

TREATMENTS

Psychotherapy

TREATMENT	DESCRIPTION
individual psychotherapy sī-kō-THĔR-ă-pē *psycho=mind* *therapy=treatment*	Treatment of emotional problems by using psychological techniques, such as talking, interpreting, listening, rewarding, problem solving, and role playing; used both for the treatment of serious mental disorders as well as a way to improve one's quality of life. Treatment may be conducted with individuals, couples, families, or as a group. Several modalities are described below.
behavior therapy	Treatment of behavioral or emotional problems by modification of maladaptive patterns of behavior and substituting new responses to given stimuli and reinforcement. Extremely useful in treating anxiety disorders and phobias, and child and adolescent behavioral disorders. Also called *behavior modification*.
cognitive behavioral therapy (CBT) KŎG-nĭ-tĭv bē-HĂV-yĕr-ĕl THĔR-ă-pē	Treatment of behavioral or emotional problems by modifying maladaptive, negative thoughts that are believed to affect the way that we feel and behave.

Psychotherapy (Continued)

TREATMENT	DESCRIPTION
play therapy	Child therapy; using games and toys to observe the behavior, affect, and interactions a child exhibits to gain insight into the thoughts, feelings, and experiences of the child that he or she may not be able to communicate in a direct manner.
psychodynamic therapy *sī-kō-dī-NĂM-ĭk*	A psychotherapy method in which the role of the past in shaping the present is emphasized with a focus on self-understanding. The purpose is to uncover underlying inner conflicts by studying the influence of past experiences on the motivation of present behavior.
psychoanalysis *sī-kō-ă-NĂL-ĭ-sĭs*	A form of psychotherapy in which the therapist analyzes and interprets a patient's unconscious thoughts using free association (free reporting of anything that comes to mind), questioning, and analyzing. This form of therapy is generally long term and time intensive.
couples/marital therapy	Treatment of two people in an intimate relationship or marriage to help them understand and resolve interpersonal conflicts.
family therapy	Treatment of an entire family to help resolve and understand conflicts and problems. Focus is on the patterns among family members that support and sustain symptoms.
group therapy	Therapy with a group of patients with similar problems to gain insight into personal issues through discussions and interaction with each other. Groups are usually facilitated by a clinician, who helps to provide structure and guidance to the group.

Other Treatments

TREATMENT	DESCRIPTION
electroconvulsive therapy (ECT) *ē-lĕk-trō-kŏn-VŬL-sĭv THĔR-ă-pē*	This treatment involves passing an electrical current through the brain to create a brief seizure in the brain. Used mainly to treat severe depression that has been unresponsive to medication (Fig. 20–4).

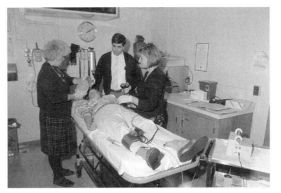

Figure 20–4 *A patient about to receive electroconvulsive therapy (ECT). (From Glod, C: Contemporary Psychiatric-Mental Health Nursing. FA Davis, Philadelphia, 1998, p. 222, with permission.)*

Other Treatments (Continued)

TREATMENT	DESCRIPTION
hypnosis *hĭp-NŌ-sĭs*	Use of an induced altered state of consciousness to increase the responsiveness to a suggestion such as a behavior change as in quitting smoking, to increase the speed of therapy, to help with the recovery of repressed memories, or to aid in pain management.
phototherapy *fō-tō-THĔR-ă-pē* *photo=light* *therapy=treatment*	The direct administration of high-intensity light treatment to combat seasonal affective disorder.
sex therapy	Treatment designed to help individuals and couples to overcome sexual dysfunction such as inhibited sexual response in women, inability for a man to achieve and/or maintain an erection, and premature ejaculation.

Pharmacology

DRUG CLASSIFICATION	THERAPEUTIC ACTION
anticonvulsants *ăn-tĭ-kŏn-VŬL-sănts*	Agents that prevent or arrest seizures; also used effectively as mood stabilizers in various mental disorders.
antidepressants *ăn-tĭ-dē-PRĔS-sănts*	Used to regulate mood and reduce symptoms of depression by affecting the amount of neurotransmitters in the brain.
tricyclic antidepressants *trī-SĪK-lĭk* *ăn-tĭ-dē-PRĔS-sănts*	Indicated for the treatment of major depression, depressed phase of bipolar disorder, and dysthymia. Some are specifically indicated for certain conditions such as obsessive compulsive disorder (OCD), borderline personality disorder, and attention deficit disorder (ADD).
monoamine oxidase inhibitors (MAO-inhibitors) *mŏn-ō-ă-MĒN ŎK-sĭ-dās* *ĭn-HĬB-ĭ-tĕrs*	Primarily reserved for treatment-resistant depression because of the potential for severe contraindications and the need for dietary restrictions.
selective serotonin reuptake inhibitors (SSRIs) *sĕ-LĔK-tĭv sĕr-ō-TŌN-ĭn* *rē-ŬP-tāk ĭn-HĬB-ĭ-tĕrs*	Indicated for the treatment of depression, dysthymia, obsessive compulsive disorder, panic disorder, and bulimia. Causes fewer side effects than tricyclics or MAO inhibitors.
antipsychotics, neuroleptics *ăn-tĭ-sī-KŎT-ĭks,* *nū-rō-LĔP-tĭks* *psycho=mind* *tics=pertaining to, relating to*	Agents that block the brain receptors responsible for psychotic behavior. Used to treat hallucination and delusion disorders.

Pharmacology (Continued)

DRUG CLASSIFICATION	THERAPEUTIC ACTION
anxiolytics and sedative hypnotics *ăng-zī-ō-LĬT-ĭks, SĔD-ă-tĭv hĭp-NŎT-ĭks*	Agents used to calm without decreasing consciousness, commonly known as *tranquilizers*.
mood stabilizers	Agents used to treat the cycles of bipolar disorder.
psychostimulants *sī-kō-STĬM-ū-lănts*	Agents used to treat attention deficit disorder (ADD) in children and adults and narcolepsy.

❖ ABBREVIATIONS

ABBREVIATION	MEANING	ABBREVIATION	MEANING
AD	Alzheimer disease, right ear (*auris dextra*)	**MRI**	magnetic resonance imaging
ADD	attention deficit disorder	**MSE**	mental status exam
CA	chronological age	**OCD**	obsessive-compulsive disorder
CBT	cognitive behavioral therapy	**PET**	positron emission tomography
CNS	central nervous system	**PTSD**	posttraumatic stress disorder
DSM	*Diagnostic and Statistical Manual of Mental Disorders*	**SAD**	seasonal affective disorder
DT	delirium tremens	**SPECT**	single photon emission computed tomography
ECT	electroconvulsive therapy	**SSRI**	selective serotonin reuptake inhibitor
IQ	intelligence quotient	**TAT**	Thematic Apperception Test
LOC	loss of consciousness	**THC**	tetrahydrocannabinol (active ingredient in marijuana)
LSD	lysergic acid diethylamide (hallucinogen)	**WAIS**	Wechsler Adult Intelligence Scale
MA	mental age	**WISC**	Wechsler Intelligence Scale for Children
MAO	monoamine oxidase		
MMPI	Minnesota Multiphasic Personality Inventory		

Activity 20–4: Clinical Application

Diagnostic Tests, Treatments, and Abbreviations

anticonvulsant
antipsychotics
anxiolytics
behavior therapy
cognitive behavior therapy (CBT)
clinical interview
computed tomography (CT)
DSM-IV
ECT
electroencephalography (EEG)
hypnosis

intelligence tests
mental status exam (MSE)
polysomnography
positron emission tomography (PET)
psychoanalysis
psychostimulants
PTSD
SAD
sex therapy
SSRI

Match the terms listed above with the definitions given in the numbered list:

1. _____ tests that measure the aptitude or potential competence of an individual.

2. _____ a clinical test designed to ascertain a person's appearance, behavior, and perception of reality.

3. _____ a critical diagnostic tool to assess current symptoms, history of present illness, cultural practices, religious beliefs, and current stressors.

4. _____ a computer analysis of brain tissue density used to detect atrophy or lesions.

5. _____ process of recording brain wave activity.

6. _____ psychotherapy in which the therapist analyzes and interprets a patient's unconscious thoughts using free association.

7. _____ an imaging procedure that provides colorimetric information about the brain's metabolic activity by detecting how quickly tissues consume radioactive isotopes; aids in the diagnosis of neuropsychiatric problems.

8. _____ an EEG performed during sleep.

9. _____ treatment of behavioral and emotional problems by modifying maladaptive, negative thoughts.

10. _____ the standard for classification of mental disorders.

11. _____ pharmacological agents used to calm a person without decreasing consciousness.

12. _____ pharmacological agents used to treat attention deficit disorder (ADD).

13. _____ seasonal affective disorder.

14. _____ agent used to control seizures.

15. _____ treatment of sexual dysfunction.

16. _____ medications to treat hallucinations and delusions.

17. _____ post-traumatic stress disorder.

18. _____ the use of a trancelike induced state to enhance therapy or uncover repressed memories.

19. _____ selective serotonin reuptake inhibitor.

20. _____ use of electric current passed through the brain to treat extreme depression that is unresponsive to medication.

Correct Answers _____ × 5 = _____ **% Score**

Activity 20–5: Build Medical Words
Diagnostic, Symptomatic, and Surgical Terms

Use *psych/o* (mind) to build medical words meaning:

1. study of the mind _____

2. abnormal condition of the mind _____

3. pertaining to the mind and body _____

4. treatment of the mind _____

Use *hypn/o* (sleep) to build medical words meaning:

5. fear of sleep _____

6. abnormal condition of sleep _____

Use *-phoria* (feeling [mental state]) to build medical words meaning:

7. feeling good _____

8. feeling bad _____

Use *-phobia* (fear) to build medical words meaning:

9. fear of strangers _____

10. fear of light _____

Correct Answers _____ × 10 = _____ **% Score**

MEDICAL RECORDS

Included in this section are psychiatry reports for three different patients who received medical treatment. You will find that these authentic reports reinforce the medical terminology related to pathological conditions, procedures and tests, pharmacology, and medical abbreviations presented in this chapter.

Reading and Dictionary Exercise

Place a check mark [✓] after you complete the exercise.

[ ] **1.** Underline the following words in the reports as you read the history and physical examination, the discharge summary, and the progress note aloud. These medical records can be found at the end of the chapter.

[ ] **2.** Use a medical dictionary, Appendix A, and Appendix F, Part 2 to complete this exercise.

Note: You are not expected to fully understand all the parts of the medical records. The important aspect of this exercise is to use all available resources to complete it. Eventually you will master the terminology and format of these reports.

>>> MEDICAL RECORD 20-1: HISTORY AND PHYSICAL EXAMINATION

Term	Pronunciation	Meaning
bipolar disorder	*bī-PŌL-ăr dĭs-ŎR-dĕr*	_____
bulimia	*bū-LĬM-ē-ă*	_____
self-mutilation	*sĕlf mū-tĭ-LĀ-shŭn*	_____
binging	*BĬN-jĭng*	_____
purging	*PŬR-jĭng*	_____
paranoia	*păr-ă-NOY-ă*	_____
Prozac	*PRŌ-zăk*	_____
Tofranil	*tō-FRĀ-nĭl*	_____
Pamelor	*PĂM-ĕ-lŏr*	_____
Cytomel	*CĪ-tō-mēl*	_____
Xanax	*ZĂN-ăks*	_____
Haldol	*HĂL-dŏl*	_____
C-section	*SĒ-sĕk-shŭn*	_____
lithium	*LĬTH-ē-ŭm*	_____
Eskalith	*ĔS-kă-lĭth*	_____

Wellbutrin	wĕl-BŪ-trĭn	_____
Zyprexa	zī-PRĔK-să	_____
Ativan	Ă-tĭv-ăn	_____
Paxil	PĂK-sĭl	_____
Ambien	ĂM-bē-ĕn	_____
normocephalic	nor-mō-sĕf-ĂL-ĭk	_____
adenopathy	ăd-ĕ-NŎP-ă-thē	_____
cyanosis	sī-ă-NŌ-sĭs	_____
bilateral	bī-LĂT-ĕr-ăl	_____
anxious	ĂNG-shŭs	_____
affect	Ă-fĕkt	_____

>>> MEDICAL RECORD 20-2: DISCHARGE SUMMARY

Term	Pronunciation	Meaning
psychiatric	sī-kē-Ă-trĭk	_____
Ativan	Ă-tĭv-ăn	_____
Desyrel	DĔS-ĭ-rĕl	_____
psychotherapy	sī-kō-THĔR-ă-pē	_____
Trazodone	TRĂZ-ŏ-dōn	_____
Premphase	PRĔM-fāz	_____
Fosamax	FŎS-ă-măks	_____

>>> MEDICAL RECORD 20-3: PHYSICIAN PROGRESS NOTE

Term	Pronunciation	Meaning
imipramine	ĭ-MĬP-ră-mēn	_____
Ritalin	RĬT-ă-lĭn	_____
attention deficit hyperactivity disorder	ă-TĔN-shŭn DĔF-ĭ-sĭt hī-pĕr-ăk-TĬV-ĭ-tē dĭ-SOR-dĕr	_____
tricyclic	trī-SĬK-lĭk	_____
group therapy	grūp THĔR-ă-pē	_____

Critical Thinking: Analysis of Psychiatry Records

This section provides experience in abstracting and analyzing information from medical records to provide a basic understanding of psychiatric care. Unlike medical reports, psychiatric reports often include a multiaxial approach to medical diagnoses. This means that in addition to the medical diagnoses, they may also include information about the factors that may contribute to the mental disorder, as well as information about the patient's current level of functioning. Before you continue, you will find it helpful to review the section previously discussed in this chapter, "Classification System of Psychiatric Disorders," which describes the multiaxial approach.

>>> MEDICAL RECORD 20-1: HISTORY AND PHYSICAL EXAMINATION

1. What problems was the patient having that indicated a need for hospital admission?

2. Which diagnoses were included in the patient's psychiatric history?

3. What was the precipitating event that triggered the patient's distress?

4. What was the patient's suicide status on admission?

5. With what method had she attempted suicide in the past?

>>> MEDICAL RECORD 20-2: DISCHARGE SUMMARY

6. How many times had this patient been hospitalized previously?

7. What event precipitated her attempted suicide?

8. How did the patient stabilize?

9. What medication was she discharged on?

_____

_____

> **>>> MEDICAL RECORD 20-3: PHYSICIAN PROGRESS NOTE**

10. Why did a physician see Eric?

_____

11. What positive behaviors did his mother report he is engaging in?

_____

_____

12. What negative behaviors did his mother report he is engaging in?

_____

Audio Practice

Listen to the audio CD-ROM to practice the pronunciation of selected medical terms from this chapter.

Medical Record 20–1. History and Physical Examination

GENERAL HOSPITAL AND MEDICAL CENTER
2211 Fifth Avenue North • Healthy City, USA 12345 • (321) 123-4567

History and Physical Examination

Patient Name: DelFuego, Cynthia
Birth Date: 10/19/xx

Patient Number: 01-63-79
Emergency Room

HISTORY

DATE OF CONSULTATION: 02-08-19xx

CHIEF COMPLAINT: Bipolar disorder

HISTORY OF PRESENT ILLNESS: The patient is a 33-year-old white female with a history of bipolar disorder and bulimia who is admitted for decompensating symptoms. The patient moved to Knoxville, TN two weeks ago to "make a new start" and subsequently became overwhelmed with the move. She began having racing thoughts and overwhelming thoughts of self-harm and self-mutilation. She also began binging and purging, which she had done in the past. She feels she has no support system in Knoxville and reports having some paranoia about other people. The patient has no active suicidal thoughts or plan at this time. Admits to difficulties sleeping, decreased level of functioning as well.

PAST PSYCHIATRIC HISTORY: Diagnoses: Bipolar disorder, bulimia. Multiple inpatient admission with the last admission in November 19xx. Previous suicidal attempts by cutting wrists. History of sexual abuse by uncle at age 6 or 7.

PAST PSCYHIATRIC MEDICATIONS: Prozac, Tofranil, Pamelor, Cytomel, Xanax, and Haldol.

PAST MEDICAL HISTORY: None

SURGERIES: C-section, tonsils and adenoids removal.

ALLERGIES: No known drug allergies.

CURRENT MEDICATIONS: Lithium, Eskalith, Wellbutrin, Zyprexa, Ativan, Paxil, and Ambien.

SOCIAL HISTORY: Patient lives with seven year old son. Denies tobacco or drug use, occasionally uses alcohol.

FAMILY HISTORY: Breast cancer, diabetes, cardiovascular disease.

REVIEW OF SYSTEMS: As above in history of present illness. Patient denies recent change in vision, hearing, speech or gait.

Continued

History and Physical Examination, page 2
Patient Name: DelFuego, Cynthia   **Patient Number:** 01-63-79

PHYSICAL EXAMINATION

VITAL SIGNS: Afebrile, pulse 94, respirations 19, blood pressure 154/84.
HEENT: Normocephalic, atraumatic, PERRLA, EOMI, oropharynx clear.
NECK: Supple without adenopathy.
HEART: Regular rate and rhythm, no murmurs, gallops, or rubs.
LUNGS: Clear to auscultation and percussion.
ABDOMEN: Soft, nontender. Positive bowel sounds. No masses, no hepatosplenomegaly.
EXTREMITIES: No clubbing, cyanosis or edema. There are multiple old scars on bilateral forearms.
NEUROLOGICAL: Cranial nerves II through XII were grossly intact.

MENTAL STATUS EXAM: Patient is alert and oriented times 3. She is neatly dressed and cooperative with exam. Patient is calm with good eye contact. Speech is clear and easy to understand. Mood anxious. Affect with full range. Thought process organized. Thought content is reality based.

IMPRESSION:
Axis I   Bipolar Disorder most recent episode depressed with suicidal ideation; Bulimia Nervosa
Axis II   Deferred
Axis III   None
Axis IV   Recent move, no family support, suicidal ideation
Axis V   GAF = 35 (at admission)

PLAN: Admit to 8 North for further evaluation and treatment per Dr. Keaton.

_____

Marilyn A. Sonders, M.D.

MAS/kje
D: 02/08/xx
T: 02/09/xx

cc: Charles Keaton, M.D.

Medical Record 20–2. Discharge Summary

GENERAL HOSPITAL AND MEDICAL CENTER
2211 Fifth Avenue North • Healthy City, USA 12345 • (321) 123-4567

Discharge Summary

Patient Name: Lapinsky, Sharon   **Patient Number:** 01-52-47
Birth Date: 09/21/xx   **Room Number:** 810

DISCHARGE DATE: 11/12/xx

REASON FOR ADMISSION: This is a 50-year-old married female, mother of two who is employed as a corporate medical officer by a large corporation. She was admitted for her first psychiatric stay via the emergency center where she was transferred from Cook County Hospital. The patient had become distraught and had taken a low dose overuse of Ativan, Desyrel and Xanax but had suicidal ideation.

SIGNIFICANT FINDINGS: The patient has been under tremendous stress with feelings of being despaired about a deteriorating marital situation that appears to be headed for divorce. After a recent attempt at reconciliation, the husband told her that the marriage of 27 years was not going to work. The patient became distraught, impulsively took an overdose of medication. She has been chronically anxious about this situation and job stress.

The patient stabilized efficiently and quickly. She dealt head on with the reality that her husband was going to leave after a meeting with the social worker and the patient confirmed his tenacity in that decision. She was seen daily for psychotherapy. Trazodone was increased, she stabilized sufficiently to shift to outpatient care.

CONDITION UPON DISCHARGE: Stabilized, markedly improved.
Axis I   Adjustment Disorder with Anxiety
Axis II   No diagnosis
Axis III   None
Axis IV   Recent news of divorce, chronic marital problems, suicidal ideation
Axis V   GAF = 65 (at discharge)

SUGGESTIONS/RECOMMENDATIONS: Trazodone 190 mg HS, Xanax 0.5 mg t.i.d., continue her Premphase 0.625 md daily, Fosamax 10 mg every AM. Calcium carbonate 1250 mg b.i.d., multivitamin daily. Follow with her family physician for general medical care. Continue counseling with either Dr. Wendy or the psychologist of her choice. Continue in partial hospitalization next week to assure continued stable status and improvement. Diet: lactose intolerant. No alcohol or any other centrally acting substances. Return to work to be decided.

_____
Luke Archbow, M.D.

LA/rd
D: 11/13/xx; T: 11/16/xx

cc: Dr. Wendy

Medical Record 20–3. Physician Progress Note

GENERAL HOSPITAL AND MEDICAL CENTER
2211 Fifth Avenue North • Healthy City, USA 12345 • (321) 123-4567

Physician Progress Note

Patient Name: Rider, Eric
Birth Date: 05/16/89

Patient Number: 02-60-98
Outpatient Clinic

DATE OF VISIT: 05/07/xx

Eric's medications are imipramine 25 mg 3 tablets q.h.s., and Ritalin 19 mg 1 tablet t.i.d.

Eric came to the office with his mother and older brother for a medication check up and to see how he is doing on his medications. When asked if he knew any information about his medicine, Eric looked at me with a blank stare and ignored any questions. He had no idea what the name, the dose, or any side effects of the medications were. These were all reviewed with mom and she reviewed Eric's dosing program with us.

When asked about school, mom said Eric is the perfect student. He listens, follows directions, although she does state that Eric still has trouble learning, he still doesn't read, he still does not speak to the teacher, but there are no unacceptable behaviors going on at school. At home, mom is a little bit concerned. He has no idea how to control his anger. She brought in a sample of the book that she had got from the library, in which he had torn all the pages and more or less ripped them to shreds. She is getting quite frustrated because he is getting bigger, and he is getting stronger than she is, and she is worried that she wont be able to control him for much longer. With that in mind, we will go ahead and increase the dose of his imipramine to 100 mg that he will take at approximately 4:30 in the afternoon.

ASSESSMENT:
Axis I   Attention Deficit Hyperactivity Disorder, combined type; Learning Disorder
Axis II   No diagnosis
Axis III   None
Axis IV   None
Axis V   GAF = 70 (current)

PLAN:
1. Will continue the Ritalin as outlined above, and he was written a prescription for #90, with no refills. His imipramine dose has changed. A prescription was written for imipramine 50 mg, #60, with 2 tablets PO q. 1630 with no refills.
2. He was advised to get an EKG and a tricyclic level in approximately one week, and those results will be faxed to us.
3. They will continue the individual and group therapy for the cause noted, and we will see him in approximately 4 weeks.

Edward A. Starkis, M.D.

EAS/rmd
D: 05/07/xx; T: 05/08/xx

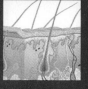
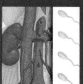

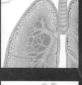

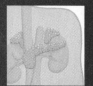

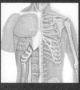

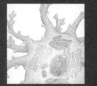
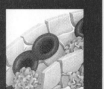

chapter

21 Medical Records

Chapter Outline

Objectives

Upon completion of this chapter, you will be able to:

- Understand the purpose of medical records in the health-care system.
- Describe the difference between the problem-oriented medical record and the source-oriented medical record.
- Describe and define the components of the history and physical examination.
- Identify and describe several types of reports found in medical records.
- Demonstrate your knowledge of this chapter by completing the activities and analysis of medical records.

Physicians treat thousands of patients during their professional careers. Without a system for recording each patient's medical care, valuable information contributing to the outcome of treatment would be lost. Establishing a medical record and maintaining its continuity ensure that the patient receives competent, comprehensive medical care. Although an introduction to medical records is included in Chapter 2, this chapter includes additional information.

THE MEDICAL RECORD

The medical record is initiated at the time of the patient's first appointment with a health-care practitioner. It is used to compile a database of relevant facts related to the patient's health history, illness, and medical treatment. The database includes various types of diagnostic reports, such as laboratory reports and imaging reports. Nonmedical information about the patient (e.g., occupation, address, telephone number, race, gender, age) is also part of the medical record. The main purpose of the medical record is summarized below:

- It is a method of communication between health-care practitioners involved in caring for the patient.
- It provides an evaluation of *symptoms* of a disease by compiling information that may be related to these symptoms.
- The *objective* documentation of medical care serves as a legal document. It provides evidence to protect the legal interests of the hospital, the health-care practitioners, and the patient in a court of law, if needed.
- It provides an assessment of the effectiveness of the patient's plan of care.
- It provides a description of exactly what happened to a patient while under the health-care practitioner's supervision.
- It provides clinical data for research and education.
- It provides a database to complete insurance claims and supports justification for maximum insurance reimbursements.

Several record management systems are available to physicians and other health-care practitioners. Two of the most commonly used systems, the *problem-oriented medical record* (POMR) and the *source-oriented medical record* (SOMR), are described here. Although the SOMR is frequently used in hospitals, both record management systems are found in clinics, private medical practices, and other health-care facilities.

Problem-Oriented Medical Record

The POMR was developed by Dr. Lawrence Weed in the l960s, and is also known as the "Weed System." The POMR system focuses on the patient's health problems and the plans to treat them. It is a record-keeping method that standardizes information and makes it quickly accessible in medical databases.

In the POMR, all information in the patient's medical record is linked to specific problems. The record includes four sections: a *database*, a *problem list*, a *plan*, and *progress notes*.

Database: The database is the first part of a POMR. This section contains the chief complaint (CC), all patient evaluations such as the patient history, physical examination, laboratory reports, dietitian assessment, as well as other documents that evaluate the patient's state of health. With these data, the physician diagnoses the illness or problem and develops a treatment plan.

Problem List: This list (Table 21–1) is attached to the front of the POMR. The list indexes information by organizing it around a problem, and includes active and inactive problems, date of onset, and the date on which the problem is resolved.

Specific problems (also listed in Table 21–1) are often numbered, defined, and then referred to throughout the record. The same number is never used twice for the same problem, even when a problem is resolved. In addition to the index list that is attached to the front of the POMR, a numbered and headed page is often added for each problem that requires diagnosis and treatment (Table 21–2). For example, a patient who has visited the office at various times with back pain, upper respiratory infection (URI), and again with back pain has a separate page for each condition. In this case, the patient has three problems, written on three pages, and all three pages are kept in one folder. Each problem page lists any other physical or psychological problems related to that particular condition.

Plan: The plan describes the method suggested to resolve each active problem. Basically, it consists of, but is not limited to, three parts: The first part, the *diagnostic plan*, contains orders for specific tests to confirm the diagnosis of a patient's disease or condition. The second part, the *therapeutic plan*, includes directions or goals for dietary, surgical, psychological, or physical treatments. The third part, *patient education*, includes instructions and information related to the patient that will help in the treatment of the illness. Table 21–2 shows three separate problem pages that include a plan for each problem. These are the three problems recorded in Joe Carson's medical record. Compare the three problem pages with the summary of these problems enumerated in Table 21–1.

Progress Notes. The progress achieved on each problem is recorded using a logical sequence called the **SOAP** format. This type of documentation, and adaptations thereof, appear to be the most commonly used type of progress note, regardless of whether a specific number is assigned to the problem. Below is an explanation of each section of SOAP.

TABLE 21-1: Problem List for Joe Carson

PROBLEM NUMBER	ONSET DATE	PROBLEM LIST	INACTIVE, RESOLVED, CONTROLLED	DATE RESOLVED
1.	1/25/xx	Back pain	Resolved	2/28/xx
2.	3/27/xx	Upper respiratory infection	Resolved	4/30/xx
3.	4/19/xx	Back pain		

Subjective — Information provided by the patient (symptoms, feelings, and comments)

Objective — Observable factual data (observations made by the physician, and results of diagnostic tests)

Assessment — An evaluation of the plan and/or success of the treatment

Plan — The decision to continue with or change the treatment

TABLE 21-2: Numbered Problem Page with Related Problems and Initial Plan for Joe Carson

EXAMPLE OF PROBLEM, PAGE 1

PROBLEM #1, 1/25/xx Back Pain
A. Cannot work as grocery stock clerk in his present position
B. Cannot sleep through the night

PLAN (Initial)
A. Physical Therapy referral for evaluation
B. Tylenol with codeine one tab qid, prn

EXAMPLE OF PROBLEM, PAGE 2

PROBLEM #2, 3/27/xx Upper Respiratory Infection
A. Coughing
B. Cannot sleep through the night.
C. Chest discomfort

PLAN (Initial)
A. Chest x-ray ordered.
B. CBC ordered.
C. Injection of Rocephin 1 gm.
D. Doxycycline 100 mg #20, one tablet bid for 3 weeks.
E. Recheck in 14 days.

EXAMPLE OF PROBLEM, PAGE 3

PROBLEM #3, 4/19/xx Back Pain
A. Back pain prevents patient from working again
B. Sleepless nights

PLAN
A. Use back support at work
B. Reevaluation of physical therapy
C. Reevaluation of exercise
D. Recheck in 12 days

In most instances, handwritten chart notes remain as permanent documents in the medical record. In other instances, handwritten chart notes become part of the patient's permanent record once they are transcribed and the health-care practitioner validates their accuracy by initialing or signing them. The handwritten notes sampled in this chapter are referred to as chart notes. See, for instance, Chart Notes 21–1 for an example of the POMR progress notes using the SOAP format.

Source-Oriented Medical Record

Unlike the POMR, the data in the source-oriented medical record (SOMR) are not organized according to patient problems. Instead, the data are systematized according to the source of information involved. Sources include, but are not limited to, physicians, nurses, laboratory technicians, social services, medical assistants, and any other health-care practitioners who may be involved with the patient. Each patient record is arranged in chronological order and is divided into sections. Each section describes the source of the document or information and may be represented by a divider and a colored tab. The section tabs are frequently labeled *medical history, physician, nursing, diagnostic reports, correspondence,* and so forth. As various information and reports are generated, they are placed behind the appropriate divider. This system is easy to use and does not require special training. For example, behind the *medical history* divider, data related to personal and family histories may be recorded on a separate form, designed specifically for this purpose, or in the allotted space on the physician's notes. Behind the *physician divider,* the physician's notes may begin with the medical history, physician orders, physician progress notes, or any other documents generated or signed by the physician. Behind the *nursing divider,* you would find the nurse's progress notes, nursing assessments, nursing care plans, or any other documents generated or signed by the nurses. Behind the *diagnostic reports* divider, you would find recorded results of laboratory and other diagnostic tests. They are usually arranged in reverse chronological order, the most recent reports and documents on the top. Laboratory slips may also be stacked using a "shingle

Chart Notes 21–1. Progress Notes Using SOAP Format

PROGRESS NOTES	Patient: *CARSON, JOE*

	DATE	FINDINGS
1	*1/23/xx*	*CC: Back pain*
2		*S: Pt states that the PT and meds*
3		*have relieved his pain; he is feeling*
4		*much better.*
5		*O: PT report indicates pt is now*
6		*able to lift wts with no stress*
7		*or pain in the back.*
8		*A: Meds offering pain relief; PT*
9		*and exercise are strengthening*
10		*the abdominal muscles.*
11		*P: Continue meds, PT, and*
12		*exercise 2 wks. Reevaluate.*
13		*M.B. Bishop, MD*

method," with one slip overlapping another. Behind the *correspondence divider* you may find correspondence from other physicians (including consultations), the patient, and others. This section excludes financial matters.

An advantage of the SOMR is that each group of professionals can easily locate the proper section of the record in which to make entries. The main disadvantage is that data are fragmented, and it is difficult to track problems chronologically because of input from different groups of health-care practitioners. In addition, the data are not organized by the patient's problems and details about a specific problem may be distributed throughout the record. Consequently, to make a comprehensive assessment of a patient's problems and devise a health-care plan, it may become necessary to locate data from several different sections of the medical record. Although the general characteristics of the SOMR are essentially the same, the specific design may vary among health-care facilities.

Activity 21–1: Competency Verification
The Two Major Types of Medical Records

1. Name two of the most commonly used record management systems in health-care facilities, and briefly state the differences between them.

_____

_____

_____

_____

2. How is information compiled in the problem-oriented medical record?

_____

_____

3. What are the four major sections of the POMR?

_____

4. What does SOAP stand for?

S: _____

O: _____

A: _____

P: _____

5. Name a major advantage and disadvantage of the source-oriented medical record.

_____

_____

_____

_____

_____

_____

Diagnostic Reports

Various types of medical reports are compiled in the medical record. Diagnostic reports, such as laboratory and imaging reports, document the results of procedures performed on the patient. The tests are ordered by the physician, and the results are used to help establish a diagnosis of a patient's condition or disease.

Laboratory Reports

Laboratory reports are a valuable diagnostic tool. They summarize documented findings of tests performed on tissue, blood, and other body fluid samples. Some of the basic laboratory tests are discussed here, but a more extensive coverage is found in Chapter 2. Note that the laboratory reports for Carol Coed have been designed by a particular hospital and do not always contain standard abbreviations.

The complete blood count shown in Medical Record 21–1 provides valuable information about the patient's state of health and is one of the most frequently ordered blood tests. It includes a white blood count (WBC), red blood count (RBC), hemoglobin (HGB), hematocrit (HCT), platelet count (plat), mean cell volume (MCV), mean cell hemoglobin (MCH), mean corpuscular hemoglobin concentration and red blood cell indices (MCHC), and red blood cell distribution width (RDW). In this case, the diagnostic test was ordered preoperatively.

Another important blood test, a chemistry profile, analyzes the chemical components of blood. It is frequently ordered as part of the patient's physical examination (PE), but it may be ordered for other reasons also. Review the chemistry profile report in Medical Record 21–2. In this case, the chemistry profile test was ordered preoperatively. Laboratory tests are discussed in greater detail in Chapter 2 and should be reviewed at this time.

Another laboratory test, a routine urinalysis (UA), analyses various physical properties and chemical components of the patient's urine. This test is illustrated in Medical Record 21–3. In this case, the physician ordered the UA preoperatively. The test is often done in preparation for a diagnostic or surgical procedure or as a screening test for a PE. To become acquainted with the various procedures of a urinalysis, review the contents of the report.

Activity 21–2: Clinical Application
Laboratory Reports

---

1. Review Medical Record 21–1 and list the names and abbreviations of at least four tests that were performed.

_____

_____

_____

_____

2. What is the purpose of the chemistry profile test shown in Medical Record 21–2?

_____

_____

3. Which of the three laboratory reports (Medical Record 21–1, 21–2, or 21–3) determines hyaline casts, bilirubin, and ketones?

_____

_____

Medical Record 21–1. Complete Blood Count

GENERAL HOSPITAL AND MEDICAL CENTER

2211 Fifth Avenue North • Healthy City, USA 12345 • (321) 123-4567

LABORATORY REPORT

January 13, xx   6 pm

Name:**COED, CAROL**   MRN:**99340465**   Loc:QC

Age:50 YRS   Sex:F

* *

CBC

* *

Procedure	WBC	RBC	HGB	HCT	PLAT
Units	X10E9/L	X10E12/L	g/dL	%	X10E9/L
Normals	4.8-10.8	3.80-5.20	11.7-16.0	35-47	149-409
Collected Date					
01/13/xx 1222*	**20.0 H**	**1.25 L**	**4.5 L***	**13.0 L**	**666 H**

Procedure	MCV	MCH	MCHC	RDW
Units	fL	pg	g/dL	%
Normals	81-100	26-33.5	32-36	11.5-14.7
Collected Date				
01/13/xx 1222*	**55 L**	**25.0 L**	**28.0 L**	**22.6 H**

*Date and time of draw

Medical Record 21–2. Chemistry Profile

GENERAL HOSPITAL AND MEDICAL CENTER

2211 Fifth Avenue North • Healthy City, USA 12345 • (321) 123-4567

LABORATORY REPORT

January 13, xx   6 pm

Name:**COED, CAROL**   MRN:**99340465**   Loc:QC
                  Age:50 YRS   Sex:F

```
***************************************************************************
                            CHEMISTRY PROFILE
***************************************************************************
```

Procedure	SODIUM	POTASSIUM	CHLORIDE	CO2	GLUCOSE
Units	mmol/L	mmol/L	mmol/L	mmol/L	mg/dL
Normals	134-146	3.5-5.0	98-109	21-30	65-110
Collected Date					
01/13/xx 1225 *	**112 L***	**3.0 L**	**99**	**25**	**125 H**

Procedure	BUN	CREATININE	CALCIUM	ALBUMIN	PROTEIN, TOTAL
Units	mg/dL	mg/dL	mg/dL	g/dL	g/dL
Normals	5-23	0.0-1.4	8.5-10.5	3.2-5.3	6.0-8.0
Collected Date					
01/13/xx 1225 *	**24 H**	**1.5 H**	**10.0**	**5.8 H**	**7.7**

Procedure	BILIRUBIN, TOTAL	ALKALINE PHOSPHATASE	AST (GOT)
Units	mg/dL	U/L	U/L
Normals	0.2-1.0	39-117	0-31
Collected Date			
01/13/xx 1225 *	**1.1 H**	**44**	**37 H**

---

*Date and time of draw

Medical Record 21 – 3. Urinalysis

GENERAL HOSPITAL AND MEDICAL CENTER

2211 Fifth Avenue North • Healthy City, USA 12345 • (321) 123-4567

LABORATORY REPORT

January 13, xx   6 pm

Name:**COED, COROL** MRN:**99340465** Loc:QC
Age:50 YRS Sex:F

****
URINALYSIS
****

Procedure	COLOR	TURBIDITY	SPECIFIC GRAVITY	PH	KETONES (URINE)
Units					Qual
Normals	STRAW/YEL	CLEAR	1.003-1.035	5-9	Negative
Collected Date					
01/13/xx 1200 *	**YELLOW**	**CLEAR**	**1.022**	**6.0**	**Negative**

Procedure	BILIRUBIN (URINE)	UROBILINOGEN	GLUCOSE (URINE)	LEUKOCYTE ESTERASE	WBC
Units	Qual	Qual	Qual	Qual	/hpf
Normals	Negative	Normal	Negative	Negative	0-5
Collected Date					
01/13/xx 1200 *	**POSITIVE**	**NORMAL**	**1+**	**1+**	**35 H**

Procedure	WBC CLUMPS	NITRITE	BLOOD/HGB	RBC	PROTEIN
Units	Qual	Qual	Qual	/hpf	Qual
Normals		Negative	Negative	0-5	Negative
Collected Date					
01/13/xx 1200 *	**FEW**	**Negative**	**1+**	**20 H**	**1+**

Procedure	HYALINE CASTS	SQUAMOUS EPITHELIUM
Units	/lpf	/hpf
Normals	0-2	0-5
Collected Date		
01/13/xx 1200 *	**2**	**4**

_____

*Date and time urine specimen was collected

Imaging Reports

Imaging reports describe findings and interpretations from radiographs or special diagnostic studies performed in a radiology department. A radiological diagnosis is summarized on the report by the radiologist who reviews the films (Medical Record 21–4. For an illustration of a mammography screening of a woman's breast, see Figure 18–6. You may also refer to Chapter 18 for a comprehensive discussion of mammography).

CONSULTATION REPORTS

These reports summarize the findings of a specialist who is requested to see a patient on a referral basis. Usually the specialist offers input or a second opinion of the medical problem to the primary physician. The consulting physician or specialist conducts an evaluation of the patient and documents the results. Particular attention is given to the consultant's area of specialization. Impressions (IMP) or diagnoses (DX) with treatment plans must be included in the report. The consultation report format varies from physician to physician. When the consultation occurs between physician offices, a business letter format is usually used. If the consultation is part of a hospitalization, the hospital usually has a standardized format that must be followed (Medical Record 21–5). See Chapter 2 for additional information about consultation reports.

DOCUMENTATION OF MEDICAL CARE

A series of authentic medical reports for Rochelle Tucker are presented to help you visualize the stages of medical care that took place during her stay at the hospital.

Rochelle Tucker's history and physical examination, her medical treatment at the hospital, her pathology report, and her discharge summary are documented in the medical record and are discussed here. Please note that the medical report is authentic, but the name is fictitious to preserve patient confidentiality.

History and Physical Examination Reports

When a patient visits a health-care facility, the physician or health-care practitioner generates a history and physical (H&P) examination report. This comprehensive document has three parts, as illustrated in Medical Record 21–6. Refer to the H&P report as you read the following information.

The *first part* of the report consists of *subjective data*, which document the patient's chief complaint, present illness, past medical history, allergies, family and social history, health habits, and a review of systems. The data provided by the patient begin with the chief complaint and conclude with the review of systems.

The *second part* of the report consists of *objective data*, which document the physical examination (PE). These are facts that the physician or health-care practitioner observes as he or she examines the patient. These observations are further supported by the accumulation of data provided by the results of various diagnostic tests. Once the subjective and objective data are recorded, the physician determines an *impression* or *diagnosis* (plural, diagnoses). The impression (IMP) or diagnosis (Dx) identifies a disease or condition by a scientific evaluation of symptoms, physical signs, history, and results of various diagnostic tests (e.g., laboratory or imaging procedures). After all data are collected, a plan of action is determined.

The *third part* of the report consists of the *conclusion*, which summarizes the *treatment plan*. Treatment plans consist of either one or more of the following: *diagnostic plan*, *operative* or *therapeutic plan*, or *patient education*. The *diagnostic* plan may contain specific orders for diagnostic testing. These tests are used to confirm suspicions of a disease or a specific condition. Examples of diagnostic tests are radiographs or laboratory tests. The *operative* and/or *therapeutic plan* includes a specific surgery or therapy for treatment such as prescriptions for specific medications.

In Rochelle Tucker's H&P, the physician recommends a total thyroidectomy (see Medical Record 21–6). Information useful to the patient regarding this procedure is included in the *patient education* section. This information can be conveyed to the patient verbally, in writing, or by video.

Some of the header styles may vary in the H&P report, depending on the nature of the illness or disease. It may also vary if a medical facility has designed a specific style that is unique to its institution.

Medical Record 21–4. Mammography Screening

GENERAL HOSPITAL AND MEDICAL CENTER

2211 Fifth Avenue North • Healthy City, USA 12345 • (321) 123-4567

NAME: Sussek, Barbara
DOB: **05/25/1936**   **62 YRS**
PHYSICIAN: **ADIUTORI,FRANK**

MR NO: **(00009)00-013967467**

EXAM	DATE	ACC NO.
76092 MAMMOGRAPHY SCREENING	**12/10/XX**	**MA-98-01408**

SCREENING MAMMOGRAM

Bilateral CC and MLO screening mammograms were obtained. There are scattered
fibroglandular densities. No masses, suspicious calcifications or areas of
architectural distortion are identified.

IMPRESSION:

There is no mammographic evidence of malignancy. No change from 7-25-XX.

BI-RADS Category I: Negative.

OVERREAD BY: ROBERT J. MELI, M.D.

                                    DAVID E. SMOCK, MD   12/11/XX
                                    DES
        TECH: E. ELLERS   ELECTRONIC SIGNATURE
        TRANS: SMC

Medical Record 21–5. Consultation

GENERAL HOSPITAL AND MEDICAL CENTER
2211 Fifth Avenue North • Healthy City, USA 12345 • (321) 123-4567

Gastroenterology Consultation

Patient Name: Joann Hill

Date: 12/14/xx

Referring Physician: Philip Day, MD

Birth Date: 5/19/xx

REASON FOR CONSULTATION: Malnutrition.

HISTORY OF PRESENT ILLNESS: This is a 58-year-old white female with end stage COPD. She has pulmonary cachexia and is unable to take adequate oral nutrition and fluids. She is currently being maintained on NG feedings. We were asked to see her to evaluate for possible percutaneous endoscopic gastrostomy. She has had some mild anorexia.

PAST MEDICAL HISTORY: The patient's past medical history is significant for severe COPD after many years of heavy smoking. She has chronic malnutrition and pulmonary hypertension, chronic anxiety disorder, and a history of alcohol abuse.

PAST SURGERIES: Include ocular surgery on the right eye and a tracheostomy in 20xx.

CURRENT MEDICATIONS: Include Theo-Dur, Solu-Medrol, Cefizox, Prevacid, Premarin, verapamil, and full strength Jevity. She uses lorazepam and Serevent on a regular basis, and Tylenol and Restoril on a PRN basis.

EXAM: Reveals a white female who appears older than her stated age. She is dyspneic at rest. She is somewhat pale but not icteric. The skin is warm and dry. The abdomen is slightly distended, soft and nontender with no mass and no hepatosplenomegaly.

LABORATORY DATA: Significant for a white blood count of 38,000. Her hemoglobin is 10.8. Platelet count is 247,000. Red cell indices are within normal limits. Liver profile is unremarkable. Her albumin is 2.0.

IMPRESSION: Pulmonary cachexia.

RECOMMENDATIONS: Percutaneous endoscopic gastrostomy was discussed with the patient in detail including the risks, benefits, and alternatives. She understands the nature of the procedure well and agrees to proceed.

Thank you for the opportunity to see your patient in consultation. We will follow with you.

_____

Charles Mathys, MD

cm:urs

d/t: 12/14/xx

Medical Record 21–6. History and Physical Examination

GENERAL HOSPITAL AND MEDICAL CENTER
2211 Fifth Avenue North • Healthy City, USA 12345 • (321) 123-4567

History and Physical Examination

Patient: Tucker Rochelle   **ID No:** 41-79-61
Birth Date: 5/19/xx   **Room No.** 1315

HISTORY

DATE OF ADMISSION: 6/12/xx

CHIEF COMPLAINT: The patient states that she is having difficulty swallowing and feels there is a lump in her throat.

HISTORY OF PRESENT ILLNESS: The patient is a previously healthy 41-year-old black female who on examination approximately twenty years ago was found to have a right thyroid nodule. She was advised to seek treatment at that time. However, she opted to observe the lesion herself. Most recently, the patient had begun having difficulty swallowing and had sensation of having a lump in her throat. Thus she sought medical treatment. The patient was placed on thyroid replacement and has been on that for approximately one year. However, her thyroid nodule appears to be getting bigger at this time. The patient denies any family history of endocrine disorders. The patient has had biopsy of the lesion on the right which was benign on two separate occasions. The patient has not had a biopsy of her thyroid nodule. However, on scan it appears as a cold nodule as well. The patient presents now for elective total thyroidectomy.

PAST MEDICAL HISTORY: Essentially unremarkable. Patient denies any history of hypertension, diabetes or heart disease. She denies any history of bleeding diathesis. Gyn patient is gravida 5 para 5 with LMP occurring approximately one month ago. Patient notes her menses are usually normal. Previous surgeries have included a tubal ligation in 3/xx. Medications at this time include Levo-T 0.075 mg po qd.

ALLERGIES: None known.

FAMILY HISTORY: Remarkable for a history of carcinoma in patient's mother and history of colitis in patient's sister. Otherwise, family history is unremarkable.

SOCIAL HISTORY: Patient is currently living in Knights Landing, Healthy City. She works as a deputy clerk for Yono County; patient is single. The patient is a Jehovah's Witness and has expressed concerns about not receiving blood transfusions during her hospitalization.

HABITS: Patient notes that she quit smoking approximately twenty years ago. Prior to that, she smoked for approximately ten years, smoking one pack per day. Alcohol—patient notes she drinks 1-2 drinks on rare occasions.

Continued

History and Physical Examination, page 2
Patient: Tucker Rochelle   **ID No:** 41-79-61

REVIEW OF SYSTEMS: GENERAL: patient denies any seizures, headaches, changes in hearing, vision, strength or sensation but does note a decreased visual acuity.
CARDIOVASCULAR: Patient denies any chest pain, edema, PND, or orthopnea.
RESPIRATORY: denies SOB, cough, sputum, hemoptysis.
GASTROINTESTINAL: denies nausea, vomiting, diarrhea, constipation, hematemesis, hematochezia or melena.
GENITOURINARY: denies hematuria, dysuria, nocturia, urgency or frequency.

PHYSICAL EXAMINATION

VITAL SIGNS: Pulse: 82. BP: 116/86. T. 99.8 degrees. Weight: 171 lbs.
GENERAL: She is a well-developed, well-nourished black female in no apparent distress.
HEENT: Traumatic, normocephalic. Eyes: PERRLA, EOMs intact. Sclera clear. Ears: Tms clear bilaterally. Nose: septum midline.
NECK: Supple with evidence of cervical lymphadenopathy in the superior aspect of the cervical chain. Additionally, the patient has an enlarged thyroid with a large approx. 3 x 4 cm nodule on the right and a smaller supraclavicular or lymphadenopathy and trachea is midline.
BACK: Without CVA or spinous tenderness.
CHEST: Clear and equal breath sounds bilaterally.
HEART: Regular rate and rhythm with normal S1, S2. There is a grade 2/6 systolic ejection murmur at the left lower sternal border.
BREASTS: Normal breasts without lumps, masses or discharge bilaterally. No evidence of axillary or lymphadenopathy bilaterally.
ABDOMEN: Soft, mildly obese, nontender. Bowel sounds present throughout. No masses or hepatosplenomegaly detected.
PELVIC: Deferred as patient states she has had this performed within the past 3-4 months and is normal by report.
RECTAL: Reveals normal sphincter tone without masses. Stool is heme negative.
EXTREMITIES: Essentially within normal limits. Pulses are 2+ and symmetrical throughout without carotid, abdominal or femoral bruits.

LABORATORY: Data pending at this time.

IMPRESSION: Patient is a 41-year-old black female with a long history of thyroid nodule who presents now with symptoms due to mass effect.

PLAN: Perform a total thyroidectomy.

_____
B. T. Hunnicone, M. D.

bth:urs
d/t: 6/12/xx

Activity 21–3: Clinical Application
History and Physical Examination

1. Define the following abbreviations and symbols that may be found in a report of this type. If you need help with the meaning, refer to Appendix A.

   a. ↓

   b. ○, ♀

   c. L

   d. VSS

2. Define the three parts of the history and physical examination report.

   _____

   _____

   _____

   _____

   _____

3. What information is used to help the health-care practitioner arrive at a diagnosis or impression?

   _____

   _____

   _____

Doctor's Order Sheet for Postoperative Care

The physician completes the doctor's order sheet for postoperative care. It becomes part of the medical record and includes the patient's diagnosis, medication(s) that is (are) to be administered, and the diagnostic tests that need to be performed after surgery (Chart Notes 21–2). As you examine this document, you will see that H. Alexander, RN, initialed the document to confirm that she had read the orders and completed them. You will note that the hour 15:10 is given in military time. Refer to Appendices A and F if you need help in interpreting the abbreviations and medications.

Operative Reports

Operative reports, also called *surgical reports*, are required for every surgical procedure. They include detailed technical descriptions of the technique(s) used to perform the surgery. Medical Record 21–7 is an example of an operative report of a total thy-

roidectomy. In addition to summarizing the surgical procedures, the report is used to assist in further patient care and to secure insurance reimbursements. The operative report serves as a legal document if needed in a court of law to support the surgeon's actions. Various state and federal laws and regulatory agencies mandate that certain components of the operative report be included in the medical record. An operative report must contain a preoperative diagnosis, a postoperative diagnosis, the name of the procedure, the reason for the operation (indications), and the findings and techniques. The operative report is also known as Description of Operation or Description of Procedures.

Informed Consent

Surgery is a special treatment and procedure for which the law requires written and informed consent. In such cases the physician must secure a signed consent form (Fig. 21–1). The American Medical Association (AMA)

Chart Notes 21–2. Postoperative Orders

GENERAL HOSPITAL AND MEDICAL CENTER
2211 Fifth Avenue North • Healthy City, USA 12345 • (321) 123-4567

DOCTOR'S ORDER SHEET FOR POSTOPERATIVE CARE

	ORDERED		
	DATE	HOUR	
1	6/13/xx	15:10	Post-op orders
2			Admit to Rec then to Ward
3			Dx: S/P total thyroidectomy
4			Cond: stable
5			Vitals: q4h X 24 then qshift
6			Allergies: NKA – No blood products
7			Activity: Ad lib – HOB @ 30°
8			Nursing: I & O
9			Diet: NPO
10			IV: D5 1/2 NS c̄ 20 mEq KCL/L @ 125 cc/hr
11			MEDS: ① MS 2-6 mg IV q1h prn pain
12			② Compazine 10 mg IM q̄6h prn N/V
13			③ Vicodin ī-īī po every 4 hours prn for pain
14			④ Colace 100 mg PO BID
15			⑤ Feosol 325 mg PO TID
16			⑥ Levo-T 0.075 mg PO qd
17			LAB: Ca⁺⁺ level ASAP BID starting in the AM
18			Call if void <300 cc/shift
19			B. T. Hunnicone, MD
20		16:30	Noted: H. Alexander, RN

recommends that this procedure be followed if a particular medical treatment either presents a recognized risk or involves hospitalization. For such a form to be binding, the patient must be of legal age (legal age varies from state to state, but usually is 18) or be an emancipated minor (a person younger than 18 who is no longer under parental care and who has been declared of legal age by the state). Regardless of the patient's age, the contents of the form should be carefully explained. If the patient is in grave danger (e.g., in a life- or limb-threatening emergency) and at the same time is unconscious or otherwise unable to respond, the physician may administer emergency treatment without signed consent forms. All other surgical procedures and special treatments require that the patient's consent be informed and in writing.

Medical Record 21–7. Operative Report

GENERAL HOSPITAL AND MEDICAL CENTER
2211 Fifth Avenue North • Healthy City, USA 12345 • (321) 123-4567

Operative Report

Patient: Tucker Rochelle

Birth Date: 06-13-xx

Age: 42

Patient Number: 41-79-61

Room Number: 1315

Surgeon: B. T. Hunnicone, M. D.

PREOPERATIVE DIAGNOSIS: Bilateral thyroid nodules

POSTOPERATIVE DIAGNOSIS: Same

PROCEDURE: Total thyroidectomy

STAFF SURGEON: T.B. Endicott, M.D.

ANESTHESIA: General endotracheal

INDICATIONS: The patient was a previously healthy 41-year-old black female who on examination approximately twenty years ago was found to have a right thyroid nodule. The patient was advised to seek treatment at that time; however, she opted to observe the lesion herself. Most recently, the patient has begun having difficulty swallowing and has sensation of having a lump in her throat, and for this she presents seeking medical therapy. The patient denies any previous radiation treatments and is now being taken to the operating room for a total thyroidectomy.

PROCEDURE: The patient was prepped and draped in the usual sterile fashion with the neck exposed. With the neck in the hyperextended position, an incision was made approximately 3 cm above the sternal notch in a curvilinear fashion following Langer's lines. The incision was carried down through the subcutaneous tissues and through the platysma. At this point, the cervical fascia was incised in the midline and the strap muscles of the neck were retracted laterally.

Initially, the right lobe of the thyroid was dissected as this contained the largest nodule, which was palpable. Additionally, the patient was palpated and two smaller nodules were found in the left thyroid. The strap muscles were dissected free of the thyroid gland and subsequently the middle thyroid vein was identified and this was serially ligated in continuity and subsequently divided using #3-0 silk sutures. At this point, the upper pole vessels of the right thyroid lobe were dissected free and these were ligated in continuity as well as divided. Further dissection was carried out then to identify the recurrent laryngeal nerve assuring not to injure them during the dissection. The vessels of the lower pole were at this point taken as the previous vessels. They were ligated in continuity and subsequently divided. Once this was accomplished, the

Continued

Operative Report, page 2
Patient: Tucker Rochelle   **Patient Number:** 41-79-61

thyroid gland was retracted medially and the isthmus of the thyroid was dissected free of the surrounding tissues in a recurrent laryngeal nerve were identified and preserved intact throughout the procedure. Once the thyroid gland was removed it was inspected and no evidence of adherent parathyroids was noted. A suture was placed in the right upper pole and the specimen was submitted to pathology. At this point, the wound was inspected for hemostasis and subsequently irrigated. Once hemostasis was felt to be satisfactory two pieces of Avitnen measuring approximately 1 × 2 cm were placed in the paratracheal gutters bilaterally. At this point, the cervical fascia was approximated in the midline with #3-0 vicryl in a running fashion and subsequently the platysma muscle was approximated with interrupted #4-0 vicryl and the skin was then closed with #5-0 Prolene in a running fashion in the subcuticular layer. Sterile dressing as well as steri-strips were applied. Final sponge and needle count was correct. Estimated blood loss was less than 50 cc.

COMPLICATIONS: None

The patient tolerated the procedure well, was extubated and transferred to the recovery room in satisfactory condition.

_____

B.T. Hunnicone, M.D.

BTH/urs

D: 06/13/xx
T: 06/14/xx

Consent to Operation

Saint Vincent Health Center
Erie, Pennsylvania

Patient _____ **Date** _____

1. I hereby authorize Dr. _____ , or a physician

   designated by him, to perform upon _____

   the following operative procedure: _____

   He is authorized to utilize in the performance of this surgical procedure the service of physicians, residents or members of the House Staff. If any unforeseen condition arises in the course of the operation calling in his judgment, for procedures in addition to or different from this now contemplated, I authorize him to do whatever he deems advisable.

2. The nature and purpose of the surgical procedure, possible alternative methods and treatment, the risks and possible consequences involved and the possibility of complication have been explained to my satisfaction. If I am a female patient, I acknowledge that any surgical procedure on my reproductive organs may REMOVE MY CAPABILITY to bear children in the future. I have discussed this with my husband and we both understand and accept this possibility. I acknowledge that no guarantee or assurance has been made as to results that may be obtained.

3. I consent to the administration of anesthesia to be administered under the direction of the Chief of the Department of Anesthesia, by one of his associates or by an individual designated by him and to the use of such anesthetics as he or she may deem advisable.

4. I consent to the administration of blood transfusions or other medications; to the disposal by authorities of Saint Vincent Health Center of any tissue or parts which may be removed; to the taking and publication of any photographs in the course of this operation and consent to the admittance of observers to the Operating Room for the purpose of advancement of medical education.

   I certify that I have read and fully understand the above consent for surgical operation and that explanations therein referred to have been made.

   Signature of Patient _____

   Signature of Patient's
   Husband or Wife _____

   Signature of person authorized
   to consent for a minor _____

   Relationship to Patient _____

Witness to Signature _____

Witness to Explanation _____

7117-3
T5387-38-SV19

Figure 21-1

Postoperative Chart Notes

Specific postoperative instructions are carried out and documented by health-care practitioners to ensure the patient's safe recovery after surgery, to minimize patient discomfort, and to prevent postoperative complications. Review Chart Notes 21–3 to see how the physician and RN documented Rochelle Tucker's progress after surgery.

Pathology Reports

Pathology reports describe the pathological or disease-related findings in a tissue sample. The tissue sample is taken during surgery, a biopsy, a special procedure, or an autopsy. The format of pathology reports may vary among institutions. The sections included in all pathology reports include the following: name of specimen submitted, gross (visible to the naked eye) description or findings, microscopic description or findings, and diagnosis. Whereas laboratory data usually concern body fluids, the pathology report focuses on disease findings related to tissue (Medical Record 21–8).

Discharge Summary Reports

A summary of a patient's hospitalization is prepared at the time of discharge. Discharge summaries include the reason for admission to the hospital, the patient's medical history, the admitting diagnosis, laboratory data, probable prognosis, and treatments performed during the hospital stay. They also contain a final diagnosis; surgical procedures performed, if any; and discharge instructions for the patient, such as when to return for follow-up visits and prescriptions. Review Medical Record 21–9 for thyroidectomy.

PRESCRIPTIONS

Prescriptions are written orders to a pharmacist. They contain specific instructions for supplying the patient with a specific drug. The drug is prepared and dispensed by the pharmacist according to the physician's written instructions on the prescription form (Fig. 21–2).

Licensing agencies in individual states mandate prescription privileges. In some states, not only the physicians but also nurse practitioners, nurse clinicians, and physician's assistants are permitted to prescribe certain types of medications. State laws specify which health-care practitioners are designated to administer medications and what kind of medications they are allowed to prescribe.

Part of the responsibility of health-care practitioners is to interpret the information on prescriptions to help patients understand how to administer medications and answer any questions either patients or pharmacists may have. This requires knowledge of prescription format, abbreviations, and medical terms. Not only are pharmaceutical symbols and abbreviations used in prescriptions, but they are also found throughout the medical record.

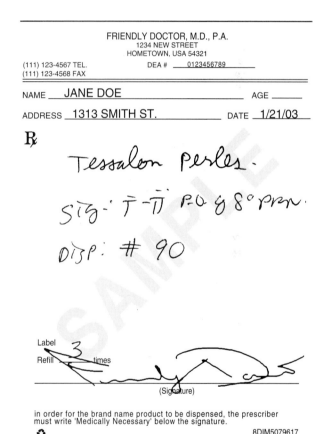

Figure 21-2

Chart Notes 21–3. Postoperative Chart Notes

GENERAL HOSPITAL AND MEDICAL CENTER
2211 Fifth Avenue North • Healthy City, USA 12345 • (321) 123-4567

SURGERY CLINIC

Chart Notes

1	6/13/xx	Post-op
2	17:15	Pt $\bar{s}$ complaints $\bar{c}$ some nausea
3		afeb VSS
4		Dsg dry
5		Voice okay
6		Doing well $\bar{p}$ OR – start diet
7		in am. Routine $\bar{p}$ op care.
8		B. T. Hunnicone, MD

9	6/13/xx	RN notes: afebrile, VSS. Ant. neck drsg dry and intact.
10	19:30	Nauseous but ø emesis this time. Spitting up white clear
11		secretions _____ H. Alexander, RN
12	23:25	Voided 300 cc. Medicated with $\bar{i}$ tablet for pain and nausea
13		with good relief. ø Δ in condition. _____ H. Alexander, RN

14	6/14/xx	Surg
15		POD#1
16		Pt $\bar{c}$ same persistent N/V this AM otherwise
17		doing well. No c/o paresthesia.
18		afeb VSS
19		Dsg dry
20		Voice okay
21		Doing well. Routine care.
22		Will check Ca^{++} level today.
23		B. T. Hunnicone, MD

Medical Record 21–8. Pathology Report

GENERAL HOSPITAL AND MEDICAL CENTER
2211 Fifth Avenue North • Healthy City, USA 12345 • (321) 123-4567

Pathology Report

Patient: Tucker Rochelle   **Pathology Report No:** 2100
Birth Date: 06-13-xx   **Patient Number:** 41-79-61
Age: 42   **Room Number:** 1315

Attending Physician: B. T. Hunnicone, M. D.

SPECIMEN: Thyroid gland, bilateral thyroid nodules,
                suture on right upper lobe, fresh

PROCEDURE PERFORMED: Total thyroidectomy on 6/13/xx

CLINICAL DIAGNOSIS: NONE PROVIDED

PREOPERATIVE DIAGNOSIS: Bilateral thyroid nodules

POSTOPERATIVE DIAGNOSIS: 1. Postoperative total thyroidectomy. 2. Anemia.

GROSS DESCRIPTION: There is a 32 gram total thyroidectomy specimen. A suture
marks the right upper pole. The right lobe measures 5 × 3 × 2.8 cm. The left lobe measures
4 × 3 × 1.7 cm. No parathyroid is identified. The right lobe shows a 2.7 × 2 × 3 cm tan
nodule on sectioning.   The nodule almost completely replaced the right lobe. The nodule
shows well circumscription but no encapsulation. Sectioning shows a hemorrhagic tan cut
surface. The left lobe shows two nodules measuring 1.5 × 1.5 × 1.5 cm and 1.3 × 1.5 × 1.5
cm.   Both nodules show well circumscription without definite encapsulation, and both
nodules show tan mucoid cut surface. The upper lobe nodule shows a small focus of
calcification. Sections are: I to VI, right lobe nodule; VII and VIII, left lower lobe nodule;
IX and X, left upper lobe nodule.

MICROSCOPIC DESCRIPTION: The right lobe nodule is composed of small follicles
lined by uniform cuboidal cells. The center of the nodule shows a focus of hemorrhage and
some fibrosis. The nodule shows a well defined thin fibrous capsule with no evidence of
capsular invasion. The left lobe nodules are composed of follicles of various size distended
with colloid. Both nodules show a thin fibrous capsule. A small focus of calcification is
identified in the capsule of the left upper lobe nodule. The involved thyroid parenchyma is
not remarkable. The findings are consistent with nodular hyperplasia.

DIAGNOSIS (Gross and Microscopic): Hyperplasia, total thyroidectomy.

_____
John H. Taiyon, M.D.

JHT/pg
D&T: 06/13/xx

ABBREVIATIONS AND SYMBOLS

Abbreviations and symbols are frequently used in medical reports. It is important to ensure the use of standardized abbreviations in the medical record so they are familiar to all health-care practitioners.

Nevertheless, many medical facilities develop their own unique list of abbreviations that may not be used elsewhere. Some of the common abbreviations are listed here, but a comprehensive list is provided in Appendix A, Part 1. Use them to verify the meanings of abbreviations in the medical records.

❖ ABBREVIATIONS

COMMON

ABBREVIATION	MEANING
A	assessment
ad lib	as desired, as much as needed, freely
CC	chief complaint; craniocaudad (radiology, view)
Dx	diagnosis
ECT	electroconvulsive therapy
EOM	extraocular movement
FH	family history
H&P	history and physical
HEENT	head, eyes, ears, nose, throat
HPI	history of present illness
IMP	impression (also known as a diagnosis)
NKA	no known allergies
NKDA	no known drug allergies
NPO	nothing by mouth
OH	occupational history
PE	physical examination, pulmonary embolism
PE, PX	physical examination
PERRLA	pupils equal, round, reactive to light and accommodation
PH	past history
PI	present illness
PMH	past medical history
POD	postoperative day
R	respiration, right
R/O	rule out
ROS	review of systems
SH	social history

COMMON

ABBREVIATION	MEANING
SOB	shortness of breath
SR	systems review, sustained release
Sx	symptom (subjective information from patient that suggests an abnormality)
TPR	temperature, pulse, and respirations
Tx	treatment
UCHD	usual childhood diseases
VSS	vital signs stable

LABORATORY

ABBREVIATION	MEANING
BUN	blood urea nitrogen
diff.	differential (white blood count)
GOT	glucose oxidase test
Hb, Hg, Hgb	hemoglobin
HCT, Hct	hematocrit
HDL	high-density lipoprotein
hpf	high-power field (microscope)
hr	hour
K	potassium (an electrolyte)
KCl	potassium chloride
L	liter, left, lumbar
LDL	low-density lipoprotein
lpf	low-power field (microscope)
mg	milligram (l/1000 gram)
mg%	milligrams percent
ml	milliliter

ABBREVIATION	MEANING	ABBREVIATION	MEANING
MLO	mediolateral oblique	RBC, rbc	red blood cells, red blood count
mm/Hg	millimeters of mercury	WBC, wbc	white blood cells, white blood count
NS	normal saline (solution)		
PLAT, PLATL	platelets		

❖ SYMBOLS

SYMBOL	MEANING	SYMBOL	MEANING
@	at	−	negative, none, without
△	change	∅	no
↓	decrease(d), down	$\dot{\tau}$	one
↑	increased	$\ddot{\pi}$	two
♀	female	$\bar{c}$	with
♂	male	$\bar{s}$	without
×	multiplied by	$\bar{p}$	after

Activity 21–4: Clinical Application
Medical Record and Prescription Abbreviations

1. Define the following abbreviations.

   a. CC _____

   b. HEENT _____

   c. IMP _____

   d. NPO _____

   e. prn _____

   f. S1, S$_1$ _____

   g. SOB _____

   h. TPR _____

   i. UCHD _____

   j. wt _____

MEDICAL RECORDS

Rochelle Tucker was diagnosed with bilateral thyroid nodules. Authentic reports are included from her medical record for analysis.

The following reading and dictionary exercise and the medical record analysis will help you develop skills to abstract information and master the terminology in the reports. Accurate interpretation is important because this type of information is used in numerous areas of the medical practice, such as initiation of treatments, evaluation of patient's progress, and completion of insurance claims.

Reading and Dictionary Exercise

Place a check mark [✓] after you complete the exercise.

[   ] **1.** Underline the following words in the reports and doctor's notes as you read the history and physical examination, postoperative orders, operative report, postoperative chart notes, pathology report, and discharge summary.

[   ] **2.** Use a medical dictionary, Appendix A, and Appendix F, Part 2 to define the terms below.

Note: You are not expected to fully understand all the parts of the medical records. The important aspect of this exercise is to use all available resources to complete it. Eventually you will master the terminology and format of these reports.

>>> MEDICAL RECORD 21–6: HISTORY AND PHYSICAL EXAMINATION

Term	Pronunciation	Meaning
biopsy	BĪ-ŏp-sē	_____
benign	bē-NĪN	_____
thyroidectomy	thī-royd-ĔK-tō-mē	_____
diathesis	dī-ĂTH-ĕ-sĭs	_____
Levo-T	LĒ-vō-tē	_____
carcinoma	kăr-sĭ-NŌ-mă	_____
colitis	kō-LĪ-tĭs	_____
orthopnea	or-THŎP-nē-ă	_____
diarrhea	dī-ă-RĒ-ă	_____
hematemesis	hĕm-ăt-ĔM-ĕ-sĭs	_____
hematochezia	hĕm-ă-tō-KĒ-zē-ă	_____
hematuria	hē-mă-TŪ-rē-ă	_____
dysuria	dīs-Ū-rē-ă	_____
nocturia	nŏk-TŪ-rē-ă	_____
bilaterally	bī-LĂT-ĕr-ăl-lē	_____
hepatosplenomegaly	hĕp-ă-tō-splē-nō-MĔG-ă-lē	_____
bruits	brwēs	_____

>>> Chart Notes 21-2: Postoperative Orders

Term	Pronunciation	Meaning
Compazine	KŎM-pă-zēn	_____
Vicodin	vī-KŌ-din	_____
Colace	CŌ-lās	_____
Feosol	FĒ-ŏ-sōl	_____

>>> Medical Record 21-7: Operative Report

Term	Pronunciation	Meaning
lesion	LĒ-zhŭn	_____
curvilinear fashion	kŭr-vĭ-LĬN-ē-ăr FĂ-shŭn	_____
subcutaneous	sŭb-kū-TĀ-nĕ-ŭs	_____
platysma	plă-TĬZ-mă	_____
palpable	PĂL-pă-bl	_____
ligated	LĪ-gā-tĕd	_____
extubated	ĔKS-tū-bā-tĕd	_____

Chart Notes 21-3: Postoperative Chart Notes

Term	Pronunciation	Meaning
afebrile	ă-FĔB-rĭl	_____
emesis	ĔM-ĕ-sĭs	_____
paresthesia	păr-ĕs-THĒ-zē-ă	_____

>>> Medical Record 21-8: Pathology Report

Term	Pronunciation	Meaning
circumscription	sĕr-kŭm-SKRĬP-shŭn	_____
encapsulation	ĕn-kăp-sū-LĀ-shŭn	_____
hemorrhagic	hĕm-ō-RĂJ-ĭk	_____
parenchyma	păr-ĔN-kĭ-mă	_____
hyperplasia	hī-pĕr-PLĀ-zē-ă	_____

>>> MEDICAL RECORD 21-9: DISCHARGE SUMMARY REPORT

Term	Pronunciation	Meaning
microcytic	*mī-krō-SĬT-ĭk*	_____
hypochromic anemia	*hī-pō-KRŌ-mĭk*	_____
hematocrit	*hē-MĂT-ō-krĭt*	_____
Os-Cal	*ŎS-kăl*	_____

Critical Thinking: Analysis of Medical Records

This section provides experience in abstracting and analyzing information from the medical records. At the same time, it reinforces the material presented in this chapter.

>>> MEDICAL RECORD 21-6: HISTORY AND PHYSICAL EXAMINATION

1. (a)   Is there a family history of endocrine disorders, hypertension, diabetes, CA, or colitis?

_____

_____

   (b)   Why didn't the doctor perform a pelvic examination?

_____

   (c)   What type of treatment did Dr. Hunnicone recommend?

_____

>>> CHART NOTES 21-2: POSTOPERATIVE ORDERS

2. Transcribe the first nine (9) lines of the doctor's order sheet for postoperative care.
Keep in mind that 15:10 hr is military time, which converts to 3:10 pm. The colon in 15:10 is used to separate the hour from the minutes. Punctuation may or may not be used to designate military time.
If you are not familiar with this conversion, seek assistance from your instructor or other sources.

Doctor's Order Sheet

Date

Line 1:   6/13/xx_____

Line 2:   _____

Line 3:   _____

Line 4:   _____

Line 5:   _____

Line 6: _____

Line 7: _____

Line 8: _____

Line 9: _____

>>> MEDICAL RECORD 21-7: OPERATIVE REPORT

3. Did the patient have any previous radiation treatments for the bilateral thyroid nodules?

_____

4. When the thyroid gland was removed, what did Dr. Hunnicone find upon inspection?

_____

_____

5. What does the statement "final sponge and needle count was correct" mean? Why is it important to do this count?

_____

_____

_____

>>> CHART NOTES 21-3: POSTOPERATIVE CHART NOTES

6. Dr. Hunnicone states that the patient was "afeb" and "VSS." What does this mean?

_____

_____

_____

7. Transcribe the first eleven (11) lines of the chart notes.

Keep in mind 17:15 is military time, which converts to 5:15 pm. If you are not familiar with this conversion, seek assistance from your instructor or other sources. The colon in 17:15 is used to separate the hour from the minutes. Punctuation may or may not be used to designate military time.

Chart Notes

Line 1: 6/13/xx_____

Line 2: _____

Line 3: _____

Line 4: _____

Line 5: _____

Line 6: _____

Line 7: _____

Line 8: _____

Line 9: _____

Line 10: _____

Line 11: _____

> >> MEDICAL RECORD 21-8: PATHOLOGY REPORT

8. Why was a total thyroidectomy performed?

_____

> >> MEDICAL RECORD 21-9: DISCHARGE SUMMARY REPORT

9. What type of anemia did Rochelle have? (You might want to review Chapter 15 to answer this question.)

_____

_____

10. What type of supplement will the patient take for anemia?

_____

Appendix A
Abbreviations and Symbols

Part 1: Abbreviations

A	assessment
A&P, P&A	auscultation and percussion
A&W	alive and well
AB, ab	abortion, antibodies
ABC	aspiration biopsy cytology
ABGs	arterial blood gases
ABO	blood groups: A, AB, B, and O
AC	air conduction
ac	before meals (ante cibum)
Acc	accomodation
ACE	angiotensin-converting enzyme (inhibitor)
ACH, Ach	acetylcholine
ACL	anterior cruciate ligament
ACLS	advanced cardiac life support
ACS	American Cancer Society
ACT	activated clotting time
ACTH	adrenocorticotropic hormone
ad lib	as desired, as much as needed, freely
AD	Alzheimer disease, right ear (*auris dextra*)
ADC	AIDS-dementia complex
ADD	attention deficit disorder
ADH	antidiuretic hormone (vasopressin)
ADHD	attention-deficit hyperactivity disorder
AFB	acid fast bacillus (TB organism)
afeb	afebrile
AFO	ankle-foot orthosis (orthopedics)
AFP	alpha-fetoprotein
Ag	antigen
AGN	acute glomerular nephritis
AH	abdominal hysterectomy
AHF	antihemophilic factor (blood coagulation factor VIII)
AHG	antihemolytic globulin
AI	artificial insemination; aortic insufficiency
AICD	automatic implanted cardioverter defibrillator
AIDS	acquired immunodeficiency syndrome
AIH	artificial insemination by husband (also called *artificial insemination, homologous*, and *artificial insemination with husband's sperm*, and *artificial insemination husband donor* and *homologous artificial insemination*)

AIHA	autoimmune hemolytic anemia
AKA	above-knee amputation
alk phos	alkaline phosphatase
ALL	acute lymphocytic leukemia
ALS	amyotrophic lateral sclerosis (also called Lou Gehrig disease)
ALT	alanine aminotransferase (elevated in liver and heart disease); new name for SGPT
am, AM	*ante meridieum* (before noon, in the morning)
AML	acute myelongenous leukemia
ANA	antinuclear antibody
angio	angiography
ANS	autonomic nervous system
ant	anterior
ANTI, anti	antibody
AP	anteroposterior
APA	American Psychiatric Association
APTT	activated partial thromboplastin time
ARC	AIDS-related complex. An outdated term that is replaced by AIDS-wasting syndrome
ARD	acute respiratory disease
ARDS	adult respiratory distress syndrome
ARF	acute renal failure
ARMD, AMD	age-related macular degeneration
AS	aortic stenosis, left ear (*auris sinistra*)
ASA	acetylsalicylic acid (aspirin)
ASC	altered state of consciousness
ASCVD	arteriosclerotic cardiovascular disease
ASD	atrial septal defect
ASHD	arteriosclerotic heart disease
AST	angiotensin sensitivity test, aspartate aminotransferase (new name for SGOT)
Ast	astigmatism
ATN	acute tubular necrosis
AU	both ears
AV	atrioventricular, arteriovenous
AVR	aortic valve replacement
AZT	zidovudine (generic name for *Retrovir*; formerly called *azidothymidine*)
Ba	barium
BaE, BE	barium enema
BAO	basal acid output

baso	basophil
BBB	bundle-branch block, blood-brain barrier
BC	bone conduction
BCC	basal cell carcinoma
B cell	lymphocyte produced in the bone marrow
BE	barium enema
BEAM	brain electrical activity mapping
bid	twice a day
BKA	below-knee amputation
BM	bowel movement
BMR	basal metabolic rate
BMT	bone marrow transplant
BNO	bladder neck obstruction
BP	blood pressure
BPH	benign prostatic hyperplasia, benign prostatic hypertrophy
BRBPR	bright red blood per rectum, hematochezia
BSE	breast self-examination
BSO	bilateral salpingo-oophorectomy; bilateral serous otitis
BUN	blood urea nitrogen
Bx, bx	biopsy
C	cervical (spine)
C&S	culture and sensitivity
c/o	complains of
C1, C2, etc.	first cervical vertebra, second cervical vertebra, etc.
Ca	calcium , cancer
CA 125	cancer cell surface antigen 125
CA	cancer, chronological age, cardiac arrest
CABG	coronary artery bypass graft
cap, caps	capsule(s)
CAD	coronary artery disease
CAPD	continuous ambulatory peritoneal dialysis
CAT	computed axial tomography; same as CT scan
Cath	catheterization, catheter
CBC	complete blood count
CBT	cognitive behavioral therapy
cc	cubic centimeter
CC	chief complaint, craniocaudad (radiology view)
CCU	coronary care unit
CDH	congenital dislocation of the hip
CEA	carcinoembryonic antigen
CF	cystic fibrosis
CGL	chronic granulocytic leukemia
CHD	coronary heart disease
chem, chemo	chemotherapy
chol	cholesterol
CHF	congestive heart failure
CIS	carcinoma *in situ*
CK	creatine kinase
CLD	chronic liver disease
CLL	chronic lymphocytic leukemia, cholesterol-lowering lipid
cm	centimeter
CML	chronic myelocytic leukemia, cell-mediated lympholysis (also called *cell-mediated lymphocytolysis*)
CMV	cytomegalovirus
CNS	central nervous system
CO	cardiac output
C/O	check out, complains of
CO1	coccygeal vertebra
CO$_2$	carbon dioxide
COLD	chronic obstructive lung disease
COPD	chronic obstructive pulmonary disease
CP	cerebral palsy
CPAP	continuous positive airway pressure
CPD	cephalopelvic disproportion
CPK	creatine phosphokinase
CPR	cardiopulmonary resuscitation
CR	complete response, complete remission
CRF	chronic renal failure
CRYPTO	cryptococcus
CS, C-section	cesarean section
CSF	cerebrospinal fluid
C-spine	cervical spine
ct	count
CT	computed tomography
CTA	clear to auscultation
CT scan, CAT scan	computerized tomography scan (x-ray images in a cross-sectional view)
CTS	carpal tunnel syndrome
CV	cardiovascular
CVA	cerebrovascular accident
CVD	cerebrovascular disease
CVS	chorionic villus sampling
c/w	consistent with
CWP	childbirth without pain
CX	cervix, chest x-ray
CXR	chest x-ray
cysto	cystoscopy
D	diopter (lens strength)
D&C	dilatation and curettage
DAW	dispense as written
DC	discharge
DDS	doctor of dental surgery
decub.	decubitus (ulcer); bedsore
derm.	dermatology

DES	diethylstilbestrol
DEXA	dual energy x-ray absorptiometry
DI	diabetes insipidus; diagnostic imaging
DIC	disseminated intravascular coagulation
diff.	differential (white blood count)
DIG	dioxin, digitalis
dil	dilute, dissolve
disc, DC	discontinue
disch	discharge(d)
disp	dispense
DJD	degenerative joint disease
dL	deciliter
DLE	discoid lupus erythematosus
DM	diabetes mellitus
DNA	deoxyribonucleic acid
DNR	do not resuscitate
DO	doctor of osteopathy
DOA	dead on arrival
DOB	date of birth
DOE	dyspnea on exertion
DPT	diptheria, pertussis, tetanus (vacinne)
DRE	digital rectal exam
drsg, dsg	dressing
DS	double strength
DSA	digital subtraction angiography
DSM	*Diagnostic and Statistical Manual of Mental Disorders*
DT	delirium tremens
DTR	deep tendon reflex
DUB	dysfunctional uterine bleeding
DVT	deep vein thrombosis
DW	distilled water
Dx	diagnosis
EAHF	eczema, asthma, and hay fever
EBV	Epstein-Barr virus
ECG, EKG	electrocardiogram
ECHO	echocardiogram, echoencephalogram
ECF	extended care facility
ECMO	extracorporeal membrane oxygenation
ECT	electroconvulsive therapy
ED	erectile dysfunction; emergency department
EDC	estimated date of confinement
EEG	electroencephalogram; electroencephalography
EGD	esophagogastroduodenoscopy
ELISA	enzyme-linked immunoadsorbent assay (AIDS test)
Em	emmetropia
EMB	endometrial biopsy
EMG	electromyography
emp	as directed

EMS	emergency medical service(s)
ENT	ear, nose, and throat
EOM	extraocular movement
EOMI	extraocular motion intact
eos	eosinophil (type of white blood cell)
Epo	erythropoietin
EQ	emotional "intelligence" quotient, educational quotient
ER	emergency room; estrogen receptor
ERCP	endoscopic retrograde cholangiopancreatography
ERS	endoscopic retrograde sphincterectomy
ERT	estrogen replacement therapy
ESR	erythrocyte sedimentation rate
ESRD	end-stage renal disease
EST	electroshock therapy
ESWL	extracorporeal shock-wave lithotripsy
ET	endotracheal, endotracheal tube
ETF	eustachian tube function
ETT	exercise tolerance test
EU	excretory urogram; same as IVP
F	fahrenheit
FACCP	Fellow of the American college of Chest Physicians
FACP	Fellow of the American College of Physicians
FACS	Fellow of the American College of Surgeons
FBS	fasting blood sugar
FDA	Food and Drug Administration
FDT	frequency doubling technology
FECG; FEKG	fetal electrocardiogram
FEF	forced expiratory flow
FEV	forced expiratory volume
FH	family history
FHR	fetal heart rate
FHT	fetal heart tone
	first sacral nerve (neurology and orthopedics)
	first sacral vertebra (neurology and orthopedics)
FISH	fluorescence in situ hybridization (newer cytogenic technique that can detect cryptic abnormalities not evident by standard cytogenic banding studies)
FRC	functional residual capacity
FROM	full range of movement/motion
FS	frozen section
FSH	follicle-stimulating hormone
FTND	full-term normal delivery
FU, F/U	follow-up
FUO	fever of unknown origin
FVC	forced vital capacity

Fx	fracture, frozen section		**H₂O**	water
G	gravida (pregnant)		**HP**	hemipelvectomy
GB	gallbladder		**hpf**	high-power field (miscroscope)
GBS	gallbladder series		**HPI**	history of present illness
GC	gonorrhea		**HPV**	human papillomavirus
G-CSF	granulocyte colony-stimulating factor		**HRT**	Heidelberg retinal tomogram
GER	gastroesophageal reflux		**hs**	at bedtime
GERD	gastroesophageal reflux disease		**HSG**	hysterosalpingography
GFR	glomerular filtration rate		**HSV**	herpes simplex virus
GGT	gamma glutamyltransferase		**HX, Hx**	history
GH	growth hormone		**I&D**	incision and drainage
GI	gastrointestinal		**I&O**	intake and output
g, gm	gram		**I/O**	input/output
GM-CSF	granulocyte macrophage colony-stimulating factor		**IBS**	irritable bowel syndrome
			ICP	intracranial pressure
GOT	glucose oxidase test		**ID**	intradermal, infectious disease
Gt, gtt	drop, drops		**IDDM**	insulin-dependent diabetes mellitus
GTT	glucose tolerance test		**IgM**	immunoglobulin M
GU	genitourinary		**IgA**	immunoglobulin A
GVHD	graft versus host disease		**IgD**	immunoglobulin D
GYN	gynecology		**IgG**	immunoglobulin G
h	hour		**IgE**	immunoglobulin E
HBOT	hyperbaric oxygen therapy		**Igs**	immunoglobulins
H&P	history and physical		**IM**	intramuscular; infectious mononucleosis
HAV	hepatitis A virus		**IMP**	impression (synonymous with *diagnosis*)
Hb, Hg, Hgb	hemoglobin		**inj**	injection
HBV	hepatitis B virus		**INR**	international normalized ratio
HCG, hCG	human chorionic gonadotropin		**I&O**	intake and output (measurement of patient's fluids)
HCl	hydrochloric acid			
HCO₃	bicarbonate		**IOL**	intraocular lens
HCT, Hct	hematocrit		**IOP**	intraocular pressure
HCV	hepatitis C virus		**IP**	inpatient
HCVD	hypertensive cardiovascular disease		**IPPB**	intermittent positive-pressure breathing
HD	hemodialysis, hip disarticulation, hearing distance		**IQ**	intelligence quotient
			IRDS	infant respiratory distress syndrome
HDL	high-density lipoprotein		**IS**	intracostal space
HDN	hemolytic disease of newborn		**ITP**	idiopathic thrombocytopenic purpura
HDV	hepatitis D virus		**IU**	international unit (measurement)
HEENT	head, eyes, ears, nose, throat		**IUD**	intrauterine device (a contraceptive device)
HEV	hepatitis E virus			
H&H	hematocrit and hemoglobin		**IUP**	intrauterine pregnancy
Histo	histoplasmosis (fungal infection seen in AIDS virus in serum)		**IUGR**	intrauterine growth rate, intrauterine growth retardation
HIV	human immunodeficiency virus (causes AIDS)		**IV**	intravenous
			IVC	intravenous cholangiography
HLA	histocompatibility locus A (system that identifies cells as "self")		**IVF**	in vitro fertilization
			IVF-ET	in vitro fertilization and embryo transfer
HMD	hyaline membrane disease		**IVP**	intravenous pyelogram; same as EU
HNP	herniated nucleus pulposus (herniated disc)		**IVPB**	intravenous piggyback (method of drug administration)
H/O	history of		**IVU**	intravenous u;rography
HOB	head of bed		**K**	potassium (an electrolyte)

KCL	potassium chloride
KD	knee disarticulation
kg	killogram
KS	Kaposi sarcoma
KS/OI	Kaposi sarcoma and opportunistic infections
KUB	kidneys, ureters, bladder
L	liter, left, lumbar
L1, L2, etc.	first lumbar vertebra, second lumbar vertebra, etc.
LA	left atrium
lat	lateral
LB	large bowel
LBBB	left bundle branch block
LBW	low birth weight
LD	lethal dose
LDH	lactate dehydrogenase
LDL	low-density lipoprotein
LDLC	low-density lipoprotein cholesterol
L-dopa	levodopa (used to treat Parkinson disease)
LEEP	loop electrocautery excision procedure
LFT	liver function test(s)
LGI	lower gastrointestinal
LH	luteinizing hormone
LLL	left lower lobe (of the lungs)
LLQ	left lower quadrant
LMP	last menstrual period
LOC	loss of consciousness
LP	lumbar puncture
lpf	low-power field (microscope)
LSD	lysergic acid diethylamide (hallucinogen)
LSO	left salpingo-ooporectomy
lt	left
LTC	long-term care
LUL	left upper lobe (of the lungs)
LUQ	left upper quadrant
LV	left ventricle
L&W	living and well
lymphos	lymphocytes
MA	mental age
MAI	*Myobacterium avium intracellulare*
MAO	maximal acid output; monoamine oxidase
MBD	minimal brain dysfunction
mcg	microgram
MCH	mean corpuscular hemoglobin, mean cell hemoglobin (average amount of hemoglobin per cell)
MCHC	mean cell hemoglobin concentration (average concentration of hemoglobin in a single red cell)

MCV	mean cell volume (average volume or size of a single red blood cell. (High MCV=macrocytic cells; Low MCV=microcytic cells)
MD	medical doctor
MEDS, meds	medications, medicines
mEq	milliequivalent
METS, mets	metastases
mg	milligram (l/1000 gram)
MG	myasthenia gravis
Mg	magnesium
Mg%	milligrams percent
MH	marital history
MHA	Mental Health Association
MI	myocardial infarction
mix astig	mixed astigmatism
Ml, ml	milliliter
MLO	mediolateral oblique
mm	millimeter
Mm/Hg	millimeters of mercury
mmol/L	millimole per liter
MMPI	Minnesota Multiphasic Personality Inventory
mono	monocyte
MR	mitral regurgitation
MRA	magnetic resonance angiogram/angiography
MRI	magnetic resonance imaging
MS	musculoskeletal, multiple sclerosis, mental status, morphine sulfate
MSE	mental status exam
MSH	melanocyte-stimulating hormone
multip	multiparous, multipara
MVP	mitral valve prolapse
Myop	myopia
N	nitrogen
Na	sodium (an electrolyte)
NB	newborn
ND	normal delivery; normal development
NED	no evidence of disease
neg	negative
NG	nasogastric
NG tube	nasogastric tube
NHL	non-Hodgkin lymphoma
NIDDM	non-insulin-dependent diabetes mellitus
NIHL	noise induced hearing loss
NIR	brand name of an artery stent, made by Medinol Ltd.
NK	natural killer
NK cells	natural killer cells
NKA	no known allergies
NKDA	no known drug allergies

NMTs	nebulized mist treatments
NPO	nothing by mouth
NS	normal saline (solution)
NSAID	nonsteroidal anti-inflammatory drug
NSR	normal sinus rhythm
NTD	neural tube defect
NTG	nitroglycerin
NTP	normal temperature and pressure
N&V	nausea and vomiting
O	oxygen
OA	osteoarthritis
OB	obstetrics
OCD	obsessive compulsive disorder
OCG	oral cholecystography
OCPs	oral contraceptive pills
OD	right eye (oculus dexter)
OH	occupational history
oint, ung	ointment
oP	outpatient, operation, operative
OR	operating room
ORTH, ortho	orthopedics
OS	left eye (oculus sinister)
otc	over the counter (referring to nonprescription drugs)
OU	each eye (oculus uterque); both eyes together (oculi unitas)
oz	ounce
P	phosphorous, pulse
P&A	percussion and auscultation
PA	posteroanterior; pernicious anemia
PAC	premature atrial contraction
PAD	peripheral arterial disease
Pap	Papanicolaou smear (test for cervical or vaginal cancer)
Para 1, 2, 3	unipara, bipara, tripara (number of viable births)
PAT	paroxysmal atrial tachycardia
Path	pathology
PBI	protein-bound iodine
PBSC	peripheral blood stem cell transplant
pc, pp	after meals (postprandial)
PCO_2, pCO_2	partial pressure carbon dioxide
PCP	*pneumocystis carinii* pneumonia
PD	progression of a disease, peritoneal dialysis
PDR	*Physician's Desk Reference*
PE tube	polyethylene ventilating tube (placed in the eardrum)
PE	physical examination, pulmonary embolism
PE, PX	physical examination
PEFR	peak expiratory flow rate
PERRLA	pupils equal, round, and reactive to light and accommodation
PET	positron emission tomography
PFT	pulmonary function test
PGH	pituitary growth hormone
PH	past history
pH	symbol for degree of acidity or alkalinity of a substance
PI	present illness
PICC	peripherally inserted central catheter
PID	pelvic inflammatory disease
PKU	phenylketonuria
PLAT, PLATL	platelets
PLT	platelet count
pm	afternoon
PMH	past medical history
PML	polymorphonuclear leukocyte(s); progressive multifocal leukoencephalopathy
PMP	previous menstrual period
PMS	premenstrual syndrome
PND	paroxysmal nocturnal dyspnea
PNS	peripheral nervous system
po	by mouth (per os)
pO_2	partial pressure oxygen
POD	postoperative day
poly, PMN, PMNL	polymorphonuclear leukocyte
POMR	problem-oriented medical record
postop	postoperative
PPD	purified protein derivative
PR	partial response, partial remission
preop	preoperatively
prep	preparation (as in preparation for surgery)
primip	primiparous, primipara
PRL	prolactin
prn	as needed, as required
procto	proctoscopy, proctology
prot	protocol
PSA	prostate specific antigen
PSS	progressive systemic scleroderma
PT	prothrombin time, physical therapy
PT, Pt, pt	patient
PTCA	percutaneous transluminal coronary angioplasty
PTH	parathyroid hormone (also called *parathormone*)
PTSD	post-traumatic stress disorder
PTT	partial thromboplastin time
PUD	peptic ulcer disease
PVC	premature ventricular contraction

PWB	partial weight bearing
q	each, every
q2h	every 2 hours
qam, qm	every morning
qd	every day
qh	every hour (This abbreviation may also contain any number
qid	four times a day
QNS	quantity not sufficient
qod	every other day
qpm, qn	every night
R	respiration, right
(R), rect	rectal
Ra	radium
r	roentgen
R/O	rule out
RA	rheumatoid arthritis, right atrium
rad	radiation absorbed dose
RAD	reactive airway disease
RAI	radioactive iodine
RAIU	radioactive iodine uptake
RBBB	right bundle branch block
RBC, rbc	red blood cell(s), red blood count
RD	respiratory disease
RDDA	recommended daily dietary allowance
RDS	respiratory distress syndrome
RDW	red cell distribution width
REM	rapid eye movement
RF	rheumatoid factor
Rh	rhesus (monkey) factor in blood
RIA	radioimmunoassay
RIG	rabies immunoglobulin
RK	radial keratotomy
RLL	right lower lobe (of lung)
RLQ	right lower quadrant
RML	right middle lobe (of lung)
RNA	ribonucleic acid
R/O	rule out
ROM	range of motion
ROS	review of systems
RP	retrograde pyelogram
RS	*Reed-Sternberg* cells
RSO	right salpingo-oophorectomy
RSV	respiratory syncytial virus
rt	right
RT	radiation therapy
RUL	right upper lobe (of lung)
RUQ	right upper quadrant
RV	residual volume, right ventricle
Rx	treatment, therapy, prescription
S	sacral

S/P	status post (refers to previous disease or surgery)
S1, S_1	first heart sound (systolic, cardiovascular)
S1, S_1, etc	first sacral nerve, first sacral vertebra, etc (neurology and orthopedics)
S2, S_2	second heart sound (diastolic, cardiovascular)
S2, S_2, etc	second sacral nerve, second sacral vertebra, etc (neurology and orthopedics)
SA	sinoatrial
SAD	seasonal affective disorder
SAH	subarachnoid hemorrhage
SaO_2	arterial oxygen saturation
SBE	subacute bacterial endocarditis
SC, sc, subcu, subq	subcutaneous (injection)
SD	shoulder disarticulation
sed rate	erythrocyte sedimentation rate
segs	segmented neutrophils
SERM	selective estrogen receptor modulator
SGOT	serum glutamic oxalo-acetic transaminase. Obsolete—now called AST
SGPT	serum glutamic-pyruvic transaminase. Obsolete—now called ALT
SH	social history
SIDS	sudden infant death syndrome
SL	sublingual
SLE	systemic lupus erythematosus
SMA 12	twelve blood chemistries
SMAS	superficial musculoaponeurotic system [flap] (plastic surgery)
SNS	sensory nervous system
SOAP	subjective, objective, assessment, and plan
SOB	shortness of breath
sono	sonogram
sos	if necessary
S/P	status post
sp.gr.	specific gravity
SPECT	single photon emission computed tomography
SR	systems review, sustained release
SSRI	selective serotonin reuptake inhibitor
ST	esotropia
stat	immediately
staph	staphylococcus (a bacterium)
strep	streptococcus (a bacterium)
STD	sexually transmitted disease, somatropin hormone
Supp, supp	suppository
SV	stroke volume

SVD	spontaneous vaginal delivery
syr	syrup
Sx	symptom (subjective information from patient that suggests an abnormality)
T	thoracic, temperature, time
T&A	tonsillectomy and adenoidectomy
T1, T2, etc.	first thoracic vertebra, second thoracic vertebra, etc
T$_3$	triiodothyronine (thyroid hormone)
T$_4$	thyroxine (thyroid hormone)
TAB	tablet
TAH	total abdominal hysterectomy
TAH-BSO	total abdominal hysterectomy with bilateral salpingo-oophorectomy
TAT	Thematic Apperception Test
TB	tuberculosis
T cells	lymphocytes produced in the thymus gland
TDM	therapeutic drug monitoring
TEE	transesophageal echocardiography
TENS	transcutaneous electrical nerve stimulation
TFT	thyroid function test
TSH	thyroid-stimulating hormone
THA	total hip arthroplasty
THC	tetrahydrocannabinol (active ingredient in marijuana)
THR	total hip replacement
TIA	transient ischemic attack
tid	three times a day
TKA	total knee arthroplasty
TKR	total knee replacement
TLC	total lung capacity
TM	tympanic membrane
TMJ	temporomandibular joint
TNM	tumor, nodes, metastases
TOH	total abdominal hysterectomy
TOT CHOL	total cholesterol
Toxo	toxoplasmosis (parasitic infection associated with AIDS)
TPR	temperature, pulse, respiration
TRAM	trans-rectus abdominis musculocutaneous
TSH	thyroid-stimulating hormone
tsp	teaspoonful
TSS	toxic shock syndrome
TT	thrombolytic therapy
TURP	transurethral resection of prostate (for prostatectomy)
TV	tidal volume
TVH	total vaginal hysterectomy
Tx	treatment
UA	urinalysis
UAO	upper airway obstruction
UC	uterine contractions
UCHD	usual childhood diseases
ud	as directed
UGI	upper gastrointestinal
UGIS	upper gastrointestinal series
umb	umbilical, umbilicus (navel)
ung, oint	ointment
U/O	urinary output
UPPP	uvulopalatopharyngoplasty
URI	upper respiratory infection
US	ultrasound
UTI	urinary tract infection
VA	visual acuity
VO	verbal order (nursing)
V$_4$, V$_5$	fourth chest (lead), fifth chest (lead)
VA	visual acuity
VC	vital capacity
VCUG	voiding cystourethrogram, voiding cystourography
VD	venereal disease
VDRL	venereal disease research laboratory
VF	visual field
VLDL	very low-density lipoprotein
VS	vital signs, versus
VSD	ventricular septal defect
VSS	vital signs stable
VT	ventricular tachycardia
w/d	well-developed
w/n	well nourished
W/O	without
WAIS	Wechsler Adult Intelligence Scale
WBC, wbc	white blood cell(s), white blood count
WDWN	well-developed, well nourished
WISC	Wechsler Intelligence Scale for Children
wt	weight
XP, XDP	xeroderma pigmentosum
XRT	radiation therapy
XT	exotropia
XX	female sex chromosomes
XY	male sex chromosomes
y/o	years old
ZDV	Zidovudine

Part 2: Symbols

@	at	±	plus or minus; either positive or negative; indefinite
āā	of each	∅	no
'	foot	#	number; following a number; pounds
"	inch	÷	divided by
c̄	with	/	divided by
Δ	change, heat	×	multiplied by; magnification
lb	pound	=	equals
p̄	after	≈	approximately equal
℞	prescription, recipe (take)	>	greater than
s̄	without	<	less than
ṫ	one	≯	not greater than
π̈	two	≮	not less than
→	to, in the direction of	°	degree
↑	increase(d), up	%	percent
↓	decrease(d), down	♀	female
+	plus, positive	♂	male
−	minus, negative		

Appendix B

Glossary of Medical Word Components

Medical Word Element	English Term	Medical Word Element	English Term
a-	without, not	aque/o	water
ab-	from, away from	-ar	pertaining to, relating to
abdomin/o	abdomen	-arche	beginning
abort/o	to miscarry	arteri/o	artery
-ac	pertaining to, relating to	arteriol/o	arteriole
acous/o	hearing	arthr/o	joint
acr/o	extremity	-ary	pertaining to, relating to
acromi/o	acromion (projection of scapula)	asbest/o	asbestos
-acusis	hearing	-asthenia	weakness, debility
ad-	toward	astr/o	star
aden/o	gland	-ate	having the form of, possessing
adenoid/o	adenoids	atel/o	incomplete, imperfect
adip/o	fat	ather/o	fatty plaque
adren/o	adrenal glands	-ation	process (of)
adrenal/o	adrenal glands	atri/o	atrium
af-	toward	audi/o	hearing
agglutin/o	clumping, gluing	audit/o	hearing
agora-	marketplace	aur/o	ear
-al	pertaining to, relating to	auricul/o	ear
albin/o	white	auto-	self, own
albumin/o	albumin (protein)	ax/o	axis, axon
-algesia	pain	azot/o	nitrogenous compounds
-algia	pain	bacteri/o	bacteria
allo-	other, differing from the normal	balan/o	glans penis
alveol/o	alveolus (pl. alveoli)	bas/o	base (alkaline, the opposite of acid)
ambly/o	dull, dim	bi-	two
amni/o	amnion (amniotic sac)	bi/o	life
-amnios	caul (the intact amniotic sac surrounding the fetus at birth)	-blast	embryonic cell
		blast/o	embryonic cell
an-	without, not	blephar/o	eyelid
an/o	anus	brachi/o	arm
ana-	against	brady-	slow
andr/o	male	bronch/o	bronchus (pl. bronchi)
aneurysm/o	widening, a widened blood vessel	bronchi/o	bronchus (pl. bronchi)
angi/o	vessel	bronchiol/o	bronchiole
aniso-	unequal, dissimilar	bucc/o	cheek
ankyl/o	stiffness, bent, crooked	calc/o	calcium
ante-	before, in front of	calcane/o	calcaneum (heel bone)
anter/o	anterior, front	-capnia	carbon dioxide (CO_2)
anthrac/o	black, coal	carcin/o	cancer
anti-	against	cardi/o	heart
aort/o	aorta	carp/o	carpus (wrist bones)
append/o	appendix	caud/o	tail
appendic/o	appendix	cauter/o	heat, burn

-cele	hernia, swelling		-cusis	hearing
-centesis	surgical puncture		cutane/o	skin
cephal/o	head		cyan/o	blue
cerebell/o	cerebellum		cycl/o	ciliary body of the eye, circular, cycle
cerebr/o	cerebrum		-cyesis	pregnancy
cervic/o	neck, cervix uteri (neck of the uterus)		cyst/o	bladder
chalic/o	limestone		cyt/o	cell
cheil/o	lip		-cyte	cell
chem/o	chemical, drug		dacry/o	tear, lacrimal sac
chlor/o	green		dactyl/o	fingers, toes
chol/e	bile, gall		de-	cessation
cholangi/o	bile vessel		dendr/o	tree
cholecyst/o	gallbladder		dent/o	teeth
choledoch/o	bile duct		derm/o	skin
chondr/o	cartilage		-derma	skin
chori/o	chorion		dermat/o	skin
choroid/o	choroid		-desis	binding, fixation (of a bone or joint)
chrom/o	color		di-	double
chromat/o	color		dia-	through, across
cine-	movement		dipl-	double, twofold
cinemat/o	things that move		dipl/o	double
circum-	around		dips/o	thirst
cirrh/o	yellow		-dipsia	thirst
-cision	cutting		dist/o	far, farthest
-clasis	to break		dors/o	back (of the body)
-clast	to break		duct/o	to lead, carry
clavicul/o	clavicle (collar bone)		-duction	act of leading, bringing, conducting
clon/o	clonus		duoden/o	duodenum
coccyg/o	coccyx (tailbone)		dur/o	dura mater, hard
cochle/o	cochlea		-dynia	pain
col/o	colon		dys-	bad, painful, difficult
colon/o	colon		-eal	pertaining to, relating to
colp/o	vagina		ec-	out, out from
condyl/o	condyle		echo-	repeated sound
coni/o	dust		-ectasis	dilation, expansion
conjunctiv/o	conjunctiva		ecto-	outside, outward
-continence	to hold back		-ectomy	excision, removal
contra-	against		-edema	swelling
core/o	pupil		ef-	away from
corne/o	cornea		electr/o	electricity
corp/o	body		-ema	state of, condition
corpor/o	body		embol/o	plug
cortic/o	cortex		-emesis	vomiting
cost/o	ribs		-emia	blood condition
crani/o	cranium, skull		emphys/o	to inflate
-crine	secrete		en-	in, within
crin/o	secrete		encephal/o	brain
cry/o	cold		end-	within
crypt/o	hidden		endo-	in, within
culd/o	cul-de-sac		enter/o	intestine (usually small intestine)
-cusia	hearing		eosin/o	dawn (rose colored)

epi-	above, upon
epididym/o	epididymis
epiglott/o	epiglottis
episi/o	vulva
erythem/o	red
erythemat/o	red
erythr/o	red
eschar/o	scab
-esis	condition
eso-	inward
esophag/o	esophagus
esthes/o	feeling
-esthesia	feeling
eu-	good, normal
ex-	out, out from
exo-	outside, outward
extra-	outside
faci/o	face
fasci/o	band, fascia (fibrous membrane supporting and separating muscles)
femor/o	femur (thigh bone)
-ferent	to carry
fibr/o	fiber, fibrous tissue
fibul/o	fibula (smaller, outer bone of lower leg)
fluor/o	luminous, fluorescence
frotteur/o	to rub
galact/o	milk
gangli/o	ganglion
ganglion/o	ganglion
gastr/o	stomach
-gen	forming, producing, origin
-genesis	forming, producing, origin
gingiv/o	gum(s)
glauc/o	gray
gli/o	glue, neuroglia tissue
-glia	glue, neuroglia tissue
-globin	protein
glomerul/o	glomerulus
gloss/o	tongue
glott/o	glottis
gluc/o	sugar, sweetness
glucos/o	sugar, sweetness
glyc/o	sugar, sweetness
-gnosis	knowing
gonad/o	gonads, sex glands
goni/o	angle
-gram	record, writing
granul/o	granule
-graph	instrument for recording
-graphy	process of recording
-gravida	pregnant woman

gynec/o	woman, female
hallucin/o	hallucination
hedon/o	pleasure
hem/o	blood
hemangi/o	blood vessel
hemat/o	blood
hemi-	one half
hepat/o	liver
hetero-	different
hidr/o	sweat
hist/o	tissue
histi/o	tissue
home/o	same, alike
homo-	same
humer/o	humerus (upper arm bone)
hydr/o	water
hyper-	excessive, above normal
hypn/o	sleep
hypo-	under, below
hyster/o	uterus, womb
-ia	condition
-iasis	abnormal condition (produced by something specified)
iatr/o	physician, medicine, treatment
-iatry	medicine, treatment
-ic	pertaining to, relating to
-ical	pertaining to, relating to
-ice	noun ending
ichthy/o	dry, scaly
-ician	specialist
-icle	small, minute, little
-icterus	jaundice
idi/o	unknown, peculiar
-ile	pertaining to, relating to
ile/o	ileum (third part of small intestine)
ili/o	ilium (lateral, flaring portion of hip bone)
im-	not
immun/o	immune, immunity
in-	in, not
-ine	pertaining to, relating to
infer/o	lower, below
infra-	under, below
inguin/o	groin
insulin/o	insulin
inter-	between
intra-	in, within
-ion	act of
irid/o	iris
-is	noun ending
isch/o	to hold back

ischi/o	ischium (lower portion of the hip bone)
-ism	condition
iso-	same, equal
-ist	specialist
-isy	state of, condition
-itic	pertaining to, relating to
-itis	inflammation
-ive	pertaining to, relating to
-ization	process (of)
jaund/o	yellow
jejun/o	jejunum
kal/i	potassium (an electrolyte)
kary/o	nucleus
kerat/o	horny tissue, hard, cornea
kern/o	kernel (nucleus)
ket/o	ketone bodies (acids and acetones)
keton/o	ketone bodies (acids and acetones)
kinesi/o	movement
-kinesia	movement
klept/o	to steal
kyph/o	hill, mountain
labi/o	lip
labyrinth/o	labyrinth, inner ear
lacrim/o	tear, lacrimal gland
lact/o	milk
-lalia	speech, babble
lamin/o	lamina (part of the vertebral arch)
-lampsia	to shine
lapar/o	abdomen
laryng/o	larynx (voice box)
later/o	side, to one side
lei/o	smooth
leiomy/o	smooth muscle (visceral)
-lepsy	seizure
leuc/o	white
leuk/o	white
lex/o	word, phrase
lingu/o	tongue
lip/o	fat
lipid/o	fat
-lith	stone, calculus
lith/o	stone, calculus
lob/o	lobe
log/o	study of
-logist	specialist in the study of
-logy	study of
-lopaxy	emptying out
lord/o	curve, swayback
-lucent	to shine, clear
lumb/o	loins (lower back)

lymph/o	lymph
lymphangi/o	lymph vessel
-lysis	separation, destruction, loosening
macro-	large
mal-	bad
-malacia	softening
mamm/o	breast
-mania	state of mental disorder, frenzy
mast/o	breast
mastoid/o	mastoid process
meat/o	opening, meatus
medi/o	middle
medull/o	medulla
-megaly	enlargement
melan/o	black
men/o	menses, menstruation
mening/o	meninges
meningi/o	meninges
ment/o	mind
meso-	middle
meta-	change, beyond
metacarp/o	metacarpus (hand bones)
metatars/o	metatarsal (foot bones)
-meter	instrument for measuring
metr/o	uterus, measure
-metry	act of measuring
mi/o	smaller, less
micr/o	small
micro-	small
mono-	one
morph/o	form, shape, structure
muc/o	mucus
multi-	many, much
muscul/o	muscle
mut/a	genetic change
my/o	muscle
myc/o	fungus
mydr/o	widen, enlarge
myel/o	bone marrow, spinal cord
myos/o	muscle
myring/o	tympanic membrane, eardrum
myx/o	mucus
narc/o	stupor, numbness, sleep
nas/o	nose
nat/o	birth
natr/o	sodium (an electrolyte)
necr/o	death, necrosis
neo-	new
nephr/o	kidney
neur/o	nerve
noct/o	night

nucle/o	nucleus	pedicul/o	louse
nulli-	none	pelv/i	pelvis
nyctal/o	night	pelv/o	pelvis
obstetr/o	midwife	pen/o	penis
ocul/o	eye	-penia	decrease, deficiency
odont/o	teeth	-pepsia	digestion
-oid	resembling	per-	through
-ole	small, minute	peri-	around
olig/o	scanty	perine/o	perineum
-oma	tumor	peritone/o	peritoneum
omphal/o	navel (umbilicus)	-pexy	suspension, fixation (of an organ)
onc/o	tumor	phac/o	lens
onych/o	nail	phag/o	swallowing, eating
oophor/o	ovary	-phagia	swallowing, eating
-opaque	obscure	phalang/o	phalanges (bones of fingers and toes)
ophthalm/o	eye	pharmaceutic/o	drug, medicine
-opia	vision	pharyng/o	pharynx (throat)
-opsia	vision	-phasia	speech
-opsy	view of	phe/o	dusky, dark
opt/o	eye, vision	-phil	attraction for
optic/o	eye, vision	-philia	attraction for
or/o	mouth	phim/o	muzzle
orch/o	testes	phleb/o	vein
orchi/o	testes	-phobia	fear
orchid/o	testes	-phonia	voice
-orexia	appetite	-phoresis	carrying, transmission
orth/o	straight	-phoria	feeling (mental state)
-ory	pertaining to, relating to	phot/o	light
-ose	pertaining to, relating to	phren/o	diaphragm, mind
-osis	abnormal condition, increase (used primarily with blood cells)	-phylaxis	protection
		-physis	growth
-osmia	smell	pil/o	hair
oste/o	bone	pituitar/o	pituitary gland
ot/o	ear	-plakia	plaque
-ous	pertaining to, relating to	plas/o	formation, growth
ovari/o	ovary	-plasia	formation, growth
ox/o	oxygen	-plasm	formation, growth
oxy-	quick, sharp	-plasty	surgical repair
palat/o	palate (roof of the mouth)	-plegia	paralysis
pan-	all	pleur/o	pleura
pancreat/o	pancreas	-pnea	breathing
-para	to bear (offspring)	pneum/o	air, lung
para-	near, beside, beyond	pneumon/o	air, lung
parathyroid/o	parathyroid glands	pod/o	foot
-paresis	partial paralysis	-poiesis	formation, production
patell/o	patella (kneecap)	poikil/o	varied, irregular
path/o	disease	poli/o	gray, gray matter (of brain or spinal cord)
-pathy	disease		
pector/o	chest	poly-	many, much
ped/i	foot, child	polyp/o	small growth
ped/o	foot, child	-porosis	porous

post-	after, behind
poster/o	back (of body), behind, posterior
-potence	power
-prandial	meal
pre-	before, in front of
presby/o	old age
primi-	first
pro-	before, in front of
proct/o	anus, rectum
prostat/o	prostate gland
proxim/o	near, nearest
pseudo-	false
psych/o	mind
-ptosis	prolapse, downward displacement
-ptysis	spitting
pub/o	pelvis bone (anterior part of the pelvic bone)
pulmon/o	lung
pupill/o	pupil
py/o	pus
pyel/o	renal pelvis
pylor/o	pylorus
pyr/o	fire
quadri-	four
rachi/o	spine
radi/o	radiation, x-ray, radius (lower arm bone on thumb side)
radicul/o	nerve root
rect/o	rectum
ren/o	kidney
reticul/o	net, mesh
retin/o	retina
retro-	backward, behind
rhabd/o	rod-shaped (striated)
rhabdomy/o	striated (skeletal) muscle
rheumat/o	discharge
rhin/o	nose
rhytid/o	wrinkle
-rrhage	bursting forth (of)
-rrhagia	bursting forth (of)
-rrhaphy	suture
-rrhea	discharge, flow
-rrhexis	rupture
rube/o	red
sacr/o	sacrum
salping/o	tube (usually fallopian or eustachian [auditory] tubes)
-salpinx	tube (usually fallopian or eustachian [auditory] tubes)
sarc/o	flesh (connective tissue)
-sarcoma	malignant tumor of connective tissue
-schisis	splitting
schiz/o	split
scler/o	hardening, sclera
scoli/o	crooked, bent
-scope	instrument to view or examine
-scopy	visual examination
scot/o	darkness
seb/o	sebum, sebaceous
semi-	one half
sequestr/o	separation
ser/o	serum
sial/o	saliva, salivary gland
sider/o	iron
sigmoid/o	sigmoid colon
silic/o	flint
sin/o	sinus, cavity
sinus/o	sinus, cavity
-sis	state of, condition
-social	society
somat/o	body
somn/o	sleep
son/o	sound
-spadias	rent (a slit, a fissure)
-spasm	involuntary contraction, twitching
sperm/o	spermatozoa, sperm cells
spermat/o	spermatozoa, sperm cells
sphygm/o	pulse
-sphyxia	pulse
spin/o	spine
spir/o	breathe
splen/o	spleen
spondyl/o	vertebrae (backbone)
squam/o	scale
staped/o	stapes
-stasis	standing still
steat/o	fat
-stenosis	narrowing, stricture
stern/o	sternum (breastbone)
steth/o	chest
stigmat/o	point
stomat/o	mouth
-stomy	forming an opening (mouth)
sub-	under, below
sudor/o	sweat
super-	upper, above
supra-	above, excessive
syn-	union, together, joined
synapt/o	synapsis, point of contact
synov/o	synovial membrane, synovial fluid
tachy-	rapid
tax/o	order, coordination
ten/o	tendon

tend/o	tendon	tubercul/o	little swelling
tendin/o	tendon	tympan/o	tympanic membrane, eardrum
-tension	to stretch	-ule	small, minute
test/o	testes	uln/o	ulna (lower arm bone on thumb side)
thalam/o	thalamus	ultra-	excess, beyond
thalass/o	sea	-um	structure, thing
thec/o	sheath (usually refers to the meninges)	umbilic/o	umbilicus, navel
thel/o	nipple	ungu/o	nail
therapeut/o	treatment	uni-	one
-therapy	treatment	ur/o	urine, urinary tract
therm/o	heat	ureter/o	ureter
thorac/o	chest	urethr/o	urethra
-thorax	chest	-uria	urine
thromb/o	blood clot	urin/o	urine, urinary tract
thym/o	thymus gland	-us	condition
-thymia	mind, emotion	uter/o	uterus, womb
thyr/o	thyroid gland	uvul/o	uvula
thyroid/o	thyroid gland	vagin/o	vagina
tibi/o	tibia (larger inner bone of the lower leg)	varic/o	dilated vein
-tic	pertaining to, relating to	vas/o	vessel, vas deferens, duct
till/o	to pull	vascul/o	vessel
-tocia	childbirth, labor	ven/o	vein
tom/o	to cut	ventr/o	belly, belly side
-tome	instrument to cut	ventricul/o	ventricle (of heart or brain)
-tomy	incision	-version	turning
ton/o	tension	vertebr/o	vertebrae (backbone)
tonsill/o	tonsils	vesic/o	bladder
-toxic	poison	vesicul/o	seminal vesicle
toxic/o	poison	vest/o	clothes
trabecul/o	trabecula (supporting bundles of fibers)	viscer/o	internal organs
		vitr/o	vitreous body (of the eye)
trache/o	trachea	vitre/o	glassy
trans-	through, across	vol/o	volume
tri-	three	voyeur/o	to see
trich/o	hair	vulv/o	vulva
trigon/o	trigone (triangular region at base of the bladder)	xanth/o	yellow
		xen/o	foreign, strange
-tripsy	crushing	xer/o	dry
-trophy	development, nourishment	xiph/o	sword
-tropia	turning	-y	condition
-tropin	stimulate		

Appendix C

Answer Key

Chapter 1 Medical Word Components

Activity 1–1: Competency Verification
Medical Word Components

1. J
2. D
3. G
4. H
5. I

6. F
7. E
8. C
9. B
10. A

Activity 1–2: Competency Verification
Word Roots, Combining Forms, Suffixes, and Prefixes

1. *mas-TEYE-tis*   m a s t / i t i s

Identify roots, combining forms (CF), suffixes, and prefixes	root	suffix
Meaning	breast	inflammation

6. *mas-TEK-toh-mee*   m a s t / e c t o m y

Identify roots, combining forms (CF), suffixes, and prefixes	root	suffix
Meaning	breast	excision, removal

2. *ton-sil-EK-toh-mee*   t o n s i l l / e c t o m y

Identify roots, combining forms (CF), suffixes, and prefixes	root	suffix
Meaning	tonsil	excision, removal

7. *ar-THREYE-tis*   a r t h r / i t i s

Identify roots, combining forms (CF), suffixes, and prefixes	root	suffix
Meaning	joint	inflammation

3. *ar-throh-sen-TEE-sis*   a r t h r / o / c e n t e s i s

Identify roots, combining forms (CF), suffixes, and prefixes	CF	suffix
Meaning	joint	surgical puncture

8. *koh-LEYE-tis*   c o l / i t i s

Identify roots, combining forms (CF), suffixes, and prefixes	root	suffix
Meaning	colon	inflammation

4. *post-NAY-tal*   p o s t / n a t / a l

Identify roots, combining forms (CF), suffixes, and prefixes	prefix	root	suffix
Meaning	after	birth	pertaining to

9. *ar-THROP-a-thee*   a r t h r / o / p a t h y

Identify roots, combining forms (CF), suffixes, and prefixes	CF	suffix
Meaning	joint	disease

5. *gas-troh-en-ter-EYE-tis*   g a s t r / o / e n t e r / i t i s

Identify roots, combining forms (CF), suffixes, and prefixes	CF	root	suffix
Meaning	stomach	intestine (usually small intestine)	inflammation

10. *koh-LEK-toh-mee*   c o l / e c t o m y

Identify roots, combining forms (CF), suffixes, and prefixes	root	suffix
Meaning	colon	excision, removal

Define and Build Medical Words

1. inflammation (of) tonsils
2. excision, removal (of) tonsils
3. pertaining to (the period) before birth
4. inflammation (of the) colon
5. instrument to view, examine the stomach
6. Rule 1: a word root is used to link a suffix that begins with a vowel.
7. Rule 2: a CF is used to link a suffix that begins with a consonant.
8. Rule 1: a word root is used to link a suffix that begins with a vowel.
9. Rule 2: a CF is used to link a suffix that begins with a consonant.
10. Rule 3: a CF is used to link multiple roots. Rule 1: a word root is used to link a suffix that begins with a vowel.
11. Rule 1: a word root is used to link a suffix that begins with a vowel.
12. Rule 3: a CF is used to link multiple roots even when a root begins with a vowel. Rule 1: a word root is used to link a suffix that begins with a vowel.
13. Rule 2: a CF is used to link a suffix that begins with a consonant.
14. Rule 2: a CF is used to link a suffix that begins with a consonant.
15. Rule 3: a CF is used to link multiple roots even when a root begins with a vowel. Rule 1: a word root is used to link a suffix that begins with a vowel.

Pronunciation Guidelines

1. long
2. short
3. hard, hard
4. hard
5. n
6. s
7. k
8. eye
9. second
10. separate

Forming Plural Words

Singular	Plural	Rule
1. sarco*ma*	sarcoma*ta*	Retain the -*ma* and add -*ta.*
2. thromb*us*	thromb*i*	Drop -*us* and add -*i.*
3. append*ix*	append*ices*	Drop -*ix* and add -*ices.*
4. diverticul*um*	diverticul*a*	Drop -*um* and add -*a.*
5. ovar*y*	ovar*ies*	Drop -*y* and add -*ies.*
6. diagno*sis*	diagno*ses*	Drop -*is* and add -*es.*
7. lum*en*	lum*ina*	Drop -*en* and add -*ina.*
8. vertebr*a*	vertebr*ae*	Retain the -*a* and add -*e.*
9. thora*x*	thora*ces*	Drop the -*x* and add -*ces.*
10. spermatozo*on*	spermatozo*a*	Drop -*on* and add -*a.*

Activity 1–6: Competency Verification

Medical Word Components

Prefix	Combining Form (s) (root + vowel)	Word Root(s)	Suffix
1.		tonsill	-ectomy
2. post-		nat	-al
3.		mast	-itis
4.	gastr/o		-scope
5.	enter/o	col	-itis
6. pre-		nat	-al
7.	oste/o	arthr	-itis
8.		append	-ectomy
9.		gastr	-ectomy
10.	arthr/o		-centesis

Activity 1–7: Competency Verification

Defining Medical Terms

1. breast
2. inflammation
3. colon
4. bone
5. after
6. joint
7. disease
8. *pre-*

9. *gastr/o*
10. *-pathy*
11. *mast/o*
12. *-scope*
13. appendix
14. intestine (usually small intestine)
15. *-centesis*

Chapter 2 Medical Specialties and Medical Records Orientation

Activity 2–1: Competency Verification

Medical Practice Information

1. What are the requirements to receive the MD degree in the United States?

Completion of 4 years of education from an accredited medical school.

2. Besides the MD degree, what are the other requirements to practice medicine?

The MD must pass a state license examination and any other requirements of the state.

3. Define *fellowship training.*

Postgraduate training following residency that focuses on clinical care (patient care) and research skills in a specialized area of medicine.

4. Define the role of the primary care provider.

The first health professional a patient usually consults. Primary care physicians tend to see patients on a regular basis for a variety of ailments and provide preventive treatments.

5. What types of specialists are considered primary care providers?

The family practitioner, internist, and pediatrician.

Medical Records

1. When is the medical record initiated?

At the time of the patient's first visit.

2. How would a medical record be advantageous as a legal document if a patient sues the physician?

Accurate, documented information provides evidence to protect the legal interests of the health-care facility, the physician, and the patient.

3. Besides medical information, what other type of information is contained in the medical record?

Nonmedical information, such as occupation, address, telephone number; demographic information, such as race, gender, and age are also part of the medical record.

4. What is the primary purpose of the history and physical?

To provide information about the patient's medical history and current physical state. The physician needs this information to make a diagnosis and prescribe a treatment plan for the patient.

5. What is a consultation report?

Written correspondence by a physician who requests, and then is provided with, further medical evaluation of patients by specialists or other physicians.

Critical Thinking: Analysis of Medical Records

>>> MEDICAL RECORD 2–2: PROGRESS NOTES

1. Does the patient have a history of hay fever or sore throat?

The patient does not have a history of hay fever; the patient does have a history of a sore throat.

2. What are the three medications prescribed to decrease inflammation and to open up the eustachian tubes?

Claritin-D, Afrin, and Flonase nasal inhaler.

>>> MEDICAL RECORD 2–3: HISTORY AND PHYSICAL EXAMINATION

3. What was the patient's CC?

The patient's CC was "difficulty breathing."

4. Does the patient suffer from nausea, diarrhea, or constipation?

No.

5. Did the physician note that there were increased breath sounds or any rales or wheezing?

In the lungs section, the physician states, "decreased breath sounds throughout; no obvious rales or wheezing noted."

6. Does the patient have any allergies?

Yes, to penicillin.

7. What was the patient's sharp pain associated with?

The sharp pain was associated with some shortness of breath.

8. What did the cardiovascular system examination reveal?

The cardiovascular examination revealed the patient to be in normal sinus rhythm without murmurs. Lungs are clinically clear.

9. Why was the imaging study ordered for Timothy Anders?

To rule out spinal cord compression.

10. What abnormalities were found?

Mild, central bulging at L5–S1 with some central flattening at the L4–5 levels.

11. What laboratory tests were performed on Joleen Smythers?

Chemistry profile and basic and microscopic urinalysis.

12. What type of sample(s) was used for the tests?

Blood and urine.

Critical Thinking: Analysis of Medical Records

1. From what organ was the biopsy sample taken?

The uterus.

2. Did the sample show evidence of carcinoma?

There was no evidence of malignancy, hyperplasia, or acute endometritis.

3. What procedure was performed on Carol Ottoman?

Laser-assisted uvulopalatoplasty, stage I.

4. Why was this procedure performed?

The patient had loud snoring and mild sleep apnea.

5. Why was the patient transferred from Smith Hospital?

Worsening shortness of breath and atrioventricular block.

6. What was done to improve the atrioventricular block?

Pacemaker implantation.

7. What was the patient's condition upon discharge?

Fair; the patient was doing reasonably well, ambulating in the hallways with oxygen and had no symptoms.

>>> MEDICAL RECORD 2-10: EMERGENCY DEPARTMENT REPORT

8. Why did Nancy Frost come to the emergency room?

She fell 4 days ago onto concrete and injured her right leg.

9. What type of fracture did the patient have?

Nondisplaced proximal fibula fracture of the right leg.

10. What treatment was she given for her injury?

Ace wrap and crutches.

Activity 2–3: Clinical Application
Medical Reports

1. Discharge Summary
2. Laboratory Report
3. Operative Report
4. Emergency Department Report
5. Progress Notes
6. Imaging Report
7. Letters
8. H&P
9. Pathology Report
10. Consultation

Activity 2–4: Clinical Application
Medical Specialists

1. cardiologist
2. orthopedist
3. pulmonologist
4. gastroenterologist
5. pediatrician
6. urologist
7. hematologist
8. dermatologist
9. ophthalmologist
10. gerontologist

Chapter 3 Suffixes and Prefixes

Activity 3–1: Competency Verification
Surgical and Diagnostic Suffixes

1. audi/o/metry
2. electr/o/cardi/o/graphy
3. col/o/stomy
4. my/o/rrhaphy
5. phleb/o/tomy
6. angi/o/gram
7. crani/o/meter
8. rhin/o/plasty
9. mast/o/pexy
10. arthr/o/desis
11. thromb/o/lysis
12. oste/o/clasis
13. col/ectomy
14. gastr/o/scopy
15. lith/o/tripsy

Surgical and Diagnostic Terms

1.	mast/ectomy	*ectomy*=excision, removal; breast
2.	rhin/o/plasty	*plasty*=surgical repair; nose
3.	my/o/rrhaphy	*rrhaphy*=suture; muscle
4.	arthr/o/centesis	*centesis*=surgical puncture; joint
5.	col/o/stomy	*stomy*=forming an opening (mouth); colon
6.	phleb/o/tomy	*tomy*=incision; vein
7.	endo/scope	*scope*=instrument to view or examine; in, within
8.	electr/o/cardi/o/graph	*graph*=instrument for recording; electricity; heart
9.	audi/o/metry	*metry*=act of measuring; hearing
10.	lith/o/tripsy	*tripsy*=crushing; stone, calculus

Pathological Suffixes

1.	neur/algia		9.	neur/o/pathy
2.	bronchi/ectasis		10.	blephar/o/spasm
3.	arteri/o/stenosis		11.	hepat/o/megaly
4.	gastr/itis		12.	oste/o/malacia
5.	carcin/oma		13.	leuk/o/penia
6.	leuk/emia		14.	hem/o/rrhage
7.	hemat/emesis		15.	cyan/osis
8.	hepat/o/cele			

Pathological Terms

1.	gastr/itis	*itis*=inflammation; stomach
2.	hepat/o/megaly	*megaly*=enlargement; liver
3.	oste/o/malacia	*malacia*=softening; bone
4.	cyan/osis	*osis*=abnormal condition; blue
5.	blephar/o/spasm	*spasm*=involuntary contraction, twitching; eyelid
6.	thyr/o/toxic	*toxic*=poison; thyroid gland
7.	dia/rrhea	*rrhea*=discharge, flow; through, across
8.	neo/plasm	*plasm*=formation, growth; new
9.	neur/algia	*algia*=pain; nerve
10.	carcin/oma	*oma*=tumor; cancer

Nouns and Adjectives

1.	adjective		6.	adjective
2.	noun		7.	noun
3.	noun		8.	noun
4.	adjective		9.	adjective
5.	adjective		10.	noun

Activity 3–6: Competency Verification

Prefixes

1. dipl/opia
2. pseudo/cyesis
3. a/mast/ia
4. hypo/glyc/emia
5. micro/cephal/y

6. tachy/pnea
7. neo/plasm
8. im/potence
9. dys/pepsia
10. brady/pnea

Activity 3–7: Competency Verification

Suffixes and Prefixes

1. hypo-
2. -ectomy
3. macro-
4. -scope
5. -malacia
6. dipl-
7. -centesis
8. -oma
9. -pathy
10. neo-
11. -lith
12. -rrhexis
13. tachy-

14. -edema
15. dys-
16. -gram
17. -megaly
18. -emesis
19. -osis
20. endo-
21. -stenosis
22. -tomy
23. -tripsy
24. -plasty
25. -dynia

Activity 3–8: Competency Verification

Medical Terms

1. macro/cephal/y
2. dys/pepsia
3. amni/o/centesis
4. gastr/o/scopy
5. tachy/pnea
6. hem/o/rrhage
7. hepat/o/cele
8. an/orexia
9. oste/o/malacia
10. carcin/oma
11. hemat/emesis
12. mast/ectomy
13. dia/rrhea

14. col/o/stomy
15. rhin/o/plasty
16. pseudo/cyesis
17. oste/o/clasis
18. thromb/o/lysis
19. leuk/emia
20. chol/e/lith/iasis
21. hyper/glyc/emia
22. bronchi/ectasis
23. audi/o/metry
24. blephar/o/spasm
25. electr/o/cardi/o/graph

Chapter 4 Body Structure

Activity 4–1: Competency Verification
Cellular Structures

1. cell membrane
2. nucleus
3. chromatin
4. nuclear membrane
5. cytoplasm
6. endoplasmic reticulum
7. ribosomes
8. mitochondrion (mitochondria, plural)
9. lysosome
10. Golgi apparatus
11. centrioles
12. cilia

Activity 4–2: Competency Verification
Word Components: Parts of the Body

1. lip/ectomy   *ectomy*=excision, removal; fat
2. spin/al   *al*=pertaining to, spine
3. chondr/oma   *oma*=tumor, cartilage
4. lumb/ar   *ar*=pertaining to; loins (lower back)
5. umbilic/al   *al*=pertaining to; umbilicus, navel
6. fibr/o/blast   *blast*=embryonic cell; fiber, fibrous tissue
7. inguin/al   *al*=pertaining to; groin
8. hist/o/logist   *logist*=specialist in the study of; tissue(s)
9. crani/o/tomy   *tomy*=incision; cranium, skull
10. thorac/ic   *ic*=pertaining to; chest

Activity 4–3: Competency Verification
Word Components: Position and Direction

1. proxim/al   *al*=pertaining to; near, nearest
2. dors/al   *al*=pertaining to; back (of body)
3. cephal/ic   *ic*=pertaining to; head
4. caud/ad   *ad*=toward; tail
5. ventr/al   *al*=pertaining to; belly, belly side
6. anter/o/later/al   *al*=pertaining to; anterior, front; side, to one side
7. infra/cost/al   *al*=pertaining to; under; below; ribs
8. hypo/derm/ic   *ic*=pertaining to; under; below; skin
9. dist/al   *al*=pertaining to; far, farthest
10. poster/o/medi/al   *al*=pertaining to; back (of body), behind, posterior; middle

Body Cavities

1. thoracic
2. abdominopelvic
3. diaphragm
4. abdominal

5. pelvic
6. cranial
7. spinal

Planes of Reference, Position, and Direction

1. medial
2. proximal
3. inferior
4. anterior
5. lateral
6. external
7. deep
8. internal
9. superficial
10. inferior

11. distal
12. superior
13. prone
14. supine
15. Fowler
16. dorsal recumbent
17. frontal (coronal)
18. transverse
19. midsagittal
20. sagittal

Areas of the Abdomen, Body Cavities, and Spinal Column

1. LUQ, left upper quadrant
2. RUQ, right upper quadrant
3. LLQ, left lower quadrant
4. umbilical
5. epigastric
6. hypogastric
7. right hypochondriac
8. left hypochondriac

9. dorsal cavity
10. ventral cavity
11. diaphragm
12. pelvic cavity
13. cervical
14. five
15. coccyx

Build Medical Words

1. medi/al
2. dist/al
3. epi/gastr/ic
4. viscer/o/megaly
5. inter/cost/al
6. umbilic/al
7. abdomin/o/pelv/ic
8. hist/o/logy
9. hypo/derm/ic
10. crani/o/tomy

11. bi/later/al
12. inguin/al
13. neur/o/logist
14. later/o/medi/al
15. anter/o/poster/ior
16. chondr/oma
17. cyt/o/logist
18. inter/vertebr/al
19. cephal/ic
20. my/o/pathy

Chapter 5 Dermatology

Activity 5-1: Competency Verification

Structures Related to the Skin, Hair Follicles, and Nails

> > > FIGURE 5-2

1. epidermis
2. stratum corneum
3. stratum germinativum
4. dermis
5. subcutaneous tissue
6. adipose tissue
7. sudoriferous gland
8. pore
9. sebaceous gland

> > > FIGURE 5-3

1. follicle
2. hair root
3. hair shaft

> > > FIGURE 5-4

1. nail root
2. lunula
3. nail bed
4. nail body
5. free edge

Activity 5-2: Competency Verification

Layers of the Skin

1. epidermis
2. basal layer
3. melanocytes
4. dermis
5. subcutaneous tissue
6. sudoriferous
7. sebaceous
8. pore(s)
9. nails, glands, hair
10. androgen

Word Components: Integumentary System

1. dermat/itis   *itis*=inflammation; skin
2. hypo/derm/ic   *ic*=pertaining to, relating to; under, below; skin
3. ichthy/osis   *osis*=abnormal condition, increase (used primarily with blood cells); dry, scaly
4. hidr/osis   *osis*=abnormal condition, increase (used primarily with blood cells); sweat
5. onych/o/malacia   *malacia*=softening; nail
6. trich/o/pathy   *pathy*=disease; hair
7. xer/o/derma   *derma*=skin; dry
8. seb/o/rrhea   *rrhea*=discharge, flow; sebum
9. lip/oma   *oma*=tumor; fat
10. sub/cutane/ous   *ous*=pertaining to; under, below; skin

Combining Forms, Prefixes, and Suffixes

1. erythr/o/cyte   *cyte*=cell; red
2. cirrh/osis   *osis*=abnormal condition, increase (used primarily with blood cells); yellow
3. xanth/o/derma   *derma*=skin; yellow
4. jaund/ice   *ice*=noun ending; yellow
5. cyan/o/derma   *derma*=skin; blue
6. melan/oma   *oma*=tumor; black
7. an/hidr/osis   *osis*=abnormal condition, increase (used primarily with blood cells); without, not; sweat
8. scler/o/derma   *derma*=skin; hardening
9. dermat/o/logy   *logy*=study of; skin
10. sub/ungu/al   *al*=pertaining to, relating to; under, below; nail

Pathological Conditions

1. ichthyosis
2. keratosis
3. dermatomycosis
4. alopecia
5. comedo
6. hyperhidrosis
7. laceration
8. xeroderma
9. pustule
10. scabies
11. onychia
12. cicatrix
13. ecchymosis
14. furuncle
15. vitiligo
16. ulcer
17. pediculosis
18. sebaceous cyst
19. hirsutism
20. erythroderma

Skin Lesions and Burns

1. ulcer
2. bulla
3. macule
4. fissure
5. thermal burn

6. wheal
7. superficial partial-thickness burn
8. chemical burns
9. tumor
10. deep partial-thickness burn

Diagnostic, Surgical, and Therapeutic Procedures

1. autograft
2. keratolytics
3. irrigation
4. antimycotics
5. cryosurgery

6. curettage
7. topical anesthetics
8. lipectomy
9. dermabrasion
10. antibacterials

Diagnostic, Symptomatic, and Surgical Terms

1. dermatitis
2. dermatologist
3. adipoma, lipoma
4. adipocyte, lipocyte
5. onychitis, onychia
6. onychoma
7. onychopathy
8. onychomalacia
9. trichopathy
10. trichosis

11. xeroderma
12. xerosis
13. leukoderma
14. cyanoderma
15. xanthoderma
16. erythrocyte
17. leukocyte
18. melanocyte
19. anhidrosis
20. hyperhidrosis

Critical Thinking: Analysis of Medical Records

> > > MEDICAL RECORD 5–1: HISTORY AND PHYSICAL EXAMINATION

1. What was Ms. Anderline's chief complaint, and what was her previous diagnosis?

The patient complained of itching on the forehead; she was diagnosed with impetigo.

2. Place a "+" in the space provided for positive findings and a "−" for negative findings. A positive finding indicates the patient had a history (Hx) of this condition; a negative finding indicates the patient did not have a history of this condition.

+high blood pressure.   −edema

−ringing in the ears   −thyroid disease or diabetes

−dysphagia   −blood clots, anemia

−chest pain   −varicose veins

3. What does the dermatologist mean when he states in the physical examination section that there is "no discharge or ulcers?

There is a rash, but it does not have any pustules or infection present.

4. What was Dr. Smith's diagnosis?

Impetigo, under investigation and treatment.

> > > MEDICAL RECORD 5-2: CONSULTATION

5. Why was the patient admitted to the hospital, and what type of treatment did she receive?

Her face was so swollen that she was almost unable to open her eyes. She was treated with IV antibiotics and was placed on Unasyn.

6. Was the patient allergic to any medication. If so, explain?

After taking Unasyn, she developed some pruritus on her feet thought to be perhaps an allergy of some sort. Her medication was changed to Cleocin and ciprofloxacin was added.

7. What was the physician's diagnosis or impression and what type of therapy was continued?

Impetigo—likely staphylococcal rather than streptococcal. The antibiotics Cleocin and ciprofloxacin were continued.

8. What body structure is the physician talking about when he suggests adding mupirocin ointment to the nares to be rid of the putative (commonly considered) staph carriage?

The nares are the nostrils. The ointment would be applied to the openings of the nostrils.

> > > MEDICAL RECORD 5-3: OPERATIVE REPORT

9. a. What type of operation was performed, and why and where was it was performed?

The patient elected cosmetic surgery for facial aging. This was an outpatient procedure (OP). Most likely, it was performed in the office's operating room.

  b. Why and where was a small stab incision made and how was the excess fat removed?

A small stab incision was made at the submental crease and excess fat from the submental region was removed by means of suction.

> > > MEDICAL RECORD 5-4: DERMATOPATHOLOGY REPORT

10. What did the clinical data indicate for several months and for many years?

There was scaly, slightly pearly plaque for several months; there was brown-pink plaque for many years.

11. What were the diagnoses for the left upper back and the left ear?

The diagnosis for the left upper back was a typical melanocytic proliferation, most compatible with malignant melanoma. The diagnosis for the left ear was a superficial squamous cell carcinoma.

12. What was the purpose of examining the 0.2 cm × 0.2 cm punch specimen?

Dr. Roff, the pathologist, examined the specimen to determine whether it was malignant or whether there was evidence of any other pathological conditions.

Chapter 6 Urology

Activity 6-1: Competency Verification

Frontal Section of Right Kidney, and Nephron with Associated Blood Vessels

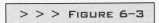 FIGURE 6-3

1. kidney
2. renal cortex
3. renal corpuscles
4. nephrons
5. renal medulla
6. renal tubules
7. renal pyramids

8. renal artery
9. renal vein
10. ureter
11. renal pelvis
12. papillary duct
13. papilla of pyramid
14. calyces

> > > FIGURE 6-4

1. proximal convoluted tubule
2. loop of Henle
3. distal convoluted tubule
4. glomerulus
5. Bowman capsule
6. renal cortex
7. renal medulla

Activity 6-2: Competency Verification

Organs of the Male Reproductive System

> > > FIGURE 6-5

1. testis
2. scrotum
3. epididymis
4. vas deferens
5. ejaculatory duct
6. urethra
7. seminal vesicles
8. prostate gland
9. bulbourethral gland or Cowper gland
10. penis
11. glans penis
12. prepuce (foreskin)
13. urethral orifice

Medical Word Components: Urinary System

1. nephr/oma   *oma*=tumor; kidney
2. cyst/o/scope   *scope*=instrument to examine; bladder
3. ureter/o/cele   *cele*=hernia, swelling; ureter
4. pyel/o/lith   *lith*=stone, calculus; renal pelvis
5. cyst/itis   *itis*=inflammation; bladder
6. urethr/o/dynia   *dynia*=pain; urethra
7. ureter/itis   *itis*=inflammation; ureter
8. glomerul/o/scler/osis   *osis*=abnormal condition, increase (used primarily with blood cells); glomerulus; hardening, sclera (outer layer of the eyeball)
9. trigon/itis   *itis*=inflammation; trigone
10. pyel/o/lith/o/tomy   *tomy*=incision; renal pelvis; stone, calculus

Activity 6–4: Competency Verification
Medical Word Components: Urine

1. ket/osis   *osis*=abnormal condition, increase (used primarily with blood cells); ketone bodies (acids and acetones)
2. ur/emia   *emia*=blood condition; urine, urinary tract
3. an/uria   *uria*=urine; without, not
4. supra/ren/al   *al*=pertaining to, relating to; above, excessive; kidneys
5. dia/lysis   *lysis*=separation, destruction, loosening; through, across
6. keton/uria   *uria*=urine; ketone bodies (acids and acetones)
7. hypo/azot/uria   *uria*=urine, under, below; nitrogenous compounds
8. urin/o/meter   *meter*=instrument for measuring; urine, urinary tract
9. poly/uria   *uria*=urine; many, much
10. hyper/kal/emia   *emia*=blood; excessive; potassium (an electrolyte)

Activity 6–5: Competency Verification
Medical Word Components: Male Reproductive System

1. orch/itis   *itis*=inflammation; testes
2. pyel/o/lith/o/tomy   *tomy*=incision; renal pelvis; stone, calculus
3. balan/o/plasty   *plasty*=surgical repair; glans penis
4. gonad/o/pathy   *pathy*=disease; gonads, sex glands
5. a/sperm/ia   *ia*=condition; without, not; spermatozoa, sperm cells
6. an/orch/ism   *ism*=condition; without, not; testes
7. balan/itis   *itis*=inflammation; glans penis
8. spermat/o/lysis   *lysis*=separation, destruction, loosening; spermatozoa, sperm cells
9. prostat/o/megaly   *megaly*=enlargement; prostate gland
10. vas/ectomy   *ectomy*=excision, removal; vas deferens, vessel, duct

Activity 6–6: Clinical Application
Pathological Conditions

1. orchitis
2. ureterolithiasis
3. balanitis
4. pyelonephritis
5. hydrocele
6. nocturia
7. azotemia
8. enuresis
9. urinary incontinence
10. cryptorchidism
11. epispadias
12. gonorrhea
13. hypospadias
14. phimosis
15. glomerulosclerosis
16. nephroma
17. ureterocele
18. hyperkalemia
19. aspermia
20. anorchism

Activity 6–7: Clinical Application
Diagnostic Tests, Treatments, and Abbreviations

1. uricosurics
2. catheterization
3. voiding cystourethrography
4. spermicidals
5. gonadotropins
6. ultrasonography
7. stent placement
8. dialysis
9. circumcision
10. KUB (kidneys, ureters, bladder)

Activity 6–8: Build Medical Words
Diagnostic, Symptomatic, and Surgical Terms

1. nephroma
2. nephrolith
3. nephrology
4. pyelogram
5. pyelectasis, pyelectasia
6. ureterocele
7. ureteroplasty
8. urethrostenosis
9. urethrodynia; urethralgia
10. urethritis
11. azoturia
12. azotemia
13. orchidectomy
14. orchidotomy
15. polyuria
16. polydipsia
17. prostatomegaly
18. prostatitis
19. vasal
20. vasectomy

Critical Thinking: Analysis of Medical Records

> > > MEDICAL RECORD 6-1. UROLOGY CONSULTATION

1. What brought Mr. Hernandez to the emergency room?

Difficulty in voiding over the last several days.

2. Place "+" in the space provided for positive findings and a "−" for negative findings. A positive finding indicates the patient had a history (Hx) of this condition: a negative finding indicates the patient did not have a history of this condition.

    − hematuria   − normal urinary flow

    + hesitancy   + enlarged prostate

    + nocturia   − dysuria

    − urinary tract infections

3. What is the purpose of a urinary catheter?

To drain urine from the bladder when the patient is unable to void it normally. It is also used to obtain a urine specimen for diagnostic evaluation.

4. Why was the patient put on the antibiotic Septra?

Septra is used in the treatment of prostatism. Septra is an antibiotic and sulfonamide anti-infective combination drug.

5. What type of surgery was advised?

Prostate obstruction surgery; TURP (transurethral resection of prostate).

> > > MEDICAL RECORD 6-2. DISCHARGE SUMMARY

6. What type of operation and special procedures did the surgeon perform?

Cystoscopy with urethral dilatation; cystolithalopaxy; transurethral resection of prostate.

7. What medication was Mr. Hernandez prescribed upon discharge from the hospital, and why was it prescribed?

Cipro (ciprofloxacin), which is used for moderate urinary tract infections (UTI)

8. What laboratory reports are pending?

Bladder calculi and chemical analysis.

9. What was his final diagnosis?

Acute urinary retention; prostatism; benign prostatic hypertrophy.

> > > MEDICAL RECORD 6-3. PATHOLOGY REPORT

10. How were the specimens labeled in the gross description, parts A and B, of the pathology report?

Part A: bladder calculi; part B: prostate tissue.

11. Were there any signs of malignancy in the biopsy performed on the prostate tissue?

Yes, the prostate tissue sample showed single occult focus of adenocarcinoma, grade 2,2 (Gleason).

12. What abnormalities were found in the bladder?

Multiple tan-yellow calculi were found in the bladder.

Chapter 7 Gastroenterology

Activity 7-1: Competency Verification

Digestive Process

> > > FIGURE 7-2

1. oral cavity
2. hard palate
3. soft palate
4. teeth
5. tongue
6. pharynx
7. uvula
8. trachea
9. esophagus
10. epiglottis

> > > FIGURE 7-3

1. gingiva
2. crown
3. neck
4. root
5. enamel
6. dentin
7. pulp cavity
8. nerve
9. blood vessels
10. cementum
11. periodontal membrane

Activity 7-2: Competency Verification

Salivary Glands and Stomach

> > > FIGURE 7-4

1. sublingual gland
2. submandibular gland
3. parotid gland

> > > FIGURE 7-5

1. lower esophageal sphincter (LES)
2. fundus
3. body
4. pylorus or antrum
5. rugae
6. pyloric sphincter
7. duodenum

Activity 7–3: Competency Verification

Small Intestine and Large Intestine

> > > FIGURE 7–6

1. duodenum
2. jejunum
3. ileum
4. stomach
5. liver
6. gallbladder
7. pancreas

> > > FIGURE 7–8

1. cecum
2. ileocecal valve
3. appendix
4. ascending colon
5. hepatic flexure
6. transverse colon
7. splenic flexure
8. descending colon
9. sigmoid colon
10. rectum
11. anal canal
12. anus

Activity 7–4: Competency Verification

Accessory Digestive Organs

> > > FIGURE 7–9

1. liver
2. gallbladder
3. common bile duct
4. right hepatic duct
5. left hepatic duct
6. hepatic duct
7. cystic duct
8. duodenum
9. pancreas
10. pancreatic duct

Activity 7–5: Competency Verification

Tracing the Route of Digestion

1. oral cavity
2. teeth
3. pharynx
4. epiglottis
5. esophagus
6. LES
7. stomach
8. pylorus
9. duodenum
10. jejunum
11. ileum
12. ascending colon
13. transverse colon
14. descending colon
15. anus

Activity 7–6: Competency Verification

Medical Word Components: Mouth, Esophagus, and Pharynx

1. dent/ist   *ist*=specialist; teeth
2. gingiv/itis   *itis*=inflammation; gums
3. esophag/itis   *itis*=inflammation; esophagus
4. stomat/o/pathy   *pathy*=disease; mouth
5. gloss/itis   *itis*=inflammation; tongue
6. orth/odont/ist   *ist*=specialist; straight; teeth
7. esophag/o/cele   *cele*=hernia, swelling; esophagus
8. cheil/osis   *osis*=abnormal condition, increase (used primarily with blood cells); lip
9. labi/al   *al*=pertaining to, relating to; lip
10. sial/o/lith   *lith*=stone, calculus; saliva, salivary gland

Medical Word Components: Stomach, Small Intestine, and Colon

1. gastr/ectomy   *ectomy*=excision, removal; stomach
2. append/ectomy   *ectomy*=excision, removal; appendix
3. jejun/o/rrhaphy   *rrhaphy*=suture; jejunum
4. enter/o/pathy   *pathy*=disease; intestine
5. colon/o/scopy   *scopy*=visual examination; colon
6. pylor/o/plasty   *plasty*=surgical repair; pylorus
7. rect/o/cele   *cele*=hernia, swelling; rectum
8. proct/o/dynia   *dynia*=pain; anus, rectum
9. col/o/stomy   *stomy*=forming an opening (mouth); colon
10. sigmoid/o/scopy   *scopy*=visual examination; sigmoid colon

Medical Word Components: Accessory Digestive Organs
Prefixes and Suffixes: Gastroenterology

1. hepat/o/megaly   *megaly*=enlargement; liver
2. chol/e/lith/iasis   *iasis*=abnormal condition (produced by something specified);
                         bile, gall; stone, calculus
3. cholecyst/ectomy   *ectomy*=excision, removal; gallbladder
4. cholangi/o/gram   *gram*=a writing, record; bile vessel
5. dys/pepsia   *pepsia*=digestion; bad, painful, difficult
6. post/prandial   *prandial*=meal; after, behind
7. sub/lingu/al   *al*=pertaining to; under, below; tongue
8. hyper/emesis   *emesis*=vomiting; excessive, above normal
9. an/orexia   *orexia*=appetite; without, not
10. hepat/oma   *oma*=tumor; liver

Pathological Conditions: Organs of Ingestion and Digestion

1. Crohn disease   6. achalasia
2. thrush   7. Hirschsprung disease
3. cheilitis   8. volvulus
4. stomatitis   9. intussusception
5. leukoplakia   10. hemorrhoids

Pathological Conditions: Accessory Digestive Organs of Digestion and Related Terms

1. steatorrhea   6. cachexia
2. flatus   7. hepatitis
3. melena   8. cholelithiasis
4. hernia   9. jaundice
5. borborygmus   10. anorexia

Diagnostic Procedures, Treatments, Abbreviations, and Pharmacology

1. barium enema (lower GI series)
2. magnetic resonance imaging (MRI)
3. anastomosis
4. endoscopic retrograde cholangiopancreatography (ERCP)
5. endoscopy
6. stool culture
7. computed tomography (CT)
8. biopsy
9. barium swallow (upper GI series)
10. lithotripsy
11. nasogastric intubation
12. antacids
13. antiemetics
14. cathartics, laxatives, purgatives
15. emetics
16. qam
17. qd
18. qid
19. stat
20. tid

Activity 7-12: Build Medical Words

Diagnostic, Symptomatic, and Surgical Terms

1. esophagitis
2. esophagoscope
3. esophagoscopy
4. gastritis
5. gastropathy
6. gastromegaly
7. duodenoscopy
8. duodenotomy
9. jejunorrhaphy
10. ileotomy
11. enteritis
12. enteropathy
13. colonoscopy
14. colorrhaphy
15. proctocele, rectocele
16. proctostenosis, rectostenosis
17. cholecystitis
18. cholelithiasis
19. hepatomegaly
20. pancreatitis

Critical Thinking: Analysis of Medical Records

> > > MEDICAL RECORD 7-1: CONSULTATION

1. What type of surgeries did this patient have in the past?

Lower abdominal surgery, including total hysterectomy and appendectomy, a bypass, and total hip surgery.

2. What is the Dr. Lee's diagnosis of this patient?

Acute cholecystitis with cholelithiasis; exogenous obesity, chronic coronary artery disease, hypercholesterolemia, status post total hip replacement surgery.

3. What findings in the physical examination led the doctor to suspect a gallbladder problem?

During examination of the abdomen the doctor found a very tender globular mass in the right upper quadrant (the location of the gallbladder). Recurrent episodes of RUQ or epigastric pain or discomfort following meals that Mrs. Waters complained of is a classic clinical finding in chronic cholecystitis with cholelithiasis.

4. Does the physician think the patient can tolerate surgery at this time?

After consulting with Dr. Stillwater, he concluded that the patient was in good shape to undergo surgery at this time.

> > > MEDICAL RECORD 7-2: OPERATIVE REPORT

5. What did the surgeon observe immediately upon opening the peritoneal cavity?

The gallbladder was quite inflamed and the omentum was packed around it.

6. What else did he observe on the medial portion of the wall?

There was a gangrenous area that showed evidence of perforation and a purulent collection of about 25 cc of material as well as fibrinous exudate.

7. What complication arose with the coagulating mechanism during surgery? Was the surgeon able to rectify the problem?

The use of the machine set off alarms from either her pacemaker or hip prosthesis; a satisfactory connection was eventually obtained and electrocoagulation proceeded in a satisfactory manner.

> > > MEDICAL RECORD 7-3: PATHOLOGY REPORT

8. What type and size of calculi did the pathologist find when he examined the excised gallbladder?

Three black spherical calculi were present within the lumen of the gallbladder varying up to approximately 1.7 cm in greatest diameter.

9. What made the pathologist conclude there was purulence present in the mucosa?

He observed that the mucosa had a patchy appearance alternating between red-brown and greenish with obvious areas of purulence present.

> > > MEDICAL RECORD 7-4: DISCHARGE SUMMARY

10. Upon discharge, what medications did the patient have to take twice a day and three times a day?

Cipro 500 mg bid; Flagyl 500 mg tid for 5 days.

11. Did the patient have an uneventful recovery?

In recovery, the patient experienced bronchospasm and a small paroxysm of atrial tachycardia.

12. Why was the patient sent home with a short prescription of iron tablets? How will the doctor know that the iron tablets were effective?

The patient developed anemia secondary to blood loss at the time of surgery. The patient is to have a CBC drawn, which will measure the hemoglobin and hematocrit levels.

Chapter 8 Pulmonology

Activity 8-1: Competency Verification
Upper Respiratory Tract and Larynx

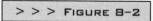
> > > FIGURE 8-2

1. nose
2. nostril
3. olfactory receptors
4. ethmoid bone
5. nasopharynx
6. soft palate
7. uvula
8. pharyngeal tonsil
9. eustachian tube
10. oropharynx
11. palatine tonsil
12. lingual tonsil
13. laryngopharynx
14. larynx
15. trachea
16. thyroid cartilage
17. epiglottis

Activity 8-2: Competency Verification
Lower Respiratory Tract

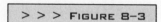
> > > FIGURE 8-3

1. trachea
2. left primary bronchus
3. right primary bronchus
4. bronchioles
5. alveolus
6. pulmonary capillary
7. right lung
8. left lung
9. mediastinum
10. apex of the lung
11. diaphragm
12. pleural membranes
13. pleural space

Activity 8-3: Competency Verification
Breathing Process

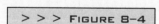
> > > FIGURE 8-4

1. lung
2. inhalation (inspiration)
3. diaphragm
4. external intercostal muscle
5. exhalation (expiration)

Activity 8–4: Competency Verification

Respiration

1. nose
2. olfactory receptors
3. pharynx
4. larynx
5. trachea

6. bronchi
7. bronchioles
8. alveoli
9. pulmonary capillaries
10. lungs

Activity 8–5: Competency Verification

Medical Word Components

1. bronch/o/spasm   *spasm*=involuntary contraction, twitching; bronchus
2. pharyng/o/scopy   *scopy*=visual examination; pharynx (throat)
3. rhin/o/plasty   *plasty*=surgical repair; nose
4. lob/ectomy   *ectomy*=excision, removal; lobe
5. pector/al   *al*=pertaining to, relating to; chest
6. pulmon/o/logist   *logist*=specialist in the study of; lung
7. thorac/o/centesis   *centesis*=surgical puncture; chest
8. trache/o/stomy   *stomy*=forming an opening (mouth); trachea
9. alveol/ar   *ar*=pertaining to, relating to; alveoli (singular, alveolus)
10. bronchi/ole   *ole*=small, minute; bronchi

Activity 8–6: Competency Verification

Prefixes and Suffixes

1. phren/o/spasm   *spasm*=involuntary contraction, twitching; diaphragm
2. eu/pnea   *pnea*=breathing; good, normal
3. anthrac/osis   *osis*=abnormal condition, increase (used primarily with blood cells); black, coal
4. tachy/pnea   *pnea*=breathing; rapid
5. an/ox/ia   *ia*=condition; without, not; oxygen (O_2)
6. brady/pnea   *pnea*=breathing; slow
7. hem/o/ptysis   *ptysis*=spitting; blood
8. atel/ectasis   *ectasis*= dilation, expansion; incomplete, imperfect
9. spir/o/metry   *metry*=act of measuring; breathe
10. pneum/o/coni/osis   *osis*=abnormal condition, increase (used primarily with blood cells); lung; dust

Activity 8-7: Clinical Application

Pathological Conditions

1. dyspnea
2. phlegm
3. hypercapnia
4. COPD
5. tachypnea
6. emphysema
7. consolidation
8. bronchiolitis
9. asphyxia
10. atelectasis
11. pulmonary embolus
12. tuberculosis (TB)
13. pleurisy
14. anoxemia
15. acute respiratory distress syndrome (ARD)
16. hydrothorax
17. adventitious
18. cystic fibrosis (CF)
19. anthracosis
20. pneumothorax

Activity 8-8: Clinical Application

Diagnostic Tests, Treatments, and Pharmacology

1. thoracotomy
2. Mantoux test
3. intubation
4. arterial blood gas (ABG)
5. pulmonary angiography
6. auscultation
7. postural drainage
8. expectorants
9. thoracentesis
10. nebulized mist treatment (NMT)

Activity 8-9: Build Medical Words

Diagnostic, Symptomatic, and Operative Terms

1. rhinorrhea
2. rhinitis
3. bronchoalveolar
4. bronchoscopy
5. broncholith
6. tracheostenosis
7. tracheotomy
8. tracheolaryngeal
9. thoracoplasty
10. thoracostomy or thoracotomy
11. pneumonopathy
12. pneumonolysis
13. pneumorrhaphy
14. pneumoconiosis
15. pneumopexy
16. pleuralgia, pleurodynia
17. pleurectomy
18. pleurocele
19. bronchiolitis
20. bronchiolectasis

Critical Thinking: Analysis of Medical Records

> > > MEDICAL RECORD 8-1: SOAP NOTE

1. What symptoms made the patient seek medical care?

Worsening asthma symptoms for 2 weeks, left-sided chest pain, severe dyspnea and some dysuria.

2. What did the doctor find upon examination of the patient?

Poor bilateral air movement with diffuse rhonchi and wheezes.

3. What does it mean that the bronchoscope was inserted transnasally?

It was inserted through the nose.

4. What was seen in the left lower bronchus?

Endobronchial friable mucosal lesion, partially occluding the entire left lower lobe bronchus.

5. What kinds of biopsy specimens were obtained during the procedure?

Transbronchial biopsies of the left lower lung area, transbronchial needle aspiration, bronchial brush biopsies, and bronchial brush washings.

6. Why was the patient admitted to the hospital?

He had severe shortness of breath with a history of chronic obstructive pulmonary disease and oxygen dependency.

7. What caused the creatinine and BUN levels to be elevated?

Acute renal failure and dehydration.

8. What contributed to the patient's episode of tachycardia and sinus arrhythmia, and what transpired to correct the problem?

It was attributed to his medication, theophylline, which was stopped because the level was above a therapeutic dose. The medication was then restarted at a lower dose and the patient's heart rate improved, and his theophylline level came back to normal.

9. Is there any indication that the patient has an excessive amount of potassium in the blood?

Yes. He was transferred to intensive care because of hyperkalemia. This was further substantiated in the initial laboratory evaluation.

10. What did the chest x-ray reveal?

35% to 40% right pneumothorax.

11. What procedure was performed to improve the patient's condition?

Thoracostomy tube placement (chest tube insertion) at the fifth intercostal space, which re-inflated the lung.

12. What complications would have occurred if this patient had not gone to the ER for treatment?

The patient's lung would have collapsed (atelectasis). If left untreated, atelectasis could result in respiratory failure.

Chapter 9 Cardiology

Activity 9–1: Competency Verification
Layers of the Heart Wall

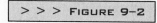

1. endocardium
2. myocardium
3. pericardium
4. epicardium
5. pericardial cavity

Activity 9–2: Competency Verification
Internal Structures of the Heart

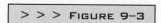

1. right atrium
2. left atrium
3. right ventricle
4. left ventricle
5. interventricular septum
6. superior vena cava
7. inferior vena cava

8. tricuspid valve
9. pulmonary valve
10. right pulmonary artery; left pulmonary artery
11. right pulmonary veins; left pulmonary veins
12. mitral valve
13. aortic valve
14. aorta

Activity 9–3: Competency Verification
Blood Flow Through the Heart

(The missing parts in the boxes of Flowchart 9–1 are given in italics)

superior and inferior *vena cava*

right *atrium*

tricuspid valve

right ventricle

right and left *pulmonary arteries*

four *pulmonary veins*

left atrium

left ventricle

aorta

Activity 9–4: Competency Verification
Coronary Arteries

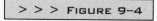

1. left coronary artery
2. right coronary artery
3. left anterior descending artery
4. circumflex artery

Activity 9–5: Competency Verification

Structures of the Blood Vessels

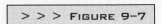

> > > FIGURE 9–6

1. artery
2. arteriole
3. capillary
4. venule
5. vein
6. valve

Activity 9–6: Competency Verification

Cardiac Conduction System

> > > FIGURE 9–7

1. SA node
2. AV node
3. bundle of His
4. right bundle branch
5. left bundle branch
6. Purkinje fibers

Activity 9–7: Competency Verification

Medical Word Components

1. phleb/itis — *itis*=inflammation; vein
2. scler/osis — *osis*=abnormal condition, increase (used primarily with blood cells); hardening, sclera
3. thromb/us — *us*=condition; blood clot
4. aort/o/tomy — *tomy*=incision; aorta
5. sphygm/o/meter — *meter*=instrument for measuring; pulse
6. arteri/o/stenosis — *stenosis*=narrowing, stricture; artery
7. tachy/cardi/ac — *ac*=pertaining to; rapid; heart
8. my/o/cardi/um — *um*=structure, thing; muscle; heart
9. electr/o/cardi/o/gram — *gram*=record, writing; electricity; heart
10. electr/o/cardi/o/graphy — *graphy*=process of recording; electricity; heart

Activity 9–8: Clinical Application

Pathological Conditions

1. hyperlipidemia
2. myocardial infarction (MI)
3. palpitations
4. aneurysm
5. thrombus
6. cardiomyopathy
7. thrombophlebitis
8. arrhythmia
9. atherosclerosis
10. coarctation
11. septal defect
12. hypertension
13. embolus
14. hemostasis
15. varicose vein
16. ischemia
17. angina pectoris
18. mitral valve prolapse
19. fibrillation
20. congestive heart failure

Diagnostic Tests, Treatments, and Pharmacology

1. lipid profile
2. echocardiography
3. cardiac catheterization
4. anticoagulants
5. angioplasty
6. Holter monitor
7. defibrillator
8. diuretics

9. angiography
10. balloon valvuloplasty
11. pacemaker
12. troponin I
13. anastomosis
14. antianginals
15. stent placement

Activity 9–10: Build Medical Words

Diagnostic, Symptomatic, and Operative Terms

1. cardial, cardiac
2. cardiomegaly
3. cardiomyopathy
4. cardialgia, cardiodynia
5. arteriorrhexis
6. arteriospasm
7. arteriosclerosis
8. venous
9. venostenosis
10. venorrhaphy

11. phlebotomy
12. phlebectomy
13. atherectomy
14. atheroma
15. arteriolitis
16. arteriolosclerosis
17. sphygmometer
18. sphygmoid
19. hemangiectasis
20. hemangioma

Critical Thinking: Analysis of Medical Records

> > > MEDICAL RECORD 9–1: EMERGENCY ROOM REPORT

1. Why did the patient call the emergency medical service or ambulance?

He had chest pain that became severe, and a tremendous feeling of weakness with some nausea.

2. What treatment did the EMS technicians administer once they arrived at the patient's home?

Three nitroglycerin and four baby aspirin.

3. What classification of drugs does nitroglycerin belong to? How does nitroglycerin relieve chest pain?

Antianginals. Nitroglycerin relieves chest pain (angina pectoris) by vasodilation of the coronary arteries.

> > > MEDICAL RECORD 9–2: LABORATORY REPORT

4. Which laboratory test results under the lipid profile are abnormal and indicate an increased risk for coronary artery disease?

High cholesterol (210), high triglycerides (301), and low HDL cholesterol (29).

5. What do the cardiac laboratory test results indicate?

Evidence of acute myocardial damage.

6. What are the significant findings of the cardiac catheterization?

Single vessel CAD with mild LV dysfunction; the large bifurcated, intermediate artery was totally occluded just beyond the origin and faintly collateralized. Ejection fraction was 53%.

7. What drugs were prescribed to the patient?

Plavix, aspirin, Lipitor.

8. Does the patient have any limitations on activity levels? If yes, what are they?

Yes; refrain from vigorous athletic activity for 3 to 4 weeks.

9. What lifestyle change is recommended for this patient to reduce his risk of future heart disease? Explain what this means.

Aggressive dietary measures. The patient should be on a strict low fat and low cholesterol diet.

10. What are the discharge diagnoses?

High lateral non-Q wave myocardial infarction with associated angina pectoris, coronary artery disease, and anxiety.

11. Which artery was found to be occluded? What procedure was then performed on it?

The intermediate artery. A stent was placed in this vessel.

Chapter 10 Endocrinology

Activity 10-1: Competency Verification

Endocrine Glands

1. pituitary gland (hypophysis)
2. thyroid gland
3. parathyroid glands
4. adrenal (suprarenal) glands
5. pancreas (islets of Langerhans)
6. ovaries
7. testes
8. pineal gland
9. thymus gland

Activity 10-2: Clinical Application

Endocrine Secretions

1. thyroid gland
2. adrenal cortex
3. parathyroid glands
4. pancreas
5. adenohypophysis
6. ovaries
7. neurohypophysis
8. adrenal medulla
9. pineal gland
10. thymus gland

Medical Word Components

1. pancreat/oma
2. parathyroid/ectomy
3. thyr/o/megaly
4. thyroid/ectomy
5. poly/dipsia
6. adren/o/pathy
7. kal/emia
8. gonad/o/pathy
9. endo/crine
10. hyper/calc/emia

oma=tumor; pancreas
ectomy=excision, removal; parathyroid glands
megaly=enlargement; thyroid gland
ectomy=excision, removal; thyroid gland
dipsia=thirst; many, much
pathy=disease; adrenal glands
emia=blood condition; potassium (an electrolyte)
pathy=disease; gonads, sex glands
crine=secrete; in, within
emia=blood condition, excessive, above normal; calcium

Activity 10–4: Clinical Application
Pathological Conditions

1. hirsutism
2. exophthalmos
3. IDDM
4. hyperkalemia
5. acromegaly
6. thyromegaly
7. polyuria
8. myxedema
9. endogenous
10. polydipsia
11. thyroid storm
12. hyperglycemia
13. hypervolemia
14. hyponatremia
15. hypogonadism

Activity 10–5: Clinical Application
Diagnostic Procedures, Treatments, and Abbreviations

1. electrolytes
2. antidiabetics
3. insulin
4. glucose tolerance test (GTT)
5. fasting blood sugar (FBS)
6. anabolic steroids
7. thyroidectomy
8. postprandial blood sugar (PPBS)
9. hypophysectomy
10. antidiuretic hormone (ADH)
11. radioiodine therapy
12. corticosteroids
13. T_3, T_4
14. hormone replacement therapy
15. thyroid scan

Activity 10–6: Build Medical Words
Diagnostic, Symptomatic, and Surgical Terms

1. adrenomegaly
2. adrenopathy
3. pancreatitis
4. pancreatopathy
5. pancreatoma
6. thyromegaly
7. thyrotomy
8. hyperglycemia
9. hypoglycemia
10. glycogenesis

Critical Thinking: Analysis of Medical Records

> > > MEDICAL RECORD 10-1. HISTORY AND PHYSICAL EXAMINATION

1. What brought Mr Jones into the ER, and what was the history of his present illness?

The patient had an infected foot with a swollen left heel. He has a long-term history of type 1 diabetes mellitus that has never been well controlled.

2. Place "+" in the space provided for positive findings and a "−" for negative findings. A positive finding indicates the patient had a history (Hx) of this condition; a negative finding indicates the patient did not have a history of this condition.

- − thyromegaly   + diabetes
- − organomegaly   + poor circulation
- + ulceration and infection of left heel   + neuropathy

> > > MEDICAL RECORD 10-2: CONSULTATION

3. Explain what "left fifth toe metatarsal head amputation" means.

The left fifth toe metatarsal bone was excised or amputated. More specifically, the proximal end of the left fifth metatarsal bone was amputated.

4. What two surgical procedures are recommended by Dr. Armani?

Either a left below- or left above-the-knee amputation and débridement of the right heel.

5. Why did the surgeon recommend these two procedures?

Because the patient has extensive gangrene, which eventually results in no circulation and complete necrosis. The right heel is infected. Débridement cleans the wound and prevents further infection.

> > > MEDICAL RECORD 10-3: OPERATIVE REPORT

6. What does it mean that the patient has not been ambulatory?

It means that the patient is not able to walk.

7. Why did the surgeon perform an above-the-knee amputation (AKA) rather than a below-the-knee amputation (BKA)?

Because of the patient's nonambulatory state and some degree of flexion contracture at the knee, as well as significant atrophy of the calf muscles, it was decided to perform AKA.

8. Explain what débridement is and whether the surgeon included débridement of the deep tissues.

Débridement is the removal of dirt, foreign objects, damaged tissue, and cellular debris from a wound or burn to prevent infection and to promote healing. The deep tissues were not débrided because the surgeon noted they may still be viable (capable of developing or growing).

9. What are the secondary diagnoses that indicate the patient has (a) an abnormally high concentration of phosphates in the circulating blood; (b) decreased osmolar concentration, especially of the blood or urine?

(a) hyperphosphatemia, (b) hyposmolarity

10. What complications did the patient experience because of his long-term, poorly controlled diabetes?

His associated complications included peripheral vascular disease with neuropathy and peripheral diabetic neuropathy.

Chapter 11 Obstetrics and Gynecology

Activity 11-1: Competency Verification
Female Reproductive System

> > > FIGURE 11-2

1. ovary	10 cervix (cervix uteri)
5. fallopian tube	13. vagina
6. fimbriae	

> > > FIGURE 11-3

1. ovary	8. fundus
2. ovarian ligament	9. body
3. graafian follicle	10. cervix
4. corpus luteum	11. myometrium
5. fallopian tube	12. endometrium
6. fimbriae	13. vagina
7. fertilization of the ovum	

Activity 11-2: Competency Verification
External Genitalia (Vulva)

> > > FIGURE 11-4

1. mons pubis	6. clitoris
2. labia majora	7. Bartholin glands
3. labia minora	8. hymen
4. urethral orifice	9. perineum
5. vaginal orifice	

Activity 11–3: Competency Verification

Mammary Glands

> > > FIGURE 11–5

1. adipose tissue
2. glandular tissue
3. lactiferous duct

4. nipple
5. areola
6. lactiferous sinus

Activity 11–4: Competency Verification

Gynecologic and Obstetrical Terms

1. fertilization
2. parturition
3. gestation
4. lactation
5. menopause

6. stage of expulsion
7. menarche
8. stage of dilation
9. estrogen
10. placental stage

Activity 11-5: Competency Verification

Medical Word Components

1. cervic/itis — *itis*=inflammation; neck, cervix uteri (neck of the uterus)
2. galact/o/rrhea — *rrhea*=discharge, flow; milk
3. amni/o/centesis — *centesis*=surgical puncture; amnion (amniotic sac)
4. mast/o/pexy — *pexy*=suspension, fixation (of an organ); breast
5. leiomy/oma — *oma*=tumor; smooth muscle (visceral)
6. vagin/itis — *itis*=inflammation; vagina
7. vulv/o/pathy — *pathy*=disease; vulva
8. episi/o/tomy — *tomy*=incision; vulva
9. colp/o/scopy — *scopy*=visual examination; vagina
10. oophor/oma — *oma*=tumor; ovary
11. salping/ectomy — *ectomy*=excision, removal; tube (usually fallopian or eustachian [auditory] tubes)
12. gynec/o/logy — *logy*=study of; woman, female
13. hyster/ectomy — *ectomy*=excision, removal; uterus, womb
14. perine/o/rrhaphy — *rrhaphy*=suture; perineum
15. ovari/o/cyesis — *cyesis*=pregnancy; ovary

Activity 11-6: Competency Verification

Prefixes and Suffixes

1. pre/nat/al — *al*=pertaining to, relating to; before, in front of; birth
2. dys/tocia — *tocia*=childbirth, labor; bad, painful difficult
3. oxy/tocia — *tocia*=childbirth, labor; quick, sharp
4. endo/metr/itis — *itis*=inflammation; in, within; uterus, womb
5. intra/uter/ine — *ine*=pertaining to, relating to; in, within; uterus
6. multi/para — *para*=to bear (offspring); many, much
7. primi/para — *para*=to bear (offspring); first
8. nulli/gravida — *gravida*=pregnant woman; none
9. multi/gravida — *gravida*=pregnant woman; many, much
10. ante/version — *version*=turning; before, in front

Activity 11–7: Clinical Application

Pathological Conditions

1. hydramnios
2. pelvic inflammatory disease (PID)
3. hydatidiform mole
4. sexually transmitted diseases (STDs)
5. placenta previa
6. endometrial cancer
7. toxic shock syndrome
8. fibrocystic breast disease
9. eclampsia
10. premenstrual syndrome (PMS)
11. breech presentation
12. endometriosis
13. carcinoma of the breast
14. polymenorrhea
15. hyaline membrane disease

Activity 11–8: Clinical Application

Diagnostic Tests, Treatments, and Abbreviations

1. pregnancy test
2. oral contraceptives
3. hysterosalpinography
4. cerclage
5. Pap smear
6. abortion
7. amniocentesis
8. oxytocins
9. dilation and curettage (D&C)
10. chorionic villus sampling (CVS)

Activity 11–9: Build Medical Words

Diagnostic, Symptomatic, and Surgical Terms

1. hysteropathy
2. hysterosalpingography
3. hysteromyoma
4. uterocervical
5. uterocele
6. uterorectal
7. oophoralgia, oophorodynia
8. oophorosalpingitis
9. oophorectomy
10. salpingitis
11. salpingopexy
12. salpingotomy
13. colposcope
14. colpostenosis
15. vaginitis
16. vaginomycosis
17. vaginolabial
18. gynecology
19. gynecologist
20. gynecopathy

Critical Thinking: Analysis of Medical Records

> > > MEDICAL RECORD 11-1: DELIVERY NOTE

1. What type of delivery did the mother have?

Spontaneous vaginal delivery from vertex occiput anterior.

2. a. What types of tears were repaired?

Periurethral and perineal.

   b. How were they repaired?

The tears were repaired with interrupted sutures of 4–0 Vicryl, one for the periurethral tear and four for the perineal tear.

3. What specific drug was used to induce labor? What classification does this drug belong to?

Pitosin. Oxytocins.

> > > MEDICAL RECORD 11-2: EMERGENCY ROOM REPORT

4. Place a "+" in the space provided for positive findings and a "−" for negative findings. A positive finding indicates the patient had these symptoms; a negative finding indicates the patient did not have the symptoms.

     − hematuria   − skin rash

     + vaginal irritation   + vaginal drainage

     − fever   + foul-smelling drainage

5. What were the diagnoses of this patient?

Probable pelvic inflammatory disease (PID), trichomoniasis, possible gonorrhea exposure.

6. What are the possible complications if the patient does not treat her STDs?

In the female, the prolonged presence or an untreated STD may result in infertility. In addition, the presence of an STD during pregnancy and childbirth could have potential negative affects on the health of the fetus and baby. The patient may also spread the STD to her sexual partner(s).

> > > MEDICAL RECORD 11-3: OPERATIVE REPORT

7. What type of surgery was performed?

Vaginal hysterectomy, bilateral salpingo-oophorectomy.

8. What position was the patient in during the surgery?

Dorsal lithotomy position.

9. How much blood did the patient lose during surgery?

Estimated blood loss was 450 cc.

> > > MEDICAL RECORD 11-4: DISCHARGE SUMMARY.

10. Why was surgery performed on the patient?

She had a pelvic mass with possible ovarian cancer.

11. What did the pathology report confirm?

Mixed epithelial borderline tumor with negative lymph nodes.

12. What were the patient's discharge instructions?

Discharged home on a soft diet, encouraged to take in fluids; discharge medications: Percocet prn, Senokot S once a day, Climara patch to be changed every week, appointment for staple removal later in the week, and she is to call the doctor about any severe abdominal pain, vaginal bleeding, or temperature greater than 100.4°F.

Chapter 12 Orthopedics

Activity 12–1: Competency Verification
Bone Tissue

> > > FIGURE 12-2

1. diaphysis
2. distal epiphysis
3. proximal epiphysis
4. compact bone
5. Haversian system
6. Haversian canal

7. osteocyte
8. medullary cavity
9. yellow bone marrow
10. spongy bone
11. periosteum
12. osteogenic layer

Activity 12–2: Competency Verification
Bones of the Skeleton

> > > FIGURE 12-3

1. crani/o
2. stern/o
3. cost/o
4. vertebr/o
5. humer/o
6. carp/o
7. metacarp/o

8. phalang/o
9. pelv/i and pelv/o
10. femor/o
11. patell/o
12. tibi/o
13. fibul/o
14. calcane/o

Activity 12–3: Competency Verification
Cranial and Facial Bones

> > > FIGURE 12-4

1. frontal bone
2. parietal bone
3. coronal suture
4. lambdoidal suture
5. occipital bone
6. temporal bone
7. mastoid process
8. external auditory meatus
9. sphenoid bone

10. ethmoid bone
11. maxilla
12. nasal bone
13. lacrimal bone
14. zygomatic bone
15. mandible
16. mandibular condyle
17. mandibular fossa of the temporal bone
18. vomer

Note: **Each leader line points to one structure.**

Activity 12–4: Competency Verification
Thorax

> > > FIGURE 1 2–5

1. sternum
2. true ribs
3. manubrium

4. costal cartilage
5. false ribs
6. floating ribs

Activity 12–5: Competency Verification
Vertebral Column

> > > FIGURE 1 2–6

1. cervical vertebrae
2. atlas
3. axis
4. thoracic vertebrae

5. lumbar vertebrae
6. sacrum
7. coccyx
8. intervertebral disks

Activity 12–6: Competency Verification
Pelvic Girdle

> > > FIGURE 1 2–7

1. ilium
2. ischium
3. pubis

4. symphysis pubis
5. sacrum
6. coccyx

Activity 12–7: Competency Verification
Actions of Muscles

> > > FIGURE 1 2–8 AND TABLE 1 2–2

1. adduction
2. supination
3. extension
4. flexion
5. dorsiflexion

6. abduction
7. plantar flexion
8. pronation
9. rotation
10. flexion

Activity 12–8: Competency Verification
Medical Word Components: Axial and Appendicular Skeleton

1. cervic/al   *al*=pertaining to, relating to; neck
2. myel/o/pathy   *pathy*=disease; bone marrow, spinal cord
3. thorac/ic   *ic*=pertaining to, relating to; chest
4. lamin/ectomy   *ectomy*=excision, removal; lamina (part of the vertebral arch)
5. spondyl/o/ptosis   *ptosis*=prolapse, downward displacement; vertebrae
6. sub/cost/al   *al*=pertaining to, relating to; under, below; ribs
7. phalang/ectomy   *ectomy*=excision, removal; phalanges (finger and toe bones)

8. pedi/algia   *algia*=pain; foot, child
9. pelv/ic   *ic*=pertaining to, relating to; pelvis
10. acromi/o/clavicul/ar   *ar*=pertaining to, relating to; acromion (projection of the scapula); clavicle (collar bone)

Activity 12–9: Competency Verification

Medical Word Components: Joints, Muscles, and Related Structures

1. tendin/itis   *itis*=inflammation; tendon
2. endo/lumb/ar   *ar*=pertaining to, relating to; in, within; loins (lower back)
3. arthr/o/desis   *desis*=binding, fixation; joint
4. rhabd/o/my/oma   *oma*=tumor; rod-shaped, (striated); muscle
5. chondr/o/malacia *malacia*=softening; cartilage
6. peri/oste/al   *al*=pertaining to, relating to; around; bone
7. synov/itis   *itis*=inflammation; synovial membrane, synovial fluid
8. ankyl/osis   *osis*=abnormal condition, increase (used primarily with blood cells); stiffness, bent, crooked
9. fasci/ectomy   *ectomy*=excision, removal; band, fascia (fibrous membrane supporting and separating muscles)
10. fibr/o/my/algia   *algia* =pain; fiber, fibrous tissue; muscle

Activity 12–10: Clinical Application

Pathological Conditions

1. gouty
2. scoliosis
3. talipes
4. lordosis
5. bunion
6. subluxation
7. strain
8. osteoporosis
9. osteoarthritis
10. sprain

11. Paget disease
12. polymyositis
13. Lyme disease
14. muscular dystrophy
15. ganglion
16. kyphosis
17. rhabdomyosarcoma
18. greenstick
19. compound
20. comminuted

Activity 12–11: Clinical Application

Diagnostic Tests, Treatments, and Abbreviations

1. EMG
2. DEXA
3. uric acid test
4. sequestrectomy
5. laminectomy

6. internal fixation devices
7. traction
8. casting
9. corticosteroids
10. calcium

Diagnostic, Symptomatic, and Surgical Terms

1. osteogenesis, osteogen
2. osteocytes
3. ostealgia, osteodynia
4. osteoarthropathy
5. osteochondroma
6. cervicobrachial
7. cervicofacial
8. sternoid
9. sternocostal
10. myelocele

11. myelomalacia
12. arthritis
13. arthroscopy
14. arthrocentesis
15. pelvimeter
16. pelvimetry
17. myopathy
18. myorrhaphy
19. myalgia, myodynia
20. myotome

Critical Thinking: Analysis of Medical Records

> > > MEDICAL RECORD 12–1: OPERATIVE REPORT

1. What type of diagnostic test verified the presence of a right rotator cuff tear?

An arthrogram.

2. What type of surgical procedure was performed to correct the rotator cuff tear?

Right shoulder open partial acromionectomy.

3. Why wasn't the rotator tear repaired?

The rotator cuff tear was too massive and was determined not to be reparable. A partial repair would have left the patient with fairly significant limitations in external motion.

4. What was done to improve the range of motion of the rotator cuff?

The joint was débrided; the spurs of the anterior surface of the acromion and over the humeral head were also débrided.

> > > MEDICAL RECORD 12–2: CONSULTATION

5. What type of previous medical treatment did the patient receive for back pain?

Laminectomy and a previous block.

6. What medication is the patient taking for his back pain?

Darvocet.

> > > MEDICAL RECORD 12–3: OPERATIVE REPORT

7. Why was a total hip arthroplasty performed?

The patient had osteoarthritis in the left hip.

8. What position was the patient in during the surgical procedure?

Right lateral decubitus.

9. What prostheses were inserted to replace the left hip?

A metal cup, two screws, and a Press-Fit 10 prosthesis.

> > > MEDICAL RECORD 12–4: EMERGENCY ROOM REPORT

10. What brought the patient into the emergency room?

She fell off a ladder onto her left hand.

11. What type of fracture does the patient have?

Comminuted, intra-articular Colles fracture of the left wrist.

12. What treatment did she receive for her injury?

Fracture reduction, a splint, and fentanyl for pain.

Chapter 13 Immunology

Activity 13–1: Competency Verification

Major Groups of Lymph Vessels and Lymph Nodes

> > > FIGURE 13–3

1. lymphatic trunks
2. right lymphatic duct
3. thoracic duct
4. left subclavian vein
5. popliteal nodes
6. inguinal nodes
7. iliac nodes
8. lumbar nodes
9. cubital nodes
10. axillary nodes
11. thoracic nodes
12. cervical nodes
13. submaxillary nodes

Activity 13–2: Clinical Application

Immune System

1. killer T cells
2. phagocytosis
3. antibodies
4. T cells
5. gamma globulins
6. macrophages
7. helper T cells
8. active humoral immunity
9. passive humoral immunity
10. autoimmune disease

Activity 13–3: Competency Verification

Medical Word Components

1. splen/o/megaly   *megaly*=enlargement; spleen
2. aden/o/pathy   *pathy*=disease; gland
3. macro/cyte   *cyte*=cell; large
4. ana/phylaxis   *phylaxis*=protection; against
5. immun/o/gen   *gen*=forming, producing, origin; immune, immunity
6. my/asthenia   *asthenia*=weakness, debility; muscle
7. lymph/aden/o/pathy   *pathy*=disease; lymph; gland

8. phag/o/cyte   *cyte*=cell; swallowing, eating
9. agglutin/ation   *ation*=process (of); clumping, gluing (together)
10. thym/oma   *oma*=tumor; thymus gland

Activity 13–4: Clinical Application

Pathological Conditions

1. lymphedema
2. cytomegalovirus (CMV)
3. elephantiasis
4. hypersensitivity
5. Kaposi sarcoma
6. lymphangioma
7. systemic lupus erythematosus (SLE)
8. acquired immunodeficiency syndrome (AIDS)
9. *Pneumocystis carinii* pneumonia (PCP)
10. AIDS-dementia complex

Activity 13–5: Clinical Application

Diagnostic Procedures and Treatments and Pharmacology

1. Western blot
2. vaccination
3. antiglobulin test
4. immunosuppressants
5. AIDS cocktail
6. bone marrow aspiration biopsy
7. tissue typing
8. immunotherapy
9. chemotherapy
10. antivirals

Activity 13–6: Build Medical Words

Diagnostic, Symptomatic, and Surgical Terms

1. adenitis
2. adenopathy
3. adenectomy
4. angiopathy
5. angiogenesis
6. angiorrhaphy
7. agglutination
8. agglutinogen
9. immunology
10. immunologist
11. immunogen
12. phagocyte
13. phagocytic
14. splenomegaly
15. splenohepatomegaly
16. thymoma
17. myasthenia
18. lymphoma
19. lymphadenopathy
20. anaphylaxis

Critical Thinking: Analysis of Medical Records

> > > MEDICAL RECORD 13–1: DISCHARGE SUMMARY

1. What type of infection does this patient have? What was the most likely mode of transmission?
She was diagnosed with human immunodeficiency virus (HIV); the most likely mode of transmission was from her husband who died from AIDS 1 year ago.

2. Place a "+" in the space provided for positive findings and a "−" for negative findings. A positive finding indicates the patient had a history (Hx) of this condition: a negative finding indicates the patient did not have a history of this condition.

+ vaginal candiasis   + Kaposi sarcoma

+ tachypnea and tachycardia   + AIDS-wasting syndrome

+ *Pneumocystis carinii* pneumonia   − bronchitis

3. How was her child affected by her disease? Is the child being monitored by a physician?

Currently the child is asymptomatic for HIV, but has failed to develop normally and is managed by a pediatric infectious disease specialist.

> > > MEDICAL RECORD 13-2: CHART NOTES

4. What are the results of her CBC? What do the results mean?

Her CBC with differential indicates profound neutropenia. Neutropenia indicates the presence of abnormally small numbers of neutrophils (responsible for much of the body's protection against infection) in the circulating blood and is the most common immune system deficiency.

5. Explain what it means when the patient complains of "floaters" in her visual field.

She has one or more spots that appear to drift in front of the eye, caused by a shadow cast on the retina by vitreous debris. Most people have these benign materials in their eyes, but the sudden onset of several floaters may indicate serious disease.

6. What was the "Plan of Care" for pneumococcal vaccination, PICC line, and Pap?

Pneumoccoccal vacination: Follow up pneumococcal immunoglobulin testing in 6 weeks to measure for adequate antibody production; PICC line: to be placed for ganciclovir therapy and ongoing monitoring of neutropenia; Pap: on the next clinic visit; not done today due to stage of menstrual cycle.

> > > MEDICAL RECORD 13-3: CLINICAL TEAM NOTE

7. What is CML? What segment of the population is most at risk for contracting this disease?

Chronic myelocytic leukemia, a proliferation of granular leukocytes, and often of megakaryocytes, in the bone marrow and bloodstream. The disease occurs most frequently in mature adults.

8. What subjective symptoms is the patient experiencing?

He has a coating on his tongue and the inside of his mouth feels rough. Otherwise, he denies pain, nausea, vomiting, fever, sweats, chills, cough, sore throat, bleeding, urinary symptoms, headaches, visual changes, and shortness of breath.

9. What abnormalities were found during the physical examination with the integumentary system?

Maculopapular erythematous rash on the entire back, upper chest, upper arms with an erythematous flush to the face. The rash involves approximately 20 to 25 percent of the body surface area.

10. What is the probable cause of the patient's integumentary problem?

Graft versus host disease, resulting from the peripheral blood stem cell transplant he received from his brother.

11. What treatment is prescribed to reduce the chances of infection while the patient is taking immunosuppressants?

The antibiotic Septra.

12. Why is the doctor performing a biopsy on Mr. Salem?

He has possible chronic graft versus host disease with involvement of the liver, mouth, and skin.

Chapter 14 Neurology

Activity 14–1: Competency Verification
Structures of the Neuron

>>> FIGURE 14–2

1. cell body
2. dendrites and dendrite
3. axon
4. axon terminals

5. synaptic end bulbs
6. myelin sheath
7. neurolemma
8. Schwann cell

Activity 14–2: Competency Verification
Pathway of the Electrochemical Impulse of the Neuron and Classification of Neurons

Pathway and Structures of Electrochemical Impulse

1. neurons, neuroglia
2. neurons
3. neuroglia
4. axon, cell body, dendrite
5. cell body
6. dendrite(s)
7. axon
8. synaptic end bulb

9. synapse
10. neurotransmitters
11. axon terminals
12. neuron
13. myelin sheath
14. gray matter
15. neurolemma or neurolemmal sheath

Classification of Neurons

16. sensory neurons, motor neurons, mixed neurons
17. afferent nerves or sensory neurons
18. efferent nerves or motor neurons

19. mixed nerves or interneurons
20. ependymal cells or ependymocytes, astrocytes, oligodendrocytes, microglia

Activity 14–3: Competency Verification
Location of the Spinal Nerves

>>> FIGURE 14-4

1. C1–C8
2. T1–T12
3. L1–L5
4. S1–S5
5. CO1

Activity 14–4: Competency Verification
Structures of the Brain

>>> FIGURE 14-5

1. brain stem
2. medulla oblongata
3. pons
4. midbrain
5. cerebellum
6. diencephalon
7. thalamus
8. hypothalamus
9. cerebrum
10. corpus callosum
11. gyri
12. sulci

Activity 14–5: Competency Verification
Lobes of the Brain

>>> FIGURE 14-6

1. frontal lobe
2. parietal lobe
3. temporal lobe
4. occipital lobe

Activity 14–6: Competency Verification
Medical Word Components

1. myel/algia   *algia*=pain; spinal cord, bone marrow
2. cortic/al   *al*=pertaining to; cortex
3. mening/itis   *itis*=inflammation; meninges
4. encephal/oma   *oma*=tumor; brain
5. medull/ary   *ary*=pertaining to; medulla
6. spin/al   *al*=pertaining to; spine
7. crani/o/faci/al   *al*=pertaining to; cranium, skull; face
8. gangl/itis   *itis*=inflammation; ganglion
9. neur/algia   *algia*=pain; nerve
10. intra/thec/al   *al*=pertaining to; in, within; sheath (usually refers to the meninges)

Prefixes and Suffixes

1. contra/later/al
2. quadri/plegia
3. an/esthesia
4. echo/lalia
5. hyper/kinesia
6. a/phasia
7. hemi/paresis
8. my/asthenia
9. dys/trophy
10. epi/lepsy

al=pertaining to; against; side, to one side
plegia=paralysis; four
esthesia=feeling; without, not
lalia=speech, babble; a repeated sound
kinesia=movement; excesssive, above normal
phasia=speech; without, not
paresis=partial paralysis; one-half
asthenia= weakness, debility ; muscle
trophy=development, nourishment; bad, painful, difficult
lepsy=seizure; above, upon

Activity 14–8: Clinical Application

Pathological Conditions

1. epidural
2. Parkinson disease
3. Huntington disease
4. shingles
5. subdural
6. Bell palsy
7. migraine
8. aura
9. TIA
10. hydrocephalus
11. meningitis
12. spina bifida
13. cerebral contusion
14. meningioma
15. aneurysm
16. multiple sclerosis (MS)
17. glioma
18. Tay-Sachs disease
19. CVA
20. myasthenia gravis
21. tremor
22. coma
23. Alzheimer disease
24. syncope
25. seizure

Activity 14–9: Clinical Application

Diagnostic Tests, Treatments, and Abbreviations

1. trephination
2. levodopa
3. EEG
4. PET
5. tractotomy
6. shunt placement
7. LP
8. folic acid
9. nerve block
10. thalamotomy

Diagnostic, Symptomatic, and Surgical Terms

1. neurologist
2. neuralgia, neurodynia
3. neuroblast
4. cerebropathy
5. cerebrospinal
6. encephalitis
7. encephalocele
8. encephaloma
9. myelorrhaphy
10. myelomalacia
11. myelosclerosis
12. meningocele
13. meningopathy
14. meningitis
15. hemiplegia, paraplegia, diplegia
16. quadriplegia
17. atrophy
18. hypertrophy
19. dysphasia
20. aphasia

Critical Thinking: Analysis of Medical Records

> >> MEDICAL RECORD 14–1: NEUROLOGY CONSULTATION

1. What was Mr. Belcourt referred for? Had he experienced these symptoms previously?

Aphasia; yes, he had previous episodes of difficulty expressing himself during the last 2 months.

2. Place a "+" in the space for positive findings and "−" for negative findings in the review of systems. A positive finding indicates the patient had a history (Hx) of this condition; a negative finding indicated the patient did not have a history of this condition.

+ aphasia   − high cholesterol

− hypertension   + cholecystitis

− cerebrovascular accident

3. How did the patient initially perform on the neurologic examination?

Initially, he did poorly on the neurological exam. He could not understand one-step (simple commands) or answer questions

4. Did his ability to complete the neurologic examination change over time?

Yes, his ability to complete the neurologic examination showed marked improvement. He was able to to do a three-step command with some difficulty (closed his eyes, squeezed doctor's hand), name objects, and was oriented to place and time. However, he still showed some impairments.

5. What was the medical plan?

Echocardiogram, carotid duplex, CT, MRI with MR angiography, increase aspirin to 650 mg twice daily, observation, and IV fluids.

6. Why did the doctor increase the daily aspirin dosage?

The doctor suspected that the patient suffered from a CVA (stroke), and aspirin aids in the prevention of CVA by inhibiting platelet aggregation.

7. What type of imaging procedure was performed?

MRI scan of the brain with gadolinium with magnetic resonance angiogram (MRA) of the vessels of the circle of Willis.

8. What was the final conclusion of the locations of the brain masses? Where in the brain were masses found?

The left parietal and temporal lobes, and right parietal lobe, with the largest in the left parietal region.

9. What procedure was recommended to confirm the diagnosis?

A brain biopsy.

>>> MEDICAL RECORD 14-3: OPERATIVE REPORT

10. What kind of brain biopsy was performed?

Stereotactic brain biopsy

>>> MEDICAL RECORD 14-4: SURGICAL PATHOLOGY REPORT

11. What was the postoperative diagnosis confirmed by microscopic evaluation?

High grade glioma, likely glioblastoma multiforme

12. Is the tumor malignant? What type of cells make up the tumor?

Yes, the tumor is the most malignant form of astrocytoma, which is composed of astrocytes.

Chapter 15 Hematology

Activity 15-1: Competency Verification

Hematologic Components and Functions

1. True
2. True
3. False. Platelets and plasma proteins initiate clot formation.
4. False. Antibodies, white blood cells, and complement proteins are contained in the blood—all of which help defend the body against foreign intruders such as bacteria and viruses.
5. true
6. globulins
7. platelets
8. erythrocyte
9. Ig
10. plasma
11. leukocytes
12. agranulocytes
13. neutrophils
14. hemoglobin

15. T cells and B cells
16. megakaryocytes
17. blood clotting
18. fibrin strands
19. embolus
20. universal recipient

Activity 15–2: Competency Verification

Medical Word Components

1. kary/o/cyte   *cyte*=cell; nucleus
2. poikil/o/cyte   *cyte*=cell; varied, irregular
3. reticul/o/cyte   *cyte*=cell; net, mesh
4. sider/o/penia   *penia*=decrease, deficiency; iron
5. thromb/o/lysis   *lysis*=separation, destruction, loosening; blood clot
6. phag/o/cyte   *cyte*=cell; swallowing, eating
7. agglutin/ation   *ation*=process (of); clumping, gluing
8. chrom/ic   *ic*=pertaining to, relating to; color
9. an/emia   *emia*=blood condition; without, not
10. erythr/o/poiesis   *poiesis*=formation, production; red (blood cells)

Activity 15–3: Competency Verification

Pathological Conditions

1. thalassemia   6. thrombocytopenia
2. purpura   7. hemolytic anemia
3. pernicious anemia   8. leukemia
4. sickle cell anemia   9. polycythemia
5. hemophilia   10. neutrophilia

Activity 15–4: Competency Verification

Diagnostic Procedures, Treatments, Pharmacology, and Abbreviations

1. blood transfusion   6. prothrombin time (PT)
2. bleeding time   7. thrombolytic enzymes
3. CBC   8. WBC differential
4. antiglobulin test   9. Hct
5. ESR   10. WBC count

Activity 15–5: Build Medical Words

Diagnostic, Symptomatic, and Surgical Terms

1. hematoma   6. thrombolysis
2. hematopoiesis   7. erythrocytes
3. hematologist   8. leukocytes, leucocytes
4. thrombectomy   9. granulocytes
5. thromboid   10. phagocytes

Critical Thinking: Analysis of Medical Records

>>> MEDICAL RECORD 15-1: OPERATIVE REPORT

1. What was the preoperative diagnosis?

Bilateral deep vein thrombosis; hypercoagulable state; status: postpulmonary embolus with contraindication to Coumadin anticoagulation.

2. What type of surgery was performed?

Insertion of inferior vena cava, infrarenal, and suprarenal Greenfield filters, inferior venacavogram.

3. What type of radiograph was performed with nonionic contrast material that showed the renal veins to be without defects?

A venacavography—a radiograph of the vena cava during the injection of a contrast medium.

4. How was the defect in the internal jugular vein controlled during surgery?

The defect in the internal jugular vein was controlled with a running suture of 5-0 cardiovascular Prolene.

>>> MEDICAL RECORD 15-2: HISTORY AND PHYSICAL EXAMINATION

5. How does a person acquire sickle cell anemia?

It is a hereditary condition and is therefore acquired from the parents.

6. What causes the severe pain in a sickle cell crisis?

The sickle-shaped erythrocytes are poorly oxygenated and clump together forming thromboses, which block small blood vessels, causing a lack of oxygen distribution.

7. What is the stated diagnosis?

1. Sickle cell crisis. 2. Rule out right lower extremity deep venous thrombosis.

8. What diagnostic test is being performed to rule out deep vein thrombosis?

Doppler studies.

>>> MEDICAL RECORD 15-3: CONSULTATION

9. What stage tumor did the patient have approximately 6 years ago?

The patient had a stage II tumor (lymph node–positive) receptor-positive breast carcinoma.

10. What type of treatment did she receive at that time?

After having a lumpectomy, she had radiation therapy to the left breast. She was also taking the chemotherapeutic drug tamoxifen.

11. Upon physical examination, was the physician able to palpate any masses?

There was no palpable lymphadenopathy or hepatosplenomegaly; no palpable breast masses.

12. What cause does the doctor attribute to the present clot formation?

He attributes her present clot to tamoxifen, which can be thrombogenic. He believed she was under-coagulated at the time of admission.

Chapter 16 Ophthalmology

Activity 16–1: Competency Verification

Accessory Structures of the Eye

>>> FIGURE 16-1

1. eyeball
2. eyelid
3. levator palpebrae superioris muscle
4. eyelashes
5. superior rectus muscle
6. inferior rectus muscle
7. lateral rectus muscle
8. inferior oblique muscle

>>> FIGURE 16-2

1. conjunctiva
2. lacrimal gland
3. lacrimal canals
4. lacrimal sac
5. nasolacrimal duct
6. nasal cavity

Activity 16–2: Competency Verification

Internal Structures of the Eyeball

>>> FIGURE 16-3

1. sclera
2. cornea
3. choroid
4. ciliary body
5. iris
6. lens
7. suspensory ligament
8. pupil
9. retina
10. fovea in macula lutea
11. optic disc
12. optic nerve
13. anterior cavity
14. canal of Schlemm
15. vitreous chamber

Activity 16–3: Competency Verification

Structures of the Eye

1. conjunctiva
2. lacrimal gland
3. choroid
4. pupil
5. retina
6. cones
7. iris
8. sclera
9. optic disc
10. aqueous humor

Activity 16–4: Competency Verification
Medical Word Components

1. core/o/plasty   *plasty*=surgical repair; pupil
2. dipl/opia   *opia*=vision; double
3. blephar/o/spasm   *spasm*=involuntary contraction, twitching; eyelid
4. ambly/opia   *opia*=vision; dull, dim
5. lacrim/al   *al*=pertaining to, relating to; tear, lacrimal gland
6. corne/itis   *itis*=inflammation; cornea
7. ophthalm/o/logist   *logist*=specialist in the study of; eye
8. choroid/o/pathy   *pathy*=disease; choroid
9. cycl/o/plegia   *plegia*=paralysis; ciliary body
10. conjunctiv/itis   *itis*=inflammation; conjunctiva

Activity 16–5: Clinical Application
Pathological Conditions

1. cataract
2. glaucoma
3. astigmatism
4. nystagmus
5. esotropia
6. monochromatism
7. hyperopia
8. hordeolum
9. exotropia
10. myopia

Activity 16–6: Clinical Application
Diagnostic Tests, Treatments, and Pharmacology

1. visual field examination
2. ophthalmoscopy
3. tonometry
4. visual acuity test
5. trabeculoplasty
6. phacoemulsification
7. radial keratotomy (RK)
8. scleral buckling
9. cycloplegics
10. beta-adrenergics

Activity 16–7: Build Medical Words
Diagnostic, Symptomatic, and Surgical Terms

1. ophthalmoscope
2. ophthalmology
3. blepharoplegia
4. blepharospasm
5. keratopathy
6. keratoplasty
7. keratome, keratotome
8. pupillometry
9. pupilloscopy
10. scleromalacia
11. sclerochoroiditis
12. amblyopia
13. diplopia
14. esotropia
15. exotropia

Critical Thinking: Analysis of Medical Records

>>> MEDICAL RECORD 16-1: OPERATIVE REPORT

1. What problems was the patient having that indicated a need for cataract surgery?

She had a progressive decrease in visual acuity due to a nuclear sclerotic cataract, and difficulty with distant vision and reading in the left eye.

2. What was the patient's vision in the left eye prior to surgery?

Her best corrected vision is 20/60.

3. What type of anesthesia was used during the surgery?

Topical with intravenous sedation.

>>> MEDICAL RECORD 16-2: OPERATIVE REPORT

4. Why does the physician use the expressions "12 o'clock position" and "1 o'clock position"?

The clock positions are used as a point of reference of where a procedure is performed in relation to the hands of a clock. In this case, the incision was made in the center and superior position of the cornea; the paracentesis track was slightly to the right of the center.

5. What is the patient's diagnosis?

Uncontrolled glaucoma.

6. What are the possible complications of uncontrolled glaucoma?

An increase in intraocular pressure leads to an inhibited blood supply to the optic neurons, which causes atrophy of the optic nerve and eventually total loss of vision.

7. How was bleeding controlled during the surgery?

The bleeding was controlled with microcautery.

8. What medications were given at the end of the surgery just before moving the patient to the recovery room?

Solu-Medrol (40 mg) and Ancef (100 mg).

>>> MEDICAL RECORD 16-3: CONSULTATION LETTER

9. What is significant in the patient's past medical history?

Amblyopia in the left eye since early childhood.

10. What type of examination was done to view the conjunctiva and cornea?

Slit lamp examination.

11. Did the fundoscopic examination reveal any abnormalities in the right eye?

Yes, dot-and-blot hemorrhage of the optic nerve.

12. What did the intravenous fluorescein angiogram reveal?

Disc edema and some ischemia of the left eye.

Chapter 17 Otolaryngology

Activity 17-1: Competency Verification
Structures of the Ear

>>> FIGURE 17-1

1. auricle
2. external auditory canal
3. tympanic membrane
4. malleus
5. incus

6. stapes
7. eustachian tube
8. vestibule
9. cochlea
10. semicircular canals

Activity 17-2: Competency Verification
Structures of the Inner Ear

>>> FIGURE 17-2

1. utricle
2. saccule
3. cochlear duct

4. semicircular canals
5. oval window
6. cochlea

>>> FIGURE 17-3

1. hair cells
2. auditory fibers of the cranial nerve VIII

Activity 17-3: Competency Verification
Tracing the Sequence of Hearing

1. auricle
2. cerumen
3. tympanic membrane
4. malleus
5. incus

6. stapes
7. oval window
8. cochlea
9. organ of Corti
10. vestibulocochlear nerve

Activity 17–4: Competency Verification

Structures of the Nose, Pharynx, and Larynx

>>> FIGURE 17-4

1. nose
2. nostril
3. conchae
4. olfactory receptors
5. ethmoid bone
6. frontal sinus
7. ethmoid sinus
8. sphenoid sinus
9. nasopharynx
10. soft palate
11. uvula
12. adenoid
13. eustachian tube
14. oropharynx
15. palatine tonsil
16. lingual tonsil
17. laryngopharynx
18. larynx
19. trachea
20. thyroid cartilage
21. epiglottis

Activity 17–5: Competency Verification

Structures of the Larynx

>>> FIGURE 17-6

1. thyroid cartilage
2. epiglottis
3. vocal cords

Activity 17–6: Competency Verification

Medical Word Components

1. pharyng/o/scopy   *scopy*=visual examination; pharynx (throat)
2. epiglott/itis   *itis*=inflammation; epiglottis
3. trache/o/stomy   *stomy*=forming an opening (mouth); trachea
4. sinus/itis   *itis*=inflammation; sinus cavity
5. tonsill/o/tome   *tome*=instrument to cut; tonsils
6. rhin/o/plasty   *plasty*=surgical repair; nose
7. staped/ectomy   *ectomy*=excision, removal; stapes
8. acous/tic   *tic*=pertaining to, relating to; hearing
9. mastoid/ectomy   *ectomy*=excision, removal; mastoid process
10. tympan/o/centesis   *centesis*=surgical puncture; tympanic membrane, eardrum

Pathological Conditions

1. labyrinthitis
2. presbycusis
3. conductive
4. serous
5. epistaxis
6. tonsillitis
7. anosmia
8. Ménière disease
9. sinusitis
10. sensorineural
11. influenza
12. thrush
13. deviated septum
14. suppurative
15. pertussis
16. nasal polyposis
17. croup
18. otitis externa
19. tinnitus
20. vertigo

Activity 17–8: Clinical Application
Diagnostic Tests and Treatments

1. antiemetic
2. Weber test
3. hearing aid
4. Rinne test
5. decongestant
6. ear lavage
7. stapedectomy
8. uvulopalatopharyngoplasty (UPPP)
9. rhinoplasty
10. tonsillectomy and adenoidectomy (T&A)

Activity 17–9: Build Medical Words
Diagnostic, Symptomatic, and Surgical Terms

1. tympanoplasty
2. tympanosclerosis
3. otalgia, otodynia
4. otoplasty
5. audiometer
6. audiogram
7. laryngostenosis
8. laryngotracheitis
9. sinusitis
10. sinusoid
11. labyrinthitis
12. labyrinthotomy
13. rhinorrhea
14. rhinopathy
15. otoscopy

Critical Thinking: Analysis of Medical Records

>>> **MEDICAL RECORD 17–1: SOAP NOTE**

1. What objective findings led to the diagnosis of sinusitis?

Moderate maxillary sinus tenderness with erythematous nasal mucosa.

2. What are the possible causes of this patient's sinusitis?

Because she does not have allergies, it could be due to bacterial or viral infection.

>>> **MEDICAL RECORD 17–2: OPERATIVE REPORT**

3. Why was the surgery performed?

The patient had recurrent ear infections with persistent fluid despite prolonged appropriate medical management.

4. What surgical procedure was performed on the patient?

Bilateral myringotomy and placement of fluoroplastic bobbin tubes.

5. What type of residue was cleaned from the left ear?

Dry wax and crust.

6. What tests were done on the mucus cultures?

Testing for aerobes and anaerobes.

7. State and describe the changes seen in the middle ear spaces.

Some polypoid changes, which indicate the presence of growths that resemble a polyp (tumor on stalk).

>>> MEDICAL RECORD 17–3: OPERATIVE REPORT

8. What instrument was used to keep the oral cavity open and the tongue retracted during surgery?

Hemi-Crowe-Davis mouth gag.

9. How was the bleeding controlled during surgery?

Prominent bleeding sites were cauterized for hemostasis and tonsil sponges were used to absorb blood.

10. Did the patient lose any blood during the surgery? If so, what was the estimated blood loss?

Yes, estimated blood loss was 40 to 50 cm³.

Chapter 18 Radiology and Nuclear Medicine

Activity 18–1: Competency Verification
Medical Word Components

1. son/o/gram	*gram*= record, writing; sound
2. ventr/al	*al*=pertaining to; belly, belly side
3. arteri/o/gram	*gram*= record, writing; artery
4. sub/stern/al	*al*=pertaining to, relating to; under, below; sternum (breastbone)
5. proxim/al	*al*=pertaining to, relating to; near, nearest
6. radi/o/graphy	*graphy*=process of recording; radiation, x-ray, radius (lower arm bone on thumb side)
7. later/al	*al*=pertaining to, relating to; side, to one side
8. fluor/o/scopy	*scopy*=visual examination; luminous, fluorescence
9. epi/gastr/ic	*ic*=pertaining to, relating to; above, upon; stomach
10. intra/ven/ous	*ous*=pertaining to, relating to; in, within; vein
11. iso/therm/al	*al*=pertaining to, relating to; same, equal; heat
12. peri/metry	*metry*=act of measuring; around
13. therapeut/ic	*ic*=pertaining to, relating to; treatment
14. medi/al	*al*=pertaining to, relating to; middle
15. echo/gram	*gram*= record, writing; a repeated sound

Activity 18–2: Competency Verification

Build Medical Words

1. inter/cost/al
2. son/o/gram
3. radi/o/log/ist
4. fluor/o/scope
5. trans/abdomin/al

6. therapeut/ic
7. ad/duction
8. medi/o/later/al or mediolateral
9. intra/ven/ous or intravenous
10. arteri/al or arterial

Activity 18–3: Clinical Application

Diagnostic Imaging Procedures

1. positron emission tomography (PET)
2. radioimmunoassay (RIA)
3. magnetic resonance imaging (MRI)
4. ultrasonography
5. cineradiography
6. Doppler

7. mammogram
8. interventional radiology
9. single photon emission computed tomography (SPECT)
10. angiography

Activity 18–4: Clinical Application

Radiologic Terminology

1. in vitro
2. head and intracranial
3. coldspot
4. oscilloscope
5. uptake
6. half-life
7. radiopharmaceutical
8. hotspot

9. scan
10. rad
11. radiopaque
12. intravenous pyelogram
13. myelogram
14. iodine
15. nonvascular interventional procedure

Critical Thinking: Analysis of Medical Records

>>> MEDICAL RECORD 18–1: RADIOLOGY REPORT: BRAIN CT WITHOUT CONTRAST

1. Why was a CT scan ordered on this patient's brain instead of a normal x-ray?

CT scans are highly sensitive in detecting abnormalities in bony structures and can provide images of internal organs that cannot be visualized with standard radiographic procedures.

2. What view was taken using the CT?

An axial view was taken, from the skull base to the vertex; displayed in brain and bone windows.

3. What abnormal findings were reported?

Several bilateral punctate areas of increased attenuation suggesting small bleed from shearing injury.

>>> MEDICAL RECORD 18–2: RADIOLOGY REPORT: RULE OUT FRACTURE, KNEES AND LEGS

4. What abnormalities are cited in this report?

There are no abnormal findings.

5. What is the recommended follow-up treatment if the patient is experiencing jaw pain? What might this indicate?

A workup with dental films or CT is recommended if there is pain in the area upon physical examination. This may indicate a possible fracture.

>>> MEDICAL RECORD 18-4: RADIOLOGY REPORT: CHEST X-RAY

6. Why was a chest x-ray performed on this patient?

To rule out injury to the chest and lungs.

>>> MEDICAL RECORD 18-5: DISCHARGE SUMMARY

7. Why was this patient seen in the ER?

He was in a motor vehicle accident.

8. What treatment was given to repair the mandibular fracture?

A dental alveolar splint was applied to the mandible and teeth.

9. Why was outpatient evaluation of cognitive language by a speech therapist suggested?

The patient scored lower than average on the cognitive test given by the speech pathologist in the hospital.

10. What are the discharge diagnoses?

Status post motor vehicle accident with positive loss of consciousness, mandibular fracture, left occipital laceration, right paresthesia at the knee and extending inferior.

Chapter 19 Oncology

Activity 19-1: Competency Verification
Oncology

1. DNA (deoxyribonucleic acid)
2. TNM staging
3. T_0
4. M_0
5. differentiated cells
6. grade 1
7. grade 4
8. carcinogenesis
9. mutation
10. undifferentiated cells

Activity 19–2: Competency Verification

Medical Word Components

1. hemat/oma   *oma*=tumor; blood
2. carcin/o/genesis   *genesis*=forming, producing, origin; cancer
3. chem/o/therapy   *therapy*=treatment; chemical, drug
4. myel/oma   *oma*=tumor; bone marrow, spinal cord
5. neo/plasm   *plasm*=formation, growth; new
6. mut/a/gen   *gen*=forming, producing, origin; genetic change
7. ana/plasia   *plasia*=formation, growth; without, not
8. sarc/oma   *oma*=tumor; flesh (connective tissue)
9. onc/o/logy   *logy*=study of; tumors
10. neur/o/blast   *blast*=embryonic cell, immature; nerve
11. cauter/ization   *ization*=process (of); heat, burn
12. leiomy/o/sarc/oma   *oma*=tumor; smooth muscle (visceral); flesh (connective tissue)
13. hyper/plasia   *plasia*=formation, growth; excessive, above normal
14. meta/stasis   *stasis*=standing still; change, beyond
15. oste/o/sarc/oma   *oma*=tumor; bone; flesh (connective tissue)

Activity 19–3: Clinical Application

Pathological Conditions, Clinical Procedures, and Laboratory Tests

1. meningioma
2. apheresis
3. PSA
4. carcinoembryonic antigen (CEA)
5. CA-125
6. leukemia
7. retinoblastoma
8. multiple myeloma
9. exfoliative cytology
10. alpha-fetoprotein (AFP)

Activity 19–4: Clinical Application

Diagnostic Tests, Treatments, and Abbreviations

1. exenteration
2. chemotherapy
3. antiemetics
4. palliative surgery
5. cryosurgery
6. immunotherapy
7. allogeneic transplant
8. antimetabolites
9. hormonal agents
10. radiation therapy

Activity 19–5: Build Medical Words

Diagnostic, Symptomatic, and Surgical Terms

1. oncology
2. oncologist
3. oncogenesis
4. oncolysis
5. carcinoma
6. carcinogenesis, carcinogen
7. carcinophobia
8. adipoma, lipoma, steatoma
9. adenoma
10. leiomyoma
11. neuroma
12. osteosarcoma
13. leiomyosarcoma
14. chondrosarcoma
15. rhabdomyosarcoma

Critical Thinking: Analysis of Medical Records

1. What laboratory test indicated that the patient had adenocarcinoma of the prostate?

The 9.7 (elevated) value for the prostate-specific antigen (PSA) test result.

2. What is a "prostatic seed implant?"

Prostatic seed implants are radioactive seeds implanted near the prostate to deliver radiation therapy directly to the area. Also known as brachytherapy.

3. Why was fluoroscopy used during the operation?

Fluoroscopy was used throughout the procedure to ensure proper positioning of the implanted seeds.

4. What did the panendoscopy reveal?

The panendoscopy revealed a normal anterior and prostatic urethra with no evidence of needles seen coming from the urethra. The bladder was investigated, and one seed was identified. It was grasped and recovered.

5. What did the chest x-ray reveal?

A suspicious mass in the left apex.

6. What diagnostic test confirmed the findings on the chest x-ray? What were the specific findings of this test?

CT scan. A 4-mm mass in the upper left lobe of the lung, cerebral atrophy, and multiple lesions of the liver, which probably represented cysts.

7. What type of biopsy was performed? What is the advantage of this type of biopsy?

A needle biopsy (under CT direction) of the left apex of the lung.

NOTE: Needle biopsy is used to sample suspicious masses that are not easily accessible, such as some growths in the breast, lung, liver, and kidney. The procedure is fast, relatively inexpensive, and easy to perform. Usually the patient experiences minimal and temporary physical discomfort. In addition, the degree to which the surrounding tissue is disturbed is kept to a minimum, thus decreasing the likelihood of cancer cell dissemination (seeding).

8. What were the biopsy findings?

Malignant cells that contain numerous extralarge nucleated cells (multinucleated cells). The biopsy was taken from the left lung.

9. What do the findings above suggest?

Giant cell adenocarcinoma of the lung.

10. What type of treatment options are available to the patient?

The doctor did not feel the patient was a good candidate for chemotherapy (probably because of his age), and suggested radiation therapy for symptomatic relief.

Chapter 20 Psychiatry

Activity 20–1: Competency Verification

The Types of Psychiatric Disorders

1. anxiety disorder
2. dementia
3. substance-related disorders
4. schizophrenia
5. sexual and gender identity disorders
6. hallucinations
7. eating disorders
8. delusion
9. somatoform disorders
10. mood disorders
11. personality disorders
12. impulse-control disorders
13. adjustment disorders
14. sleep disorders
15. factitious disorder

Activity 20–2: Competency Verification

Medical Word Components

1. hallucin/o/gen   *gen*=forming, producing, origin; hallucination
2. hypn/osis   *osis*=abnormal condition, increase (used primarily with blood cells); sleep
3. psych/iatr/ist   *ist*=specialist; mind; physician, medicine, treatment
4. ment/al   *al*=pertaining to, relating to; mind
5. schiz/o/phren/oid   *oid*=resembling; split; diaphragm, mind
6. neur/osis   *osis*=abnormal condition; nerve
7. ped/o/philia   *philia*=attraction for; foot, child
8. klept/o/mania   *mania*=state of mental disorder, frenzy; to steal
9. xen/o/phobia   *phobia*=fear; foreign, strange
10. eu/phoria   *phoria*=feeling (mental state); good, normal

Activity 20–3: Clinical Application

Pathological Conditions

1. euphoria
2. Munchausen syndrome
3. primary insomnia
4. anorexia nervosa
5. seasonal affective disorder (SAD)
6. fetishism
7. bipolar disorder
8. social phobia
9. narcissistic personality disorder
10. pedophilia
11. conduct disorder
12. trichotillomania
13. kleptomania
14. delirium tremens (DT)
15. separation anxiety disorder
16. encopresis
17. panic attack
18. anhedonia
19. sleepwalking
20. hypochondriasis

Activity 20–4: Clinical Application

Diagnostic Tests, Treatments, and Abbreviations

1. intelligence tests
2. mental status exam (MSE)
3. clinical interview
4. computed tomography (CT)
5. electroencephalography (EEG)
6. psychoanalysis
7. positron emission tomography (PET)
8. polysomnography
9. cognitive behavior therapy (CBT)
10. DSM-IV
11. anxiolytics
12. psychostimulants
13. SAD
14. anticonvulsant
15. sex therapy
16. antipsychotics
17. PTSD
18. hypnosis
19. SSRI
20. ECT

Activity 20–5: Build Medical Words

Diagnostic, Symptomatic, and Surgical Terms

1. psychology
2. psychosis
3. psychosomatic
4. psychotherapy
5. hypnophobia
6. hypnosis
7. euphoria
8. dysphoria
9. xenophobia
10. photophobia

Critical Thinking: Analysis of Medical Records

> > > MEDICAL RECORD 20–1: HISTORY AND PHYSICAL EXAMINATION

1. What problems was the patient having that indicated a need for hospital admission?

She was having decompensating symptoms, racing thoughts, and thoughts of self-harm and self-mutilation.

2. Which diagnoses were included in the patient's psychiatric history?

Bipolar disorder and bulimia.

3. What was the precipitating event that triggered the patient's distress?

A recent move to a place where the patient has no support system.

4. What was the patient's suicide status upon admission?

She had no active suicidal thoughts or plan at admission.

5. With what method had she attempted suicide in the past?

She had attempted suicide by cutting her wrists.

> > > MEDICAL RECORD 20–2: DISCHARGE SUMMARY

6. How many times had this patient been hospitalized previously?

None, this was her first psychiatric hospitalization.

7. What event precipitated her attempted suicide?

Her husband of 27 years told her the marriage was not going to work, even after a recent attempt at reconciliation.

8. How did the patient stabilize?

She stabilized quickly and efficiently by facing the reality of her impending divorce head on in psychotherapy.

9. What medication was she discharged on?

She was discharged on Trazodone, Xanax, Premphase, Fosamax, calcium carbonate, and a multivitamin.

> >>> MEDICAL RECORD 20-3: PHYSICIAN PROGRESS NOTE

10. Why did a physician see Eric?

He was seen for a medication check up and to see how he is doing on the medications.

11. What positive behaviors did his mother report he is engaging in?

His mother reported that Eric listens and follows directions at school and generally has been an excellent student lately.

12. What negative behaviors did his mother report he is engaging in?

At home, Eric tore a library book apart and has trouble controlling his anger.

Chapter 21 Medical Records

Activity 21-1: Competency Verification
The Two Major Types of Medical Records

1. Name two of the most commonly used record management systems in health-care facilities, and briefly state the difference between them.

The problem-oriented medical record (POMR) and the source-oriented medical record (SOMR). The POMR is organized according to patient problems whereas the SOMR is organized according to the source of information (doctor, nurse, etc.) or the document (lab report, pathology report, etc.) involved.

2. How is information compiled in the problem-oriented medical record?

All patient information is linked to specific problems. The record includes four sections: a database, a problem list, a plan, and progress notes.

3. What are the four major sections of the POMR?

Database, problem list, plan, progress notes.

4. What does SOAP stand for?

> ***S****ubjective: information provided by the patient (symptoms, feelings, and comments)*
>
> ***O****bjective: observable factual data (observations made by the physician, and results of diagnostic tests)*
>
> ***A****ssessment: an evaluation of the plan and/or success of the treatment*
>
> ***P****lan: the decision to continue with or change the treatment*

5. Name a major advantage and disadvantage of the source-oriented medical record.

Advantages: Each group of health-care professionals can easily locate the proper section of the record in which to make entries; it does not require special training to understand the system.

Disadvantages: Data are fragmented, and it is difficult to track problems chronologically because of input from different groups of health-care professionals. The data are not organized by the patient's problems, and details about a specific problem may be distributed throughout the record. Consequently, to make a comprehensive assessment of a patient's problems and devise a health-care plan, it may become necessary to locate data from several different sections of the medical record.

Activity 21–2: Clinical Application
Laboratory Reports

1. Review Medical Record 21–1 and list the names and abbreviations of at least four tests that were performed.

White blood count (WBC), red blood count (RBC), hemoglobin (HGB), hematocrit (HCT), and platelet count (PLAT), mean corpuscular volume (MCV), mean corpuscular hemoglobin (MCH), mean corpuscular hemoglobin concentration (MCHC), and red blood cell distribution width (RDW).

2. What is the purpose of the chemistry profile test shown in Medical Record 21–2?

It is a blood test to analyze the chemical components of the patient's blood. In this case it was ordered before the patient had surgery (preoperatively).

3. Which of the three laboratory reports (Medical Records 21–1, 21–2, or 21–3) determines hyaline casts, bilirubin, and ketones?

> *Medical Record 21–2, Chemistry Profile: bilirubin*
>
> *Medical Record 21–3, Urinalysis: hyaline casts, bilirubin, ketones*

Activity 21–3: Clinical Application
History and Physical Examination

1. Define the following abbreviations and symbols in the report.

a. ↓	decrease(d), down
b. ○, ♀	female
c. L	liter, left, lumbar
d. VSS	vital signs stable

2. Define the three parts of the History and Physical Examination Report.

Part 1 includes subjective data (begins with the chief complaint and concludes with the review of systems.

Part 2 contains objective data (begins with the physical examination and includes observations and data provided by various tests).

Part 3 is the conclusion (it may list an impression; it summarizes a plan for treatment).

3. What information is used to help the physician, or health-care practitioner, arrive at a diagnosis or impression?

Subjective and objective information is collected, and the physician or practitioner determines an impression (IMP) or diagnosis by a scientific evaluation of symptoms, physical signs, history, and the results of various diagnostic tests.

Activity 21–4: Clinical Application

Medical Record and Prescription Abbreviations

a.	CC	chief complaint, craniocaudad (radiology view)
b.	HEENT	head, eyes, ears, nose, throat
c.	IMP	impression (also known as *diagnosis*)
d.	NPO	nothing per mouth
e.	prn	as needed, as required
f.	S1, S$_1$	first heart sound (systolic, cardiovascular), first sacral nerve (neurology and orthopedics), first sacral vertebra (neurology and orthopedics)
g.	SOB	shortness of breath
h.	TPR	temperature, pulse, respiration
i.	UCHD	usual childhood disease
j.	wt	weight

Critical Thinking: Analysis of Medical Records

>>> MEDICAL RECORD 21–6: HISTORY AND PHYSICAL EXAMINATION

1. (A)   Is there a family history of endocrine disorders, hypertension, diabetes, CA or colitis?
Patient denies any history of endocrine disorders, hypertension, or diabetes. There is a history of carcinoma in patient's mother and history of colitis in patient's sister.

(B)   Why didn't the doctor perform a pelvic examination?
Patient stated she had a pelvic examination 3 to 4 months ago and it was normal.

(C)   What type of treatment did Dr. Hunnicane recommend?
He recommended a total thyroidectomy.

>>> CHART NOTES 21–2: POSTOPERATIVE ORDERS

2. Transcribe the first nine (9) lines of the Doctor's Order Sheet for Postoperative Care.

Doctor's Order Sheet

Line 1:   6/13/xx 3:10 pm Postoperative orders.

Line 2:   Admit to recovery then to ward.

Line 3:   Diagnosis: status post (refers to previous disease or surgery) total thyroidectomy.

Line 4:   Condition: stable.

Line 5: Vitals: every 4 hours times 24; then every shift.

Line 6: Allergies: no known allergies—No blood products.

Line 7: Activity: as desired, as much as needed, freely; head of bed at 30 degrees.

Line 8: Nursing inputs/outputs.

Line 9: Diet: nothing by mouth.

>>> MEDICAL RECORD 21-7: OPERATIVE REPORT

3. Did the patient have any previous radiation treatments for the bilateral thyroid nodules?

The patient denies any previous radiation treatments.

4. When the thyroid gland was removed, what did Dr. Hunnicone find upon inspection?

Once the thyroid gland was removed, it was inspected and no evidence of adherent parathyroids were noted.

5. What does the statement "final sponge and needle count was correct" mean? Why is it important to do this count?

The final sponge and needle count agreed with the number of items counted at the beginning of the surgery. This is a double check to be sure there was nothing left inside of the patient before closing the incision site.

>>> CHART NOTES 21-3: POSTOPERATIVE CHART NOTES

6. Dr. Hunnicone states that the patient was "afeb" and "VSS." What does this mean?

Afeb *means* afebrile *or without a fever;* Rochelle does not have an elevated temperature, it is within normal limits; VSS stands for vital signs stable, which means her temperature, blood pressure, pulse, and respirations were stable and within normal limits.

7. Transcribe the first eleven (11) lines of the doctor's order sheet for postoperative care.

Chart Notes

Line 1: 6/13/xx Postoperative.

Line 2: 5:15 pm Patient without complaints with some nausea.

Line 3: afebrile; vital signs stable.

Line 4: Dressing dry.

Line 5: Voice okay.

Line 6: Doing well after operating room—start diet.

Line 7: in am; routine after operative care.

Line 8: B. T. Hunnicone, MD.

Line 9: 6/13/xx RN notes: afebrile, vital signs stable. Anterior neck dressing dry and intact.

Line 10: 7:30 pm Nauseous but no emesis this time. Spitting up white clear.

Line 11: secretions—H. Alexander RN.

8. Why was a total thyroidectomy performed?

There were bilateral thyroid nodules present.

9. What type of anemia did Rochelle have? (You might want to review Chapter 15 to understand the answer to this question).

Microcytic hypochromic anemia. The red blood cells are small and lack normal amount of hemoglobin.

10. What type of supplement will the patient take for anemia?

Iron sulfate, 325 milligrams by mouth every day.

Appendix D

Index of Genetic and Congenital Disorders

Appendix E

Index of Diagnostic Imaging Procedures

Appendix F

Index of Pharmacology

Part 1: Drug Classifications

Part 2: Medications Listed in Medical Records

You are not expected to know the names of medications, nor have the ability to distinguish between generic and trade names. The purpose of this appendix is to provide a "user-friendly" table to complete the dictionary exercises in the medical records sections and to help you distinguish between generic and brand name drugs (also called trade name drugs). The table also provides a means of understanding the therapeutic classifications of drugs and their common indications, or their general use.

As you examine medical records, you will find that health-care practitioners generally document medications by brand name and capitalize the brand name; generic names are usually documented in lowercase letters.

The table below is an alphabetical listing of medications as they appear in the medical records. The chapters in which the medical record and medication are found are enclosed in parenthesis. Brand name medications are capitalized and appear in regular type; generic medications are given in lowercase boldface.

The generic name of a drug is the official drug name assigned by the United States Adopted Names (USAN) Council in the United States and by the World Health Organization (WHO) in other countries. In this table, generic names are followed by a pronunciation key. Although drugs can be classified in a variety of ways, this table lists them only according to their therapeutic classification. The common indications are the general usages for the drug.

Medication	Generic Name	Brand Name	Therapeutic Classifications	Common Indications
Accupril (2)	**quinapril** KWĬN-ă-prĭl	Accupril	Antihypertensive	Hypertension, heart failure management
Actigall (13)	**ursodiol** ŭr-sō-DĪ-ōl	Actigall, URSO	Anticholelithic	Gallstone dissolution; treatment of primary biliary cirrhosis
Adalat (2)	**nifedipine** nī-FĔD-Ĭ-pēn	Adalat, Procardia	Antianginal	Angina, hypertension
Afrin (2, 17)	**oxymetazoline** ŏks-ĭ-mĕth-ĂZ-ō-leen	Afrin, Allerest, Dristan	Decongestant, vasoconstrictor	Nasal congestion
albuterol (8)	**albuterol** ăl-BŪ-tĕr-ōl	Proventil, Ventolin, Volmox	Bronchodilator	Prevention and treatment of bronchospasm
Aldactone (7)	**spironolactone** spēr-ō-nō-LĂK-tōn	Aldactone	Edema management, antihypertensive	Edema, hypertension
Ambien (20)	**zolpidem tartrate** ZŌL-pĭ-dĕm TĂR-trāt	Ambien	Hypnotic	Insomnia
amoxicillin (2,17)	**amoxicillin** ă-mŏks-ĭ-SĬL-ĭn	Augmentin, Clavulin	Antibiotic	Lower respiratory infections, otitis media, sinusitis, skin infections, urinary tract infections
Ancef (5, 16)	**cefazolin** sĕf-Ă-zō-lĭn	Ancef	Antibiotic	Serious respiratory, skin, joint, and bone infections

Medication	Generic Name	Brand Name	Therapeutic Classifications	Common Indications
Ativan (20)	**lorazepam** *lor-ĂZ-ĕ-păm*	Ativan	Anxiolytic sedative-hypnotic	Anxiety, agitation, tension
Azmacort (17)	**triamcinolone** *trī-ăm-SĬN-ō-lōn*	Azmacort, Nasacort	Anti-inflammatory, antiasthmatic	Steroid-dependent asthma, rhinitis, allergic disorders
AZT (13)	**zidovudine** *zī-DŌ-vū-dēn*	AZT, Retrovir	Antiviral	HIV infection, AIDS
Bactrim (13)	**trimethoprim/ sulfamethoxazole** *trī-MĔTH-ō-prĭm/ sŭl-fă-mĕth-ŎKS-ă-zōl*	Bactrim, Septra	Antibiotic	Urinary tract infection, otitis media, *Pneumocystis carinii* pneumonia, bronchitis, diarrhea
Benadryl (5, 17)	**diphenhydramine** *dī-fĕn-HĪ-dră-mēn*	Benadryl, Nytol, Sominex	Antihistamine, antiemetic, sedative, topical anesthetic	Rhinitis, allergies, motion sickness, insomnia, sedation, nonproductive cough
Betadine (5, 9, 10, 15)	**povidone-iodine** *PŌV-ĭ-dōn Ī-ō-dĭn*	Betadine, Efodine	Antiseptic, germicidal	Preoperative skin preparation
Cefizox (2, 21)	**ceftizoxime** *sĕf-tĭ-ZŎKS-ēm*	Cefizox	Antibiotic	Bacteremia, septicemia, meningitis, pelvic inflammatory disease
Cipro (6, 7)	**ciprofloxacin** *sĭp-rō-FLŎKS-ă-sĭn*	Cipro	Antibiotic	Urinary tract infection, diarrhea; respiratory, bone, or joint infection
ciprofloxacin (5)	**ciprofloxacin** *sĭp-rō-FLŎKS-ă-sĭn*	Cipro	Antibiotic	Urinary tract infection, diarrhea; respiratory, bone, and joint infection
Claritin-D (2)	**loratadine** and **pseudoephedrine** *lor-Ă-tă-dēn, soo-dō-ĕ-FĔD-rĭn*	Claritin-D	Antihistamine and decongestant	Seasonal allergic rhinitis
Cleocin (5)	**clindamycin** *klĭn-dă-MĪ-sĭn*	Cleocin	Antibiotic	Serious infections of the skin, respiratory tract, and abdomen (intra-abdominal)
Climara (11)	**estradiol** *ĕs-tră-DĪ-ōl*	Climara, Estrace, Estraderm	Astrogen replacement	Atrophic vaginitis, dystrophy of vulva, hypogonadism

Medication	Generic Name	Brand Name	Therapeutic Classifications	Common Indications
Colace (21)	**docusate** *DŎK-ū-sāt*	Colace, Modane	Emollient laxative	Stool softener
Combivent (2)	**albuterol** and **ipratropium bromide** *ăl-BŪ-tĕr-ōl, ĭ-pră-TRŌ-pē-ŭm BRŎ-mĭd*	Combivent	Antiasthmatic, bronchodilator	Prevention and treatment of bronchospasm
Compazine (21)	**prochlorperazine** *prō-klor-PAIR-ă-zeen*	Compazine	Antipsychotic, antiemetic, anxiolytic	Nausea, vomiting, anxiety, psychosis
Cordarone (2)	**amiodarone** *ăm-ē-Ō-dă-rōn*	Cordarone	Ventricular antiarrhythmic	Ventricular fibrillation, tachycardia, angina
Coumadin (2, 15)	**warfarin** *WĂR-fă-rĭn*	Coumadin	Anticoagulant	Pulmonary emboli, thrombosis, myocardial infarction
cyclosporine (13)	**cyclosporine** *SĪ-klō-spor-ēn*	Neoral, Sandimmune	Immunosuppressant	Prophylaxis of organ and tissue rejection
Cytomel (20)	**liothyronine** *lī-ō-THĪ-rō-nēn*	Cytomel, Triostat	Thyroid hormone replacement	Hypothyroidism, myxedema, goiter
Darvocet (7, 12, 15)	**acetaminophen** and **propoxyphene** *ă-sēt-ă-MĬN-ō-fĕn, prŏ-PŎKS-ĭ-fēn*	Darvocet	Narcotic analgesics	Pain relief
Demerol (8)	**meperidine** *mĕ-PĔR-ĭ-dēn*	Demerol	Narcotic analgesic	Pain relief
Desyrel (20)	**trazodone** *TRĂZ-ō-dōn*	Desyrel	Antidepressant	Depression, insomnia
Detrol (19)	**tolterodine tartrate** *tōl-TĔR-ō-dēn tăr-TRĀT*	Detrol	Anticholinergic	Overactive bladder
digoxin (2, 8)	**digoxin** *dĭ-JŎKS-ĭn*	Lanoxin	Antiarrhythmic	Heart failure, atrial fibrillation, tachycardia
dopamine (2)	**dopamine** *DŌP-ă-mēn*	Intropin	Vasopressor	Adjunct in shock to increase cardiac output and blood pressure, severe heart failure

Medication	Generic Name	Brand Name	Therapeutic Classifications	Common Indications
doxycycline (11)	**doxycycline** *dŏks-Ĭ-SĪ-klēn*	Vibramycin, Doryx, Monodox	Antibiotic	Variety of bacterial infections, particularly traveler's diarrhea, and sexually transmitted diseases
Dulcolax (11)	**bisacodyl** *bĭs-ă-KŌ-dĭl*	Bisacolax, Dulcolax, Fleet Bisacodyl	Stimulant laxative	Constipation, preparation for rectal or bowel procedures
Duricef (5)	**cefadroxil** *sĕf-ă-DRŎKS-ĭl*	Duricef	Antibiotic	Urinary, skin, and soft tissue infection
Epogen (13)	**erythropoietin** *ĕ-rĭth-rō-PŌ-ĕ-tĭn*	Epogen, Procrit	Antianemic	Anemia
erythromycin (5)	**erythromycin** *ĕ-rĭth-rō-MĪ-sĭn*	Ilosone, Erythrocin	Antibiotic	Acute pelvic inflammatory disease, endocarditis, penicillin alternative
Eskalith (20)	**lithium** *LĬTH-ē-ŭm*	Eskalith, Carbolith, Lithane	Antimanic, antipsychotic	Symptoms of mania and depression, especially for bipolar disease
fentanyl (12)	**fentanyl** *FĔN-tă-nĭl*	Duragesic, Fentanyl Oralet	Narcotic analgesic	Pain relief
Feosol (21)	**iron preparation** *Ī-ĕrn*	Feosol	Iron supplement	Anemia
5-fluorouracil (16)	5-fluorouracil *fĭv-floor-ō-ŪR-ă-sĭl*	Adrucil, Efudex, 5-FU	Antineoplastic	Used alone or in combination with other modalities in the treatment of certain types of cancer
Flagyl (7, 11)	**metronidazole** *mĕ-trō-NĬ-dă-zōl*	Flagyl	Antibacterial	Abscess, bacterial infections, postoperative infection, peptic ulcer
Flomax (19)	**tamsulosin** *tăm-SOO-lō-sĭn*	Flomax	Treatment of benign prostatic hyperplasia	Signs and symptoms of benign prostatic hypertrophy
Flonase (2)	**fluticasone propionate** *floo-TĬ-kă-sōn PRŌ-pē-ō-nāt*	Cutivate, Flonase, Flovent	Topical/inhalation anti-inflammatory	Dermatosis-related inflammation, allergic rhinitis, asthma

Medication	Generic Name	Brand Name	Therapeutic Classifications	Common Indications
Fosamax (20)	**alendronate** *ă-LĔN-drōn-āt*	Fosamax	Antiosteoporotic	Postmenopausal osteoporosis, Paget's disease of bone
ganciclovir (13)	**ganciclovir** *găn-SĪ-klō-vĭr*	Cytovene, Vitrasert	Antiviral	Cytomegalovirus
Haldol (20)	**haloperidol** *hă-lō-PĔR-Ĭ-dōl*	Haldol	Antipsychotic	Psychotic disorders
hydrocodone (17)	**hydrocodone** *hī-drō-KŌ-dōn*	Hycodan, Robidone	Antitussive	Cough suppressant, pain relief
imipramine (20)	**imipramine** *ĭm-ĬP-ră-mēn*	Tofranil, Impril, Novopramine	Antidepressant	Depression, childhood enuresis
Isordil (2)	**isosorbide** *ī-sō-SOR-bĭd*	Isordil, Sorbitrate, Titradose	Antianginal, vasodilator	Angina, ischemic heart disease, heart failure
kanamycin (9)	**kanamycin** *kăn-ă-MĪ-sĭn*	Kantrex	Antibiotic	Endocarditis prophylaxis, staphylococci infections when penicillin is contra-indicated
lamivudine (13)	**lamivudine** *lă-MĬ-vū-dēn*	Epivir, 3TC	Antiviral	HIV infection, hepatitis B
Lasix (8)	**furosemide** *fŭr-Ō-sĕ-mīd*	Lasix	Antihypertensive	Edema, pulmonary edema, hypertension
Levaquin (19)	**levofloxacin** *lĕv-ō-FLŎKS-ă-sĭn*	Levaquin	Broad-spectrum antibacterial	Acute sinusitis, acute exacerbation of bronchitis, pneumonia, skin infection
Levo-T (21)	**levothyroxine** *lē-vō-thī-RŎKS-ēn*	Levo-T, Levothroid, Synthroid	Thyroid hormone replacement	Hypothyroidism, myxedema, treatment of some types of thyroid cancer
lidocaine (11, 15)	**lidocaine** *LĪ-dō-kān*	Xylocaine	Ventricular antiarrhythmic, local anesthetic	Ventricular arrhythmia, epileptic seizure, local anesthesia of skin or mucous membranes particularly for medical procedures

Medication	Generic Name	Brand Name	Therapeutic Classifications	Common Indications
Lipitor (9)	**atorvastatin** *ă-TOR-vă-stăt-ĭn*	Lipitor	Antilipemic	Elevated total cholesterol, low-density lipopro-teins, and triglyc-erides
lithium (20)	**lithium** *LĬTH-ē-ŭm*	Eskalith, Lithane, Lithotabs	Antimanic, antipsychotic	Mania and depres-sion especially in bipolar, major depressive, schizo-affective, and schizophrenic disorders
lorazepam (21)	**lorazepam** *lor-ĂZ-ĕ-păm*	Ativan	Anxiolytic, sedative-hypnotic	Anxiety, tension, agitation, irritabil-ity, insomnia
Marcaine (5, 16, 17)	**bupivacaine** *byoo-PĬ-vĭ-kān*	Marcaine	Local anesthetic	Local or regional anesthesia, analge-sia for surgery
Maxitrol (18)	**dexamethasone neomycin and polymyxin** *dĕks-ă-MĔTH-ă-sōn nē-ō-MĪ-sĭn and pŏl-ĭ-MĬKS-ĭn*	Maxitrol	Ophthalmic steroid and antibiotic	Bacterial eye infec-tions and swelling; prophylaxis for cataract and other eye surgeries
Micro-K (2)	**potassium chloride** *pō-TĂS-ē-ŭm KLŌ-rīd*	K-Dur, Micro-K, Micro-K ExtenCaps	Electrolyte balance	Hypokalemia, potassium replace-ment
Monistat (11)	**miconazole** *mī-KŎN-ă-zōl*	Monistat, Micatin	Antifungal	Fungal infection, especially vaginal
mupirocin (5)	**mupirocin** *myoo-PĔR-ō-sĭn*	Bactroban	Topical antibacterial	*Staphylococcus* or *Streptococcus* topical bacterial infection
Naprosyn (17)	**naproxen** *nă-PRŎK-sēn*	Aleve, Anaprox, Naprelan, Naprosyn	Nonnarcotic analgesic, anti-pyretic, anti-inflammatory	Musculoskeletal or soft tissue irrita-tion, pain from dysmenorrhea
Nasonex (17)	**mometasone** *mō-MĔT-ă-sōn*	Nasonex	Locally acting anti-inflammatory	Decreases symp-toms of allergic rhinitis, nasal polyps
nelfinavir (13)	**nelfinavir** *nĕl-FĬN-ă-vēr*	Viracept	Antiviral	HIV infection

Medication	Generic Name	Brand Name	Therapeutic Classifications	Common Indications
Neupogen (13)	**filgrastim** *fĭl-GRĂ-stĭm*	Neupogen	Colony stimulating factor	Decreases infection after cancer chemotherapy or bone marrow transplantation; neutropenia, agranulocytosis, leukemia
Nitro-Bid (7)	**nitroglycerin** *nī-trō-GLĬ-sĕr-ĭn*	Nitro-Bid, Nitrol	Antianginal, vasodilator	Anginal attacks, acute hypertension from surgery, heart failure, myocardial infarction
nitroglycerin (9)	**nitroglycerin** *nī-trō-GLĬ-sĕr-ĭn*	Nitro-Bid, Nitrol	Antianginal, vasodilator	Anginal attacks, acute hypertension from surgery, heart failure, myocardial infarction
Norvasc (12)	**amlodipine** *ăm-LŌ-dĭ-pēn*	Norvasc	Antianginal, antihypertensive	Angina, hypertension
Ocuflox (16)	**ofloxacin** *ō-FLŎKS-ă-sĭn*	Ocuflox, Floxin	Antibiotic	Conjuntivitis, bronchitis, sexually transmitted disease, urinary tract infection
Os-Cal (21)	**calcium** *KĂL-sē-ŭm*	Os-Cal, Caltrate	Calcium supplement, therapeutic drug for electrolyte balance	Hypocalcemia, hyperkalemia, hypermagnesemia
Pamelor (20)	**nortriptyline** *nor-TRĬP-tĭ-lēn*	Pamelor, Aventyl	Antidepressant	Depression
Paxil (2, 20)	**paroxetine** *păr-ŎKS-ĕ-tēn*	Paxil	Antidepressant	Depression; obsessive compulsive, panic, or social anxiety disorder
Percocet (11)	**acetaminophen** and **oxycodone** *ă-sēt-ă-MĬN-ō-fĕn* and *ŏks-Ĭ-KŌ-dōn*	Percocet	Narcotic analgesic	Pain
Pitocin (11)	**oxytocin** *ŏks-ĭ-TŌ-sĭn*	Pitocin, Syntocinon	Oxytocic, lactation stimulator	Induction or augmentation of labor
Plavix (9)	**clopidogrel** *klō-PĬ-dō-grĕl*	Plavix	Anitplatelet agent	Reduction of atherosclerotic events such as stroke, myocardial infarction, peripheral vascular disease

Medication	Generic Name	Brand Name	Therapeutic Classifications	Common Indications
prednisone (2, 8)	**prednisone** PRĔD-nĭ-sōn	Deltasone, Meticorten	Immunosuppressant, anti-inflammatory	Severe inflammation, undesirable immune response
Premarin (21)	**estrogen** ĔS-trō-jĕn	Premarin	Estrogen replacement	Abnormal uterine bleeding, osteoporosis
Premphase (20)	**estrogen** and **medroxyprogesterone** ĔS-trō-jĕn and mĕ-DRŎKS-ē prō-JĔS-tĕr-ōn	Premphase	estrogen and progesterone replacement	Treatment of menopause symptoms, including vaginal dryness, and osteoporosis
Prevacid (21)	**lansoprazole** lăn-SŌ-pră-zōl	Prevacid	Antiulcerative	Duodenal ulcer, esophagitis, gastric ulcer
Prilosec (12)	**omeprazole** ŏ-MĔP-ră-zōl	Prilosec	Gastric acid suppressant	Duodenal ulcer, esophagitis, gastric esophageal reflux disease (GERD)
Propulsid (12)	**cisapride** SĬS-ă-prĭd	Propulsid	Digestive agent	Reduces symptoms of nocturnal heartburn associated with GERD
Proventil (2)	**albuterol** ăl-BYOO-tĕr-ōl	Proventil, Ventolin	Bronchodilator	Bronchospasms
Prozac (15, 20)	**fluoxetine** floo-ŎKS-ŭ-tēn	Prozac	Antidepressant	Primarily used for depression, but is also used to treat panic disorder, bipolar disorder, obsessive-compulsive disorder
Relafen (17)	**nabumetone** nă-BYOO-mĕ-tōn	Relafen	Antiarthritic	Rheumatoid arthritis, osteoarthritis
Restoril (21)	**temazepam** tĕm-ĂZ-ă-păm	Restoril	Sedative-hypnotic	Insomnia
Ritalin (20)	**methylphenidate** mĕth-ĭl-FĔN-Ĭ-dāt	Ritalin, Concerta, Methylin	Stimulant	Attention deficit hyperactivity disorder
Senokot (11)	**senna** SĔ-nă	Black-Draught, Senexon, Senokot	Stimulant laxative	Constipation, preparation for medical procedures involving the intestines

Medication	Generic Name	Brand Name	Therapeutic Classifications	Common Indications
Septra (6)	**trimethoprim/ sulfamethoxazole** *trī-MĔTH-ō-prĭm/ sŭl-fă-mĕth-ŎKS-ă-zōl*	Septra, Bactrim	Antibiotic	Urinary tract infection, otitis media, *Pneumocystis carinii* pneumonia, bronchitis, diarrhea
Serevent (21)	**salmeterol** *săl-MĔ-tĕ-rōl*	Serevent	Bronchodilator	Asthma, bronchospasm, chronic obstructive pulmonary disease, emphysema
Solu-Medrol (2, 8, 16, 21)	**methylprednisolone** *mĕth-ĭl-prĕd-NĬS-ō-lōn*	Solu-Medrol	Glucocorticoid	Multiple sclerosis, inflammation, shock
Suprax (11)	**cefixime** *sĕ-FĬKS- ēm*	Suprax	Antibiotic	Otitis media, bronchitis, tonsillitis, urinary tract infection, gonorrhea
Sustiva (13)	**efavirenz** *ĕ-FĂV-ĭ-rĕnz*	Sustiva	Antiretroviral	HIV infection
Synthroid (7)	**levothyroxine** *lē-vō-thī-RŎKS-ēn*	Eltroxin, Levoxyl, Synthroid	Thyroid hormone replacement	Congenital hypothyroidism, myxedema coma, thyroid hormone replacement
tetracycline (17)	**tetracycline** *tĕ-tră-SĪ-klēn*	Panmycin, Sumycin	Antiobiotic	Infections, especially those associated with sexually transmitted diseases, acne, Lyme disease
Theo-Dur (21)	**theophylline** *thē-ŎF-ĭ-lĭn*	Theo-Dur, Aerolate	Bronchodilator	Long-term control of asthma and chronic obstructive pulmonary disease
3TC (13)	**lamivudine** *lă-MĬ-vū-dēn*	3TC, Epivir	Antiretroviral	HIV infection
Theophylline (8)	**theophylline** *thē-ŎF-ĭ-lĭn*	Theophylline	Bronchodilator	Long-term control of asthma and chronic obstructive pulmonary disease
Tofranil (20)	**imipramine** *ĭm-ĬP-ră-mēn*	Tofranil	Antidepressant	Depression
trazodone (20)	**trazodone** *TRĂZ-ō-dōn*	Desyrel	Antidepressant	Depression, insomnia
Triaminic (6)	**codeine syrup combination** *KŌ-dēn*	Triaminic	Decongestant	Nasal and eustachian tube decongestant

Medication	Generic Name	Brand Name	Therapeutic Classifications	Common Indications
Tylenol (21)	**acetaminophen** *ă-sēt-ă-MĬN-ō-fĕn*	Tylenol	Nonnarcotic analgesic	Mild pain, fever, anti-infammatory
Unasyn (5)	**ampicillin** and **sulbactam** *ăm-pĭ-SĬL-ĭn* and *sŭl-BĂK-tăm*	Unasyn	Antibiotic	Systemic infections, urinary tract infection, meningitis, gonorrhea
vancomycin (17)	**vancomycin** *văn-kō-MĪ-sĭn*	Vancocin, Vancoled	Antibiotic	Staphylococcal infection, endocarditis prophylaxis for dental and medical procedures
Vasocidin (17)	**prednisolone** and **sulfacetamide** *prĕd-NĬS-ō-lōn* and *SŬL-fă-sĕt-ă-mĭd*	Vasocidin, Blephamide	Ophthalmic steroid and antibiotic	Bacterial eye infections
verapamil (21)	**verapamil** *vĕr-ĂP-ă-mĭl*	Calan, Isoptin, Verelan	Antianginal, antihypertensive, antiarrhythmic	Angina, arrhythmias, tachycardia, hypertension
Versed (8)	**midazolam** *mĭ-DĂZ-ō-lăm*	Versed	General anesthetic	Preoperatively to produce sedation and amnesia; may be used alone for anesthesia
Vicodin (21)	**acetaminophen** and **hydrocodone** *ă-sēt-ă-MĬN-ō-fĕn* and *hī-drō-KŌ-dōn*	Vicodin	Narcotic analgesic	Pain relief
Viracept (13)	**nelfinavir** *nĕl-FĬN-ă-vēr*	Viracept	Antiviral	HIV infection
Wellbutrin (2, 20)	**bupropion** *byoo-PRŌ-pē-ŏn*	Wellbutrin, Zyban	Antidepressant, non-nicotine smoking cessation aid	Depression, nicotine addiction
Xanax (2, 9, 12, 20)	**alprazolam** *ăl-PRĂ-zō-lăm*	Xanax	Anxiolytic	Anxiety, panic disorder, agoraphobia
Xylocaine (5, 16)	**lidocaine** *LĪ-dō-kān*	Xylocaine	Ventricular antiarrhythmic, local anesthetic	Ventricular arrhythmia, epileptic seizure, local anesthesia of skin or mucous membranes particularly for medical procedures
Zestril (2)	**lisinopril** *līs-ĬN-ō-prĭl*	Zestril, Prinivil	Antihypertensive	Hypertension, heart failure, myocardial infarction

Medication	Generic Name	Brand Name	Therapeutic Classifications	Common Indications
zidovudine (13)	**zidovudine** *zī-DŌ-vū-dēn*	Retrovir, AZT	Antiviral	HIV infection, AIDS-related complex, maternal-fetal HIV transmission
Zithromax (11)	**azithromycin** *ā-ZĬTH-rō-mī-sĭn*	Zithromax	Antibiotic	Bacterial infections and exacerbations
Zyprexa (20)	**olanzapine** *ō-LĂN-ză-pēn*	Zyprexa	Antipsychotic	Signs and symptoms of psychotic disorders

Index